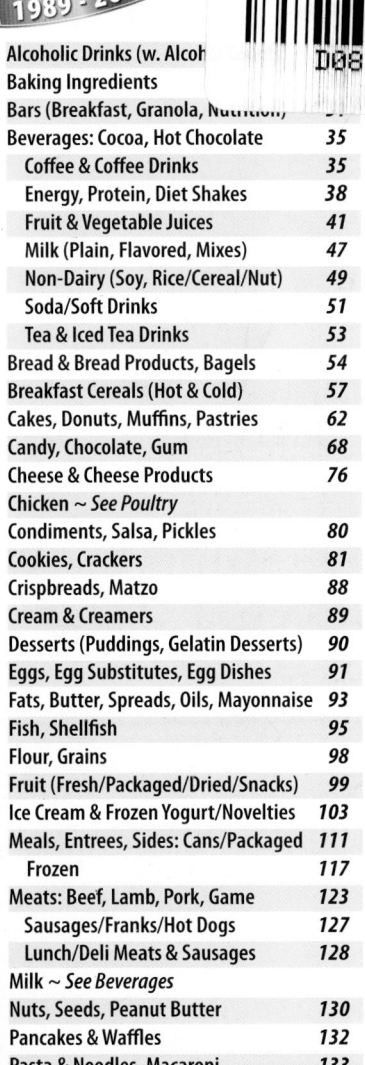

# Weight Control Tips

## ✅ Eat & Drink Sensibly

- Avoid fad diets. Eat 3 sensible portion-controlled meals daily.
- Limit fats, high-fat foods/snacks and sugar. Eat adequate fresh fruit & vegetables.
- Limit soft drinks, energy drinks, fruit juice and alcohol. Quench your thirst on water. *(See Sample Meal Plan ~ Page 11)*

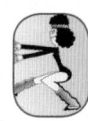

## ✅ Exercise Daily

- Aim for at least 30 minutes daily – even in 5-10 minute lots. For motivation, find an exercise buddy, personal trainer or join a gym. *(Extra Notes ~ Page 12)*

## ✅ Reshape Eating Behaviors

- Be aware of eating and shopping behaviors that lead to overeating.
- Also focus on social and emotional situations that may trigger compulsive eating. *(Extra Notes ~ Page 14)*

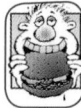

## ✅ Keep a Food & Exercise Journal

- A journal helps you see exactly what you eat and drink, and how much you exercise. *(Extra Notes ~ Page 15)*
- An excellent motivator and proven weight loss aid. Keeps you honest!

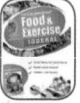

## ✅ Arrange Moral Support

- Gain the support of family and friends.
- Get extra professional help if required, from your doctor, dietitian, psychologist, exercise trainer, or slimming group.
- Beware of family saboteurs who discourage you from adopting a healthier lifestyle!

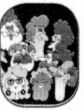

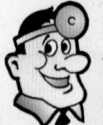

**DOCTOR CHECK-UP**
*Ask your doctor to check your blood pressure, blood sugar and blood cholesterol levels.*

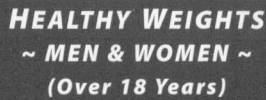

**HEALTHY WEIGHTS**
**~ MEN & WOMEN ~**
**(Over 18 Years)**

Based on weights with least risk of disease or death from heart disease, diabetes, stroke and cancer.

Based on Body Mass Index of 20-25

BMI calculated as: $\dfrac{\text{Weight (kg)}}{\text{Height (m)}^2}$

| Height (No Shoes) Ft Ins | | Healthy Weight Range (Pounds) |
|---|---|---|
| 4'7" | ~ | 86-108 |
| 4'8" | ~ | 88-110 |
| 4'9" | ~ | 92-114 |
| 4'10" | ~ | 97-121 |
| 4'11" | ~ | 99-123 |
| 5'0" | ~ | 101-127 |
| 5'1" | ~ | 105-132 |
| 5'2" | ~ | 110-136 |
| 5'3" | ~ | 112-140 |
| 5'4" | ~ | 114-145 |
| 5'5" | ~ | 119-149 |
| 5'6" | ~ | 123-156 |
| 5'7" | ~ | 127-158 |
| 5'8" | ~ | 129-162 |
| 5'9" | ~ | 134-167 |
| 5'10" | ~ | 138-173 |
| 5'11" | ~ | 143-178 |
| 6'0" | ~ | 145-182 |
| 6'1" | ~ | 149-187 |
| 6'2" | ~ | 156-193 |
| 6'3" | ~ | 158-198 |
| 6'4" | ~ | 162-202 |
| 6'5" | ~ | 170-211 |
| 6'6" | ~ | 172-215 |
| 6'7" | ~ | 175-220 |

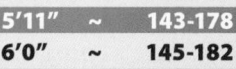

### Body Fat Distribution & Health

Moderate amounts of body fat do not compromise health. However, excess fat above the hips carries a far greater health risk than fat on or below the hips - better to be a 'pear-shape' than an 'apple-shape'.

**Abdominal obesity** greatly increases the risk of developing diabetes, heart disease, high blood fats, hypertension, stroke, sleep apnea, arthritis and some cancers. So-called 'cellulite' carries no extra health risk.

**Waist Circumference** directly reflects the increased health risk of abdominal obesity. Waist size associated with a high health risk: **Men** ~ Over 40 inches   **Women** ~ Over 35 inches

### Body Mass Index (BMI)

BMI is a general (but not specific) indicator of body fatness. Although BMI alone is not diagnostic, the higher the BMI, the greater the health risk of developing diabetes, high blood pressure and heart disease. BMI does not apply to heavily muscled persons. BMI is used in a different way for children.

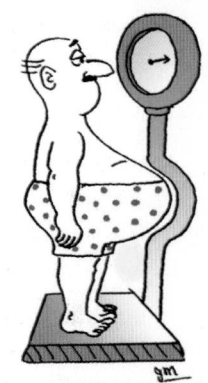

*Abdominal obesity greatly increases the risk of ill-health and earlier death.*

**Check Your BMI:** Find your height (no shoes) - look across the row to the weight nearest your own. Then track down to BMI.

| Ht | | WEIGHT (LBS) ~ ADULTS | | | | | | | | | | | | |
|---|---|---|---|---|---|---|---|---|---|---|---|---|---|---|
| 5'1" | 100 | 106 | 111 | 116 | 122 | 127 | 132 | 137 | 143 | 148 | 153 | 158 | 185 | 211 |
| 5'2" | 104 | 109 | 115 | 120 | 126 | 131 | 136 | 142 | 147 | 153 | 158 | 164 | 191 | 218 |
| 5'3" | 107 | 113 | 118 | 124 | 130 | 135 | 141 | 146 | 152 | 158 | 163 | 169 | 197 | 225 |
| 5'4" | 110 | 116 | 122 | 128 | 134 | 140 | 145 | 151 | 157 | 163 | 169 | 174 | 204 | 232 |
| 5'5" | 114 | 120 | 126 | 132 | 138 | 144 | 150 | 156 | 162 | 168 | 174 | 180 | 210 | 240 |
| 5'6" | 118 | 124 | 130 | 136 | 142 | 148 | 155 | 161 | 167 | 173 | 179 | 186 | 216 | 247 |
| 5'7" | 121 | 127 | 134 | 140 | 146 | 153 | 159 | 166 | 172 | 178 | 185 | 191 | 223 | 255 |
| 5'8" | 125 | 131 | 138 | 144 | 151 | 158 | 164 | 171 | 177 | 184 | 190 | 197 | 230 | 262 |
| 5'9" | 128 | 135 | 142 | 149 | 155 | 162 | 169 | 176 | 182 | 189 | 196 | 206 | 236 | 270 |
| 5'10" | 132 | 139 | 146 | 153 | 160 | 167 | 174 | 181 | 188 | 195 | 202 | 207 | 243 | 278 |
| 5'11" | 136 | 143 | 150 | 157 | 165 | 172 | 179 | 186 | 193 | 200 | 208 | 215 | 250 | 286 |
| 6'0" | 140 | 147 | 154 | 162 | 169 | 177 | 184 | 191 | 199 | 206 | 213 | 221 | 258 | 294 |
| 6'1" | 144 | 151 | 159 | 166 | 174 | 182 | 189 | 197 | 204 | 212 | 219 | 227 | 265 | 302 |
| 6'2" | 148 | 155 | 163 | 171 | 179 | 186 | 194 | 202 | 210 | 218 | 225 | 233 | 272 | 311 |
| 6'3" | 152 | 160 | 168 | 176 | 184 | 192 | 200 | 208 | 216 | 224 | 232 | 240 | 279 | 319 |
| 6'4" | 156 | 164 | 172 | 180 | 189 | 197 | 205 | 213 | 221 | 230 | 238 | 246 | 287 | 328 |

| BMI | 19 | 20 | 21 | 22 | 23 | 24 | 25 | 26 | 27 | 28 | 29 | 30 | 35 | 40 |

**BMI Classification:**

**BMI Below 19**
Underweight

**BMI 19-24.9**
Healthy Weight
(Low Health Risk)

**BMI 25-29.9**
Overweight
(Moderate Health Risk)

**BMI 30-40**
Obese (High Health Risk)

**BMI Over 40**
Morbid Obesity
(Very High Risk)

Interactive BMI Calculator
www.calorieking.com

# Calories & Weight Loss

## Calories in Food

Calories in food are derived from protein, fat and carbohydrate. Alcohol also provides calories. Vitamins, minerals and water provide no calories.

### Calorie Values Per Gram

| Fat/Oil | ~ 9 Calories |
|---|---|
| Carbohydrate | ~ 4 Calories |
| Protein | ~ 4 Calories |
| Alcohol | ~ 7 Calories |

Note that fats have over double the calories of protein and carbohydrate. The higher the fat content of food, the higher the calories.

### Sample Calculation

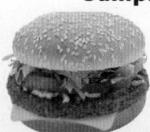

**QUARTER POUNDER®
WITH CHEESE**
has 510 calories
derived from:

| | | |
|---|---|---|
| 26g Fat (x 9 cals/gram) | = | 234 |
| 40g Carbohyd.(x 4 cals/gram) | = | 160 |
| 29g Protein (x 4 cals/gram) | = | <u>116</u> |
| Total Calories | = | 510 |

## Calorie Levels for Weight Loss

Start with a calorie-controlled diet that allows a moderate weight loss of ½ - 1 pound per week. Weight loss is usually much greater in the first few weeks due to extra fluid losses.

Note: It is better to increase exercise rather than lessen food calories too drastically.

### Suggested Calories for Weight Loss

| | | |
|---|---|---|
| **Women:** | Non-active | 1000 - 1200 |
| | Active | 1200 - 1500 |
| **Men:** | Non-active | 1200 - 1500 |
| | Active | 1500 - 1800 |
| **Teenagers:** | | 1200 - 1800 |

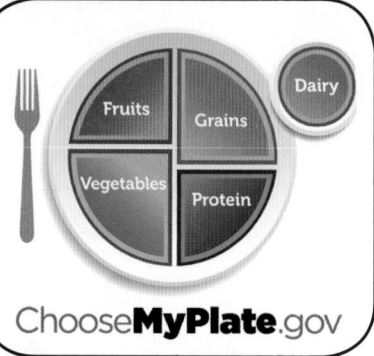

## ChooseMyPlate.gov

The MyPlate symbol represents the recommended proportion of foods from each food group. It focuses on the importance of making smart food choices in every food group, every day. Daily physical activity is also important. *(More info: www.ChooseMyPlate.gov)*

## Examples of Single Serving Sizes

**Grains (Eat 6 servings per day):**
- 1 slice wholegrain bread (1 oz)
- ½ bun, small bagel or English muffin
- 4 small crackers or 1 tortilla
- 1 oz ready-to-eat wholegrain cereal
- ½ cup cooked cereal, rice or pasta

**Vegetables (Eat 3-5 servings per day):**
- 1 cup raw leafy vegetables
- 1½ cups raw chopped vegetables
- ½ cup cooked vegetables
- ½ - ¾ cup vegetable juice

**Fruit (Eat 3-5 servings per day):**
- 1 medium apple, orange, banana
- ½ cup canned fruit (in own juice)
- ¼ cup dried fruit
- ½ cup fruit juice (unsweetened)
- ¼ medium avocado

**Protein (2-3 servings per day):**
- 2-3 oz (cooked) lean meat/poultry/fish
- 2 eggs **or** 6 oz tofu **or** ¼ cup nuts
- 1 cup (cooked) dried beans **or** chickpeas

**Dairy (2-3 servings per day):**
- 1 cup (8 fl.oz) milk/soy (enriched)/yogurt
- 1½ oz cheese or ½ cup cottage cheese

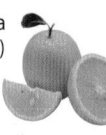

## Portion Size Counts!

Food portion size is critical to controlling calorie intake for weight control.

Super-sized food servings have become more common when eating out and in the home. This can mean a day's worth of calories being consumed in one meal; or a snack being equivalent to a full meal.

It is easy to underestimate portion size of foods and drinks, and unwittingly consume excess calories – even if the fat content is low or even zero!

To more accurately estimate portion size of different foods, weigh and measure your food with food scales, measuring spoons and cups. Better control of calories will result.

**For a visual idea of portion sizes, visit www.CalorieKing.com.au** See examples (fries and cola) on this page.

## Allow for Extra Calories in Packaged Food

The actual weight of packaged foods is usually 5-10% more than the label net weight (the minimum legal weight) – and in some cases up to 50% more. However, manufacturers calculate the calories based on the net weight. For actual calories, weigh the product and calculate the extra calories.

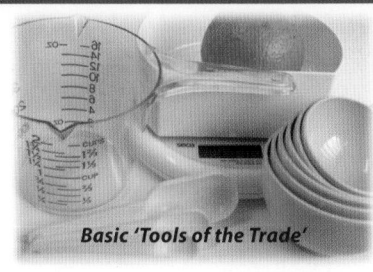

*Basic 'Tools of the Trade'*

**CALORIEKING PORTION WATCH**

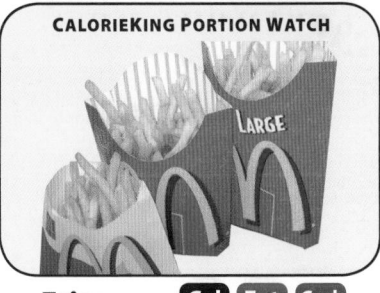

| Fries | Cal | Fat | Carb |
|-------|-----|-----|------|
| Small | 230 | 11 | 29 |
| Medium | 380 | 19 | 48 |
| Large | 500 | 25 | 63 |

**CALORIEKING PORTION WATCH**

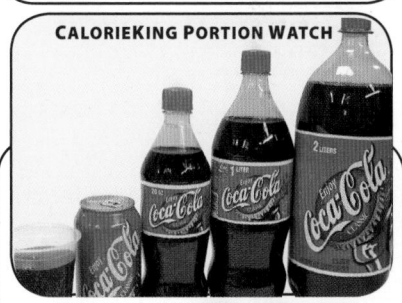

| Cola | Cal | Fat | Carb |
|------|-----|-----|------|
| 8 fl.oz Cup | 100 | 0 | 25 |
| 12 fl.oz Can | 150 | 0 | 37 |
| 20 fl.oz Bottle | 250 | 0 | 63 |
| 1 Liter Bottle | 400 | 0 | 100 |
| 2 Liter Bottle | 800 | 0 | 200 |

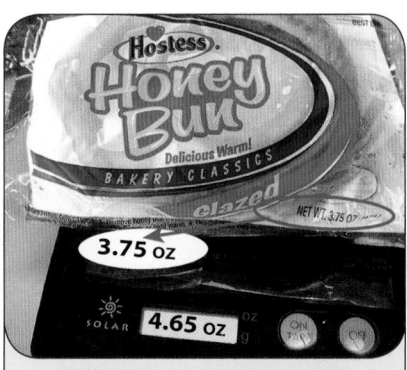

Actual weight of this bun is 24% more than the stated net weight.

# Recommended Fat Intake

## ▶ Fat in the Diet

Fats in the diet are essential for good health. However, too much fat can contribute to obesity and a higher risk of heart disease, high blood pressure, diabetes, gallstone and certain cancers.

Dietary fat and oils have over double the calories of carbohydrates and protein. (Example: Changing from whole-milk to non-fat milk halves the calories.)

| MAXIMUM DESIRABLE FAT INTAKE (DAILY) | |
| --- | --- |
| Calories | Fat |
| 1200 cals | 30g fat |
| 1500 cals | 40g fat |
| 1800 cals | 50g fat |
| 2000 cals | 60g fat |
| 2200 cals | 70g fat |
| 2500 cals | 80g fat |
| 3000 cals | 110g fat |

### ZERO GRAMS TRANS FAT

*Don't be fooled by **Zero Grams Trans Fat** boldly displayed on some high-fat snacks. They are still high in fat and calories.*

*Examples: Cheetos 99c pkg ~ 24g fat, 380 cals*
*Lay's Chips (2¾ oz pkg) ~ 27g fat, 430 calories*

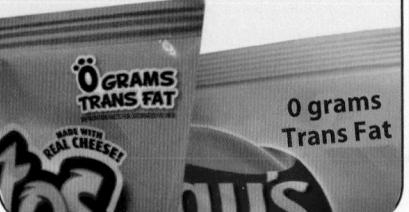

0 grams
Trans Fat

## ▶ Beware low-fat foods

It is a mistake to think that eating low-fat or fat-free foods allows you to eat double the quantity. You can end up with even more calories than eating smaller amounts of regular-fat products.

Food products which are fat-free but high in calories include soda drinks, fruit juices, beer, alcoholic spirits, sugar and candy. Bread, rice and pasta also have negligible fat but need to be eaten in controlled amounts.

Ultimately, **it is food portion size as well as total calories that count** whether from fat, carbohydrate or protein. Remember, cows get fat on grass!

*Reduced fat and fat-free foods are not necessarily low calorie. Portion size is still important.*

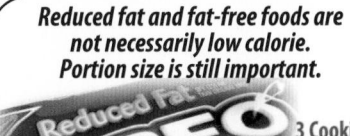

3 Cookies
140 Calories

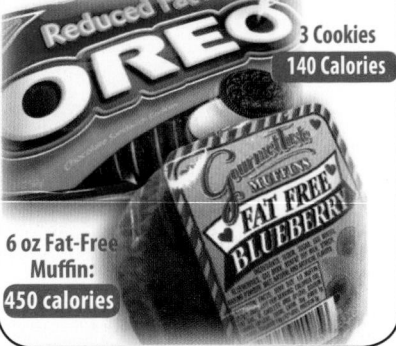

6 oz Fat-Free Muffin:
450 calories

### FOOD LABEL MEANINGS

**FDA Nutrition Claim Definitions**
(All are on a Per Serving Basis)

*Low Calorie:* 40 Calories or less

*Light or Lite:* One third fewer calories or, 50% or less fat than regular product

*Fat-Free:* Less than half a gram of fat

*Low-Fat:* 3 grams or less of fat

*Reduced Fat:* 25% less fat than regular product

*Fewer or Less Calories:* At least 25% fewer calories than regular product

### ▶ Meats, Poultry, Fish

- **Choose lean cuts** of meat with little marbling. **Trim all visible fat** from meat and remove the skin from poultry. Removal of fat after cooking, is okay (to prevent dryness). Choose 'extra lean' ground beef.

- **Avoid high-fat meat products** such as salami, bacon, sausage and franks.

- **Broil or bake. Avoid frying in oil.** Allow casseroles to cool and skim off surface fat.

- **Avoid fried fish,** frozen fish in batter and canned fish in oil.

### ▶ Fats & Oils

- **Use minimal amounts** of all types of fat and oil. All are high in calories.

- **Choose** 'light' and 'reduced fat' spreads but still use sparingly.

- Use minimal amounts of oil when stir-frying. Use no-stick sprays like Pam.

### ▶ Salad Dressings & Sauces

- **Avoid regular mayonnaise and oil dressings.** Choose 'light', 'reduced fat' or 'fat-free' brands.

- **Choose low-fat or fat-free sauces** (mainly tomato-based). Avoid 'pesto', 'alfredo', 'cheese' and 'creamy' sauces.

### ▶ Milk, Cheese

- **Choose low-fat or nonfat milks and yogurts.** Avoid full-cream milk, cream, Half & Half.

- **Cheese:** Choose fat-free, and low-fat cheese. Part-skim ricotta is still high in fat. Low-fat cottage cheese is a good choice. Cheese substitutes can still be high in fat.

### ▶ Snacks, Cookies, Candy

- **Avoid** high-fat snacks such as potato chips, corn/tortilla chips, cheese puffs, buttered popcorn, chocolate and carob bars.

### ▶ Desserts/Sweets

- **Avoid high-fat desserts,** such as cake, pie, pastries, cheesecake, full-fat puddings.

- **Choose** fresh fruits, fresh fruit salad, canned fruit in water pack, low-fat ice cream. Use low-fat yogurt in place of cream.

### ▶ Fast-Foods & Take-Out

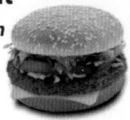

*Check the Fast-Foods Section of this book for actual fat and calorie counts.*

- **Avoid deep-fried foods such as** chicken, french fries and onion rings.

- **Pizzas:** Avoid sausage/pepperoni. Choose vegetarian topping and modest quantity of cheese. Eat a moderate serving. Eat extra salad and fresh fruit.

- **Hamburgers:** Choose medium size, lower fat burgers. Avoid bacon. Have a side salad (with fat-free dressing).

- **Delis:** Choose sandwiches/bread rolls, pitas with low-fat fillings and plain salad. Limit meat/cheese to small portions.

- **Coffees:** Avoid large sizes of latte and frappuccino. Request nonfat milk and no whipped cream. Avoid cookies and pastries.

*Extra Information: www.CalorieKing.com*

---

## FRYING ADDS FAT!

*The greater the surface are of potato exposed to fat or oil, the higher the fat content and calories.*

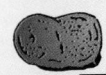 **Whole Potato (3 oz)**
**0g Fat**    65 Cals

 **Roasted Potato (3 oz)**
**5g Fat**    155 Cals

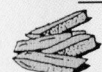 **Fries (Large cut, 3 oz)**
**12g Fat**    220 Cals

 **Fries (Small, 3 oz)**
**15g Fat**    265 Cals

 **Potato Chips (3 oz)**
**30g Fat**    450 Cals

## Naturally-Friendly Carbs

- **Carbohydrate foods in their more natural forms** (not overly processed) are essential to good health. They are the main source of fuel for the body, and also provide important vitamins, minerals, antioxidants and fiber – all of which help protect against heart disease, diabetes, hypertension, constipation-related ailments and many other diseases.

- Carbohydrates even help the body produce serotonin, the 'feel good' brain chemical that helps control appetite and overeating. Too little serotonin can lead to mood swings and depression.

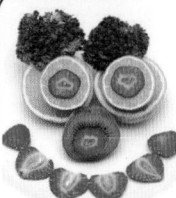

*Carbohydrate foods (minimally processed) are essential to good health.*

*Be sure to eat adequate fruit (2 servings) and vegetables (5 servings) every day.*

## Carbohydrates are found in different forms in food as:

- Sugars in fruit, sugar cane, milk
- Starches in whole grains, legumes, nuts, seeds and vegetables
- Dietary fiber (See Fiber Guide ~ Page 264)

*Glycemic Index & Diabetes ~ Page 21*

### RECOMMENDED CARBOHYDRATE INTAKE

| Calories (Daily) | Carbohydrate (Grams) | Percent Carbohydrate Calories |
|---|---|---|
| 1200 cals | 120g | 40% |
| 1500 cals | 170g | 45% |
| 1800 cals | 210g | 47% |
| 2000 cals | 250g | 50% |
| 2500 cals | 345g | 55% |
| 3000 cals | 450g | 60% |

## How Much Do We Need?

- As shown in the chart, well-balanced diets above 2000 calories contain 50-60% of total calories from carbohydrates.

- At lower calorie levels used for weight control (1200-1500 calories), carbohydrates account for as little as 40% of total calories. This is because protein calories have nutritional priority.

- Carbohydrates & Diabetes ~ *See Page 21*

## Low-Carbohydrate Diets

- Popular low-carbohydrate diets are extreme in their recommendations to initially cut carb intake to as little as 20 grams per day – the amount in 1 thick slice of bread, or 1 medium apple, or 1 small potato.

  This greatly increases the risk of nutritional deficiencies and compromises health, particularly if fat intake is excessive through fatty meats, high-fat dairy products, and fried foods.

- While overweight Americans do need to reduce carbohydrate intake, it should be done **sensibly as part of reducing portion size and total calories.**

- Simply eating 'low-carb' food products without regard to portion size, calories or fats, will do little to promote weight loss or good health.

- **Low-carb diets (and indeed any diet) only work if total calories are reduced.**

- Refined sugars should be one of the first targets in reducing carb intake.

**FAT MATTERS CARBS COUNT BUT CALORIES ARE KING!**

*Extra Info ~ www.CalorieKing.com*

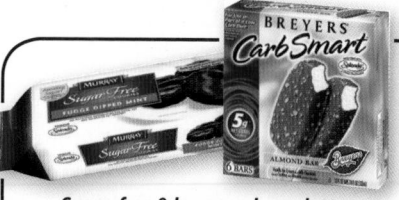

*Sugar-free & lower carb products may still be high in calories and fat.*

- Many overweight, inactive people consume over 500 calories of refined sugars per day, either self-added or as part of food products. This is equivalent to over 30 level teaspoons – a significant amount in weight control terms. Halving this amount would be reasonable and worthwhile.

**Note:** Naturally occurring sugars in fruits, vegetables and milk are fine when consumed in normal recommended amounts. These foods are also rich in other nutrients.

Refined sugar is referred to as having 'empty calories' because it supplies calories but negligible nutrients and no fiber.

- **Most sugar in our diet is 'hidden'** in processed foods such as soft drinks, fruit drinks, candy, cookies, cake, jam, sauces, ice cream, desserts, canned foods, and breakfast cereals.

Certainly enjoy moderate quantities of these foods, but for serious weight control, look for 'low calorie', 'diet' or 'sugar-free'.

- **However, be careful not to substitute sugar-rich foods with high-fat foods which might boost calories even more!**

- Be aware that sugar comes in different forms such as sucrose, glucose, fructose, malt, high-fructose corn syrup, molasses, honey and maple syrup. Check the label.

- **Sugar alcohols such as sorbitol,** mannitol and maltitol are carb-based and have ½ - ¾ the calories of regular sugar. While not counted as sugar on food labels, they do add to the carb count. Excess amounts can cause bloating, gas and diarrhea.

- **Sugar-free sweeteners** such as *Equal, DiabetiSweet, NutraSweet, Splenda, Sweet'n Low* and *Stevia* make it easy to reduce sugar in drinks and recipes. Use only in moderation. Note: Most recipes can be adapted to contain less sugar with little effect on taste or quality.

*Extra Info ~ www.CalorieKing.com*

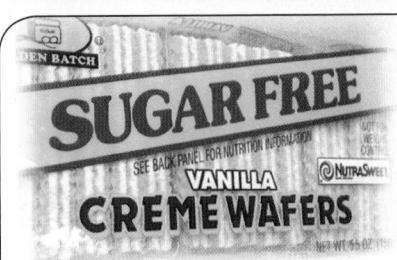

*Sugar-free snacks and foods may be higher in fat and calories than the regular product.*

| Example | ~ Creme Wafers (3): |
| --- | --- |
| Regular | ~ 115 cals, 6g fat |
| Sugar-Free | ~ 160 cals, 10g fat |

## SUGAR CONTENT OF SOME COMMON FOODS

### Teaspoons of Sugar

| | |
| --- | --- |
| *Coca Cola* or *Pepsi,* 12 fl.oz | 10 |
| 20 fl.oz size | 17 |
| Iced Tea, sweetened, 12 fl.oz | 8 |
| Chocolate Milk, 12 fl.oz | 6 |
| *Honey Smacks* Cereal, ¾ cup, 1 oz | 4 |
| Popcorn, caramel, 1 cup | 3.5 |
| Chocolate Bar, 1.5 oz | 6 |
| M&M's 1.7 oz pkg | 7 |
| Muffin, large, 4 oz | 6 |
| Choc Chip Cookie, 1 oz | 2 |
| Donut, iced | 6 |
| Apple Pie, 1 piece | 7 |
| *Jell-O,* ½ cup | 4.5 |
| Jam, 1 Tbsp, ¾ oz | 2.5 |
| Syrup, maple, 1 Tbsp | 3 |

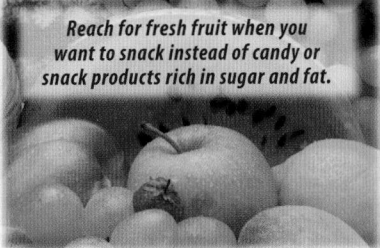

*Reach for fresh fruit when you want to snack instead of candy or snack products rich in sugar and fat.*

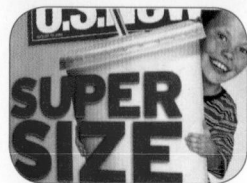

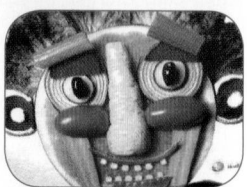

### The XL Generation

Some 15% of American kids and adolescents are overweight; and childhood obesity has doubled over the last 20 years. Diabetes, high blood pressure and high cholesterol are major problem areas for overweight children and adolescents, as are depression, low self-esteem, sleep apnea and bone joint problems.

To address this problem, cooperation is required between kids, parents, schools and government. Weight control is a family and community affair.

### *Five Simple Tips To Get Started:*

### ❶ Watch Soda Intake

Limit soda and sugary drinks to one serving on the weekends. Soda should not be an everyday beverage – water should be. When at restaurants or using a soda fountain, choose small servings with ice or choose diet soda instead. Schools should provide water and restrict access to soda as should parents when eating out or in the home!

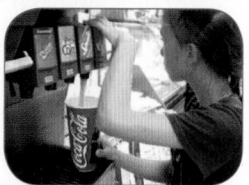

### ❷ Cut back on Fast-Foods and Eating Out

Many more calories are consumed when you eat out. Healthy meals prepared at home are best for the whole family.

### ❸ Say "No" to Super-Sizing

When meals are upsized, loads more calories are consumed. Choose sensible portion sizes when eating out and at home. Use smaller plates and choose smaller packages.

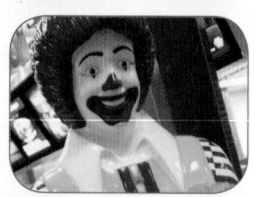

### ❹ Limit Between-Meal Snacking

Watch out for high-fat and high-calorie snacks – they can have more calories than a meal! Keep your eye on portion sizes and limit salty snack foods and candy to parties and special occasions. Choose fresh fruit, vegetables, nuts and low-fat milk instead.

### ❺ Get Moving ~ Watch Less TV

Kids need at least 60 minutes of physical activity every day. It's critical for their fitness, and greatly lessens the risk of obesity.

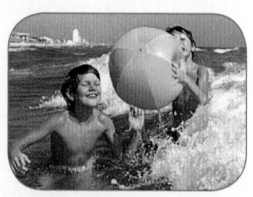

Encourage kids to be active out of school hours. Wearing a pedometer can be highly motivational for kids to move more – as can playing dance video games such as *Dance Dance Revolution*. *Dance Central* (XBox360) and *Wii Fit (Nintendo)* are also excellent fitness motivator.

**Limit TV and non-active computer games** to just one hour per day. Also limit the accompanying snacks! Include exercise in family activities.

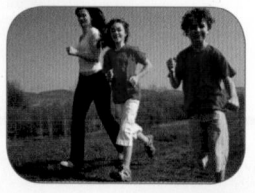

*Extra information and tips ~ www.CalorieKing.com*

**For Healthy, Overweight Persons ~ Not for Persons With Any Medical Condition**
**~ Please Check With Your Doctor & Dietitian ~**

## Breakfast (approx. 300 cal)

| | 1 Small Fruit or ½ oz Dried Fruit |
|---|---|
| Plus | Cereal: 1½ oz Dry (high fiber) |
| | or 1 cup cooked Oatmeal |
| Plus | ½ oz Almonds/Seeds |
| Plus | Milk (from daily allowance) or Yogurt (low-fat) |

**Daily Milk Allowance (approx.160 calories)**
2 cups Non-Fat Milk or 1½ cups Low-fat (1%) Milk
or equivalent Soy Drink, Yogurt, Cheese, Tofu

**Fat Allowance (140 calories; 15g Fat)**
4 tsp Fat or 6-8 tsp Diet Margarine or 3 tsp Oil
or 1½ Tbsp Mayonnaise or ½ medium Avocado
or 1½ Tbsp Peanut Butter or 30g Nuts/Seeds

## Lunch (approx. 440 calories)

| | 2 slices Wholegrain Bread (2 oz) |
|---|---|
| | or 4 Crispbreads/Crackers or 6" Pita |
| Plus | 2 oz lean Meat, Chicken or Turkey |
| | or 3½oz Tuna (in water) or 2½ oz Salmon |
| | or 1 oz Cheese or ½ cup (4 oz) Cottage Cheese |
| | or ½ cup (4 oz) Ricotta Cheese (low-fat) |
| | or ½ cup (4 oz) Fruit Yogurt (low-fat) |
| | or ½ cup (4 oz) Bean Salad |
| Plus | Large Salad (Oil-free dressing) |
| Plus | 1 small Fruit or ½ oz Dried Fruit |

## Dinner (approx. 360 calories)

| | Soup (fat-free) |
|---|---|
| Plus | 3 oz lean Meat (cooked weight) |
| | or 4 oz Chicken Breast (no skin) |
| | or 3 oz Chicken Thigh/Leg (no skin) |
| | or 5 oz Fish (grilled, no fat) |
| | or ¾ cup (6 oz) Beans (Soy, Kidney, Pinto etc)/Lentils |
| | or Low-fat Entree (e.g. Lean Cuisine) |
| Plus | 1 small Potato or ½ cup Rice/Pasta/Sweet Corn |
| | or 1 slice Wholegrain Bread |
| Plus | 2-3 servings Vegetables/Salad |
| Plus | 1 small Fruit + Diet Gelatin Dessert |

## Breakfast ~ Choice 2

| | 1 Small Fruit |
|---|---|
| Plus | 2 Eggs (no added fat) |
| | or 2 oz Cheese (low-fat) |
| | or 4 oz Cottage Cheese (low-fat) |
| | or 2 oz Lean/Canadian Bacon |
| Plus | 1 Tomato |
| Plus | 1 Slice Wholegrain Toast |

## Between Meals

Water, Coffee, Tea, Diet drinks,
Fruit from main meals; Raw vegetable
pieces, Milk from Daily Allowance

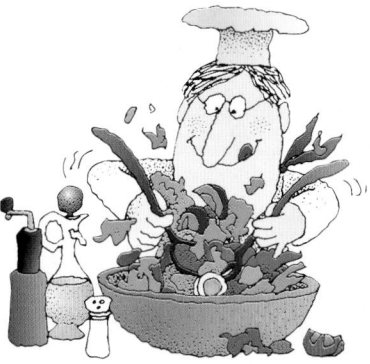

- Persons who exercise regularly lose more weight and keep it off longer than non-exercisers.
- Exercise also improves general health and well-being. Mood, confidence and self-esteem are enhanced by a sense of control and accomplishment.
- **Exercise increases the metabolic rate** of the body even for hours after exercise – a good way to 'wake up' a sluggish metabolism and burn extra fat.

  Exercise compensates for any decrease in metabolic rate with increasing age and also in some heavy smokers who stop smoking.
- **Strength training** further builds muscle and aids body reshaping. You can also eat a little more food!

  Note: Each extra pound of muscle burns an extra 50 calories daily ~ even while you sleep! Weight from exercised muscles is okay. It is surplus fat (particularly abdominal fat) that is potentially harmful to health.
- **Avoid injury** by beginning with walking, low impact aerobics, or weight-supported exercise (e.g. swimming, cycling). Avoid competitive sports.
- **How Much?** Start with 10 - 20 minutes/day and progress to 30 - 60 minutes/day.

  Also walk up stairs instead of using elevators. Take a brisk walk at lunch. Use an exercise bike, treadmill or stair machine while watching TV. Walk the dog.
- **How Often?** While aerobic fitness requires only 3 - 4 sessions weekly, **weight control is a daily event which requires daily exercise.**

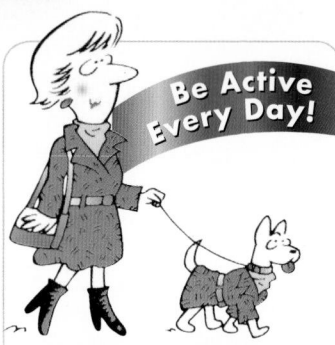

**Be Active Every Day!**

*Brisk walking each day is a safe and effective way to keep trim and fit. Try it – you'll like it!*

*Strength-training with light weights helps to retain or rebuild muscle tissue. It enhances weight control.*

### FATNESS VS FITNESS

*An overweight but fit person can be healthier than a thin, unfit person.*

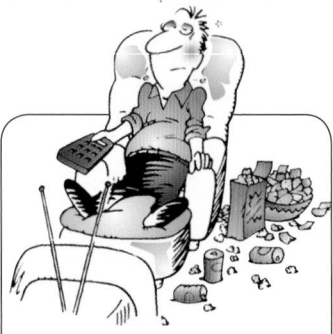

### TV CAN BE FATTENING!

- **Many adults and children spend over 20 hours per week watching TV or at the computer (playing games or 'surfing') – at the same time as eating high-calorie snacks and drinks.**
- **Are you a TV couch potato or computer addict? Limit your TV and computer hours and plan healthy physical activities.**
- **At home, limit kids to just one hour daily for TV and computers. Kids need at least 60 minutes of physical activity every day.**

*Too little exercise and too much food are the main contributors to middle-age spread.*

*Daily exercise and sensible eating can minimize middle-age spread. Include some strength-training to retain or build muscle.*

# Calories Used in Exercise

| LIGHT | MODERATE | HEAVY |
|---|---|---|
| 130 lbs ~ 3 Cals/Min | 130 lbs ~ 5 Cals/Min | 130 lbs ~ 8 Cals/Min |
| 170 lbs ~ 4 Cals/Min | 170 lbs ~ 6 Cals/Min | 220 lbs ~ 12 Cals/Min |
| 220 lbs ~ 5 Cals/Min | 220 lbs ~ 7 Cals/Min | 170 lbs ~ 10 Cals/Min |

| LIGHT | MODERATE | HEAVY |
|---|---|---|
| Walking, slow | Walking, brisk | Walking (power), Jogging |
| Cycling, light | Cycling, moderate | Cycling (vigorous), Spinning |
| Frisbee playing | Swimming, crawl | Swimming, strenuous |
| Gardening, light | Weight-training, light | Weight-training, heavy |
| Golf, social | Tennis, moderate | Wrestling/Judo, advanced |
| Tennis, doubles | Racquetball, beginners | Racquetball, advanced |
| Housework, cleaning | Aerobics, light | Tae Bo, Kick Boxing |
| Calisthenics, light | Football, touch | Football, training |
| Bowling | Basketball, Baseball | Basketball (Pro) |
| Ping-pong, social | Walking Downstairs | Climbing Stairs |
| Ice Skating, light | Snow Skiing (downhill) | Skipping Rope |
| Aquarobics, light | Shovelling snow | Skiing (cross country) |
| Skate Boarding | Dancing (ballroom) | Aquarobics, advanced |
| Line/Square Dancing | Rowing, moderate | Dancing (strenuous), Zumba |
| Tai Chi, Yoga | Volleyball, competitive | Rowing, vigorous |
| Volleyball | | Martial Arts |

Note: Only those sports or activities that are sustained over a period of time (e.g running)
qualify for heavy exercise. Stop-start sports such as tennis are considered 'moderate'.

## Interactive Calculations ~ www.CalorieKing.com/tools

### WALKING PROGRAM

#### USE DISTANCE, STEPS OR TIME

| Weeks | Distance | Steps Pedometer | Time |
|---|---|---|---|
| 1-2 | 1 mile | 2000 | 20 mins |
| 3-5 | 1.5 miles | 3000 | 28 mins |
| 6-8 | 2 miles | 3500 | 35 mins |
| 9-10 | 2.5 miles | 4500 | 45 mins |
| 11+ | 3.5 miles | 6000 | 60 mins |

### 10,000 STEPS PER DAY

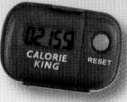

A pedometer can motivate you to be more active. It clips to your belt or waist band and registers each step.

Aim for 8,000 - 10,000 steps per day, instead of an average of only 3,000 - 4,000 steps.

For Extra Information:
www.CalorieKing.com

# Reshaping Eating Behaviors

- Eating is a behavior that is largely controlled by people with whom we live or socialize, places in which we carry out our lives, and our emotions. Become aware of those situations that commonly lead to extra food being eaten.

- We may also be unaware of 'bad' eating habits that can lead to excess calorie intake; e.g. eating quickly, large mouthfuls, eating when tense or bored, finishing a large serving of food when not hungry.

**Tips to help uncover and correct those 'bad' or problem eating habits:**

- **Don't eat while engaged in other activities;** for example, watching TV, reading. Eat only at the table, not at the fridge or while standing.

- **Don't eat quickly.** Chewing slowly allows time to register a feeling of fullness. Don't use fingers, only utensils. Cut food into smaller pieces. Don't load your fork until the previous mouthful is finished.

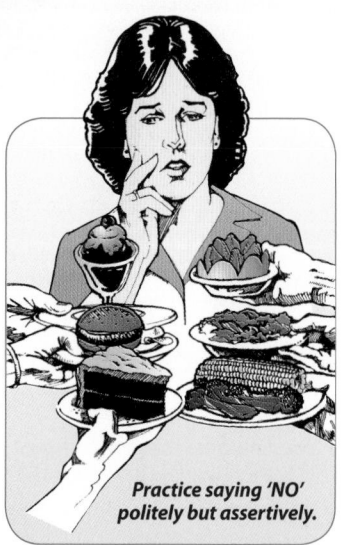

*Practice saying 'NO' politely but assertively.*

- **Don't purchase problem high calorie foods.** Shop from a set list to prevent impulse buying. Avoid shopping with children.

- **Buy snack foods** in the smallest package. The larger the serving size or package, the more you are likely to eat or drink.

- **Plan meals in advance. Stick to a set menu.**

- **Plan a strategy to avoid uncontrolled eating** and drinking at social events, or when your emotions urge you to binge.

    Rehearse repeatedly in your mind exactly what you will do in such situations. Remind yourself several times each day that you are in charge of your actions and that you can be strong-willed. Seek counseling or coaching on various strategies.

- **Distract yourself** when you feel the urge to snack impulsively. Engage in some activity that will distract you from thinking about food. Examples: go for a walk, brush your teeth, phone a friend.

    If you eat out of boredom, find some new hobby or interest that gets you out of the house. Even enrol in an adult education class.

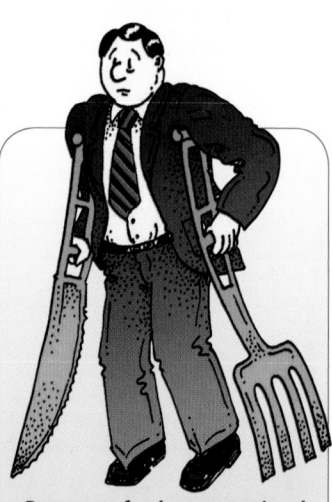

*Do you use food as an emotional crutch? If so, professional counseling may be helpful.*

**The food journal is the most powerful proven aid for dieters.** Persons who keep a food and exercise journal not only lose more weight, they also keep it off. Here are some of the reasons:

- **Recording your eating and exercise habits** jolts you into realizing just what you do eat and drink each day; and also whether you exercise sufficiently.

- **Helps you identify problem foods** and drinks with excessive calories and fat.

- **Helps identify moods,** situations and events that lead to excessive eating of unwanted calories. You can then plan to overcome or avoid them.

- **Prevents 'calorie amnesia',** the forgetfulness that leads to rebound weight gain after successful weight loss. Recording puts you back on the right track.

- **Helps you develop greater self-discipline.** You will think twice about overindulging if you have to record it - especially if someone checks your journal regularly. It certainly keeps you honest!

- **Motivates you** to carefully plan your meals and to exercise each day.

- **Serves as a check system** for your doctor, dietitian or counselor to assess your progress and make recommendations.

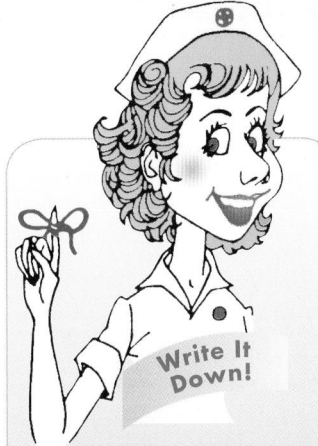

*Write It Down!*

*"Keeping a journal gives me feedback on exactly what I eat and drink each day.*

*It helps prevent 'calorie amnesia' and reminds me to exercise each day.*

*It's a 'must' for successful weight control!"*

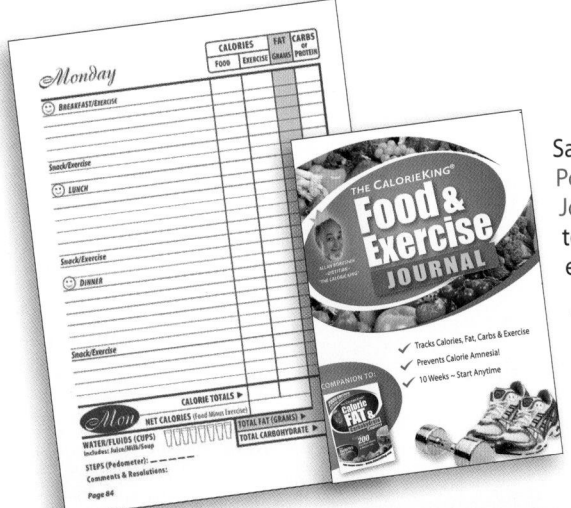

Sample Page from The Pocket Food & Exercise Journal, a 10-week journal to record food and exercise.

At day's end, exercise calories are deducted from food calories.

Includes Weekly Summary Page & Progress Checklist.

## What is Diabetes?
**Diabetes occurs when the body has difficulty processing glucose sugar in the blood.**

- **After digestion,** sugar and starches are changed into **glucose** – the simplest form of sugar vital for body energy and growth.
- Insulin is the hormone which acts like a key that opens the door to body cells and allows glucose to enter.
- **Without enough insulin,** glucose builds up in the blood and passes into the urine. High blood glucose levels lead to frequent urination, extreme thirst, and tiredness.
- **Untreated diabetes increases the risk of damage to nerves and blood vessels.** This, in turn, increases the risk of heart disease, stroke, blindness, kidney damage, foot ulcers and gangrene (with amputation), impotence and other complications.

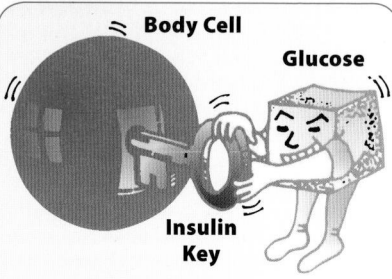

*Insulin acts like a key.
It opens the door to body cells
and allows glucose to enter.*

*People with type 1 diabetes and some
with type 2 have too few or no keys and
require insulin injections.*

*Others (primarily type 2) make enough
insulin but the body doesn't use it as well as
it should – particularly if obese and inactive.*

### SYMPTOMS OF DIABETES

- Frequent urination
- Extreme thirst
- Unusual hunger
- Rapid weight loss
- Extreme fatigue
- Blurred vision
- Skin infections that are slow to heal
- Tingling/numbness in feet

**DON'T IGNORE DIABETES**

*IT'S A SERIOUS DISEASE!*

*Note: Diabetes can be present even with no symptoms.*

### TYPE 2 DIABETES

- Occurs in 90% of diabetes cases
- Occurs mainly in adults - particularly in overweight and inactive persons
- Insulin is produced but body cells resist its action and glucose cannot enter cells
- Usually treated with meal planning and physical activity. Sometimes requires medication (pills or insulin)

### TYPE 1 DIABETES

- Occurs in 10% of diabetes cases
- Usually in children and young adults
- Pancreas produces little or no insulin. Daily insulin injections (or use of an insulin pump) are necessary, as well as:
  - matching pre-meal insulin to the amount of carbohydrate eaten
  - weight control and regular physical activity

### GESTATIONAL DIABETES

- Occurs in some women during pregnancy. It usually disappears after the baby's birth.
- Women who have had gestational diabetes still have a high risk of developing type 2 diabetes within 5 to 10 years.
- Requires weight control, a healthy lifestyle and regular medical checks

## Are You At Risk for Diabetes?

*Pre-Diabetes ~ An Early Warning!*

Pre-diabetes means that your blood glucose levels are higher than normal, but not high enough to be called diabetes.

**If you have pre-diabetes, you have a higher risk for getting diabetes later on.**

The good news is that you can start taking steps to prevent diabetes by making healthy lifestyle changes – such as losing weight if overweight, and being more physically active.

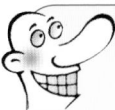

### WHAT'S YOUR RISK?

*Find out if you're at risk for diabetes by answering the following questions:*

☐ I have been told I have pre-diabetes

☐ I have a family history of diabetes

☐ I am African American, Latino American, Asian American, Native American or a Pacific Islander

☐ I have had gestational diabetes (diabetes during pregnancy)

☐ I am over age 45

☐ I am overweight

☐ I get little or no physical activity

☐ My waist is larger than: 35 inches (for a woman) or 40 inches (for a man)

☐ My blood pressure is higher than 130 over 85

☐ My HDL (good cholesterol) is too low

☐ My triglycerides (blood fats) are too high

### ✔ CHECK YOUR RESULT

• If you've put a check mark in two or more of the boxes, you may be more likely to develop type 2 diabetes.

• Talk with your healthcare provider to see if you should have a blood test for diabetes.

### BLOOD GLUCOSE CLASSIFICATION OF DIABETES

| | |
|---|---|
| **Normal:** | **Below 100 mg/dl*** |
| **Pre-Diabetes:** | 100-125 mg/dl* |
| **Diabetes:** | **Over 125 mg/dl*** |

*(\*Fasting Blood Glucose)*

#### KNOW YOUR BGL

*(Blood Glucose Level)*
*Everyone over the age of 45 should have a blood glucose test every three years*

## Importance of Weight Control

• **Type 2 diabetes** is more common in people who are overweight.

• **Being overweight** means that your insulin doesn't work as well to control blood glucose levels.

• **Losing just 10 to 20 pounds** can help you better manage your diabetes and lower your risk for heart disease.

• **Keys to weight control include:**

• Following a healthy eating plan

• Controlling food portions

• Being physically active most days of the week

• Keeping food records

• Setting realistic goals

• **Work with a registered dietitian** who can help you reach a weight that's ideal for you.

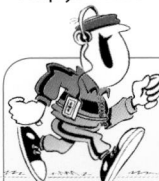

### KEEP MOVING!

*Every day, do at least 30 minutes of moderate intensity exercise.*
*(even in 5-minute sets)*

*It's the key to improving insulin action.*
*Add muscle strength training 3-4 times a week to double the benefits.*

## Managing Diabetes

Don't battle diabetes alone. Establish a partnership with your doctor, dietitian, certified diabetes educator, and pharmacist.

**Extra Support:** • *Joslin Diabetes Center*
• *American Diabetes Association*
• *American Association of Diabetes Educators*
• *Juvenile Diabetes Research Foundation*
• *National Diabetes Education Program*

### Hints to keep blood glucose within safe limits:

• **Control your food intake.** Know what and when you will eat. Seek referral to a dietitian for expert advice.

• **Exercise regularly.** It assists weight control and can improve sensitivity of body cells to insulin. Plan physical activity into your daily routine.

• **Monitor your blood glucose** at home and work with a blood glucose meter. It will help you become familiar with your blood glucose patterns, and the effects of food, activity and medication.

• T**ake insulin or oral medication as prescribed.** If on insulin, know what action to take if hypoglycemia (low blood glucose) occurs. Also educate your family and friends. More Info: www.joslin.org

### Be Heart Smart ~ Know Your ABC's

If you have diabetes, you are at a higher risk for heart attack and stroke than someone without diabetes. But you can fight back!

### Be smart about your heart!

Take control of the ABC's of diabetes and live a long and healthy life. Talk to your healthcare provider about your ABC targets.

**Ⓐ is for A1C**
The A1C (A-one-C) test – short for hemoglobin A1C. It reflects your average blood glucose (sugar) over the last 3 months.
Suggested Target: Below 7%

**Ⓑ is for Blood Pressure**
High blood pressure makes your heart work too hard.
**Suggested Target: Below 130/80**

**Ⓒ is for Cholesterol**
Bad cholesterol, or LDL, can build up and clog your arteries. **Suggested Target: Below 100**

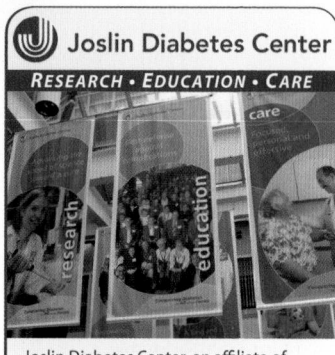

**Ⓤ Joslin Diabetes Center**

**RESEARCH • EDUCATION • CARE**

Joslin Diabetes Center, an affiliate of Harvard Medical School, is the world's largest diabetes research center, diabetes clinic and provider of diabetes education.

**MORE INFORMATION**
www.joslin.org or call 800-344-4501

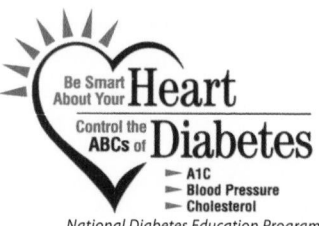

Be Smart About Your **Heart**
Control the **Diabetes**
ABCs of
➤ A1C
➤ Blood Pressure
➤ Cholesterol
*National Diabetes Education Program*

***Be smart about your heart!***

***Take control of the ABC's of diabetes and live a long and healthy life.***

***Talk to your healthcare provider about your ABC targets.***

***Take action now to lower your risk for heart attack, stroke and other diabetes problems.***

**\* \* \***

◀ *Note: These targets are suggested by the National Institutes for Health and the American Diabetes Association*

**Guidelines for choosing a healthy diet apply equally to people with or without diabetes.** Eating a wide variety of foods that are mainly low in fat, low in refined sugars, and high in fiber, is recommended.

However, actual food quantities, as well as when you eat, will also influence control of blood glucose. Your dietitian will individualize a meal plan to suit your food preferences, lifestyle and medical status.

### Here are a few tips:

- **Maintain a healthy weight.** If overweight, even a modest weight loss plus daily physical activity can help manage blood glucose in type 2 diabetes.

- **Don't skip meals.** If you take insulin or an oral hypoglycemic agent, regular meals are important.

  **If on insulin,** eat meals at the same time each day. Eat a similar amount of food at each meal. Eating about the same amount of carbohydrate over the day will make best use of insulin and prevent wide variations in blood glucose levels.

- **Know which foods contain carbohydrate;** and learn how to check the *Nutrition Facts Label* on foods. Check the serving size, total fat and total carbohydrate – not just the sugar content. All carbohydrate breaks down to sugars after digestion.

- **Choose wholegrain breads, cereals and pasta.** Eat fresh fruits, vegetables and legumes. These foods contain more fiber and slow the release of glucose into your blood after a meal.

- **Limit foods high in saturated fat, trans fat and cholesterol.** Enjoy fish, soy foods, and other foods rich in omega-3 fats. *(Extra Notes: Page 259)*

- **Limit sugars and foods high in added sugar** particularly if overweight. Small amounts of sugar as part of a meal may occasionally be okay. Check with your dietitian. *(Extra Notes: Page 9)*

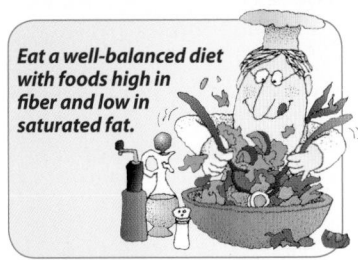

*Eat a well-balanced diet with foods high in fiber and low in saturated fat.*

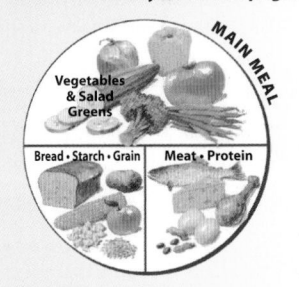

*The Plate Method is an easy way to eat healthfully. (See next page)*

MAIN MEAL

Vegetables & Salad Greens

Bread · Starch · Grain

Meat · Protein

## ALCOHOL TIPS

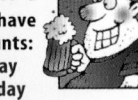

- **If you drink alcohol, have only moderate amounts:**
  **Men ~ 1-2 drinks/day**
  **Women ~ 1 drink/day**
  For some people, safe drinking will mean no alcoholic drinks at all.

  *(Also see Alcohol Guide ~ Page 23)*

- **Drink along with your food** – especially if you use insulin or diabetes pills.

- **Do not omit any carb food** in exchange for an alcoholic drink. However, non-alcoholic beers (12 fl oz) count as one carb exchange.

- **Alcohol increases the risk of hypoglycemia** (low blood sugar) and drug interactions if you take insulin and certain types of diabetes pills.

- **Check with your doctor and dietitian.**
  *Extra Info: www.joslin.org*

## The Plate Method – An Easy Way to Eat Healthfully

The plate method is a helpful tool to guide your food choices until you see a dietitian for your own meal plan.

### For a healthy meal:

- Fill half of your plate with non-starchy vegetables (broccoli, green beans, carrots).
- Fill a quarter of your plate with carbohydrate (wholegrain bread, pasta, potato, brown rice).
- Fill the other quarter of your plate with 3-4 ounces of lean meat, poultry, or fish.
- Use 1-2 teaspoons of tub margarine or a heart-healthy vegetable oil.
- Add a small piece of fruit or 8 ounces of skim/low-fat milk or yogurt.

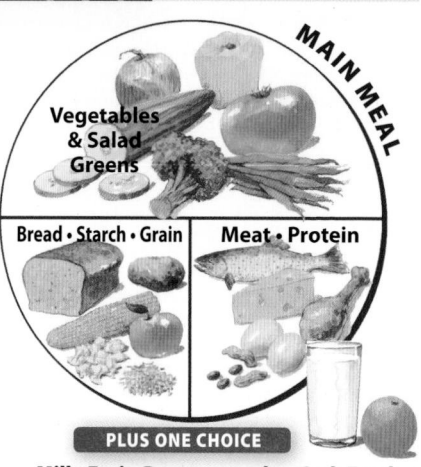

MAIN MEAL

**Vegetables & Salad Greens**

**Bread • Starch • Grain**  |  **Meat • Protein**

**PLUS ONE CHOICE**

**Milk, Fruit, Dessert or other Carb Food**

## How Much Carbohydrate Should You Eat?

A dietitian can best determine how much carbohydrate you need at each of your meals, based on your lifestyle, food preferences, and overall diabetes control.

Until you see a dietitian, aim to keep the amount of carbohydrate you eat the same at each of your meals.

### CARB CHOICES MEAL PLAN
#### One Carb Choice = 15 Grams of Carb

**The amount in:** 1 slice Bread **or** ¾ cup Cereal (unsweetened) **or** 1 small Potato **or** 1 small Fruit

### Breakfast
- Eat 2-3 carb choices (30-45 grams)
- Include a low-fat protein source such as egg whites or skim milk.

### Lunch and Dinner
- Eat 3-4 carb choices (45-60 grams carb)
- Include fruit and non-starchy vegetables. Choose small portions of low-fat protein foods.

**Snacks:** If needed, eat 1-2 carb choices (15-30 grams carb).

*Note: Above plan is for adults. Carbohydrate amounts will vary with physical activity level.*

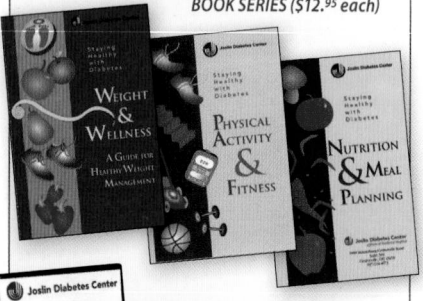
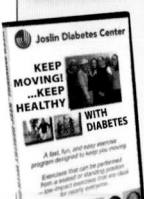

## Carb Type Affects Blood Glucose

The various forms of carbohydrate affect blood glucose levels in different ways. It is difficult to predict the effect of particular foods, sugars, or meals, simply by their carbohydrate content.

Thus the same amount of carbohydrate from different foods may affect blood sugar levels very differently. Many factors affect the rate of digestion and absorption such as:

- the type of sugar, starch, and fiber
- the degree of processing and cooking (which increases digestion rate)
- the amount of protein and fat (which slow stomach emptying and digestion).

## Glycemic Index (GI)

**The GI is a method of ranking carbohydrate foods on a scale (0-100)** according to how they affect blood glucose levels. (See next column.)

The higher the GI value, the greater the food's ability to rapidly raise blood glucose levels, and the more insulin needed by the body (not desirable).

**Eating low-GI foods may lead to better control of blood glucose and insulin levels** (which in turn lowers the risk of damage to blood vessels and nerves). The slower digestion of low-GI foods may also help to delay hunger pangs and benefit weight control.

## Cautionary Notes on GI

**Choosing low-GI foods is not a license to eat unlimited amounts.** Calorie restriction and portion control for weight control is of prime importance.

**Also remember, Low-GI foods are carbohydrate foods** and must still be counted as part of any dietetic carbohydrate plan.

GI is not meant to be used by itself without regard to portion size, and other dietary recommendations for healthy eating. Foods are not good or bad on the basis of their GI.

While GI may be a helpful tool for some people with diabetes, what is most important is to control the total amount of carbohydrate that you eat.

## LOWER-GLYCEMIC FOODS

### Slower-Acting Carbohydrates

These foods are more slowly digested and absorbed. They help maintain more even blood glucose levels, as long as excessive amounts are not eaten. Use these foods regularly but still limit portion size for weight control.

*Examples:*

- Dried beans, peas, lentils
- Nuts and seeds
- Wholegrain breads
- Bran cereals, oats
- Sweet corn, barley, buckwheat
- Wholegrain pasta, basmati rice
- Fresh fruit: apples, avocados, bananas (firm), cherries, grapefruit, grapes, olives, oranges, peaches, pears, plums. Fresh juices.
- Vegetables: broccoli, yam, sweet potatoes, salad greens
- Milk, yogurt, soy drinks
- Dark chocolate
- Sugar alcohols (sorbitol, maltitol)

## HIGHER-GLYCEMIC FOODS

### Quicker-Acting Carbohydrates

These foods more rapidly raise blood glucose levels. Eat only in moderation.

- White bread, rice cakes, bagels, croissants, doughnuts
- Low-fiber cereals: Cornflakes, *Rice Krispies, Froot Loops*
- White potatoes, white rice
- Watermelon, ripe bananas, cantaloupe, pineapple
- Soda, sugar-sweetened sports and energy drinks
- Sugar, candy, popcorn (plain)
- Ice cream (low-fat), frozen yogurt

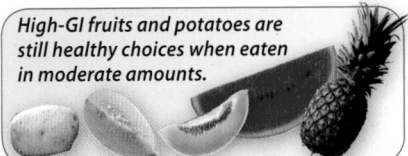

*High-GI fruits and potatoes are still healthy choices when eaten in moderate amounts.*

» Calorie and fat values have been rounded off.
**Calories** ~ to the nearest 5 or 10 calories.
**Fat** ~ to nearest half gram. **Note:** Trace amounts of fat (less than 0.3 grams) have been treated as zero.

» **Carbohydrate figures** in this book are for total carbohydrate, and not **Net Carbs** (which deducts fiber, polydextrose and sugar alcohols from total carbs).

» Because manufacturers' figures on labels are rounded off, figures in this book may differ slightly from the label. Serving sizes may also vary.

## IMPORTANT DISCLAIMER

\* The authors and publishers of this book are not physicians and are not licensed to give medical advice. This book is not a substitute for professional advice. Users should consult their medical professional before making any health, medical or other decisions based on the material contained herein.

\* This book is a compilation of original material from other sources intended for educational purposes only. Because food manufacturers constantly change their products, only they are the authoritative source for food's most current nutritional information.

\* Persons using the information herein for any medical purposes, such as matching insulin dosage to carbohydrate intake, should not rely solely on the accuracy of figures herein and should independently check food labels or contact the food manufacturer for the latest data.

\* Because nutrition data for food products is subject to change, users should consult the most recent edition of this book, and the author's website www.calorieking.com for the most up-to-date information.

## \* WARRANTY DISCLAIMER:

THE AUTHOR AND PUBLISHER DISCLAIM ANY LIABILITY ARISING DIRECTLY OR INDIRECTLY FROM THE USE OF THIS BOOK. THE INFORMATION HEREIN IS PROVIDED "AS IS" AND WITHOUT ANY WARRANTY EXPRESSED OR IMPLIED. ALL DIRECT, INDIRECT, SPECIAL, INCIDENTAL, CONSEQUENTIAL OR PUNITIVE DAMAGES ARISING FROM ANY USE OF THIS INFORMATION IS DISCLAIMED AND EXCLUDED.

This information is also provided subject to Family Health Publications' Terms and Conditions found at the website, www.calorieking.com/terms and incorporated herein.

---

**C** ~ **Calories**
**F** ~ **Fat (grams)**
**Cb** ~ **Carbohydrate (grams)**

### Abbreviations

| | |
|---|---|
| tsp | = teaspoon |
| Tbsp or T | = Tablespoon |
| oz | = ounce(s) |
| c | = cup |
| fl.oz | = fluid ounce(s) |
| g | = gram(s) |
| avg | = average |
| pkg | = package |

### Volume Measures

(All measures are level)
3 tsp = 1 Tbsp
2 Tbsp = 1 fl.oz
½ cup = 4 fl.oz
1 cup = 8 fl.oz
2 cups = 1 Pint
2 Pints = 1 Quart

Note: 8 oz weight is not the same as 8 fl oz volume (space occupied). Dense foods weigh more per set volume. Examples:
1 cup popcorn weighs ½ oz
1 cup milk weighs 8½ oz
1 cup pudding weighs 10 oz

### Metric Conversion

½ oz = 14 grams
1 oz = 28.4 grams
2 oz = 57 grams
3½ oz = 100 grams
1 fl.oz = 30 mls
1 cup (8 fl.oz) = 240 mls
33 fl.oz = 1 liter (volume)

## INFORMATION SOURCES

• U.S. Dept. of Agriculture
• Food Manufacturers
• Food Industry Boards & Councils
• Author extrapolations

## FEEDBACK WELCOME!

Please contact the author with your queries and suggestions.
feedback@calorieking.com

- **Health Hazards: Excessive alcohol intake** contributes to obesity, high blood pressure, stroke, heart and liver disease, some cancers, and even impotence. **Concentration and short-term memory** are reduced as well as athletic performance.

  **Other alcohol hazards include:** Fetal Alcohol Syndrome, stomach upsets, menstrual problems, depression, snoring, sleep problems, work absenteeism, impaired judgement, and social/family problems.

- **Alcohol contributes to obesity:** Through its high calories and by lessening the body's ability to burn fat. Fat storage is promoted, particularly in the belly – a health danger zone. Alcohol can also stimulate the appetite.

- **Alcohol is potentially more harmful while dieting:** Blood sugar levels may drop with resultant fatigue and further impairment of concentration, reflexes and driving skills – and maybe even the dieter's resolve!

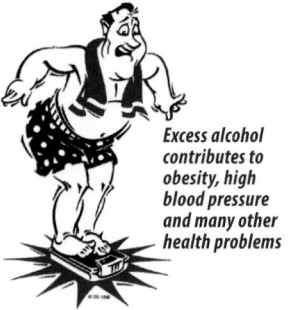

*Excess alcohol contributes to obesity, high blood pressure and many other health problems*

## LOWER RISK ALCOHOL LIMITS

 **WOMEN:**
No more than
**1 drink** per day

 **MEN:**
No more than
**2 drinks** per day
(Over 65 y.o. ~ 1 drink)

(At least 2 days a week should be alcohol-free)

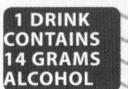

**1 DRINK CONTAINS 14 GRAMS ALCOHOL**

➤ 12 fl.oz Regular Beer (5% Alc.)
➤ OR 14 fl.oz Light Beer (4.2% Alc.)
➤ OR 5 fl.oz Wine (12% Alc.)
➤ OR 1½ fl.oz Spirits (80 Proof)

Note: You cannot save daily drinks for one occasion.
Binge drinking is particularly harmful:
4 drinks for males or 3 drinks for females (within 2 hours).

## HOW TO CALCULATE ALCOHOL CONTENT

Percent alcohol on label refers to alcohol volume (ml alcohol/100ml).
Note: 100ml = 3½ fl.oz

To convert to grams (weight) of alcohol, multiply the percent volume by 0.8 – since 1 ml of alcohol weighs only 0.8 grams.

*EXAMPLE:*
*12 fl.oz Can Beer*
*(5% alcohol)*
5% alc. volume
= 5% of 12 fl.oz = 0.6 fl.oz
= 18ml alcohol (Note: 1 fl.oz = 30ml)
Weight (18ml x 0.8) = 14.4g alcohol

For some people, safe drinking means no alcohol at all. Even one drink may impair driving skills, particularly if tired. For women who drink frequently, breast cancer risk is increased by 9% for each drink after the first drink.

**It is advisable not to drink at all if you are:**
- pregnant, trying to conceive or breastfeeding
- taking medication or have liver or heart disease (unless approved by your doctor or pharmacist)
- planning to drive, use machinery or play sports
- studying or needing to concentrate
- a child or adolescent

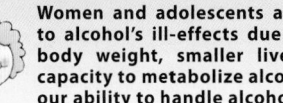 **Women and adolescents are more prone to alcohol's ill-effects due to their lower body weight, smaller livers and lesser capacity to metabolize alcohol. As we age, our ability to handle alcohol decreases.**

## GOVERNMENT WARNINGS!

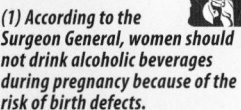

*(1) According to the Surgeon General, women should not drink alcoholic beverages during pregnancy because of the risk of birth defects.*

*(2) Consumption of alcoholic beverages impairs your ability to drive a car or operate machinery, and may cause health problems.*

### EXTRA INFORMATION
Alcohol & Diabetes ~ See Page 21
Alcohol & The Heart ~ See Page
Tips to Avoid Harmful Drinking ~ Page

## Quick Guide    **Alc** ~ Alcohol (Grams)

**Beer**    **Cb** ~ Carbohydrate

**Beer Contains Zero Fat**

| | **C** | **Alc** | **Cb** |
|---|---|---|---|
| **Regular Beer (5% Alc. Vol.):** | | | |
| 7 fl.oz Glass | 80 | 8.5 | 4 |
| 12 fl.oz Bottle/Can/Glass | 140 | 14 | 10 |
| 16 fl.oz Bottle/Can | 185 | 19 | 13 |
| 22 fl.oz Bottle | 260 | 26 | 18 |
| 24 fl.oz Can | 280 | 28 | 20 |
| 32 fl.oz Bottle | 370 | 38 | 28 |
| 40 fl.oz Bottle | 470 | 47 | 35 |
| 50 fl.oz Football | 590 | 59 | 50 |
| **Light Beer (4.2% Alc. Vol.):** | | | |
| 7 fl.oz Glass | 65 | 7 | 4 |
| 12 fl.oz Bottle/Can/Glass | 110 | 12 | 7 |
| 16 fl.oz Bottle/Can | 145 | 16 | 9 |
| 22 fl.oz Bottle | 200 | 22 | 13 |
| 24 fl.oz Can | 220 | 24 | 14 |
| **Non-Alcoholic Brews:** | | | |
| (Less than 0.5% alcohol by volume) | | | |
| Average all Brands, 12 fl.oz | 70 | 1 | 14 |

## Beer Brands

*Note: Figures shown are for the United States except for the states of Utah, Colorado, Kansas and Oklahoma who have certain restrictions limiting the alcohol content to not more than 4% by volume (3.2% by weight).*

*Per 12 fl.oz Serving*
*Percentage alcohol listed is by volume - not by weight.*    **Alc** ~ Alcohol (Grams)

| | **C** | **Alc** | **Cb** |
|---|---|---|---|
| **Amstel,** Light (3.5%) | 95 | 10 | 5 |
| **Anchor:** Porter (5.6%) | 210 | 15 | 23 |
| Steam (4.9%) | 165 | 14 | 14 |
| **Asahi:** Kuronama (5.3%) | 165 | 14 | 14 |
| Select (4.7%) | 140 | 13 | 11 |
| Super Dry (4.9%) | 150 | 14 | 11 |
| **Bass,** Pale Ale (5.1%) | 155 | 14 | 12 |
| **Beck's:** Original (5%) | 145 | 14 | 12 |
| Premier Light (2.3%) | 65 | 7 | 4 |
| **Big Sky:** Original IPA (6.2%) | 195 | 18 | 17 |
| Moose Drool (5.3%) | 175 | 15 | 16 |
| Scape Goat (4.7%) | 155 | 14 | 14 |
| Trout Slayer Ale ( 4.7%) | 145 | 14 | 12 |
| **Blatz:** Original (4.6%) | 145 | 13 | 13 |
| Light (3.9%) | 110 | 11 | 8 |
| **Blue Moon:** Belgian (5.4%) | 165 | 15 | 13 |
| Grand Cru Ale (8.2%) | 230 | 21 | 19 |
| Harvest Pumpkin Ale (5.8%) | 180 | 17 | 14 |
| Spring Ale (5.7%) | 180 | 16 | 15 |
| Summer Ale (5.2%) | 150 | 15 | 13 |
| Winter Abbey Ale (5.7%) | 180 | 16 | 14 |
| **Bohemia** (4.73%) | 140 | 8 | 12 |

## Brands (Cont)    **Alc** ~ Alcohol (Grams)

*Per 12 fl.oz Serving*

| | **C** | **Alc** | **Cb** |
|---|---|---|---|
| **Bud:** Bud Light (4.2%) | 110 | 12 | 7 |
| Chelada Light (4.2%) | 150 | 12 | 16 |
| Dry (5%) | 130 | 14 | 8 |
| Ice (5.5%) | 150 | 16 | 9 |
| Ice Light (4.1%) | 110 | 12 | 7 |
| Light Lime (4.2%) | 115 | 12 | 8 |
| Light Platinum (6%) | 140 | 17 | 5 |
| **Budweiser:** Pale Lager (5%) | 145 | 14 | 11 |
| American Ale (5.3%) | 180 | 15 | 18 |
| Chelada (5%) | 185 | 14 | 20 |
| Select (4.3%) | 100 | 12 | 3 |
| Select 55 (2.4%) | 55 | 6 | 2 |
| **Busch:** Original (4.6%) | 120 | 13 | 7 |
| Ice (5.9%) | 135 | 17 | 4 |
| Light (4.1%) | 95 | 12 | 3 |
| **Carlsberg,** Pilsner (5%) | 135 | 14 | 10 |
| **Carta Blanca** (4.6%) | 145 | 13 | 11 |
| **Castlemaine XXXX,** | | | |
| Bitter (4.6%) | 140 | 14 | 10 |
| **Cerveza,** Aguila (4%) | 125 | 11 | 11 |
| **Colt 45,** Malt Liquor (5.6%) | 155 | 16 | 11 |
| **Coors:** Banquet (5%) | 150 | 14 | 12 |
| Extra Gold (5%) | 150 | 14 | 13 |
| Light (4.2%) | 100 | 12 | 5 |
| **Corona:** Extra (4.6%) | 150 | 13 | 14 |
| Light (4.1%) | 100 | 12 | 5 |
| **Dos Equis XX:** Amber (4.6%) | 145 | 13 | 12 |
| Lager (4.6%) | 140 | 13 | 11 |
| **Fosters:** Lager (5%) | 145 | 14 | 11 |
| Premium Ale (5.5%) | 145 | 16 | 12 |
| **Genesee:** Lager (4.5%) | 150 | 13 | 14 |
| Genny Light Lager, (3.6%) | 95 | 10 | 6 |
| **George Killian's,** Irish Red (5%) | 160 | 14 | 15 |
| **Grolsch:** Blonde (2.8%) | 120 | 18 | 16 |
| Light (3.6%) | 95 | 11 | 6 |
| Premium (5%) | 145 | 14 | 10 |
| **Guinness:** Draught (4%) | 125 | 12 | 10 |
| Extra Stout (6%) | 175 | 17 | 14 |
| **Hamm's:** Original (4.7%) | 145 | 13 | 12 |
| Special Light (3.9%) | 110 | 12 | 8 |
| **Harp,** Pale Lager (5%) | 150 | 13 | 12 |
| **Heineken:** Lager (5%) | 150 | 14 | 12 |
| Special Dark (5%) | 165 | 14 | 15 |
| Premium Light (3.5%) | 100 | 10 | 7 |
| **Hurricane:** Malt Liquor (5.9%) | 135 | 17 | 4 |
| High Gravity (8.1%) | 185 | 23 | 6 |
| **Icehouse:** Pale Lager (5%) | 135 | 14 | 9 |
| Light (5.9%) | 125 | 14 | 7 |
| **Keystone:** Ice (5.9%) | 140 | 17 | 6 |
| Light (4.2%) | 105 | 12 | 5 |
| **Killian's,** Irish Red (5%) | 165 | 14 | 14 |
| **King Cobra** (6%) | 135 | 17 | 5 |

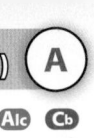

## Brands (Cont)     Alc ~ Alcohol (Grams)

**Beer Contains Zero Fat:**
*Per 12 fl.oz Serving*

| | C | Alc | Cb |
|---|---|---|---|
| **Kirin:** Ichiban (5%) | 145 | 14 | 10 |
| Light (3.2%) | 95 | 9 | 8 |
| **Labatt:** Blue (4.7%) | 135 | 14 | 10 |
| Blue Light (4%) | 110 | 11 | 8 |
| **Landshark,** Lager (4.7%) | 150 | 13 | 14 |
| **Leinenkugel's:** Orig. (4.6%) | 150 | 13 | 14 |
| Summer Shandy (4.2%) | 130 | 12 | 12 |
| **Lone Star:** Pale Lager (4.7%) | 135 | 13 | 12 |
| Light (3.9%) | 110 | 11 | 9 |
| **Lowenbrau,** Original (5%) | 140 | 14 | 12 |
| **Magic Hat,** #9 (5.1% alc) | 155 | 15 | 14 |
| **Magnum,** Malt Liquor (5.6%) | 160 | 16 | 11 |
| **Michelob:** Original Lager (5%) | 165 | 14 | 15 |
| Golden Draft (4.7%) | 125 | 13 | 8 |
| Golden Draft Light (4.1%) | 110 | 12 | 7 |
| Honey Lager (4.9%) | 175 | 14 | 16 |
| Light (4.3%) | 125 | 12 | 9 |
| Pale Ale (5.6%) | 185 | 16 | 9 |
| Porter (5.9%) | 185 | 17 | 16 |
| Ultra (4.2%) | 95 | 12 | 3 |
| Ultra Amber (5%) | 95 | 12 | 3 |
| Ultra Fruit Varieties (4%) | 95 | 12 | 6 |
| **Mickey's,** Malt Liquor (5.6%) | 160 | 16 | 11 |
| **Miller:** Chill, 100 Cal, (4.2%) | 100 | 12 | 4 |
| Genuine Draft: (4.7%) | 145 | 13 | 13 |
| High Life (4.7%) | 145 | 13 | 13 |
| High Life Light (4.2%) | 110 | 12 | 7 |
| Lite (4.2%) | 95 | 12 | 3 |
| **Milwaukee's Best:** | | | |
| Premium (4.3%) | 130 | 12 | 11 |
| Ice (5.9%) | 145 | 17 | 7 |
| Light (4.2%) | 100 | 12 | 4 |
| **Minnesota's Best,** Original (4.9%) | 140 | 14 | 10 |
| **Modelo,** Especial (4.4%) | 145 | 13 | 13 |
| **Molson:** Canadian/Golden (5%) | 135 | 14 | 11 |
| Ice (5.6%) | 160 | 16 | 12 |
| Light (4%) | 115 | 11 | 10 |
| Molsons XXX (7.3%) | 200 | 21 | 11 |
| **Moosehead,** Lager (5%) | 140 | 14 | 11 |
| **Natural:** Ice (5.9%) | 130 | 17 | 4 |
| Light (4.2%) | 95 | 12 | 3 |
| **Negra Modelo** (5.4%) | 170 | 15 | 15 |
| **Newcastle,** Brown Ale (4.7%) | 140 | 13 | 10 |
| **Old English"800",** Malt (5.9%) | 160 | 17 | 11 |
| **Old Milwaukee:** Lager (4.5%) | 150 | 13 | 15 |
| Light (4.3%) | 125 | 12 | 10 |
| Ice (5.5%) | 150 | 16 | 10 |
| **Old Style:** Lager (4.7%) | 145 | 13 | 12 |
| Light (4.2%) | 115 | 12 | 7 |
| **Olympia Gold,** Light (2.1%) | 70 | 6 | 6 |
| **Pabst:** Blue Ribbon (4.7%) | 145 | 13 | 12 |
| Light (3.9%) | 110 | 11 | 8 |

## Cb ~ Carbohydrate

| | C | Alc | Cb |
|---|---|---|---|
| **Pacifico,** Clara (4.4%) | 145 | 13 | 13 |
| **Pete's,** Wicked Ale (5.3%) | 175 | 15 | 18 |
| **Piels,** Lager (4.3%) | 125 | 12 | 9 |
| **Pilsner Urquell,** Lager (4.4%) | 155 | 13 | 16 |
| **Point:** Amber Classic (4.7%) | 160 | 14 | 11 |
| Special Lager (4.6%) | 150 | 13 | 9 |
| 2012 Black Ale (4.6%) | 150 | 13 | 9 |
| **Red Dog,** Lager (5%) | 150 | 14 | 14 |
| **Red Hook:** ESB (5.8%) | 185 | 16 | 16 |
| India Pale Ale (7%) | 190 | 13 | 19 |
| **Red Stripe,** Jamaican Ale (5%) | 155 | 14 | 14 |
| **Rolling Rock,** Extra Pale Ale (4.5%) | 130 | 13 | 10 |
| **Samuel Adams:** | | | |
| Boston Lager (4.9%) | 175 | 14 | 19 |
| Summer Ale (5.3%) | 160 | 15 | 13 |
| **Sam Adams,** Light Lager (4%) | 125 | 13 | 9 |
| **Sapporo,** Premium Lager (4.9%) | 140 | 14 | 10 |
| **Schaefer:** Lager (4.6%) | 145 | 13 | 12 |
| Light (3.9%) | 110 | 11 | 8 |
| **Schell's:** Deer (4.8%) | 135 | 14 | 8 |
| Light (4%) | 100 | 11 | 7 |
| **Schlitz:** Pale Lager (4.6%) | 145 | 13 | 12 |
| Light (3.8%) | 110 | 11 | 8 |
| **Schmidt's:** Pale Lager (4.6%) | 145 | 13 | 13 |
| Light (3.8%) | 110 | 11 | 8 |
| **Sheaf,** Stout (5.8%) | 190 | 16 | 19 |
| **Shock Top,** Belgian White (5.2%) | 165 | 15 | 15 |
| **Sierra Nevada:** Bigfoot (9.6%) | 330 | 28 | 32 |
| Pale Ale (5.6%) | 175 | 16 | 14 |
| Glissade Golden Bock (6.4%) | 205 | 18 | 18 |
| Porter (5.6%) | 195 | 16 | 18 |
| **Sol** (4.2%) | 130 | 12 | 11 |
| **Southpaw,** Light (5%) | 125 | 14 | 7 |
| **St Pauli Girl,** Lager (5%) | 135 | 14 | 9 |
| **Sparks:** Lager (6%) | 255 | 17 | 35 |
| Flavors ~ see page 27 | | | |
| **Steel Reserve:** | | | |
| High Gravity Malt Liquor (8.1%) | 220 | 23 | 16 |
| Steel 6 (6%) | 160 | 17 | 11 |
| **Stella Artois,** Pale Lager (5.2%) | 155 | 15 | 12 |
| **Stroh's :** Pale Lager (4.6%) | 145 | 13 | 12 |
| Light (3.9%) | 115 | 11 | 7 |
| **Tecate:** Pale Lager (4.6%) | 140 | 13 | 11 |
| Light (4%) | 110 | 10 | 8 |
| **Trader Jose:** Per 11.2 fl.oz | | | |
| Premium Lager (5%) | 145 | 14 | 14 |
| Light (5%) | 105 | 14 | 8 |
| **Victoria,** (4%) | 135 | 12 | 14 |
| **Warsteiners,** Verum (4.8%), 11.2 fl.oz | 140 | 13 | 12 |
| **Weinhard's:** Private Reserve (4.8%) | 150 | 14 | 13 |
| Hefeweizen (4.86%) | 150 | 14 | 13 |
| **Widmer,** Hefeweizen (4.9%) | 165 | 14 | 13 |
| **Zeigenbock,** Amber (4.9%) | 145 | 14 | 11 |

**Home-Brewed Beer:**
Similar to regular beers, according to alcohol content.

# A  Alcohol ~ Cider ◆ Wine

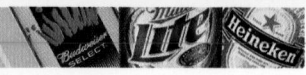

**Alc** ~ Alcohol (Grams)   **Cb** ~ Carbohydrate

## Non-Alcoholic Brews

*Less Than 0.5% Alcohol*
*Average All Brands:*
(Busch NA, Coors NA, Haake Beck,
Kaliber, Kingsbury, O'Douls,
Old Milwaukee NA, Pabst NA,
Stroh's NA, Texas Select):

| | | |
|---|---|---|
| 12 fl.oz Can/Bottle | 70 | 1 | 14 |
| **O'Doul's,** Amber, 12 fl.oz | 90 | 1 | 18 |
| **Sharp's,** 12 fl.oz | 60 | 1 | 12 |

## Cider ~ *Alcoholic*

*Per 12 fl.oz*

| | C | Alc | Cb |
|---|---|---|---|
| **Ace Cider:** (5%), av. all flavors | 155 | 14 | 12 |
| Ace Joker (6.9%) | 135 | 19 | 12 |
| **Hornsby's:** Draft Cider (6%) | 170 | 16 | 16 |
| Hard Apple Cider (5.5%) | 200 | 15 | 27 |
| **Woodchuck:** Amber (5%) | 200 | 14 | 21 |
| Dark & Dry (5%) | 180 | 14 | 16 |
| Granny Smith (5%) | 160 | 14 | 11 |
| Pear (4%) | 150 | 12 | 18 |
| Raspberry (4%) | 170 | 12 | 22 |
| **Wyder's:** Apple (5%) | 150 | 14 | 14 |
| Pear (4%) | 140 | 12 | 22 |
| Raspberry (4%) | 120 | 12 | 17 |

## Quick Guide

**Table Wines**
*Average All Varieties (11.5% Alc.)*
*(Wine Contains Zero Fat)*

| | C | Alc | Cb |
|---|---|---|---|
| **4 fl.oz,** 1 small wine glass OR ½ large wine glass | 100 | 12 | 3 |
| **6 fl.oz,** (3/4 large wine glass) | 145 | 18 | 5 |
| **8 fl.oz,** (1 large wine glass) | 195 | 25 | 7 |
| **½ Carafe/Bottle,** 12 fl.oz | 295 | 37 | 10 |
| **1 Bottle,** 750ml, 25.4 fl.oz | 620 | 78 | 20 |

## Table Wines

| | C | Alc | Cb |
|---|---|---|---|
| **Red:** *Per 4 fl.oz* | | | |
| Burgundy/Cabernet/Merlot, av. | 100 | 11 | 4 |
| **White:** *Per 4 fl.oz* | | | |
| Dry (Chenin; Fume Blanc; Chardonnay) | 95 | 11 | 4 |
| Sparkling, 4 fl.oz | 95 | 11 | 4 |
| Zinfandel Sweet (Moselle/Sauterne), 4 fl.oz | 85 | 11 | 2 |

## Table Wines (Cont)

| | C | Alc | Cb |
|---|---|---|---|
| **Champagne:** *Per 4 fl.oz Serving* | | | |
| Average 1 glass, | 85 | 11 | 2 |
| with Orange Jce (3:1 orange) | 75 | 8 | 4 |
| with Orange Jce (1:1 orange) | 65 | 5 | 7 |
| Cold Duck 4 fl oz | 110 | 11 | 8 |
| Korbel (12%): Brut | 90 | 11 | 3 |
| Extra Dry | 90 | 11 | 4 |
| **Mulled Wine** *(Gluhwein),* 4 fl.oz | 180 | 14 | 20 |
| **Non-Alcoholic Wine,** avg., 4 fl.oz | 50 | 0 | 12 |
| **Reduced Alcohol Wine** (6%): | | | |
| Average all types, 4 fl.oz | 50 | 6 | 12 |
| **Sake** *(Gekkeikan),* (16%), 4 fl.oz | 120 | 15 | 5 |

## Flavored Wines

*Average All Brands (6% alcohol)*
(Examples: Arbor Mist, Wild Vines, Boones)

| | | | |
|---|---|---|---|
| 1 small wine glass, 4 fl.oz | 80 | 6 | 10 |
| 1 large wine glass, 8 fl.oz | 160 | 11 | 20 |
| 1 bottle, 750 ml (25.4 fl.oz) | 510 | 35 | 64 |

## Dessert Wines

| | | | |
|---|---|---|---|
| **Madeira** (18%), 2 oz | 85 | 9 | 5 |
| **Marsala** (18%), 2 oz | 110 | 9 | 11 |
| **Port,** Muscatel (18%), 2 oz | 85 | 9 | 5 |
| **Sherry** (15%), 2 oz | | | |
| Dry, 1 Sherry glass | 90 | 7 | 7 |
| Sweet/Cream, average | 90 | 7 | 8 |
| **Vermouth** *(Martini & Rossi):* | | | |
| Extra Dry (18%), 2 oz | 65 | 9 | 2 |
| Martini Rosso (16%), 2 oz | 90 | 10 | 8 |

## Cooking Wines

| | | | |
|---|---|---|---|
| **Holland House:** | | | |
| **Marsala,** (14%), 2 T., 1 fl.oz | 45 | 4 | 4 |
| **Red/White,** (10%), 2 T., 1 fl.oz | 20 | 2 | 1 |
| 1 cup, 8 fl.oz | 160 | 24 | 8 |
| **Sherry,** (17%), 2 Tbsp, 1 fl.oz | 45 | 5 | 2 |

## COOKING WITH WINE

For alcohol to evaporate, sufficient heat and cooking time (at least 30 minutes) is required.

**Red and white table wines** would then contain negligible residual calories.

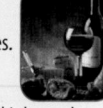

**Sweetened wines** (marsala/sherry) would contain 10 calories per 1 fl.oz.

**Flambé Desserts:** Only surface alcohol is burned off, so negligible reduction in alcohol or calories.

## Quick Guide    Alc ~ Alcohol (Grams)

**Spirits/Liquors:**
*Includes Bourbon, Brandy, Gin, Rum, Scotch, Tequila, Vodka, Whiskey.*
Note: All spirits with same alcohol proof have similar calories and zero fat.

| *Average All Brands* | C | Alc | Cb |
|---|---|---|---|
| **80 Proof (40% Alcohol by Volume):** | | | |
| 1 fl.oz | 65 | 9.5 | 0 |
| 1½ fl.oz (1 shot) | 100 | 14 | 0 |
| 3 fl.oz (Double shot) | 195 | 28 | 0 |
| ½ Bottle, 350 ml | 770 | 113 | 0 |
| 1 Bottle, 700 ml (24 fl.oz) | 1540 | 227 | 0 |
| **86 Proof (43% Alc):** 1 fl.oz | 70 | 10 | 0 |
| 1½ fl.oz (1 shot) | 105 | 15 | 0 |
| 1 Bottle, (24 fl.oz) | 1670 | 244 | 0 |
| **100 Proof (50% Alc):** 1½ fl.oz | 125 | 18 | 0 |
| **Shochu (Soju) ~ Izakaya Lounges:** | | | |
| Average all types (25% alc), 2 fl.oz | 65 | 12 | 0 |

### Flavored Spirits

| | C | Alc | Cb |
|---|---|---|---|
| **Captain Morgan:** *Per 1½ fl.oz* | | | |
| Original (35%) | 85 | 12 | 0.5 |
| Black Label (40%) | 100 | 14 | 0 |
| Parrot Bay (21%), average | 95 | 7.5 | 11 |
| Silver Spiced (35%) | 95 | 12 | 2 |
| **Malibu Rum:** *Per 1½ fl.oz* | | | |
| Original/Banana (21%) | 80 | 7.5 | 30 |
| Pineapple (21%) | 75 | 7.5 | 22 |
| **Southern Comfort**, (35%), 1½ fl.oz | 100 | 12 | 3 |

### Hard Lemonade & Sodas

| | C | Alc | Cb |
|---|---|---|---|
| **Margaritaville,** | | | |
| Spiked Lemonade/Tea (5.5%), 12 fl.oz | 225 | 15 | 30 |
| **Mike's Hard Lemonade:** *Per 11.2 fl.oz* | | | |
| Original (5%), av. all flavors | 220 | 14 | 33 |
| Light (4%) | 110 | 11 | 14 |
| Mike's Harder (8%) av., 16 fl.oz | 395 | 22 | 22 |
| Mike's Margarita (5.5%), 11.2 fl.oz | 235 | 15 | 34 |
| Mike's Hard Punch (5.5%), 11.2 fl.oz | 230 | 15 | 33 |
| **Sparks:** *Per 12 fl.oz (Half of 24 oz Can)* | | | |
| Blackberry; Iced Tea (8%), av. | 295 | 23 | 34 |
| Lemonade (8%) | 275 | 23 | 29 |
| Original (6%) | 260 | 17 | 35 |
| **Tilt:** *Per 16 fl.oz Can* | | | |
| Blue/Green/Purple (6%), av. | 340 | 23 | 45 |
| Pink (6%) | 320 | 23 | 41 |
| Red/Yellow (6%) | 280 | 23 | 30 |
| **Twisted Tea:** Light (4%), 12 fl.oz | 115 | 11 | 9 |
| Original (5%) av., all flavors, 12 fl.oz | 210 | 14 | 31 |

## Coolers & Premix Cocktails

| **Ready-To-Drink:** | C | Alc | Cb |
|---|---|---|---|
| *Zero Fat Unless Indicated* | | | |
| **Bacardi Silver:** *Per 12 fl.oz* | | | |
| Lemonade/Sangria, av. (6%) | 270 | 17 | 41 |
| Raz/Strawberry (5%) | 240 | 14 | 36 |
| Mojito: Original (5%) | 230 | 14 | 34 |
| Mango (5%) | 235 | 14 | 35 |
| **Bacardi:** *Per 4 fl.oz* | | | |
| **Party Drinks (Ready To Pour):** | | | |
| Bahama Mama; Mai Tai (10%) | 130 | 9 | 16 |
| Mojito (15%) | 160 | 14 | 16 |
| Rum Island Ice Tea (12.5%) | 150 | 12 | 16 |
| **Bartles & Jaymes:** *Per 11.2 fl.oz* | | | |
| **Malt Based Coolers** (3.6%): | | | |
| Exotic Berry | 195 | 10 | 31 |
| Fuzzy Navel | 215 | 10 | 36 |
| Margarita | 245 | 10 | 43 |
| Pina Colada | 250 | 10 | 45 |
| Pomegranate Raspberry | 205 | 10 | 34 |
| Strawberry Daiquiri | 205 | 10 | 34 |
| **Captain Morgan's,** | | | |
| Parrot Bay (4.1%), av. all flav., 11.2 fl.oz | 210 | 10 | 35 |
| **Daily's** (6.9%): | | | |
| Bag-In-Box Cocktails, 4 fl.oz | 110 | 6 | 15 |
| Single Serve Bottles, all flav., 8 fl.oz | 220 | 12 | 30 |
| **Jack Daniels**, Country Cocktails (5%), | | | |
| average all flavors, 10 fl.oz | 245 | 12 | 40 |
| **Jose Cuervo:** | | | |
| **Margaritas:** | | | |
| Classic Lime (10%), 6 fl.oz | 210 | 14 | 29 |
| Golden (12.7%), 4.7 fl.oz | 170 | 14 | 19 |
| **Seagram's:** | | | |
| **Escapes Coolers (3.2%):** | | | |
| Bahama Mama, 12 fl.oz | 150 | 9 | 39 |
| Strawberry Daiquiri, 12 fl.oz | 170 | 9 | 44 |
| **Smirnoff:** Ice (4.5%), 11.2 fl.oz | | | |
| Original/Grape, average | 205 | 12 | 37 |
| Apple/Stawb Acai, average | 235 | 12 | 36 |
| Mango | 225 | 12 | 33 |
| Pomeg./Raspb./Triple Black | 225 | 12 | 37 |
| **TGI Friday's:** *Per 6 fl.oz* | | | |
| **On The Rocks:** | | | |
| Margarita (7.5%) | 180 | 6 | 28 |
| Long Island Ice Tea (15%) | 245 | 12 | 27 |
| Mudslide (10%) | 355 | 8 | 30 |
| **Blenders** (12.5% alc), | | | |
| average all flavors | 435 | 10 | 51 |

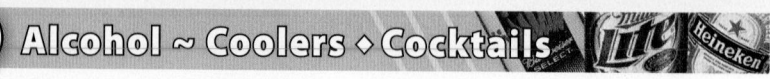
## Coolers & Premix Cocktails (Cont)

**Ready-To-Drink:**

| The Club Premix Cocktails: Per 3.4 oz Serving (½ can) | C | Alc | Cb |
|---|---|---|---|
| Censored on Beach; Margarita (7.5%) | 105 | 6 | 17 |
| Gin/Vodka Martini, av. (21%) | 155 | 17 | 0.2 |
| Long Island Ice Tea(15%) | 145 | 12 | 17 |
| Manhattan (17%) | 115 | 13 | 5 |
| Mudslide/Pina Colada (10%) av. | 200 | 8 | 16 |
| Screwdriver (7.5%) | 95 | 6 | 14 |
| Whiskey Sour (10%) | 95 | 8 | 11 |

### Shooters
Alc ~ Alcohol (Grams)

| | C | Alc | Cb |
|---|---|---|---|
| Alabama Slammer | 110 | 14 | 2 |
| Amaretto Sour | 120 | 6 | 19 |
| B52 | 145 | 14 | 11 |
| Beam Me Up Scotty | 145 | 13 | 13 |
| Blue Tequila | 160 | 18 | 6 |
| Jager Bomb | 205 | 8 | 30 |
| Jager Bomb (w. Sugar-Free Red Bull) | 155 | 8 | 18 |
| Jell-O Shot, 3 oz (w.1½ oz Vodka) | 180 | 14 | 19 |
| With Diet Jell-O, 3 oz | 110 | 14 | 0 |
| Kamikaze | 75 | 8 | 3 |
| Kool-Aid | 160 | 15 | 14 |
| Orgasm | 100 | 12 | 6 |
| Peppermint Patty | 195 | 8 | 11 |
| Stinger | 170 | 18 | 12 |
| Surfer on Acid | 90 | 7 | 11 |

### Cocktail Mixers ~ Non-Alcoholic

| Bacardi: Per 8 fl.oz Prepared from 2 fl.oz concentrate | C | Alc | Cb |
|---|---|---|---|
| Daiquiris, Rum runner | 120 | 0 | 32 |
| Margarita | 90 | 0 | 25 |
| Mojito | 110 | 0 | 30 |
| Pina Colada | 170 | 0 | 36 |
| **Baja Bob's** (Sugar Free): Per 4 fl.oz | | | |
| Cranberry Cosmo Martini | 10 | 0 | 2 |
| Pina Colada | 30 | 0 | 4 |
| **Jose Cuervo,** | | | |
| Margaritas, av. all flav, 4 fl.oz | 115 | 0 | 28 |
| **Mr & Mrs T:** | | | |
| Bloody Mary: Original, 5 oz | 30 | 0 | 7 |
| Bold & Spicy, 4 oz | 35 | 0 | 7 |
| Mai Tai | 130 | 0 | 32 |
| Margarita | 100 | 0 | 26 |
| Pina Colada | 170 | 0 | 44 |
| Strawberry Daiquiri | 180 | 0 | 46 |
| **TGI Fridays:** | | | |
| Mudslide, 2.3 fl.oz | 110 | 0 | 3 |
| Cosmo; Berrytini, 2 fl.oz | 80 | 0 | 20 |
| Strawb. Daiquiri; Marg., 4 fl.oz | 190 | 0 | 46 |

## Cocktails
Alc ~ Alcohol (Grams)

**Made to Standard Recipes (Standard Size):**
(Main Reference: The New American Bartender's Guide)

| Zero Fat Unless Indicated | C | Alc | Cb |
|---|---|---|---|
| Bacardi & Coke (w/ 1½ oz Bacardi) | 160 | 14 | 17 |
| Bellini, av., 4.5 fl.oz | 95 | 11 | 7 |
| Bloody Mary (w/ 1½ oz Vodka) | 125 | 10 | 7 |
| Blushin' Russian (20g fat) | 405 | 14 | 23 |
| Bourbon & Soda (w. 2 oz Bourbon) | 130 | 19 | 0 |
| Brandy Alexander (10g fat) | 300 | 20 | 15 |
| Chi Chi's: Long Island Iced Tea, 4 fl.oz | 145 | 12 | 17 |
| Mexican Mudslide, 4 fl.oz (8g fat) | 240 | 1.5 | 42 |
| Mojito, 4 fl.oz | 160 | 11 | 21 |
| Pina Colada 4 fl.oz (6g fat) | 240 | 4 | 42 |
| White Russian 4 fl.oz (7g fat) | 245 | 1.5 | 43 |
| Chupa Naranjas (w/ 1½ oz Tequila) | 150 | 16 | 8 |
| Cosmopolitan | 215 | 24 | 12 |
| Daiquiri (w/ 2 oz Rum) avg. all types | 140 | 19 | 4 |
| Frozen Daiquiri (w. 2 oz Rum): | | | |
| Without fruit | 155 | 19 | 6 |
| With fruit (w/ 1½ oz Rum) | 145 | 19 | 11 |
| Gin Martini (w/ 2 oz alcohol) | 140 | 19 | 0 |
| Grasshopper | 260 | 17 | 28 |
| Harvey Wallbanger (2 oz Alc.) | 200 | 19 | 17 |
| Highball (1½ oz Whiskey) | 100 | 14 | 0 |
| Irish Coffee (contains 10g fat) | 205 | 14 | 2 |
| Kahlua Mudslide: W/ milk (3g fat) | 145 | 11 | 12 |
| With cream (12g fat) | 230 | 11 | 10 |
| Lemon Drop, 4 fl.oz | 130 | 14 | 10 |
| Long Island Iced Tea (w/ 3 oz Cola) | 270 | 19 | 32 |
| With 3 oz Diet Cola | 235 | 19 | 22 |
| Mai Tai (with 2 oz Rum) | 290 | 24 | 33 |
| Manhattan | 130 | 17 | 5 |
| Margarita | 160 | 18 | 7 |
| Mint Julep (w/ 2½ oz Bourbon) | 180 | 24 | 4 |
| Moscow Mule | 185 | 14 | 24 |
| Pina Colada (10g fat) | 325 | 19 | 26 |
| Red Bull & Vodka | 210 | 14 | 28 |
| With Sugar Free Red Bull | 105 | 14 | 3 |
| Screwdriver | 160 | 14 | 15 |
| Sex On The Beach | 235 | 19 | 25 |
| Spritzer (with 3 oz Wine) | 65 | 8 | 2 |
| Tequila Sunrise | 200 | 14 | 25 |
| Tom Collins (with 2 oz Gin) | 210 | 19 | 18 |
| Vodka Soda (with 1½ oz Vodka) | 100 | 14 | 0 |
| Vodka Tonic (with 1½ oz Vodka) | 165 | 14 | 18 |
| Whiskey Sour (with 2 oz Whiskey) | 155 | 19 | 7 |
| White Russian (10g fat) | 240 | 19 | 7 |

| Non-Alcoholic: | C | Alc | Cb |
|---|---|---|---|
| Cinderella | 45 | 0 | 11 |
| Shirley Temple (w/ 6 oz Ginger Ale) | 140 | 0 | 34 |

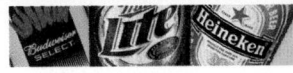

## Liqueurs/Cordials **C** **Alc** **Cb**

*Per 1 fl.oz*

| | C | Alc | Cb |
|---|---|---|---|
| Advocaat (36 Proof; 2g fat) | 85 | 4 | 9 |
| Alizé, Cognac (80 Proof) | 70 | 9 | 2 |
| Gold/Red Passion (32 Proof) | 105 | 4 | 11 |
| Amaretto (56 Proof) | 100 | 7 | 14 |
| Baileys Irish Cream (34 Proof; 5g fat) | 95 | 4 | 3 |
| Benedictine (80 Proof) | 90 | 9 | 5 |
| Chambord (33 Proof) | 105 | 4 | 11 |
| Chartreuse (80 Proof) | 100 | 9 | 9 |
| Cherry Brandy (48 Proof) | 80 | 6 | 9 |
| Coffee Liqueur (53 Proof) | 115 | 0.5 | 16 |
| Cointreau (80 Proof) | 95 | 9 | 7 |
| Creme de Cacao (54 Proof) | 100 | 6 | 15 |
| Creme de Menthe (72 Proof) | 125 | 9 | 14 |
| Curacao (70 Proof) | 95 | 8 | 6 |
| Drambuie (80 Proof) | 105 | 9 | 9 |
| Frangelico (40 Proof) | 65 | 5 | 12 |
| Galliano (86 Proof) | 100 | 10 | 8 |
| Grand Marnier (80 Proof) | 100 | 9 | 7 |
| Kahlua (40 Proof) | 85 | 5 | 14 |
| Kirsch (68 Proof) | 80 | 8 | 6 |
| Midori (42 Proof) | 80 | 5 | 11 |
| Ouzo (80 Proof) | 105 | 9 | 11 |
| Pernod (80 Proof) | 75 | 9 | 11 |
| Sambuca (84 Proof) | 100 | 10 | 11 |
| Schnapps (100 Proof) | 115 | 12 | 9 |
| Southern Comfort (70 Proof) | 65 | 8 | 3 |
| *Starbucks Liqueur:* | | | |
| Cream (30 Proof) | 85 | 3 | 9 |
| Tia Maria (53 Proof) | 120 | 9 | 15 |
| Triple Sec (48 Proof) | 60 | 6 | 10 |

## Liqueur Coffee & Hot Drinks

*Per Standard Drink*

| | C | Alc | Cb |
|---|---|---|---|
| **Liqueur Coffee,** avg. all types | 200 | 10 | 10 |
| Hot Toddy, with 1½ oz liquor, av. all | 170 | 9 | 19 |
| Irish Coffee, 1½ oz Whiskey & 1 oz whip | 205 | 9 | 4 |
| Mulled Wine (Glühwein), 4 fl.oz, av | 195 | 14 | 25 |

*"The doctor told him to cut down to just one glass a day."*

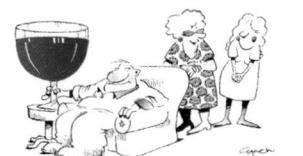

## TEN HINTS TO AVOID HARMFUL DRINKING

1. **Add up the alcohol** you typically drink each day and on social occasions. How does this compare with 'low risk' amounts? (*See page 23*)

2. **Compare the alcohol content** of different drinks and select the lowest. Request half ounces of alcohol in cocktails and mixed drinks. Dilute them and keep topping off with non-alcoholic drinks.

3. **Go easy on 'Light' beers.** At 4% alcohol, on average, they are still high in alcohol compared to regular beer (5% alcohol).

4. **Try low alcohol or non-alcohol** alternatives such as fruit juices and mineral water. Take your own to parties.

5. **Before drinking alcohol,** quench your thirst with water and non-alcoholic drinks – particularly after vigorous exercise or sports.

6. **Slow the rate of drinking.** Chugging or drinking fast is the major cause of illness and death from alcohol poisoning.

7. **Avoid drinking in 'rounds'.**

8. **Have a non-alcoholic 'spacer'** between drinks (e.g. mineral water, orange juice).

9. **Don't drink on an empty stomach.** Food slows the rate of alcohol absorption.

10. **Keep track of the number of drinks** and know when to stop. Stick to a set limit.

*Note: Alcohol can be very dangerous when taken with prescription or street drugs, or when you are very tired.*

***Extra Info: www.CalorieKing.com***

## Cocktail Mixers & Extracts

| | C | Alc | Cb |
|---|---|---|---|
| Angostura Bitters, ¼ tsp | 2 | 0 | 0.5 |
| Grenadine, ½ tsp | 6 | 0 | 2 |
| Lime/Lemon Juice, 2 Tbsp, 1 oz | 10 | 0 | 2 |
| Maraschino Cherry, 1 small | 8 | 0 | 2 |
| Simple Syrup, 1 Tbsp, av. | 50 | 0 | 14 |
| Sweet & Sour Mix, 2 Tbsp, 1 oz | 30 | 0 | 7 |
| Tonic Water, 8 fl.oz | 80 | 0 | 22 |
| **Flavor Extracts** (McCormick): | | | |
| Pure Lemon (83%), 1 tsp | 0 | 3.5 | 0 |
| Pure Vanilla (35%), 1tsp | 0 | 1.5 | 0 |

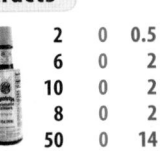
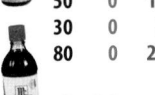

## Baking Ingredients

| | C | F | Cb |
|---|---|---|---|
| **Almond Paste**, (*Marzipan*), 2 Tbsp | 170 | 7 | 24 |
| **Apple Pie Filling**, Sweetened, 9.4 oz | 240 | 0 | 60 |
| **Also** ~ *See Page 134* | | | |
| Baking Powder: Regular, 1 tsp | 5 | 0 | 2 |
| Cream of Tartar, 1 tsp | 10 | 0 | 2 |
| **Baking Mix** (*Bisquick*) : | | | |
| Original, ⅓ cup, 1½ oz | 160 | 5 | 26 |
| Heart Smart, ⅓ cup, 1½ oz | 140 | 2.5 | 27 |
| **Batter Mix** (*Golden Dipt*), ¼ cup | 100 | 0 | 23 |
| **Blueberries**, 1 cup, 5 oz | 85 | 0.5 | 21 |
| **Butter/Margarine**, ½ cup, 4 oz | 815 | 92 | 1 |
| Stick (*Land O' Lakes*), ½ oz | 100 | 11 | 0 |
| **Carob Flour**, ½ cup | 115 | 0.5 | 46 |
| **Chocolate Baking Bars:** *Average all Brands* | | | |
| **Sweet** (*Baker's*): | | | |
| 1 oz portion | 120 | 7 | 16 |
| 4 oz bar | 470 | 28 | 64 |
| Semi-sweet, 1 oz | 140 | 9 | 16 |
| Bittersweet, 1 oz | 140 | 12 | 14 |
| White Baking, 1 oz | 160 | 9 | 16 |
| Unsweetened: 1 oz | 140 | 14 | 8 |
| Grated, 1 cup, 4½ oz | 660 | 69 | 39 |
| **Chocolate Baking Chips:** *Average all Brands* | | | |
| Milk Choc./Semi Sweet 1 oz | 140 | 8 | 18 |
| ½ cup, 3 oz | 420 | 24 | 54 |
| 1 cup, 6 oz | 840 | 48 | 108 |
| Mini Kisses (*Hershey*), 1 piece | 5 | 0.5 | 1 |
| **Cocoa Powder:** (*Nestle*), 1 Tbsp | 15 | 1 | 3 |
| ⅓ cup, 1 oz | 85 | 5 | 17 |
| *Hershey's*, 1 Tbsp | 20 | 0.5 | 3 |
| ⅓ cup, 1 oz | 115 | 3 | 17 |
| **Coconut, dried:** | | | |
| Unsweetened, 1 oz | 190 | 18 | 7 |
| Sweetened/flaked, 1 oz | 130 | 8 | 15 |
| ½ cup, 1.3 oz | 195 | 12 | 22 |
| Toasted (*Baker's*), 1 oz | 170 | 13 | 13 |
| **Coconut Cream/Milk** ~ *See Page 89* | | | |
| **Coconut Manna** (*Nutiva*), 1 Tbsp | 100 | 9 | 3 |
| **Cornstarch**, 1 Tbsp | 30 | 0 | 7 |
| **Eggs:** Large (1) | 75 | 5 | 0 |
| Jumbo (1) | 90 | 6 | 0.5 |
| **Egg White:** 1 Egg White | 15 | 0 | 0 |
| ½ cup (4 egg whites), 4 oz | 60 | 0 | 1 |
| **Flour:** White: 1 Tbsp, 0.3 oz | 25 | 0 | 5.5 |
| 1 cup, 4.2 oz | 400 | 1 | 88 |
| Whole Wheat, 1 cup, 4.2 oz | 400 | 2 | 84 |

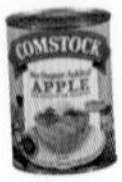

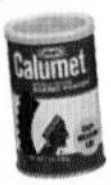

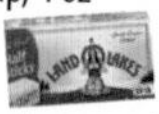

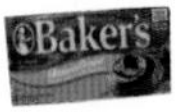

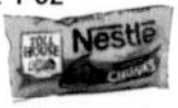

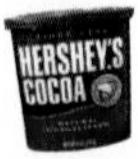

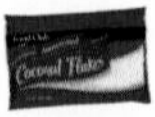

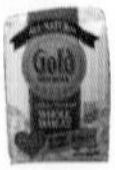

| | C | F | Cb |
|---|---|---|---|
| **Flavor Extracts:** *Average all Brands* | | | |
| Imitation, 1 tsp | 10 | 0 | 2 |
| Pure Extract, 1 tsp | 10 | 0 | 0.5 |
| Almond, Vanilla, 1 tsp | 10 | 0 | 0.5 |
| **Fruit Pectin:** Swtnd, 1/4 tsp | 5 | 0 | 1 |
| Unsweetened, ¼ tsp | 0 | 0 | 0 |
| **Gelatin**, dry, ¼ oz pkg | 20 | 0 | 0 |
| **Glaze** (*Duncan Hines*): Choc. 2 Tbsp | 150 | 7 | 21 |
| Vanilla, 2 Tbsp | 140 | 6 | 22 |
| *Golden Dipt*, Batter Mix | | | |
| ¼ cup, 1 oz | 100 | 0 | 23 |
| **Honey**, ½ cup, 6 oz | 515 | 0 | 140 |
| **Lemon/Orange Peel**, ¼ cup | 25 | 0 | 6 |
| **Lighter Bake** (*Sunsweet*) (Butter & Oil replacement) | | | |
| 1 Tbsp, ½ oz | 35 | 0 | 9 |
| ¼ Cup, 2.7 oz | 140 | 0 | 36 |
| **Milk:** Whole, 1 cup, 8 fl.oz | 150 | 8 | 12 |
| 2%, 1 cup, 8 fl.oz | 120 | 5 | 12 |
| 1%, 1 cup, 8 fl.oz | 100 | 2.5 | 12 |
| Fat-Free, 1 cup, 8 fl.oz | 90 | 0.5 | 13 |
| **Pastry** ~ *See Page 134* | | | |
| **Pie Crusts** ~ *See Page 134* | | | |
| **Pie Fillings: Fruits** ~ *See page 134* | | | |
| Lemon Creme, ⅓ cup | 130 | 1.5 | 28 |
| Mincemeat, 3½ oz | 190 | 5 | 45 |
| Pumpkin, 1 cup, 9.3 oz | 270 | 1.5 | 60 |
| **Prune Puree**, ¼ cup, 3 oz | 220 | 0 | 55 |
| **Raisins**, ½ cup, 2.8 oz | 240 | 0.5 | 63 |
| **Rennin**, 1 pkg (11g) | 10 | 0 | 2 |
| **Soy Milk** ~ *See Pages 49-50* | | | |
| **Sprinkles**, all types, 1 tsp | 20 | 1 | 3 |
| **Sugar:** 1 Tbsp, ½ oz | 55 | 0 | 14 |
| 1 oz | 110 | 0 | 28 |
| 1 cup, 7 oz | 775 | 0 | 195 |
| 1 lb, 16 oz | 1760 | 0 | 454 |
| **Sweeteners & Sugar Substitutes** ~ *See Page 156* | | | |
| **Vinegar**, average all types, 1 oz | 5 | 0 | 1 |
| **Whey**, sweet, dry, 1 oz | 100 | 0.5 | 21 |
| **Yeast:** Active, dry, ¼ oz pkg | 21 | 0 | 3 |
| Bakers, compressed, 1 oz | 30 | 0.5 | 5 |
| *Fleischmann's*, 0.6 oz pkg | 0 | 0 | 0 |

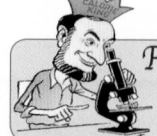

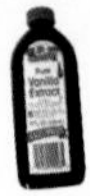

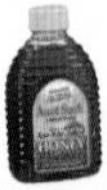

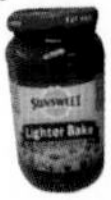

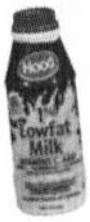

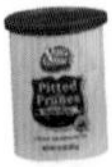

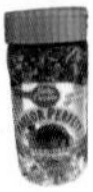

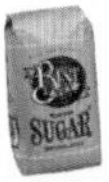

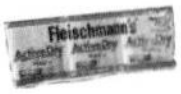

*F*or Full Nutritional Data & Product Updates
~ *See Author's Website*
www.CalorieKing.com

Note: Actual weight of bars is usually 5-10% more than label Net Weight. Weigh bar and allow extra calories.

## Breakfast Bars    C F Cb

*Per Bar*

**Atkins:** *Per 1.23 oz Bar*

| | | | |
|---|---|---|---|
| **Day Break:** Apple Crisp | 130 | 5 | 17 |
| Choc. Chip Crisp; Cranb. Almond, av. | 145 | 6 | 16 |
| Peanut Butter Fudge Crisp | 150 | 7 | 14 |
| **Barbara's Bakery:** | | | |
| Nature's Choice, av., 1.3 oz | 145 | 2 | 29 |
| Fruit & Yogurt, av., 1.48 oz | 150 | 3 | 29 |
| **Corazonas,** Oatmeal Squares, | | | |
|   average all varieties, 1 bar, 1.75 oz | 185 | 6 | 28 |
| **dotFIT:** *Per 2 oz Bar* | | | |
| **Iced Oatmeal:** Blueb. | 220 | 5 | 29 |
| Peanut Butter Delight | 190 | 6 | 26 |

Note: Carb figures include 11 grams of sorbitol & maltitol sweetners

| | | | |
|---|---|---|---|
| **Fresh & Easy,** Cereal Bars, | | | |
|   Mixed Berry, 1.3 oz | 140 | 2.5 | 27 |
| **General Mills:** *Per 1.6 oz Bar* | | | |
| **Milk 'n Cereal Bars:** Cinn Toast Crunch | 180 | 4 | 33 |
|   Honey Nut Cheerios | 160 | 4 | 28 |
| **Great Value** *(Walmart):* | | | |
| 90 Calories, av. all, 0.81 oz | 90 | 1.5 | 19 |
| Chewy: Hi Fibre Oats, av., 1.4 oz | 145 | 4 | 29 |
|   Sweet & Salty P'nut Butter, 1.4 oz | 200 | 7 | 29 |
| Toaster Pastries, all flavors, 1.8 oz | 200 | 5 | 37 |
| **Health Valley:** | | | |
| Cobbler Cereal Bars, all flav., 1.3 oz | 130 | 2.5 | 27 |
| Toaster Tarts, all flavors, 1.4 oz | 150 | 3 | 29 |
| **Kashi,** TLC Cereal Bars, av., 1.2 oz | 125 | 3 | 24 |
| **Kellogg's:** | | | |
| Cinnabon Bars, all flavors,1.3 oz | 150 | 4.5 | 26 |
| Fiber Plus, Antiox., av. all, 1.26 oz | 125 | 5 | 25 |
| **Pop Tarts:** *Per 1.8 oz* | | | |
|   Fruit/Frosted | 200 | 5 | 36 |
|   Low-Fat, all flavors | 185 | 3 | 39 |
| **Market Pantry,** 1.4 oz | 140 | 3 | 26 |
| **Nature's Path,** | | | |
|   Toaster Pastries, av.,1.8 oz | 210 | 5 | 40 |
| **Nutri-Grain** *(Kellogg's):* *Per 1.3 oz Bar* | | | |
| Cereal Bars, all flavors | 120 | 3 | 24 |
| Yogurt Bar, Strawberry | 130 | 3.5 | 25 |
| **Quaker,** B'fast Cookies (1), av., 1.7 oz | 175 | 4.5 | 33 |
| **Granola Bars** ~ *See Page 33* | | | |
| **Special K** *(Kellogg's),* | | | |
|   Cereal Bars, av., 0.8 oz | 90 | 1.5 | 18 |
| **Toaster Strudel** *(Pillsbury):* *Per 1.9 oz* | | | |
| Fruit flavors, all varieties | 170 | 7 | 25 |
| Boston Cream Pie | 170 | 7 | 25 |
| Cream Cheese , average | 185 | 9 | 24 |
| **Trader Joe's:** Fig, 1.3 oz | 120 | 2 | 24 |
|   Average other fruit flavors, 1.3 oz | 140 | 2.5 | 27 |

## Sports & Diet Bars    C F Cb

*Per Bar*

| | | | |
|---|---|---|---|
| **ABB,** Steel Bar, average, 2.3 oz | 255 | 5 | 35 |
| **AdvantEdge** ~ *See EAS* | | | |
| **Annie's Homegrown:** | | | |
| **Organic Granola Bars:** *Per 1 oz Bar* | | | |
|   Berry Berry | 120 | 3 | 20 |
|   Chocolate Chipper | 120 | 4 | 19 |
|   Peanutty | 120 | 4 | 17 |
| **Anytime Health:** | | | |
| Meal Replacement Bars, 2.8 oz | 310 | 9 | 42 |
| Snack Bars, av., 1.75 oz | 190 | 6 | 26 |
| **Apex,** Fix Crisp Bars, average | 155 | 4 | 22 |
| **Atkins:** | | | |
| **Advantage:** Alm. Coconut Crunch | 190 | 15 | 16 |
| Caramel varieties, average, 1.55 oz | 170 | 10 | 21 |
| Chocolate Peanut Butter, 2.1 oz | 240 | 12 | 22 |
| Dark Chocolate Decadence, 1.55 oz | 150 | 6 | 23 |
| Granola flavors, av., 1.7 oz | 210 | 9 | 18 |
| Mudslide, 1.7 oz | 210 | 10 | 19 |
| Sweet and Salty Alm. | 200 | 15 | 14 |
| **Endulge:** Caramel Nut Chew, 1.2 oz | 130 | 8 | 17 |
| Choc. C'mel Mousse, 1.2 oz | 120 | 4.5 | 23 |
| Nutty Fudge Brownie, 1.4 oz | 170 | 12 | 18 |
| Peanut Caramel Cluster | 140 | 9 | 12 |
| **Attune Bars:** | | | |
| **Probiotic Wellness Bars:** *Per 0.7 oz Bar* | | | |
|   Dark Chocolate | 80 | 6 | 11 |
|   Milk Chocolate Crisp | 90 | 6 | 12 |
|   Mint Chocolate | 90 | 6 | 12 |
| **Balance:** *Per 1.76 oz Bars* | | | |
|   Original; Bare, average | 200 | 7 | 21 |
|   Carb Well, average | 195 | 8 | 23 |
|   Gold, average | 200 | 7 | 23 |
| **Barbara's Bakery,** | | | |
|   Crunchy Granola (2), av., 1.5 oz | 195 | 9 | 27 |
| **Bariatrix Proti-Bar** *(15g Protein),* | | | |
|   Crisp; Layered, av. all, 1.4 oz | 160 | 5.5 | 15 |
| **Cascadian Farms** *(General Mills),* | | | |
|   Chewy Granola, av. all | 140 | 4 | 25 |
| **Clif Bars:** | | | |
| Original, av., 2.4 oz | 240 | 3.5 | 45 |
| Builder's, av., 2.4 oz | 270 | 8 | 30 |
| Kid, ZBar, av., 1.25 oz | 130 | 3.5 | 23 |
| Mojo, av., 1.59 oz | 195 | 10 | 20 |

Note: Actual weight of bars is usually 5-10% more than label Net Weight. Weigh bar and allow extra calories.

### Sports & Diet Bars (Cont)

| Per Bar | C | F | Cb |
|---|---|---|---|
| **Detour:** | | | |
| **Original,** Caramel Peanut, 3 oz | 350 | 11 | 32 |
| **Biker,** average all varieties, 1¾ oz | 210 | 6 | 27 |
| **Lean Muscle:** Av. all var. 1.6 oz | 190 | 7 | 14 |
| Average all varieties, 3.2 oz | 395 | 15 | 33 |
| **Lower Sugar:** Av. all var., 1.5 oz | 170 | 5.5 | 16 |
| Average all varieties, 3 oz | 345 | 10 | 32 |
| **Oatmeal,** av. all varieties, 4.28 oz | 460 | 10 | 60 |
| **Runner,** av. all varieties, 1.75 oz | 205 | 5.5 | 28 |
| **Yoga,** Blueberry Acai,1.6 oz | 170 | 2 | 28 |
| **Doctor's,** CarbRite Diet, av., 2 oz | 195 | 3.5 | 23 |
| **dotFIT,** Breakfast Bars ~ See Page 31 | | | |
| **dotSTICK,** (12 g Protein), | | | |
| **Iced,** all varieties, 1.75 oz | 190 | 6 | 26 |
| **EAS:** | | | |
| **AdvantEDGE:** | | | |
| Carb Control: Crisp Bars, av., 2.1 oz | 240 | 8 | 27 |
| Average other varieties, 2.1 oz | 230 | 8 | 27 |
| **Myoplex:** | | | |
| Carb Control, average, 2.46 oz | 260 | 8 | 27 |
| Mass, Chocolate Chunk, 3.17 oz | 390 | 20 | 29 |
| Nutrition: Strength Formula, | | | |
| average, 2.65 oz | 280 | 8 | 35 |
| Lite, av. all, 1.9 oz | 190 | 4.5 | 28 |
| **Elevate Me!:** Strawb. Pie, 2.33 oz | 250 | 4.5 | 38 |
| Average other varieties, 2.33 oz | 235 | 4.5 | 35 |
| **Extend Bar:** Crunch, av., 1.4 oz | 155 | 3 | 30 |
| Sugar Free varieties, 1.4 oz | 150 | 3 | 21 |
| (Carbs include 4-5g sugar alcohol) | | | |
| **Fiber One:** Chewy, average, 1.4 oz | 145 | 4 | 29 |
| 90-Calorie Bars, average, 0.8 oz | 90 | 3 | 18 |
| **FiberPlus** (Kellogg's), Antioxidants: | | | |
| Chocolate Chip, 1.27 oz | 120 | 4 | 26 |
| Other Varieties, 1.27 oz | 130 | 5 | 24 |
| **Fresh & Easy:** | | | |
| Grain/Fruit: Cranb. Orange, 1.4 oz | 160 | 5 | 29 |
| Pomegranate Cherry, 1.4 oz | 150 | 6 | 22 |
| Granola, | | | |
| P'nut Butter & Choc. Chip, 1.23 oz | 170 | 7 | 22 |
| **Full Bar:** Regular, av. all, 1.59 oz | 170 | 4 | 28 |
| Fit (15g Protein), average, 1.76 oz | 180 | 4 | 24 |
| **GeniSoy:** Average, 2.2 oz | 240 | 5.5 | 32 |
| Organic, all varieties, 1.6 oz | 160 | 3 | 25 |
| Protein Crunch, average, 1.6 oz | 150 | 5 | 18 |

| Per Bar | C | F | Cb |
|---|---|---|---|
| **Glenny's,** | | | |
| **100 Calorie,** Brownies, 1.45 oz | 100 | 4 | 15 |
| **Glucerna:** Meal Bars, av., 2 oz | 220 | 7 | 34 |
| Snack Bars, average, 1.4 oz | 145 | 4 | 23 |
| Mini Snack Bar, average, 0.7 oz | 75 | 2.5 | 12 |
| **GNC:** | | | |
| **Pro Performance:** | | | |
| Pro Crunch, average, 2.3 oz | 255 | 6 | 35 |
| Lite, 1.2 oz | 140 | 6 | 14 |
| **Lean Bar,** average, 1.6 oz | 150 | 5 | 18 |
| (Carbs include 5g sugar alc.) | | | |
| **Gnu Foods:** Per 1.6 oz Bar | | | |
| Banana Walnut | 140 | 4 | 30 |
| Cinn. Raisin; Orange Cranb. | 130 | 3 | 32 |
| Choc. Brownie; P'B | 140 | 4.5 | 30 |
| **Great Value** (Walmart): | | | |
| Granola: Choc Chunk, 0.84 oz | 90 | 2 | 18 |
| Choc Chip; PB; Smores, av., 0.81 oz | 100 | 3 | 19 |
| Peanut, 1.23 oz | 180 | 9 | 19 |
| Sweet & Salty, Almond, 1.24 oz | 160 | 8 | 20 |
| **Health Valley,** Chewy Granola, av. | 110 | 1.5 | 22 |
| **Herbalife,** Protein Deluxe!, 1.25 oz | 140 | 4 | 15 |
| **HMR,** Benefit Bars, average, 1.4 oz | 155 | 4 | 23 |
| **Jenny Craig:** S'mores, 1.23 oz | 130 | 4 | 22 |
| Chocolatey Caramel P'nut, 1.23 oz | 140 | 5 | 19 |
| Choc Chip Snack Bar, 1.21 oz | 140 | 3 | 23 |
| **Joy Ride,** | | | |
| Protein Bars, average, 2.8 oz | 340 | 12 | 27 |
| **Kashi:** | | | |
| **GoLean:** Snack size, av., 1.94 oz | 195 | 4.5 | 32 |
| Crunchy!: Choc. Peanut, 1.76 oz | 180 | 5 | 30 |
| Average others, 1.58 oz | 155 | 4 | 27 |
| Roll!, average, 1.95 oz | 190 | 5 | 28 |
| **TLC:** Crunchy Granola (2), av.,1.4 oz | 170 | 5.5 | 26 |
| Chewy Granola, average, 1.23 oz | 135 | 4 | 20 |
| **Keebler,** | | | |
| Granola Fudge, average, 1.23 oz | 150 | 6 | 25 |
| **Kellogg's Bars** ~ see page 31 | | | |
| **Kind:** Per 1.4 oz Bar Unless Indicated | | | |
| **Fruit & Nut:** Almond & Apricot | 190 | 11 | 22 |
| Apple Cinnamon & Pecan | 180 | 10 | 23 |
| Macadamia & Apricot | 190 | 12 | 22 |
| Nut Delight | 210 | 16 | 14 |
| Peanut Butter & Strawberry | 190 | 11 | 18 |
| Sesame & Peanuts with Chocolate | 240 | 17 | 16 |
| Walnut & Date | 170 | 9 | 22 |
| **In Yogurt,** | | | |
| average, 1.58 oz | 215 | 12 | 26 |
| **Plus:** | | | |
| Cranberry Almond + Antioxidants | 190 | 13 | 20 |
| Almond Cashew w/ Flax & Omega 3 | 180 | 10 | 20 |
| Alm. Walnut Macadamia + Protein | 190 | 12 | 15 |

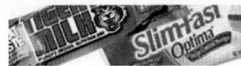

### Sports & Diet Bars (Cont)

| Per Bar | C | F | Cb |
|---|---|---|---|
| **Kudos:** Choc. Chip; P. Butter, av., 1 oz | 125 | 5 | 19 |
| M&M's; Snickers, average, 0.84 oz | 100 | 3 | 17 |
| **Larabar:** | | | |
| Apple Pie, 1.6 oz | 190 | 10 | 24 |
| Cherry Pie, 1.7 oz | 200 | 8 | 30 |
| Choc. Chip Brownie, 1.6 oz | 200 | 9 | 31 |
| Peanut Butter & Jelly, 1.7 oz | 210 | 10 | 27 |
| Tropical Fruit Tart, 1.6 oz | 210 | 11 | 27 |
| **Lean Body:** | | | |
| **Cookie Roll Bars:** Per 2.82 oz Bar | | | |
| Chocolate Chip | 330 | 11 | 34 |
| Cinn. Bun; Iced Brownie, average | 300 | 9 | 34 |
| **Hi-Protein Meal Repl. Bars:** | | | |
| Cookies & Cream, 2.4 oz | 290 | 9 | 28 |
| Peanut Butter Cup, 2.4 oz | 315 | 14 | 22 |
| **Lindora,** average, 1.6 oz | 155 | 5 | 17 |
| **Luna:** | | | |
| **Bars For Women,** average, 1.7 oz | 180 | 4.5 | 27 |
| **Protein,** average, 1.6 oz | 185 | 7 | 20 |
| **Marathon** (Snickers): | | | |
| **Energy:** Chewy, 2 oz | 215 | 7 | 26 |
| Crunchy, av.,1.56 oz | 150 | 4.5 | 22 |
| **Protein,** average, 2.8 oz | 285 | 10 | 38 |
| **Smart Stuff,** average, 1.23 oz | 140 | 4 | 22 |
| **Market Pantry** (Target): | | | |
| Crunchy Granola, Oat & Honey,1.5 oz | 190 | 6 | 30 |
| **Mariana:** Cranberry, 1.4 oz | 180 | 10 | 20 |
| Granola | 160 | 6 | 25 |
| Sesame | 200 | 14 | 16 |
| Trail Mix | 190 | 12 | 18 |
| **Medifast:** Crunch, average, 1.13 oz | 110 | 3 | 12 |
| Maintenance, average, 1.5 oz | 160 | 4.5 | 21 |
| **Met-Rx:** Per 3.53 oz Bar Unless Indicated | | | |
| **Big 100,** average all varieties | 375 | 6 | 49 |
| **Big 100 Colossal:** | | | |
| Brownie, average | 395 | 13 | 41 |
| Chocolate Toasted Almond | 410 | 13 | 46 |
| Crispy Apple Pie | 400 | 10 | 47 |
| **Protein Plus,** Mud Pie, 3 oz | 300 | 9 | 32 |
| **MLO:** Bio Protein Bar, av., 2.85 oz | 315 | 6.5 | 43 |
| Xtreme Bar, Chocolate, 3.2 oz | 320 | 6 | 44 |
| **Mojo Bars** ~ See Clif | | | |
| **Muscle Milk:** Regular, av.,2.57 oz | 295 | 11 | 29 |
| Light, all flavors, 1.59 oz | 170 | 6 | 18 |
| **Muscle Tech:** | | | |
| **Nitro-Tech Hardcore,** all varieties, 2.8 oz | 310 | 8 | 29 |
| **Smart Protein:** Triple Choc.: 2.2 oz | 270 | 9 | 26 |
| Peanut Caramel Crunch: 2.2 oz | 290 | 12 | 26 |

| Per Bar | C | F | Cb |
|---|---|---|---|
| **Nabisco,** 100 Calorie Fruit Crisps, all varieties, 2 crisps, 0.88 oz | 100 | 2 | 20 |
| **Nature's Path:** | | | |
| Granola Bars, average, 1.23 oz | 150 | 5 | 26 |
| Optimum Energy Bars, av., 1.98 oz | 220 | 5.5 | 37 |
| **Nature Valley:** | | | |
| **Crunchy Granola Bars:** | | | |
| Apple Crisp (2), 1.48 oz | 160 | 6 | 26 |
| Cinnamon (2), 1.48 oz | 180 | 6 | 29 |
| **Chewy,** Yog. coating, av., 1.23 oz | 140 | 3.5 | 26 |
| **Trail Mix,** average, 1.23 oz | 135 | 3.5 | 25 |
| **Nutiva:** Hempseed, 1.4 oz | 210 | 15 | 14 |
| Hemp Choc.; Flax & Raisin, 1.4 oz | 200 | 13 | 16 |
| **Nutrigrain** (Kellogg's), Cereal Bars, av. all flav., 1.3 oz | 120 | 3 | 24 |
| **Nutrilite** (Amway Global): | | | |
| **Meal Bars:** Blueb. Crunch, 1.8 oz | 200 | 7 | 26 |
| Cherry Almond, 1.8 oz | 200 | 6 | 26 |
| Chocolate Crisp, 1.8 oz | 190 | 6 | 26 |
| Lemon Twist, 1.8 oz | 200 | 7 | 27 |
| **Snack Bar:** Caramel Creme, 0.9 oz | 100 | 2.5 | 16 |
| Cranberry Crunch, 0.9 oz | 100 | 3 | 15 |
| Fudgy Brownie w/ Almonds, 0.9 oz | 100 | 3.5 | 9 |
| **NutriSystem:** | | | |
| **Dessert Bars:** Blueberry Lemon | 160 | 5 | 25 |
| Chocolate Peanut Butter | 170 | 8 | 17 |
| **Odwalla:** Per 2 oz Bar | | | |
| Energy: Berries GoMega | 210 | 6 | 36 |
| Blueberry Swirl | 200 | 3 | 41 |
| Choc. Chip Peanut | 230 | 8 | 33 |
| Choc. Chip Trail Mix | 200 | 7 | 28 |
| Choco-walla | 210 | 5 | 39 |
| Dark Chocolate Chip Walnut | 220 | 7 | 36 |
| Strawberry Pomeganate | 200 | 2 | 42 |
| Superfood, Original | 200 | 3.5 | 39 |
| **Oh Yeah!** (ISS), P'nut var., av., 3 oz | 375 | 17 | 31 |
| **One Way,** Protein, 3 oz | 340 | 12 | 29 |
| **Optifast,** 800 Bars, av., 1.6 oz | 165 | 4 | 20 |
| **PowerBar:** | | | |
| **Energy Bars:** Fruit Smoothie, all var. | 220 | 3.5 | 43 |
| Harvest, average, | 245 | 4.5 | 42 |
| Nut Naturals, all varieties, 1.6 oz | 210 | 10 | 20 |
| Performance, average, 2.1 oz | 230 | 3 | 41 |
| Pria Bars, 110 Plus, av., 1.7 oz | 110 | 3 | 16 |
| Protein Plus, av. | 300 | 7 | 37 |
| Pure & Simple, av. | 135 | 3 | 23 |
| Triple Threat, average, 1.94 oz | 225 | 7.5 | 31 |

## Sports & Diet Bars (Cont)

| Per Bar | C | F | Cb |
|---|---|---|---|
| **PR Bar:** Double Chocolate, 1.8 oz | 200 | 6 | 22 |
| Yogurt Berry, 1.8 oz | 210 | 7 | 22 |
| Granola, Peanut Butter, 1.75 oz | 200 | 7 | 22 |
| **Premier Nutrition:** | | | |
| Protein, av., 2.53 oz | 280 | 7 | 24 |
| Titan, av., 2.8 oz | 325 | 13 | 32 |
| **Promax:** | | | |
| Cookies 'N Cream, 2.64 oz | 270 | 4.5 | 39 |
| Chocolate Peanut Crunch, 2.64 oz | 300 | 8 | 37 |
| Double Fudge Brownie, 2.6 oz | 280 | 7 | 37 |
| **Lower Sugar,** Energy, av., 2.4 oz | 220 | 7 | 33 |
| **Proti Bars** (Bariatrix), | | | |
| Crisp; Layered, av., 1.4 oz | 160 | 5.5 | 16 |
| **Pure Protein:** | | | |
| 1.75 oz Bars, av. | 180 | 5 | 18 |
| 2.75 oz Bars, average | 300 | 8 | 30 |
| **PureFit,** average, 2 oz | 220 | 7 | 25 |
| **Quaker:** | | | |
| **Chewy Granola Bars:** | | | |
| Regular, av., 0.85 oz | 100 | 3 | 18 |
| Dipps, Caramel Nut | 140 | 6 | 21 |
| Fiber/Omega-3, PB. Choc, 1.25 oz | 150 | 5 | 25 |
| 25% Less Sugar, Choc. Chip, 0.85 oz | 100 | 3.5 | 17 |
| 90 Calories, all varieties, 1 oz | 90 | 2 | 19 |
| SmashBar, 0.84 oz | 90 | 2 | 18 |
| True Delights, average, 1.25 oz | 135 | 4.5 | 23 |
| **Rebar:** Original, 1.75 oz | 160 | 0 | 38 |
| Perfect 10 Energy, Lemon, 1.75 oz | 210 | 12 | 24 |
| Elev8me, Banana Nut Bread, 2.3 oz | 230 | 4.5 | 34 |
| **Revival Soy Bars** (Direct): | | | |
| Chocolate Temptation | 270 | 7 | 32 |
| Apple Cinnamon; Marshm. Krunch | 225 | 3 | 30 |
| Peanut Pal | 240 | 6 | 28 |
| **Low Carb,** average all flavors | 235 | 8 | 31 |
| (Contains 22g sugar alc. & 3g fiber) | | | |
| **Slim-Fast Bars:** | | | |
| **Meal Bars:** Chewy Chocolate Crisp | 200 | 6 | 26 |
| Chocolate Peanut Caramel | 200 | 7 | 23 |
| Sweet & Salty Chocolate Almond | 200 | 8 | 23 |
| **Snack Bars:** | | | |
| Chocolate Nougat Gone Nuts | 100 | 5 | 14 |
| Chocolatey Vanilla Blitz | 100 | 2.5 | 17 |
| Double-Dutch Choc. | 100 | 3.5 | 16 |

| Per Bar | C | F | Cb |
|---|---|---|---|
| **SoyJoy Bars,** av., 1 oz | 135 | 6 | 16 |
| **Solo,** GI, average, 1.75 oz | 200 | 7 | 26 |
| **Special K:** | | | |
| Blueberry; Rasp. Ch.cake, av., 0.8 oz | 90 | 2 | 18 |
| Protein Meal, average, 1.6 oz | 180 | 5 | 25 |
| Protein Snack Bars, average, 0.9 oz | 110 | 3 | 16 |
| **Steel Bar** (ABB), average, 2.47 oz | 260 | 5 | 34 |
| **Supreme Protein:** | | | |
| Caramel Nut Choc., 3.38 oz | 400 | 15 | 36 |
| Carb Conscious, PB Crunch, 3 oz | 390 | 18 | 26 |
| **thinkThin:** | | | |
| Protein: | | | |
| 1.76 oz Bars, average | 200 | 7 | 23 |
| 2.1 oz Bars, average | 235 | 8 | 24 |
| Bites, average, 0.88 oz | 100 | 4 | 12 |
| (Contains between 5-14g Sugar Alc) | | | |
| **Tiger's Milk:** | | | |
| Protein Rich, 1.2 oz | 140 | 5 | 18 |
| Peanut Butter, 1.2 oz | 150 | 6 | 18 |
| King Size, average, 1.9 oz | 225 | 9 | 28 |
| **Trader Joe's:** | | | |
| **Chewy Granola Bars, 6-Packs:** | | | |
| Chocolate Chip, 1.23 oz | 150 | 4 | 26 |
| Vanilla Almond, 1.23 oz | 150 | 6 | 22 |
| Peanut Butter, 1.23 oz | 170 | 8 | 19 |
| **Granola Bars, 6-packs:** | | | |
| Fruit & Nut Trek Mix, 1.23 oz | 130 | 2.5 | 25 |
| Trail Mix, 1.23 oz | 150 | 5 | 23 |
| **Tri-O-Plex:** | | | |
| **High Protein,** Ban. Walnut, 4.2 oz | 440 | 16 | 45 |
| **Duo:** Caramel Peanut Butter, 3.5 oz | 340 | 8 | 45 |
| Peanut Butter & Jelly, 3.5 oz | 360 | 11 | 41 |
| **U-Turn,** Protein Bars, 2.8 oz | 300 | 8 | 26 |
| **Usana:** | | | |
| Nutrition Bar: Oatmeal Raisin, 2 oz | 170 | 3 | 30 |
| Peanut Butter Crunch, 1.5 oz | 160 | 5 | 19 |
| **Vyo-Pro** (AST), Choc. Brownie, 2.2 oz | 220 | 7 | 27 |
| **Wheaties,** Fuel Energy Bars: | | | |
| Chocolate Peanut Butter, 2.25 oz | 290 | 12 | 30 |
| Double Chocolate, 2.25 oz | 280 | 10 | 34 |
| **Zoe's,** Omega-3's, Choc. Delight | 190 | 7 | 27 |
| **Zone Perfect:** | | | |
| **Classic,** av., 1.76 oz | 210 | 7 | 24 |
| **Cookie Dough,** average, 1.58 oz | 185 | 6 | 23 |
| **Dark Chocolate,** average, 1.58 oz | 190 | 6 | 22 |
| **Fruitified,** average, 1.75 oz | 195 | 5 | 25 |
| **Sweet & Salty,** average, 1.58 oz | 200 | 7 | 22 |

## Cocoa & Hot Chocolate

| | C | F | Cb |
|---|---|---|---|
| **Cocoa:** (8 fl.oz cup): | | | |
| With Whole Milk | 205 | 8.5 | 22 |
| With Nonfat Milk | 145 | 1 | 23 |
| Tall (12 fl.oz): With Whole Milk | 280 | 12 | 26 |
| With Nonfat Milk | 185 | 1 | 28 |
| **Hot Chocolate:** | | | |
| 8 fl.oz cup: With Whole Milk | 180 | 7 | 26 |
| With Nonfat Milk | 140 | 2 | 17 |
| Tall (12 fl.oz): With Whole Milk | 260 | 10 | 36 |
| With Nonfat Milk | 190 | 2 | 37 |
| **Cinnabon,** Mochalatta Chill, 16 oz | 420 | 17 | 63 |
| **Swiss Miss,** Mixes, av., 1 packet | 120 | 2.5 | 22 |

## Cocoa - Chocolate Mixes

*Add extra cals/fat/carbohydrate for milk*
**Carnation Breakfast Drinks** ~ *See Page 38*

| **Carnation:** *Per 3 Tbsp* | C | F | Cb |
|---|---|---|---|
| Malted Milk: Original | 90 | 2 | 15 |
| Chocolate | 90 | 1 | 18 |
| **Ghirardelli:** | | | |
| Choc. Mocha, 4 Tbsp, 1.2 oz | 135 | 1.5 | 33 |
| Double Chocolate, 4 Tbsp, 1.4 oz | 140 | 1.5 | 34 |
| White Mocha, 2 Tbsp, 0.8 oz | 100 | 0 | 24 |
| **Hershey's,** Cocoa, | | | |
| Natural, 1 Tbsp, 0.18 oz | 10 | 0.5 | 3 |
| **Horlicks,** Orig. Malt Powder, 1.1 oz | 180 | 4 | 27 |
| **Land O Lakes,** | | | |
| Mint/Raspberry/Supreme, 1.25 oz | 140 | 3.5 | 26 |
| **Nestle:** *Per Single ½ Serve Package* | | | |
| Dark Milk Chocolate | 80 | 1 | 17 |
| Carb Select: Fat-Free Hot Cocoa | 25 | 0 | 5 |
| With Marshmallows | 35 | 0 | 8 |
| Rich Milk Chocolate | 80 | 3 | 15 |
| No Sugar Added | 50 | 0 | 10 |
| Supreme Cocoa, 1 oz | 120 | 2 | 22 |
| **Nesquik Powder:** *Per 2 Tbsp* | | | |
| Choc.; Strawberry, 25% less sugar | 60 | 0 | 15 |
| Chocolate; Strawb., No Added Sugar | 35 | 1 | 7 |
| **Ovaltine,** Cocoa Mixes, av., 4 T. | 80 | 0 | 19 |
| **Swiss Miss:** *Per Single Serve Envelope* | | | |
| Breakfast Blends: Great Start | 60 | 1 | 1 |
| Pick Me Up | 110 | 2 | 23 |
| Milk Chocolate: Made with water | 120 | 2 | 23 |
| Made with milk | 210 | 6 | 31 |
| French Vanilla | 115 | 2 | 23 |
| Marshmallow | 110 | 2 | 23 |
| Marshmallow Lovers | 120 | 2.5 | 23 |
| Rich Chocolate | 120 | 2 | 23 |
| Fat-Free: Original | 50 | 0 | 10 |
| Marshmallow Lovers | 70 | 0 | 13 |

## Instant Coffee

| | C | F | Cb |
|---|---|---|---|
| **Powder/Granules:** *Regular or Decaffeinated,* | | | |
| 1 level tsp | 2 | 0 | 0.5 |
| 1 rounded tsp | 4 | 0 | 1 |
| **Ground,** 3 tsp | 7 | 0 | 1 |
| **Brewed/Percolated,** 1 cup, 8 fl.oz | 4 | 0 | 1 |
| **Coffee With Milk/Cream/Creamers:** *Per 8 oz Cup* | | | |
| **Black:** | 4 | 0 | 1 |
| With Whole Milk: Dash, 1 Tbsp | 15 | 0.5 | 2 |
| 2 Tbsp, 1 fl.oz | 25 | 1 | 2 |
| With 2% Milk, 2 Tbsp | 20 | 0.5 | 2 |
| With 1% Milk, 2 Tbsp | 20 | 0.5 | 3.5 |
| With Fat Free Milk, 2 Tbsp | 15 | 0 | 3 |
| With Half & Half: 2 Tbsp | 50 | 3 | 2 |
| With, ¼ cup, 2 fl.oz | 90 | 6 | 3 |
| With Cream (light coffee), 2 Tbsp | 65 | 6 | 2 |
| With Coffee Mate: Liquid, reg., 1 T. | 20 | 1 | 2 |
| Liquid Fat Free, 1 Tbsp | 25 | 0 | 5 |
| Powder, 1 heaping tsp | 15 | 1 | 2 |
| **Sugar ~ Add Extra:** 1 heaping tsp | 25 | 0 | 6 |
| Single portion, 1 package | 25 | 0 | 6 |
| **Sweeteners,** Equal/Splenda/Sweet N Low, | | | |
| Powder, 1 package | 0 | 0 | 0 |

## Flavored Coffee Mixes

| **Chicory:** | C | F | Cb |
|---|---|---|---|
| Instant Coffee, 1 tsp | 5 | 0 | 1 |
| Coffee Essence, 1 tsp | 15 | 0 | 4 |
| **Caffé D'Vita:** Mixes, 3 tsp | 60 | 1.5 | 11 |
| Sugar Free Mixes, 2 tsp | 35 | 2 | 3 |
| **General Foods International:** | | | |
| Average, ½ oz | 60 | 3 | 10 |
| Sugar-free, av,. 1 tsp | 30 | 2.5 | 2 |
| Cappuccino Coolers, ½ oz | 60 | 0 | 15 |
| **Hills Bros,** | | | |
| Cappuccino, Fr. Vanilla, 3 Tbsp, 1 oz | 120 | 4.5 | 19 |
| **Nescafé,** Latte; Mocha, av. 1oz | 115 | 3.5 | 21 |
| **Starbucks,** VIA® Iced Coffee, 1 stick | 100 | 0 | 24 |

## Coffee Shops/Restaurants

*Per 8 fl.oz Cup (Unless Indicated)*

| | C | F | Cb |
|---|---|---|---|
| **Coffee,** Regular/Percolated/Filtered | 5 | 0 | 0 |
| **Americano Drip Coffee,** 1 cup | 7.5 | 0 | 1 |
| **Cafe Au Lait:** 1 cup, 8 fl.oz | 60 | 3.5 | 5 |
| Nonfat Milk, 1 cup, 8 fl.oz | 35 | 0 | 5 |
| **Caffe Latté:** | | | |
| 8 fl.oz cup: With Whole Milk | 110 | 6 | 9 |
| With 2% Milk | 100 | 3.5 | 9 |
| With Nonfat Milk | 70 | 0 | 10 |
| 12 fl.oz: With Whole Milk | 180 | 9 | 14 |
| With Nonfat Milk | 100 | 0 | 15 |
| 16 fl.oz: With Whole Milk | 220 | 11 | 18 |
| With Nonfat Milk | 130 | 0 | 19 |
| **Cafe Mocha (Mochaccino):** 8 fl.oz | 150 | 6 | 20 |
| 12 fl.oz | 230 | 9 | 31 |
| 16 fl.oz | 290 | 12 | 41 |
| **Cappuccino:** | | | |
| 8 fl.oz cup: With Whole Milk | 90 | 3.5 | 7 |
| With 2% Milk | 80 | 3 | 8 |
| With Nonfat Milk | 50 | 0 | 8 |
| 12 fl.oz: With Whole Milk | 110 | 6 | 9 |
| With 2% Milk | 90 | 3.5 | 9 |
| With Nonfat Milk | 60 | 0 | 9 |
| 16 fl.oz: With Whole Milk | 140 | 7 | 11 |
| With 2% Milk | 120 | 3.5 | 11 |
| With Nonfat Milk | 80 | 0 | 12 |
| **Mocha** *(with cream):* | | | |
| 8 fl.oz: With Whole Milk | 200 | 11 | 22 |
| With Nonfat Milk | 160 | 6 | 22 |
| 12 fl.oz: Whole Milk | 290 | 15 | 33 |
| With Nonfat Milk | 230 | 8 | 34 |
| **Iced Mocha** *(without cream):* | | | |
| 12 fl.oz: With Whole Milk | 170 | 6 | 26 |
| With Nonfat Milk | 130 | 2 | 27 |
| **Espresso:** Single (Solo) | 5 | 0 | 1 |
| Doppio (Double) | 10 | 0 | 2 |
| **Espresso con Panna,** | | | |
| (with dollop whipped cream), solo | 30 | 2.5 | 2 |
| **Espresso Macchiato,** solo | 10 | 0 | 1 |
| **Frappuccino:** Tall, 12 fl.oz | 180 | 2.5 | 37 |
| Grande, 16 fl.oz | 240 | 3 | 48 |
| **Frappuccino Mocha,** | | | |
| (with Cream): Tall, 12 fl.oz | 280 | 11 | 43 |
| Grande, 16 fl.oz | 380 | 15 | 57 |

**Iced Latte**: *Similar to Caffe Latte*

**McCafe (McDonald's)** ~ *See Fast Food Section ~ Page 216*

**Starbucks** ~ *See Fast-Foods Section ~ Page 243*

## Coffee Substitute Mixes

| | C | F | Cb |
|---|---|---|---|
| **Roasted Cereal Beverages ~** *(No Caffeine)* | | | |
| **Cafix,** Instant Beverage, 1 tsp | 5 | 0 | 1 |
| **Kaffree,** Roma (Morn. Farms) 1 tsp | 10 | 0 | 2 |
| **Teeccino Caffe,** 1 tsp | 10 | 0 | 2 |

## Irish & Liqueur Coffees

| | C | F | Cb |
|---|---|---|---|
| **Irish Coffee,** without sugar | 175 | 10 | 0 |
| **Liqueur Coffee,** | | | |
| with cream, average, 1 fl.oz | 100 | 5 | 7 |

## Coffee Extras

| | C | F | Cb |
|---|---|---|---|
| Chocolate (Cocoa) Topping, ½ tsp | 5 | 0 | 1 |
| Flavored Syrups: Regular, 2 Tbsp | 80 | 0 | 20 |
| Sugar-free, 2 Tbsp | 0 | 0 | 0 |
| Half & Half Cream: 2 Tbsp | 40 | 3.5 | 1 |
| Single serve pkg, ⅜ fl.oz | 15 | 1.5 | 0.5 |
| Light Whipped Cream, 2 Tbsp | 15 | 1.5 | 1 |
| Marshmallows, miniature (2) | 5 | 0 | 1 |
| **Sugar:** 1 single portion package | 20 | 0 | 5 |
| 1 level tsp | 15 | 0 | 4 |
| 1 heaping tsp | 25 | 0 | 6 |
| *Equal/Splenda/Sweet 'N Low* | 0 | 0 | 0 |

## Coffee Shop ~ Cakes, Cookies

| | C | F | Cb |
|---|---|---|---|
| **Cookies:** | | | |
| Biscotti, 1 oz | 140 | 6.5 | 18 |
| Chocolate Chip, 3 oz | 350 | 15 | 54 |
| Oatmeal Raisin, 3 oz | 350 | 12 | 56 |
| Peanut Butter, 3 oz | 410 | 25 | 39 |
| White Chocolate Macadamia, 3⅓ oz | 420 | 20 | 55 |
| **Cakes/Pastries:** | | | |
| Almond Croissant, 5 oz | 620 | 35 | 67 |
| Apple Danish, 5 oz | 450 | 18 | 67 |
| Banana Walnut, 4½ oz | 410 | 17 | 60 |
| Brownie, 3 oz | 390 | 24 | 42 |
| Bundt, Chocolate, 4 oz | 440 | 21 | 61 |
| Carrot Cake, 4 oz | 400 | 22 | 45 |
| Chocolate Cake, 5 oz | 530 | 28 | 65 |
| Crumble Coffee Cake, 4½ oz | 500 | 25 | 65 |
| Cupcake, 3 oz | 330 | 16 | 43 |
| Pound Cake, av., 3 oz | 330 | 17 | 40 |
| **Cinnamon Roll,** 6 oz | 500 | 15 | 83 |
| **Donuts:** | | | |
| Sugared, 1¾ oz | 220 | 11 | 27 |
| Glazed, 2 oz | 250 | 12 | 34 |
| **Pretzel,** large, 4 oz | 290 | 5 | 52 |

**Starbucks Bakery Items** ~ *See Page 244*

## Bottled Coffee (Chilled)

| Ready-To-Drink: | C | F | Cb |
|---|---|---|---|
| **Adina:** *Per 8 fl.oz Can* | | | |
| Double XXpresso | 100 | 2 | 18 |
| Mayan Mocha | 130 | 2.5 | 24 |
| Mocha Madness | 110 | 2.5 | 20 |
| **Coffee Bean & Tea Leaf,** | | | |
| Cafe Latte/Mocha/Vanilla, 9.5 fl.oz | 200 | 3 | 33 |
| **Full Throttle Coffee & Energy** ~ *See Page 38* | | | |
| **Java Monster Energy** ~ *See Page 39* | | | |
| **Kahlua,** Cappuccino Shake, 10.5 fl.oz | 130 | 2 | 24 |
| **Shock Coffee:** Triple Latte, 8fl.oz | 150 | 3.5 | 28 |
| Triple Mocha, 8 fl.oz can | 150 | 3.5 | 28 |
| **Starbucks:** *Per Bottle* | | | |
| **Frappuccino:** | | | |
| Coffee, 9.5 fl.oz | 200 | 3 | 37 |
| Mocha, 9.5 fl.oz | 180 | 3 | 33 |
| Vanilla: 9.5 fl.oz | 200 | 3 | 37 |
| Light, 9.5 fl.oz | 100 | 3 | 12 |
| **DoubleShot:** | | | |
| Coffee, 6.5 fl.oz | 140 | 6 | 18 |
| Light, 6.5 fl.oz | 70 | 4 | 6 |
| **Starbucks Coffee & Energy** ~ *See Page 40* | | | |
| **Trader Joes,** | | | |
| Caffe Latte; Caffe Mocha, 6.5 fl.oz | 120 | 1.5 | 25 |

---

## CALORIE KING TIP!

### Reduce the Calories in Your Coffee Drinks:

- Request non-fat milk in place of whole or 2% milk
- Downsize to 8 fl.oz or 12 fl.oz
- Avoid cream on frappuccinos
- Replace sugar with *Equal, Splenda Stevia* or *Sweet 'N Low*
- Avoid syrup add-ons

---

## CAFFEINE COUNTER

Moderate caffeine intake is not harmful to healthy adults. However, frequent large amounts (over 350mg/day) may cause dependency ('caffeinism') and adversely affect health. To be safe, limit caffeine to 200mg/day. Avoid if pregnant, breast feeding, a child under 8, have sleep problems, an overactive bladder or heart arrhythmia.

| **Caffeine** (mg) | |
|---|---|
| **Coffee:** Instant, weak, 1 level teaspoon | 30 |
| Medium, 1 rounded teaspoon | 60 |
| Strong, 1 heaping teaspoon | 100 |
| **Decaffeinated**, 1 round teaspoon | 2 |
| **Bags (Folgers)**, 1 bag (6-8 fl.oz) | 115 |
| **Ground**, 1 Tbsp, 0.2 oz | 60 |
| **Bottled (Ready-To-Drink)**, 9.5 fl.oz | 70 |
| **Coffee Shop:** Brewed, 8 fl.oz | 110-150 |
| **Cappuccino**: 1 cup, 8 fl.oz | 75 |
| **Tall**, 12 fl.oz | 110 |
| **Large**, 16 fl.oz | 150 |
| **Decappuccino**, decaffeinated | 5 |
| **Espresso**: Regular/Solo | 75 |
| **Double (Doppio)** | 150 |
| **Iced Coffee**, 12 fl.oz | 140 |
| **Latte**, 1 cup, 8 fl.oz | 75 |
| **Mocha**, 1 cup, 8 fl.oz | 90 |
| **Hot Chocolate**, 8 fl.oz | 15 |
| **Tea (Black/Green)**: Weak, 1 cup | 20 |
| Medium Strength, 1 cup | 40 |
| Strong, 1 cup | 70 |
| Decaffeinated Tea | 0-5 |
| Herbal Tea | 0 |
| **Iced Tea**, tall glass/can, 12 fl.oz | 25-30 |
| **Soft Drinks:** *Per 12 fl.oz Can* | |
| Coca-Cola, Pepsi (Regular/Diet) | 35 |
| Diet Coke; TAB; RC Cola (Regular) | 45 |
| Dr. Pepper, Sunkist Orange | 40 |
| Pepsi One; Mountain Dew; Mellow Yellow; Surge | 55 |
| Pepsi Max (Regular/Diet) Sun Drop (Reg/Diet) | 70 |
| 7-Up, Fanta, Sprite, Fresca, Diet Rite Cola | 0 |
| **Energy Drinks (with added caffeine):** | |
| (AMP, Adrenaline Rush, Full Throttle Monster, No Fear, Red Bull, Rockstar) | |
| Average all brands: 8 fl.oz | 80 |
| 16 fl.oz | 160 |
| **NOS Energy**, 16 fl.oz | 260 |
| **Chocolate Bars:** Milk Chocolate, 2 oz | 20 |
| Dark Chocolate, 2 oz | 30 |
| **Choc Chip Cookies**, 2 medium, 2 oz | 6 |
| **Chocolate Syrup**, 2 Tbsp, 1.4 oz | 5 |
| **Medicinals:** Excedrin, Extra Strength (2) | 130 |
| NoDoz Maximum, 1 tablet | 200 |

## Energy/Protein Drinks

| | C | F | Cb |
|---|---|---|---|
| **5-hour Energy**, 2 fl.oz | 4 | 0 | 1 |
| **ABB:** | | | |
| **Anytime,** Turbo Tea, 18 fl.oz | 150 | 0 | 38 |
| **Energy:** Speed Shot, 8.5 fl.oz | 0 | 0 | 0 |
|   Ripped Force, 18 fl.oz | 90 | 0 | 23 |
| **Hi-Pro:** | | | |
|   Pure Pro Shake, Chocolate, 12 fl.oz | 160 | 0.5 | 5 |
|   Pure Pro 50, 14.5 fl.oz | 240 | 1.5 | 7 |
| **Recovery,** | | | |
|   Maxx Recovery, Grape, 18 fl.oz | 480 | 0.5 | 6 |
| **AdvantEDGE** *(EAS)*, | | | |
|   Carb Control, average, 11 fl.oz | 110 | 3 | 4 |
| **AllSport,** | | | |
|   Body Quencher, all flav., 20 fl.oz | 150 | 0 | 40 |
| **AMP:** *Per 16 fl.oz Can* | | | |
| Elevate | 230 | 0 | 58 |
| Energy Drink | 220 | 0 | 58 |
| Average other varieties | 225 | 0 | 58 |
| **Anytime Health:** | | | |
| **Performance Powder:** | | | |
|   Green Apple/Lemonade, | | | |
|     2 scoops, 1 pkt, 1.73 oz | 160 | 0 | 30 |
| **Whey Protein Isolate,** | | | |
|   all flavors, 1 oz | 105 | 0 | 1 |
| **Arizona:** AM Awake Fast Shot, 2 fl.oz | 10 | 0 | 3 |
|   Caution Energy, 11 fl.oz | 160 | 0 | 40 |
| **Atkins,** Advantage Shakes, av., 11 oz | 160 | 10 | 4 |
| **Bally Total Fitness:** | | | |
| Whey Pro, Vanilla, 1 scoop | 115 | 1.5 | 3 |
| Blast, Sugar Free, 8.3 oz | 10 | 0 | 3 |
| **Bariatrix:** Pudding Shakes (1), av. | 100 | 2 | 7 |
|   Ready To Serve Drinks, average | 110 | 4 | 4 |
| **Bawls,** Guarana, 10 fl.oz | 120 | 0 | 32 |
| **Biggest Loser:** *Per 11.2 fl.oz ctn* | | | |
| **Shakes:** Crmy Vanilla | 180 | 5 | 24 |
|   Milk Chocolate | 190 | 5 | 26 |
| **Blue Sky,** | | | |
|   Blue Energy, 8.3 fl.oz | 120 | 0 | 29 |
| **Body Fuel** *(w. NutraSweet)*, | | | |
|   1 scoop | 80 | 0 | 20 |
| **Bolthouse:** *Per 8 fl.oz* | | | |
| Perfectly Protein: | | | |
|   Mocha Cappuccino | 180 | 3 | 31 |
|   Vanilla Chai Tea | 160 | 3 | 25 |
| **Boost:** High Protein, 8 fl.oz | 240 | 6 | 33 |
|   Glucose Control, 8 fl.oz | 190 | 7 | 16 |
|   Nutritional Energy, 8 fl.oz | 240 | 4 | 41 |
|   Plus, 8 fl.oz | 360 | 14 | 45 |
|   Kid Essentials, 8.25 fl.oz | 245 | 9 | 33 |

| | C | F | Cb |
|---|---|---|---|
| **Carnation Breakfast Essentials:** | | | |
| Powder: All flav., 1 envelope, 1.3 oz | 130 | 1 | 27 |
|   No Sugar Added, average, 0.7 oz | 60 | 1 | 12 |
|   Ready-To-Drink, average, 11.5 fl.oz | 260 | 5 | 41 |
| **Celebrity Juice Diet,** 4 fl.oz | 60 | 0 | 14 |
| **CeraSport,** EX1, 8.45 fl.oz | 20 | 0 | 5 |
| **Champion Lyte,** Sports Drink | 0 | 0 | 0 |
| **Champion Nutrition:** | | | |
| Heavyweight Gainer 900, 4 scps, 5.4 oz | 630 | 10 | 101 |
| Ultramet: Original, 1 packet, 2.7 oz | 280 | 2 | 24 |
|   Lite, 1 packet, 2 oz | 190 | 1 | 17 |
|   Low Carb, 1 packet, 2 oz | 230 | 6.5 | 6 |
| **Clif Shot,** Energy Gel, 1.1 oz pkt | 100 | 0 | 24 |
| **Cocaine,** Energy, 8.4 fl.oz can | 70 | 0 | 18 |
| **Curves Protein Drink:** | | | |
| Chocolate; Vanilla, 2 scoops,1 oz | 120 | 1 | 12 |
|   Made with skim milk, 8 fl.oz | 210 | 2 | 24 |
| **CytoSport,** Muscle Milk, 2 scoops | 300 | 12 | 16 |
| **Drank,** Anti Energy, 8 fl.oz | 110 | 0 | 27 |
| **EAS ~ See AdvantEdge/Myoplex** | | | |
| **Endura** *(Unipro)*, 2 scoops, 1.3 oz | 120 | 0 | 30 |
| **Ensure:** | | | |
| High Protein Shakes, 14 fl.oz | 210 | 2.5 | 23 |
|   Immune Health, 8 fl.oz | 250 | 6 | 42 |
|   Plus, average, 8 fl.oz bottle | 350 | 11 | 50 |
| **Enterex,** Diabetic, 8 fl.oz | 235 | 9 | 27 |
| **FRS,** Energy, Orange Cream, 12 fl.oz | 190 | 2.5 | 11 |
| **Fruit₂O** *(Veryfine)* | 0 | 0 | 0 |
| **Full Throttle:** *Per 16 fl.oz* | | | |
| Energy, Citrus | 220 | 0 | 58 |
| Coffee & Energy: | | | |
|   Caramel | 230 | 0 | 58 |
|   Mocha | 270 | 7 | 50 |
| **Fuze:** Slenderize, 8 fl.oz | 10 | 0 | 2 |
|   Refresh, 8 fl.oz | 95 | 0 | 25 |
|   Vitalize, 8 fl.oz | 100 | 0 | 25 |
| **Gatorade:** | | | |
| **Thirst Quencher/Perform:** | | | |
| (Lemon/Lime, AM, Fierce, Rain) | | | |
|   1 cup, 8 fl.oz | 50 | 0 | 14 |
|   12 fl.oz bottle | 75 | 0 | 20 |
|   20 fl.oz bottle | 125 | 0 | 32 |
|   24 fl.oz bottle | 150 | 0 | 41 |
|   32 fl.oz bottle | 200 | 0 | 52 |
| **Carbohydrate Energy,** | | | |
|   12 fl.oz bottle | 330 | 0 | 82 |
| **Endurance,** *(Powder)*, made up, 8 fl.oz | 50 | 0 | 14 |
| **G2,** *(Low Calorie)*: 1 cup, 8 fl.oz | 25 | 0 | 7 |
|   20 fl.oz bottle | 70 | 0 | 17 |
| **Nutrition Shake,** all flav., 11 oz | 360 | 8 | 54 |
| **Prime 01 Pre-game,** 4 fl.oz pouch | 100 | 0 | 25 |
| **Protein Recovery Shake,** 8 fl.oz | 200 | 1 | 33 |

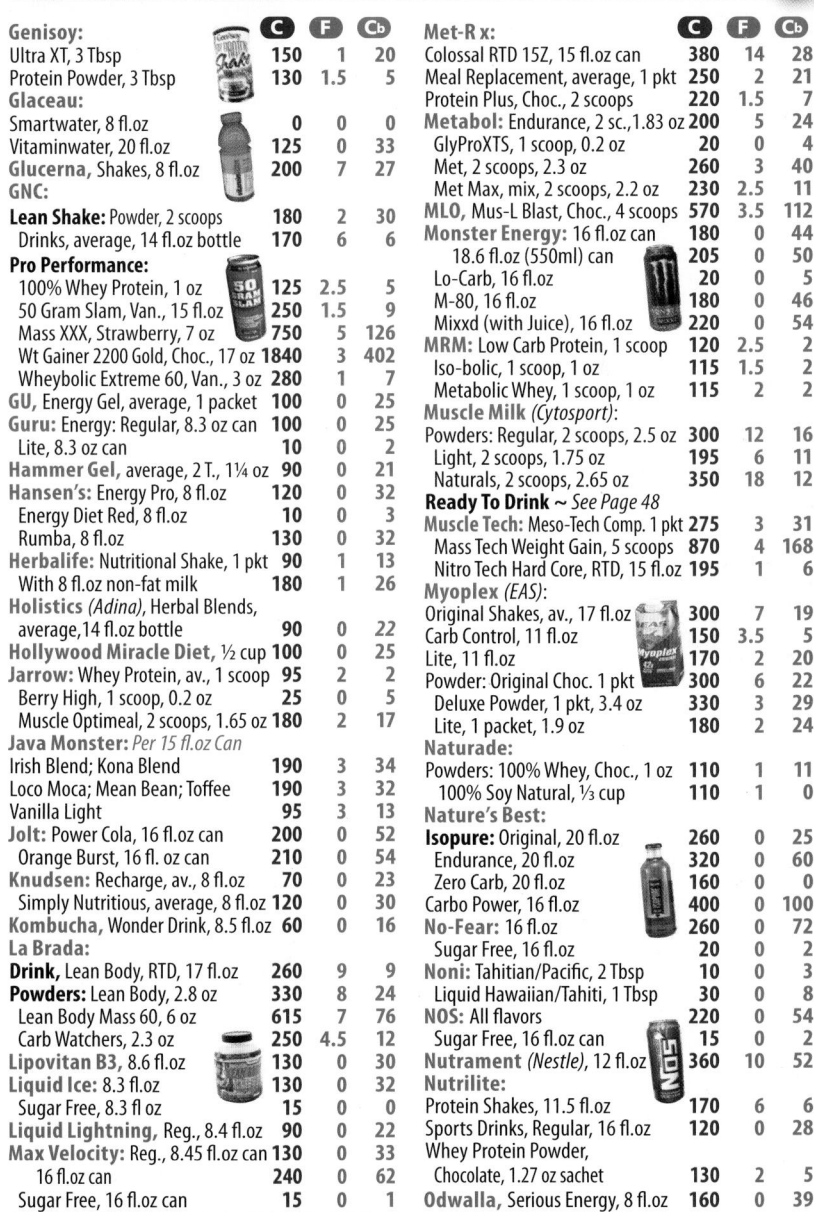

| | C | F | Cb |
|---|---|---|---|
| **Genisoy:** | | | |
| Ultra XT, 3 Tbsp | 150 | 1 | 20 |
| Protein Powder, 3 Tbsp | 130 | 1.5 | 5 |
| **Glaceau:** | | | |
| Smartwater, 8 fl.oz | 0 | 0 | 0 |
| Vitaminwater, 20 fl.oz | 125 | 0 | 33 |
| **Glucerna,** Shakes, 8 fl.oz | 200 | 7 | 27 |
| **GNC:** | | | |
| **Lean Shake:** Powder, 2 scoops | 180 | 2 | 30 |
| Drinks, average, 14 fl.oz bottle | 170 | 6 | 6 |
| **Pro Performance:** | | | |
| 100% Whey Protein, 1 oz | 125 | 2.5 | 5 |
| 50 Gram Slam, Van., 15 fl.oz | 250 | 1.5 | 9 |
| Mass XXX, Strawberry, 7 oz | 750 | 5 | 126 |
| Wt Gainer 2200 Gold, Choc., 17 oz | 1840 | 3 | 402 |
| Wheybolic Extreme 60, Van., 3 oz | 280 | 1 | 7 |
| **GU,** Energy Gel, average, 1 packet | 100 | 0 | 25 |
| **Guru:** Energy: Regular, 8.3 oz can | 100 | 0 | 25 |
| Lite, 8.3 oz can | 10 | 0 | 2 |
| **Hammer Gel,** average, 2 T., 1¼ oz | 90 | 0 | 21 |
| **Hansen's:** Energy Pro, 8 fl.oz | 120 | 0 | 32 |
| Energy Diet Red, 8 fl.oz | 10 | 0 | 3 |
| Rumba, 8 fl.oz | 130 | 0 | 32 |
| **Herbalife:** Nutritional Shake, 1 pkt | 90 | 1 | 13 |
| With 8 fl.oz non-fat milk | 180 | 1 | 26 |
| **Holistics** (Adina), Herbal Blends, | | | |
| average,14 fl.oz bottle | 90 | 0 | 22 |
| **Hollywood Miracle Diet,** ½ cup | 100 | 0 | 25 |
| **Jarrow:** Whey Protein, av., 1 scoop | 95 | 2 | 2 |
| Berry High, 1 scoop, 0.2 oz | 25 | 0 | 5 |
| Muscle Optimeal, 2 scoops, 1.65 oz | 180 | 2 | 17 |
| **Java Monster:** Per 15 fl.oz Can | | | |
| Irish Blend; Kona Blend | 190 | 3 | 34 |
| Loco Moca; Mean Bean; Toffee | 190 | 3 | 32 |
| Vanilla Light | 95 | 3 | 13 |
| **Jolt:** Power Cola, 16 fl.oz can | 200 | 0 | 52 |
| Orange Burst, 16 fl. oz can | 210 | 0 | 54 |
| **Knudsen:** Recharge, av., 8 fl.oz | 70 | 0 | 23 |
| Simply Nutritious, average, 8 fl.oz | 120 | 0 | 30 |
| **Kombucha,** Wonder Drink, 8.5 fl.oz | 60 | 0 | 16 |
| **La Brada:** | | | |
| **Drink,** Lean Body, RTD, 17 fl.oz | 260 | 9 | 9 |
| **Powders,** Lean Body, 2.8 oz | 330 | 8 | 24 |
| Lean Body Mass 60, 6 oz | 615 | 7 | 76 |
| Carb Watchers, 2.3 oz | 250 | 4.5 | 12 |
| **Lipovitan B3,** 8.6 fl.oz | 130 | 0 | 30 |
| **Liquid Ice:** 8.3 fl.oz | 130 | 0 | 32 |
| Sugar Free, 8.3 fl oz | 15 | 0 | 0 |
| **Liquid Lightning,** Reg., 8.4 fl.oz | 90 | 0 | 22 |
| **Max Velocity:** Reg., 8.45 fl.oz can | 130 | 0 | 33 |
| 16 fl.oz can | 240 | 0 | 62 |
| Sugar Free, 16 fl.oz can | 15 | 0 | 1 |

| | C | F | Cb |
|---|---|---|---|
| **Met-R x:** | | | |
| Colossal RTD 15Z, 15 fl.oz can | 380 | 14 | 28 |
| Meal Replacement, average, 1 pkt | 250 | 2 | 21 |
| Protein Plus, Choc., 2 scoops | 220 | 1.5 | 7 |
| **Metabol:** Endurance, 2 sc.,1.83 oz | 200 | 5 | 24 |
| GlyProXTS, 1 scoop, 0.2 oz | 20 | 0 | 4 |
| Met, 2 scoops, 2.3 oz | 260 | 3 | 40 |
| Met Max, mix, 2 scoops, 2.2 oz | 230 | 2.5 | 11 |
| **MLO,** Mus-L Blast, Choc., 4 scoops | 570 | 3.5 | 112 |
| **Monster Energy:** 16 fl.oz can | 180 | 0 | 44 |
| 18.6 fl.oz (550ml) can | 205 | 0 | 50 |
| Lo-Carb, 16 fl.oz | 20 | 0 | 5 |
| M-80, 16 fl.oz | 180 | 0 | 46 |
| Mixxd (with Juice), 16 fl.oz | 220 | 0 | 54 |
| **MRM:** Low Carb Protein, 1 scoop | 120 | 2.5 | 2 |
| Iso-bolic, 1 scoop, 1 oz | 115 | 1.5 | 2 |
| Metabolic Whey, 1 scoop, 1 oz | 115 | 2 | 2 |
| **Muscle Milk** (Cytosport): | | | |
| Powders: Regular, 2 scoops, 2.5 oz | 300 | 12 | 16 |
| Light, 2 scoops, 1.75 oz | 195 | 6 | 11 |
| Naturals, 2 scoops, 2.65 oz | 350 | 18 | 12 |
| **Ready To Drink ~** See Page 48 | | | |
| **Muscle Tech:** Meso-Tech Comp. 1 pkt | 275 | 3 | 31 |
| Mass Tech Weight Gain, 5 scoops | 870 | 4 | 168 |
| Nitro Tech Hard Core, RTD, 15 fl.oz | 195 | 1 | 6 |
| **Myoplex** (EAS): | | | |
| Original Shakes, av., 17 fl.oz | 300 | 7 | 19 |
| Carb Control, 11 fl.oz | 150 | 3.5 | 5 |
| Lite, 11 fl.oz | 170 | 2 | 20 |
| Powder: Original Choc. 1 pkt | 300 | 6 | 22 |
| Deluxe Powder, 1 pkt, 3.4 oz | 330 | 3 | 29 |
| Lite, 1 packet, 1.9 oz | 180 | 2 | 24 |
| **Naturade:** | | | |
| Powders: 100% Whey, Choc., 1 oz | 110 | 1 | 11 |
| 100% Soy Natural, ⅓ cup | 110 | 1 | 0 |
| **Nature's Best:** | | | |
| **Isopure:** Original, 20 fl.oz | 260 | 0 | 25 |
| Endurance, 20 fl.oz | 320 | 0 | 60 |
| Zero Carb, 20 fl.oz | 160 | 0 | 0 |
| Carbo Power, 16 fl.oz | 400 | 0 | 100 |
| **No-Fear:** 16 fl.oz | 260 | 0 | 72 |
| Sugar Free, 16 fl.oz | 20 | 0 | 2 |
| **Noni:** Tahitian/Pacific, 2 Tbsp | 10 | 0 | 3 |
| Liquid Hawaiian/Tahiti, 1 Tbsp | 30 | 0 | 8 |
| **NOS:** All flavors | 220 | 0 | 54 |
| Sugar Free, 16 fl.oz can | 15 | 0 | 2 |
| **Nutrament** (Nestle), 12 fl.oz | 360 | 10 | 52 |
| **Nutrilite:** | | | |
| Protein Shakes, 11.5 fl.oz | 170 | 6 | 6 |
| Sports Drinks, Regular, 16 fl.oz | 120 | 0 | 28 |
| Whey Protein Powder, | | | |
| Chocolate, 1.27 oz sachet | 130 | 2 | 5 |
| **Odwalla,** Serious Energy, 8 fl.oz | 160 | 0 | 39 |

## Energy/Protein Drinks (Cont)

| | C | F | Cb |
|---|---|---|---|
| **Optifast 800:** | | | |
| Ready To Drink Shakes, 8 fl.oz | 160 | 3 | 20 |
| Powder 800 Formula, 1 pkg | 160 | 3 | 20 |
| High Protein Powder, 1 pkg | 200 | 6 | 10 |
| **Optimum Nutr.:** 100% Whey, 1 oz | 120 | 1 | 3 |
| 100% Oats & Whey, 1 sc., 1.85 oz | 200 | 1.5 | 22 |
| 100% Soy Protein, 1.1 oz Scoop | 120 | 1.5 | 1 |
| **Piranha Energy**, 8.4 oz | 140 | 0 | 35 |
| **PowerAde ION4:** | | | |
| Average all flavors: 12 fl.oz | 75 | 0 | 23 |
| 20 fl.oz bottle | 125 | 0 | 35 |
| PowerAde Zero | 0 | 0 | 0 |
| **PowerBar:** | | | |
| Endurance, 1 scoop, 0.7 oz | 70 | 0 | 17 |
| Power Gel, average, 1.5 oz package | 110 | 0 | 27 |
| Pro-Cal 100 (R-Kane), 1 packet | 100 | 1.5 | 7 |
| **Propel Enhanced Water,** | | | |
| all flavors, 20 fl.oz | 25 | 0 | 5 |
| **Red Bull Energy:** 8.4 fl.oz | 110 | 0 | 28 |
| 12 fl.oz can | 160 | 0 | 40 |
| Sugar-Free, 8.4 fl.oz | 10 | 0 | 3 |
| Shots: 2 fl.oz | 25 | 0 | 6 |
| Sugar Free, 2 fl.oz | 2 | 0 | 0 |
| **Resource** (Nestle): Breeze, 8 fl.oz | 250 | 0 | 54 |
| Diabetishield, 8 fl.oz | 150 | 0 | 30 |
| Health Shake: 4 fl.oz | 200 | 4 | 35 |
| No Added Sugar, 4 fl.oz | 200 | 9 | 22 |
| Shake Plus, 8 fl.oz | 480 | 16 | 69 |
| Shake, Thickened, 6 fl.oz | 270 | 6 | 45 |
| **Revenge** (Champion Nutrition): | | | |
| Pro-Score 100, Choc., 2 scoops, 1.4 oz | 150 | 2 | 3 |
| Sport, 1 scoop, 0.9 oz | 90 | 0 | 23 |
| **Revival:** Soy Mix, unsweetened: | | | |
| Plain, 2 scoops, 0.8 oz | 90 | 1 | 0.5 |
| Chocolate Day Dream, 1 package | 120 | 2.5 | 7 |
| Av. other varieties, 1 package | 115 | 2 | 4 |
| **Rhino's Energy Drink**, 100ml | 50 | 0 | 11 |
| **Rip It,** Energy Fuel, Citrus X, 16 fl.oz | 260 | 0 | 66 |
| **Rockstar:** Per 16 fl.oz Can | | | |
| Energy Drink: Regular | 280 | 0 | 62 |
| Sugar Free | 20 | 0 | 0 |
| Punched | 260 | 0 | 62 |
| **Rush:** Per 8 fl.oz | | | |
| Energy Drink: Regular | 140 | 0 | 31 |
| Lite | 0 | 0 | 0 |
| **Slim-Fast:** Per 10 fl.oz | | | |
| **Shake** (Ready To Drink): | | | |
| Cappuccino; High Protein, av | 190 | 6 | 25 |
| Lower Carb Diet, average | 180 | 9 | 3.5 |
| **Powder Shake Mix:** Average, 0.9 oz | 110 | 3 | 18 |
| With 8 fl.oz fat-free milk | 200 | 5 | 30 |

| | C | F | Cb |
|---|---|---|---|
| **Snapple,** LYTe Water, | | | |
| average all flavors, 8 fl.oz | 0 | 0 | 0 |
| **SoBe:** Per Can/Bottle | | | |
| Energize, Citrus Energy, 20 fl.oz | 270 | 0 | 67 |
| Lifewater: All flavors, 20 fl.oz | 100 | 0 | 42 |
| O-Cal, all flavors | 0 | 0 | 6 |
| Lizard Fuel, 20 fl.oz | 300 | 0 | 75 |
| Power, 20 fl.oz | 250 | 0 | 63 |
| Tsunami, 20 fl.oz | 250 | 0 | 63 |
| **Vita Boom:** Per 20 fl.oz | | | |
| Cranberry Grapefruit | 260 | 0 | 66 |
| Orange-Carrot | 220 | 0 | 57 |
| **Spiru-Tein,** Powder, av., 1.2 oz | 100 | 0 | 10 |
| **Starbucks,** Doubleshot, | | | |
| Energy & Coffee , 15 fl.oz | 205 | 3 | 37 |
| **Steaz:** Energy, 12 fl.oz | 135 | 0 | 35 |
| Zero Calorie, Berry, 12 fl.oz | 0 | 0 | 0 |
| **The Sports Club/LA:** | | | |
| PTS Protein Powder, | | | |
| Choc; Mocha; Van., 2 scoops, 1.4 oz | 130 | 4 | 7 |
| **Trader Joe's,** | | | |
| Enhanced Water, 33.8 oz | 0 | 0 | 0 |
| **Twin Lab:** | | | |
| Endurance Fuel, 1 sc., 1.1 oz | 110 | 0 | 20 |
| Energy Fuel, 250ml can | 0 | 0 | 0 |
| **Ukon,** Energy, 3.4 fl.oz bottle | 30 | 0 | 7 |
| **Vault:** Citrus; Red Blitz, 20 fl.oz | 290 | 0 | 78 |
| Vault Zero, 8 fl.oz | 0 | 0 | 0 |
| **Venom:** Energy, av., 16.9 fl.oz | 25 | 0 | 60 |
| Low Carb, 16.9 fl.oz | 60 | 0 | 8 |
| **Verve,** Energy, 8.3 fl.oz can | 70 | 0 | 18 |
| Sugar Free | 5 | 0 | 1 |
| **Vitamin Water** ~ See Glaceau | | | |
| **Weider (Powders):** | | | |
| Creatine ATP, ½ cup, 1.7 oz | 210 | 0 | 37 |
| Mega Mass 4000, average,1½ cups | 570 | 3.5 | 105 |
| Muscle Builder, 1½ cup | 170 | 1 | 22 |
| Pure Pro Shake: Chocolate, 11.5 fl.oz | 170 | 0.5 | 7 |
| Vanilla, 11.5 fl.oz | 160 | 0 | 6 |
| Ultra Whey Pro, ⅓ cup, 1 oz | 110 | 1.5 | 6 |
| Weight Gainer, 4 scoops, 3.4 oz | 380 | 2 | 71 |
| **Worldwide:** Carbo Rush, 20 fl.oz | 270 | 0 | 68 |
| **Pure Protein Shakes,** | | | |
| 35g Protein, 11 fl.oz | 165 | 1 | 3 |
| **Worx Energy,** | | | |
| Original; Extra Strength, 2 fl.oz | 0 | 0 | 0 |
| **XS** (Quixtar), Energy Drink, 8.4 oz | 10 | 0 | 1 |
| **Zico,** Coconut Water, all flav., 11 fl.oz | 60 | 0 | 13 |
| **Zola Acai,** Original Juice, 12 fl.oz | 185 | 3 | 39 |

## Quick Guide — C F Cb

### Orange Juice
*Average ~ Fresh*

| | C | F | Cb |
|---|---|---|---|
| ½ Cup, 4 fl.oz | 55 | 0 | 13 |
| Small Glass, 6 fl.oz | 85 | 0 | 19 |
| Regular Glass, 8 fl.oz | 110 | 0.5 | 26 |
| 8¾ fl.oz Box | 120 | 0.5 | 28 |
| 10 fl.oz Bottle | 140 | 0.5 | 32 |
| 11½ fl.oz Can | 160 | 0.5 | 37 |
| 16 fl.oz Bottle | 225 | 1 | 52 |
| 20 fl.oz Bottle | 280 | 1 | 64 |
| 64 fl.oz, ½ Gallon | 895 | 4 | 206 |

### Juices ~ Generic

*Average All Brands:*

| | C | F | Cb |
|---|---|---|---|
| Aloe Vera Juice, unsweetened, 2 oz | 10 | 0 | 0 |
| Apple Juice: 8 fl.oz | 120 | 0 | 29 |
| 10 fl.oz Bottle | 145 | 0.5 | 36 |
| 16 fl.oz | 235 | 0.5 | 58 |
| Carrot Juice: Fresh, 6 fl.oz | 35 | 0 | 8 |
| Sweetened, 6 fl.oz | 75 | 0 | 17 |
| Coconut Water, 8 fl.oz | 50 | 0.5 | 9 |
| Cranberry Juice, Cocktail/Blend | 140 | 0 | 34 |
| Fruit Blends, average, 8 fl.oz | 110 | 0 | 27 |
| Fruit Nectars, average, 8 fl.oz | 140 | 0 | 36 |
| Grape Juice, 8 fl.oz | 155 | 0 | 38 |
| Grapefruit Juice, 8 fl.oz | 95 | 0 | 22 |
| Lemon/Lime Juice: 1 Tbsp | 3 | 0 | 1 |
| 1 cup, 8 fl.oz | 50 | 0.5 | 16 |
| Concentrate, 1 tsp | 0 | 0 | 0 |
| Noni Juice: Tahitian, 2 Tbsp, 1 fl.oz | 5 | 0 | 1 |
| Tahiti Traders, 1 fl.oz | 20 | 0 | 5 |
| Passion Fruit Juice (Fresh): | | | |
| Purple, 1 cup, 8 fl.oz | 125 | 0 | 34 |
| Yellow, 1 cup, 8 fl.oz | 80 | 1.5 | 14 |
| Papaya/Peach Nectar, av., 8 fl.oz | 140 | 0 | 36 |
| Pear Nectar, 8 fl.oz | 150 | 0 | 40 |
| Pineapple Juice, 8 fl.oz | 130 | 0 | 32 |
| Pomegranate Juice, 8 fl.oz | 160 | 0 | 40 |
| Prune Juice, 8 fl.oz | 180 | 0 | 45 |
| Strawb./Raspberry Juice, 8 fl.oz | 100 | 0 | 23 |
| Tangerine Juice, 8 fl.oz | 105 | 0.5 | 25 |
| Tomato Juice, 8 fl.oz | 40 | 0 | 10 |
| Vegetable Juice, 8 fl.oz | 45 | 0 | 11 |
| Wheat Grass Juice: 1 fl.oz 'Shot' | 5 | 0 | 1 |
| 2 fl.oz 'Shot' | 15 | 0 | 2 |

## Quick Guide — C F Cb

### Fruit Smoothies (Jamba Juice; Smoothie King)
*Average All Brands*

| | C | F | Cb |
|---|---|---|---|
| Fruit Only: 8 fl.oz | 115 | 0.5 | 29 |
| 12 fl.oz | 175 | 1 | 43 |
| 16 fl.oz | 230 | 1 | 58 |
| 24 fl.oz | 350 | 1 | 78 |
| Fruit + Non-Fat Milk/Soy: | | | |
| 12 fl.oz | 135 | 0 | 29 |
| 16 fl.oz | 155 | 0 | 37 |
| 24 fl.oz | 265 | 1 | 59 |
| Fruit + Non-Fat Frozen Yogurt/Sherbet: | | | |
| 12 fl.oz | 200 | 0.5 | 47 |
| 16 fl.oz | 265 | 1 | 63 |
| 24 fl.oz | 395 | 1.5 | 95 |

### Juice Brands — C F Cb

*Per 8 fl.oz Unless Indicated*

| | C | F | Cb |
|---|---|---|---|
| **Apple & Eve:** | | | |
| Naturally Cranberry | 130 | 0 | 32 |
| Cranberry Grape | 140 | 0 | 34 |
| Fruitables, average, 6.75 fl.oz | 70 | 0 | 16 |
| **Bolthouse:** | | | |
| 100% Juices: Carrot | 70 | 0 | 14 |
| Clementine | 110 | 0 | 29 |
| **Fruit Smoothies:** *Per 15.2 fl.oz Bottle* | | | |
| Berry Boost | 245 | 2 | 57 |
| Blue Goodness | 325 | 0 | 78 |
| C-Boost | 285 | 0 | 70 |
| Green Goodness | 265 | 0 | 63 |
| Strawberry Banana | 230 | 0 | 55 |
| **Bom Dia:** | | | |
| Acai: Original | 100 | 0 | 26 |
| Coconut Splash | 60 | 0 | 16 |
| Pomegranate | 160 | 0.5 | 39 |
| Superblend | 120 | 0 | 29 |
| **Bossa Nova:** *Per 10 fl.oz Bottle* | | | |
| Acai Juice, Original | 130 | 0 | 33 |
| Acerola/Goji/Mangostein, average | 105 | 0 | 26 |
| **Bright & Early** *(Minute Maid),* | | | |
| Orange Juice (Chilled/Frozen) | 110 | 0 | 29 |
| **Campbell's:** | | | |
| Tomato Juice: 5.5 fl.oz can | 30 | 0 | 7 |
| 8 fl.oz | 50 | 0 | 10 |
| **Capri Sun:** *Per 6.75 fl.oz* | | | |
| Juice Drinks (25% Less Sugar): | | | |
| Average all flavors | 70 | 0 | 19 |
| 100% Juice, average, 6.75 fl.oz | 100 | 0 | 24 |

## Juice Brands (Cont)   C   F   Cb

*Per 8 fl.oz Unless Indicated*

| | C | F | Cb |
|---|---|---|---|
| **Chiquita Smoothies:** | | | |
| Average all flavors: | | | |
| 4 oz concentrate (8 oz reconst'd) | 120 | 0 | 28 |
| 12 oz Can (concentrate) | 360 | 0 | 84 |
| **Clamato,** | | | |
| Tomato Cocktail, average | 50 | 0 | 11 |
| **Crystal Geyser:** | | | |
| *Juice Squeeze: Per Bottle (12 fl.oz)* | | | |
| Blackberry Pomegranate | 170 | 0 | 43 |
| Ruby Grapefruit | 150 | 0 | 36 |
| Average other flavors | 140 | 0 | 32 |
| **Dannon:** | | | |
| Frusion Smoothie, av., 7 fl.oz | 180 | 2.5 | 35 |
| Light & Fit, 7 fl.oz bottle | 70 | 0 | 14 |
| **Dole:** | | | |
| **Chilled, 100%:** | | | |
| Orange Peach Mango | 120 | 0 | 29 |
| Pina Colada | 120 | 0 | 29 |
| Pineapple Juice | 130 | 0 | 30 |
| Pineapple-Orange Banana | 120 | 0 | 30 |
| Strawberry Kiwi | 120 | 0 | 31 |
| Average other flavors | 120 | 0 | 29 |
| **Frozen Concentrates 100%,** | | | |
| average all flavors, ¼ cup | 125 | 0 | 31 |
| **Five Alive** *(Minute Maid)*, | | | |
| Frozen Concentrate, | | | |
| prepared, 8 fl.oz | 110 | 0 | 29 |
| **Florida's Natural:** | | | |
| Apple Juice | 120 | 0 | 29 |
| Cranberry Ruby Red | 130 | 0 | 32 |
| Orange, Original | 110 | 0 | 26 |
| Orange Mango | 110 | 0 | 27 |
| Orange Pineapple | 130 | 0 | 31 |
| Orange Strawberry | 110 | 0 | 26 |
| Raspberry Lemonade | 110 | 0 | 28 |
| Ruby Red Grapefruit, Original | 90 | 0 | 22 |
| **Fuze:** *Per 16.9 fl.oz* | | | |
| Original, all flavors | 160 | 0 | 38 |
| Slenderize, all flavors | 230 | 0 | 52 |

*Per 8 fl.oz Unless Indicated*

| | C | F | Cb |
|---|---|---|---|
| **Goya:** | | | |
| **100% Natural,** | | | |
| av. all flavors, 16 fl.oz | 200 | 0 | 50 |
| **5% Juice:** *Per 12 fl.oz* | | | |
| Guanabana | 230 | 0 | 57 |
| Passion & Pineapple | 220 | 0 | 55 |
| **Mango Nectar,** 12 fl.oz | 230 | 0 | 56 |
| **Hansen's:** | | | |
| **Juice Slam:** *Per 6.75 fl.oz Box* | | | |
| Awesome Apple | 90 | 0 | 23 |
| Strawberry Banana | 110 | 0 | 27 |
| Other flavors | 100 | 0 | 24 |
| **Junior Juice,** | | | |
| **100% Juice,** all flav., 4.23 oz box | 60 | 0 | 15 |
| **Natural,** (64 fl.oz Bottles): *Per 8 fl.oz* | | | |
| Apple | 120 | 0 | 28 |
| Apple Strawberry | 110 | 0 | 27 |
| Grape | 120 | 0 | 33 |
| Ruby Red Grapefruit Cocktail | 100 | 0 | 25 |
| White Grape | 140 | 0 | 36 |
| **Smoothie Nectar,** av., 12 fl.oz | 180 | 0 | 44 |
| **Hawaii's Own:** *Per 8 fl.oz Prepared* | | | |
| Frozen Concentrate, | | | |
| 10% Juice, average all varieties | 110 | 0 | 28 |
| **Hi-C Juice Drinks:** | | | |
| 6.75 fl.oz box, average | 90 | 0 | 26 |
| Blast, 6.75 fl.oz pouch | 100 | 0 | 26 |
| **Hood:** Apple, 8 fl.oz | 120 | 0 | 31 |
| Fruit Punch; Orange | 120 | 0 | 30 |
| **Jamba Juice** ~ *See Fast-Foods Section* | | | |
| **Juicy Juice** *(Nestle): Per 6.75 fl.oz Box* | | | |
| Average all flavors | 100 | 0 | 24 |
| 4.23 fl.oz box, average | 60 | 0 | 15 |
| **Kerns:** | | | |
| **Nectars:** *Per 11.5 fl.oz Can* | | | |
| Pear | 220 | 0 | 54 |
| Pineapple Coconut | 280 | 8 | 53 |
| Average other flavors | 215 | 0 | 52 |
| **Kool Aid:** | | | |
| Bursts, 6.75 fl.oz, av. | 35 | 0 | 9 |
| Jammers, 6.75 fl.oz, av. | 90 | 0 | 24 |
| Jammers 10 | 10 | 0 | 2 |
| **Kroger/Ralph's Smoothies:** | | | |
| Active Lifestyle *(Ralph's)*, average | 130 | 0 | 25 |
| Regular, average all flavors | 200 | 2.5 | 38 |
| **L & A:** *Per 8 fl.oz* | | | |
| All Cherry | 180 | 0 | 45 |
| All Prune Juice | 180 | 0 | 41 |
| Mixed Berry | 120 | 0 | 30 |

| Juice Brands (Cont) | C | F | Cb |
|---|---|---|---|

*Per 8 fl.oz Unless Indicated*
**Lakewood Organic:** *Per 8 fl.oz*

| | C | F | Cb |
|---|---|---|---|
| Acai Amazon Berry | 125 | 3.5 | 28 |
| Banana Strawberry | 115 | 0 | 30 |
| Blueberry Blend | 110 | 0 | 27 |
| Cranberry Lemonade | 75 | 0 | 20 |
| Fruit Garden: Summer Gold, av. | 100 | 0 | 20 |
| Blue/Purple/Red Pomegr., average | 110 | 0 | 24 |
| Goji | 90 | 0 | 20 |
| Lemonade | 80 | 0 | 20 |
| Pomegranate Blend | 125 | 0 | 31 |
| Pure: Apple | 110 | 0 | 27 |
| Blueberry | 90 | 0 | 22 |
| Carrot | 80 | 0 | 19 |
| Pink Grapefruit | 90 | 0 | 22 |
| Prune | 170 | 0 | 42 |
| Super Veggie | 55 | 0 | 13 |
| **Light:** Lemonade | 40 | 0 | 10 |
| Average other flavors | 60 | 0 | 21 |

(Note: Carbs include Erythritol natural sweetener)

**Langers:** *Per 8 fl.oz*
**100% Juice** *(No Sugar Added):*

| | | | |
|---|---|---|---|
| All Pomegranate | 140 | 0 | 34 |
| Apple Cider | 120 | 0 | 28 |
| Apple Juice | 120 | 0 | 28 |
| Mixed Berry | 120 | 0 | 30 |
| Pineapple Coconut | 140 | 3 | 28 |
| Red/White Grape Juice | 160 | 0 | 40 |
| **Diet Low-Carb** *(25-50% Juice):* | | | |
| Apple Juice Cocktail | 60 | 0 | 14 |
| Cranberry | 30 | 0 | 8 |
| Pomegranate | 40 | 0 | 9 |
| **Juice Cocktails** *(27% Juice):* | | | |
| Blueberry Cranberry | 135 | 0 | 34 |
| Cranberry Berry | 135 | 0 | 34 |
| Cranberry Grape | 165 | 0 | 41 |
| Cranberry Raspberry | 150 | 0 | 36 |
| Pomegranate | 140 | 0 | 34 |
| Pomegranate Blueb./Cranberry | 140 | 0 | 34 |
| Strawberry Peach (20% Juice) | 120 | 0 | 30 |
| White Cranberry | 120 | 0 | 28 |
| White Cran-Raspberry | 120 | 0 | 28 |
| **Martinellli's,** Sparkling Apple Juice, | | | |
| 10 fl.oz bottle | 180 | 0 | 43 |

*Per 8 fl.oz Unless Indicated*
**Minute Maid:**

| | C | F | Cb |
|---|---|---|---|
| Apple Juice, 15.2 fl.oz bottle | 210 | 0 | 52 |
| Cranb. Apple, Rasp.,15.2 fl oz bottle | 230 | 0 | 63 |
| Orange Juice: | | | |
| 100% Original: 8 fl.oz | 110 | 0 | 27 |
| 15.2 fl.oz bottle | 210 | 0 | 51 |
| Light, 42%, 8 fl.oz | 50 | 0 | 12 |
| Fruit Punch, 6.75 fl.oz | 100 | 0 | 24 |
| Pineapple Orange, Apple | 120 | 0 | 29 |
| Kids+Orange Juice, 6.75 fl.oz | 100 | 0 | 23 |
| **Enhanced:** *Per 8 fl.oz* | | | |
| Pomegranate Blueberry | 120 | 0.5 | 31 |
| Pomegranate Lemonade | 110 | 0 | 31 |
| **Boxed Juices,** av., 6.75 fl.oz | 100 | 0 | 22 |
| **Soft Frozen,** Limeade, 3 fl.oz | 70 | 0 | 19 |
| **MonaVie:** | | | |
| **Acai Blends,** | | | |
| Original; Active, 4 fl.oz | 120 | 2 | 20 |
| **Mott's:** | | | |
| **100% Original Juice:** Apple | 120 | 0 | 29 |
| All other varieties, 6.75 fl.oz | 100 | 0 | 25 |
| **Garden Blend** | 45 | 0 | 9 |
| **Natural Juice,** Apple | 110 | 0 | 27 |
| **Medley Juice:** Apple & Carrot | 110 | 0 | 25 |
| Average other varieties | 140 | 0 | 33 |
| **Mott's For Tots:** *Per 47-54% Juice* | | | |
| All varieties: 6.75 fl.oz | 50 | 0 | 13 |
| 8 fl.oz | 60 | 0 | 15 |
| **Mott's Plus For Kids:** | | | |
| 100%: Apple | 130 | 0 | 32 |
| Apple Punch | 120 | 0 | 30 |
| **Plus Light,** Apple | 60 | 0 | 15 |
| **Naked Juice:** | | | |
| **Antioxidants:** | | | |
| Pomegranate Acai | 160 | 1 | 36 |
| Pomegranate Blueberry | 150 | 0 | 36 |
| **Probiotics,** Tropical Mango, 10 fl.oz | 180 | 0 | 43 |
| **Protein Zone:** Mango | 220 | 1 | 35 |
| Pineapple, Coconut & Banana | 220 | 2 | 34 |
| **Pure Juice (100%):** O-J | 110 | 0 | 27 |
| Coconut Water, 11 fl.oz | 60 | 0 | 14 |
| **Well Being:** Berry Blast | 130 | 0 | 29 |
| Mighty Mango | 150 | 0 | 36 |
| Orange Carrot | 120 | 0 | 29 |
| Orange Mango | 130 | 0 | 31 |
| Strawberry Banana | 130 | 0 | 31 |

## Juice Brands (Cont)  C  F  Cb

*Per 8 fl.oz Unless Indicated*

**Naked Juice (Cont):**

**Superfood Smoothies:** *Per 15.2 fl.oz*

| | C | F | Cb |
|---|---|---|---|
| Acai Machine | 305 | 5 | 58 |
| Berry Veggie | 245 | 1 | 70 |
| Blue Machine | 320 | 0 | 76 |
| Gold/Green Machine, av. | 265 | 0 | 63 |
| Power C Machine | 230 | 0 | 55 |
| Red Machine | 320 | 8 | 58 |

**Nantucket Nectars:**

**Juice Cocktails:** *Per 17.5 fl.oz Bottle*

| | C | F | Cb |
|---|---|---|---|
| Big Cranberry | 285 | 0 | 70 |
| Carrot Orange Mango | 260 | 0 | 60 |
| Grapeade | 305 | 0 | 72 |
| Average other varieties | 260 | 0 | 65 |

**100% Juice:** *Per 17.5 fl.oz Bottle*

| | C | F | Cb |
|---|---|---|---|
| Peach Orange | 285 | 0 | 70 |
| Pineapple Orange Banana | 305 | 0 | 74 |
| Pomegranate Cherry | 265 | 0 | 63 |
| Premium Orange Juice | 240 | 0 | 57 |
| Pressed Apple | 260 | 0 | 65 |
| **Nectar,** Squeezed Lemonade | 240 | 0 | 61 |

**Newman's Own:**

| | C | F | Cb |
|---|---|---|---|
| Lemonade: Regular; Pink, 8 fl.oz | 110 | 0 | 27 |
| Limeade, 8 fl.oz | 140 | 0 | 34 |
| **Fruit Juice Cocktail:** Gorilla Grape | 140 | 0 | 34 |
| Orange Mango Tango | 130 | 0 | 33 |

**Northland:**

**100% Juice:**

| | C | F | Cb |
|---|---|---|---|
| Cranberry; Blackberry; Raspberry | 140 | 0 | 34 |
| Cranberry Grape | 140 | 0 | 36 |

**Ocean Spray:**

**Juice Cocktails:**

| | C | F | Cb |
|---|---|---|---|
| Cranberry Juice Cocktail | 120 | 0 | 30 |
| With Calcium | 130 | 0 | 31 |
| Ruby Tangerine | 120 | 0 | 31 |
| Ruby Red Grapefruit | 110 | 0 | 28 |

**100% Juice Blends:**

| | C | F | Cb |
|---|---|---|---|
| Cranberry & Concord Grape | 150 | 0 | 37 |
| Cranberry Blueberry | 140 | 0 | 36 |
| Cranberry Blends | 140 | 0 | 35 |

**Juice Drinks:**

| | C | F | Cb |
|---|---|---|---|
| CranApple | 130 | 0 | 32 |
| CranGrape | 120 | 0 | 31 |
| CranRaspberry/Strawberry | 110 | 0 | 27 |
| **Light Juice Drinks,** all flav. | 40 | 0 | 10 |

**Diet Juice Drinks:**

| | C | F | Cb |
|---|---|---|---|
| Cranberry Spray | 5 | 0 | 2 |
| Cranberry Grape Spray | 5 | 0 | 2 |

*Per 8 fl.oz Unless Indicated*

**Odwalla:** *Per 12 fl.oz Bottle*  C  F  Cb

| | C | F | Cb |
|---|---|---|---|
| Blueberry B | 210 | 0.5 | 50 |
| Carrot Juice | 100 | 0.5 | 22 |
| Mo'Beta | 170 | 0 | 40 |
| Pink Poetry | 210 | 0 | 48 |
| PomaGrand, Pomeg. Limeade | 180 | 0 | 44 |
| Protein Monster, Chocolate | 320 | 6 | 40 |
| Strawberry C Monster | 240 | 0 | 56 |
| Super Food, Original | 190 | 0.5 | 40 |
| Super Protein, Original | 290 | 1 | 52 |
| Tropical Energy | 240 | 0 | 59 |

**Orange Julius:**

**Originals,** Orange:

| | C | F | Cb |
|---|---|---|---|
| Small, 16 fl.oz | 230 | 0.5 | 62 |
| Medium, 20 fl.oz | 290 | 0 | 77 |
| Large, 32 fl.oz | 470 | 0 | 123 |

**Smoothies ~** *See Fast-Foods Section*

**Pom Wonderful:**

**100% Juice:**

| | C | F | Cb |
|---|---|---|---|
| Pomegranate: Blueberry | 160 | 0 | 39 |
| Cherry | 150 | 0 | 38 |
| Kiwi | 150 | 0 | 36 |
| Mango | 140 | 0 | 36 |
| Nectarine | 130 | 0 | 31 |

**R.W. Knudsen:**

| | C | F | Cb |
|---|---|---|---|
| **Natural Juices:** 100% Apple | 120 | 0 | 30 |
| Cranberry Raspberry | 130 | 0 | 32 |
| Grape | 150 | 0 | 37 |
| Hibiscus Cooler | 100 | 0 | 25 |
| Kiwi Strawberry | 120 | 0 | 29 |
| Mango Peach | 120 | 0 | 31 |
| Razzleberry | 120 | 0 | 30 |
| Rio Red Grapefruit | 140 | 0 | 35 |
| Other varieties, average | 120 | 0 | 30 |
| **Just Juice:** Just Black Currant | 100 | 0 | 15 |
| Just Black Cherry | 160 | 0 | 37 |
| Just Blueberry | 100 | 0 | 24 |
| **Simply Nutritious:** Mega C | 140 | 0 | 34 |
| Average other varieties | 125 | 0 | 30 |
| **Sparkling Essence,** average all varieties, 10.5 fl.oz | 0 | 0 | 0 |

**Spritzers, 100% Juice:** *Per 12 fl.oz Bottles*

| | C | F | Cb |
|---|---|---|---|
| Black Cherry | 180 | 0 | 46 |
| Mango | 170 | 0 | 42 |
| Red Raspberry; Tangerine | 200 | 0 | 47 |
| **Very Veggie,** Orig, 8 fl.oz | 50 | 0 | 11 |

### Juice Brands (Cont) | C | F | Cb

*Per 8 fl.oz Unless Indicated*

**ReaLemon – ReaLime:**
Lemon/Lime Juice (from concentrate)

| | C | F | Cb |
|---|---|---|---|
| 1 teaspoon | 0 | 0 | 0 |
| 2 Tbsp, 1 fl.oz | 8 | 0 | 2.5 |

**Santa Cruz:**
**100% Juice:**

| | | | |
|---|---|---|---|
| Apple Juice | 120 | 0 | 30 |
| Concord Grape; White Grape | 160 | 0 | 40 |
| Orange Mango | 130 | 0 | 32 |
| Strawberry Kiwi | 120 | 0 | 30 |

**25% Juice Drink Boxes:**

| | | | |
|---|---|---|---|
| Lemon | 120 | 0 | 29 |
| Orange; Grape, average | 100 | 0 | 24 |
| Tropical | 110 | 0 | 27 |

**Champagne Style:**

| | | | |
|---|---|---|---|
| Sparkling Lemonade | 110 | 0 | 27 |
| Sparkling Limeade | 100 | 0 | 26 |
| **Nectars:** Cranberry | 110 | 0 | 27 |
| Passionfruit | 150 | 0 | 40 |
| Average other varieties | 120 | 0 | 30 |

**Sparkling Beverages:** *Per 10.5 fl.oz Can*

| | | | |
|---|---|---|---|
| Lemon Lime | 130 | 0 | 32 |
| Root Beer | 130 | 0 | 32 |

**Seismic:**
**Super Juices:** *Per 10 fl.oz Bottle*

| | | | |
|---|---|---|---|
| Citrus; Berry | 180 | 0 | 44 |
| Low Sugar Cherry | 100 | 0 | 26 |

**Simply Orange:**

| | | | |
|---|---|---|---|
| Lemonade; Limeade | 120 | 0 | 30 |
| Orange Juice, av., all varieties | 110 | 0 | 26 |

**Snap·E· Tom,**

| | | | |
|---|---|---|---|
| Tomato & Chili Cocktail, 8 fl.oz | 50 | 0 | 11 |

**Snapple:**
**Juice Drink Blends:**

| | | | |
|---|---|---|---|
| Grapeade; Orangeade | 100 | 0 | 26 |
| Average other flavors | 110 | 0 | 27 |
| **Diet:** Cranberry Raspberry | 10 | 0 | 2 |
| 100% Juiced, (added vitamins), 11.5 fl.oz | 170 | 0 | 40 |

**Ssips,** Juice Drinks,

| | | | |
|---|---|---|---|
| average, 6.75 fl.oz box | 105 | 0 | 26 |

**Stonyfield Farm:** *Per 10 fl.oz Bottle*

| | | | |
|---|---|---|---|
| Peach Smoothie | 230 | 3 | 41 |
| Berry; Strawberry Smoothie | 230 | 3 | 39 |

*Per 8 fl.oz Unless Indicated*

**SunnyD:** | C | F | Cb

**Baja Juice:** *Per 12 fl.oz Bottle*

| | | | |
|---|---|---|---|
| Orange | 190 | 0 | 46 |
| Orange Berry | 190 | 0 | 46 |
| Orange Pineapple | 190 | 0 | 46 |
| Red Punch | 170 | 0 | 43 |

**SunnyD Blends,**

| | | | |
|---|---|---|---|
| Orange Fused, all flavors, 8 fl.oz | 80 | 0 | 20 |

**SunnyD Original:**

| | | | |
|---|---|---|---|
| Smooth/Tangy Style | 90 | 0 | 22 |
| Fruit Punch | 80 | 0 | 21 |
| Mango | 90 | 0 | 22 |
| Reduced Sugar | 60 | 0 | 15 |

**SunnyD Smoothies,**

| | | | |
|---|---|---|---|
| Orange Whirl; Strawberry Swirl | 140 | 0 | 34 |

**Sunsweet,**

| | | | |
|---|---|---|---|
| Prune Juice/with Pulp | 180 | 0 | 43 |
| **Tampico:** Citrus Punch | 110 | 0 | 25 |
| Mango/Tropical Fruit Punch | 110 | 0 | 28 |

**Tang:**
**Pouches,** average all flavors (1)

| | | | |
|---|---|---|---|
| | 90 | 0 | 24 |

**Mix:** *Prepared as Directed*

| | | | |
|---|---|---|---|
| Regular (2 Tbsp dry), 6 fl.oz | 110 | 0 | 27 |
| Sugar Free, 8 fl.oz | 5 | 0 | 0 |

**Trader Joe's:**
**Refrigerated:** *Per 15.2 fl.oz Bottle Unless Indicated:*

| | | | |
|---|---|---|---|
| Carrot Juice, 16 fl.oz | 160 | 2 | 32 |
| Coconut Water, 14.7 fl.oz | 110 | 0 | 26 |
| Mango Smoothie | 140 | 0 | 34 |
| Organic Acai, 10.5 fl.oz | 190 | 3.5 | 39 |
| Protein with Pzazz | 420 | 4 | 65 |
| Strawberry Smoothie | 230 | 0 | 55 |
| Watermelon Juice | 150 | 0 | 38 |

**Organic,** 32/64 fl.oz Bottle: *Per 8 fl.oz*

| | | | |
|---|---|---|---|
| 100% Pomegranate | 140 | 0 | 35 |
| Apple Juice | 120 | 0 | 30 |
| Concord Grape Juice | 160 | 0 | 39 |
| Cranberry | 70 | 0 | 18 |
| Grapefruit Sunset; Lemonade | 120 | 0 | 30 |
| Mango Nectar | 130 | 0 | 32 |
| Pink Lemonade | 130 | 0 | 32 |
| Strawberry Lemonade | 120 | 0 | 29 |
| White Grape Juice | 160 | 0 | 40 |

**All Natural Pasteurized,** 32/64 fl.oz Bottle: *Per 8 fl.oz*

| | | | |
|---|---|---|---|
| 100% Cranberry | 70 | 0 | 18 |
| Blueberry Pomegranate | 140 | 0 | 34 |
| Just Blueberry | 100 | 0 | 24 |
| Just Pomegranate | 150 | 0 | 37 |
| Mango PassionFruit | 130 | 0 | 32 |
| Omega Orange Carrot | 110 | 0 | 26 |

| **Juice Brands (Cont)** | **C** | **F** | **Cb** |
|---|---|---|---|

*Per 8 fl.oz Unless Indicated*
**Trader Joe's (Cont):**
**Joe's Kids:** *Per 6.75 oz Box*

| | C | F | Cb |
|---|---|---|---|
| 100% Juice: Apple | 90 | 0 | 23 |
| Apple Grape | 100 | 0 | 24 |
| White Grape | 120 | 0 | 30 |
| 10% Juice, Lemonade | 90 | 0 | 22 |

**Sparkling Juices:** *Per 8 fl.oz*

| | C | F | Cb |
|---|---|---|---|
| Blueberry | 120 | 0 | 30 |
| Cranberry | 140 | 0 | 35 |
| Pomegranate | 130 | 0 | 31 |

**Tree Top:**
**100% Juice From Concentrates:**

| | C | F | Cb |
|---|---|---|---|
| Apple Berry/Grape | 120 | 0 | 31 |
| Apple Pear, 6.75 fl.oz | 100 | 0 | 25 |
| Apple/Spiced Cider | 120 | 0 | 29 |
| Kiwi Strawberry, 10 fl.oz | 130 | 0 | 32 |
| Mango Peach, 10 fl.oz | 160 | 0 | 39 |
| Ochango, 10 fl.oz | 170 | 0 | 42 |
| Orange, 6.75 fl.oz | 110 | 0 | 27 |
| Orange Passionfruit | 110 | 0 | 26 |
| Pineapple Orange | 120 | 0 | 29 |

**100% Juice Fresh Pressed,**

| | C | F | Cb |
|---|---|---|---|
| 3 Apple Blend | 120 | 0 | 30 |
| **Fiber Rich:** Apple | 140 | 0 | 35 |
| Apple Apricot | 160 | 0 | 37 |
| **Trim,** average all flavors | 60 | 0 | 16 |

**Tropicana:**

| | C | F | Cb |
|---|---|---|---|
| **Chilled:** Pure Prem. Orange Juice | 110 | 0 | 26 |
| Light Drinks, all flavors | 10 | 0 | 2 |
| Punches, average all flavors | 125 | 0 | 31 |
| **Non-Refrigerated**: 100% Juice, | | | |
| average all varieties | 115 | 0 | 22 |
| Trop50 (50% less sugar,) av all flav. | 50 | 0 | 12 |
| Tropics, average all flavors | 120 | 0 | 30 |
| Twisters, average, 8 fl.oz | 120 | 0 | 29 |

**V8® Juices & Drinks:**
V8 100% Vegetable Juice:

| | C | F | Cb |
|---|---|---|---|
| 5.5 fl.oz can | 35 | 0 | 7 |
| 8 fl.oz cup | 50 | 0 | 10 |
| 11.5 fl.oz can | 70 | 0 | 14 |
| 12 fl.oz bottle | 75 | 0 | 15 |
| V8 Spicy Hot, 12 fl.oz | 70 | 0 | 14 |
| V8 Splash, average, 8 fl.oz | 70 | 0 | 19 |
| V8 Splash Smoothies: Strawberry | 90 | 0 | 20 |
| Tropical Colada, 8 fl.oz | 100 | 0 | 21 |
| Diet V8 Splash, all flavors, 8 fl.oz | 10 | 0 | 3 |

*Per 8 fl.oz Unless Indicated*
**V8® Juices & Drinks (Cont):**

| | C | F | Cb |
|---|---|---|---|
| **V-Fusion:** Grape Raspberry, 8 fl.oz | 140 | 0 | 35 |
| Average other flavors, 8 fl.oz can | 110 | 0 | 27 |
| 12 fl.oz bottle | 165 | 0 | 40 |
| Light varieties; Green Tea, 8 fl.oz | 50 | 0 | 13 |
| Smoothies, av. all flavors, 8 fl.oz | 125 | 0 | 31 |

**Veryfine:**

| | C | F | Cb |
|---|---|---|---|
| Apple Juice (100%) | 120 | 0 | 29 |
| Orange Juice (100%) | 120 | 0 | 30 |

**Walnut Acres:**
**Organic:**

| | C | F | Cb |
|---|---|---|---|
| **Organic:** Apple | 110 | 0 | 29 |
| Apricot; Raspberry | 130 | 0 | 32 |
| Cherry | 140 | 0 | 34 |
| Cranberry | 110 | 0 | 26 |
| Incredible Vegetable | 50 | 0 | 12 |
| Mango Nectar | 120 | 0 | 29 |

**Welch's:**

| | C | F | Cb |
|---|---|---|---|
| 100% Juice: Red Grape | 170 | 0 | 43 |
| White Grape Cherry | 140 | 0 | 35 |
| White Grape Peach | 160 | 0 | 39 |

**Cocktails** *(Refrigerated, 64 fl.oz Ctn):*

| | C | F | Cb |
|---|---|---|---|
| Guava Pineapple | 140 | 0 | 35 |
| Mango Twist | 150 | 0 | 38 |
| Strawberry Breeze | 130 | 0 | 33 |
| **Light Juice** *(52 fl.oz Bottle),* | | | |
| Grape | 45 | 0 | 12 |
| **Sparkling Juice Cocktail** | 160 | 0 | 40 |
| **Concentrates** *(100% Juice),* | | | |
| All flavors, ¼ cup, 2 fl.oz | 160 | 0 | 41 |

**Zola:** *Per 12 fl.oz Bottle*

| | C | F | Cb |
|---|---|---|---|
| Acai: Original | 185 | 2 | 44 |
| With Blueberry Juice | 120 | 2 | 25 |

**CALORIEKING PORTION WATCH**

| **ORANGE JUICE** | **C** | **Cb** |
|---|---|---|
| 8 fl.oz | 110 | 26 |
| 16 fl.oz | 220 | 52 |
| 24 fl.oz | 330 | 78 |
| 32 fl.oz | 440 | 104 |

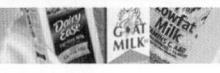

## Quick Guide

| | **C** | **F** | **Cb** |
|---|---|---|---|
| **Cow's Milk** ~ *Average All Brands* | | | |
| **Whole (3.25% fat):** | | | |
| 2 Tbsp, 1 fl.oz | 20 | 1 | 1.5 |
| 1 Cup, 8 fl.oz | 150 | 8 | 12 |
| 1 Large Glass, 12 fl.oz | 220 | 12 | 17 |
| 1 Pint, 16 fl.oz | 295 | 16 | 22 |
| 1 Quart, 946 ml | 590 | 32 | 44 |
| **Reduced-Fat (2% fat):** | | | |
| 2 Tbsp, 1 fl.oz | 15 | 0.5 | 1.5 |
| 1 Cup, 8 fl.oz | 120 | 5 | 12 |
| 1 Large Glass, 12 fl.oz | 180 | 7.5 | 18 |
| 1 Pint, 16 fl.oz | 245 | 10 | 23 |
| 1 Quart, 946 ml | 490 | 20 | 46 |
| **Light/Low-Fat (1% fat):** | | | |
| 2 Tbsp, 1 fl.oz | 13 | 0.3 | 1.5 |
| 1 Cup, 8 fl.oz | 100 | 2.5 | 12 |
| 1 Large Glass, 12 fl.oz | 150 | 4 | 18 |
| 1 Pint, 16 fl.oz | 205 | 5 | 25 |
| 1 Quart, 946 ml | 410 | 10 | 49 |
| **Fat Free/Skim:** | | | |
| 2 Tbsp, 1 fl.oz | 10 | 0 | 1.5 |
| 1 Cup, 8 fl.oz | 90 | 0.5 | 13 |
| 1 Pint, 16 fl.oz | 180 | 1 | 26 |
| Protein Fortified 1 cup | 100 | 0.5 | 14 |
| **Buttermilk:** *Average All Brands* | | | |
| Reduced-Fat (2%), 1 cup, 8 fl.oz | 120 | 5 | 10 |
| Low-Fat (1%), 1 cup, 8 fl.oz | 100 | 2.5 | 12 |
| **Lactose-Free:** *Per 8 fl.oz* | | | |
| *Dairy Ease:* Whole | 160 | 9 | 11 |
| 2% Reduced-Fat | 130 | 5 | 12 |
| Fat-Free | 90 | 0 | 12 |
| *Lactaid 100:* Whole | 150 | 8 | 12 |
| 2% Reduced-Fat | 130 | 5 | 12 |
| 1% Low-Fat | 110 | 2.5 | 13 |
| Fat-Free; Calcium Fort. | 80 | 0 | 13 |
| *Real Goodness:* 2% Fat | 120 | 5 | 7 |
| Fat Free 0% | 80 | 0 | 7 |
| *Smart Balance,* FF + Omega-3s & Vit. E | 110 | 1 | 14 |
| **Lower Calorie Dairy Drinks:** *Per 8 fl.oz Cup* | | | |
| *Calorie Countdown (Hood):* | | | |
| 2% Reduced-Fat | 90 | 5 | 3 |
| 2% Reduced-Fat, Chocolate | 90 | 5 | 5 |
| Fat-Free | 45 | 0 | 3 |

## Goat/Sheep Milk, Kefir

| | **C** | **F** | **Cb** |
|---|---|---|---|
| **Goat's Milk (Meyenberg):** | | | |
| Whole, 1 cup, 8 fl.oz | 140 | 7 | 11 |
| Light/Low-Fat (1%), 8 fl.oz | 100 | 2.5 | 11 |
| Evaporated, reconst., 8 fl.oz | 150 | 8 | 11 |
| **Kefir (Cultured Milk):** Per 8 fl.oz | | | |
| *Lifeway:* Original | 150 | 8 | 12 |
| Greek Style | 210 | 14 | 12 |
| Green | 170 | 2 | 25 |
| Lowfat, average all flavors | 140 | 1.5 | 20 |
| *Nancy's:* Plain | 110 | 3 | 14 |
| Fruit flavors, average | 180 | 2.5 | 34 |
| *Trader Joe's:* Plain | 110 | 2.5 | 8 |
| Strawberry | 160 | 2 | 21 |
| **Sheep's Milk,** Whole, 1 cup | 265 | 17 | 13 |

## Canned & Dried Milk

| | **C** | **F** | **Cb** |
|---|---|---|---|
| **Condensed:** Reg. 2 Tbsp, 1 fl.oz | 130 | 3 | 23 |
| Low-Fat (*Eagle*), 2 Tbsp | 120 | 1.5 | 23 |
| Fat-Free (*Eagle*), 2 Tbsp | 110 | 0 | 24 |
| **Evaporated:** Whole, 2 Tbsp | 40 | 3 | 3 |
| Whole, ½ cup, 4 fl.oz | 170 | 10 | 13 |
| Low-Fat (*Carnation*): 2 Tbsp, 1 oz | 25 | 0.5 | 3 |
| ½ cup, 4 fl.oz | 115 | 2.5 | 14 |
| Fat-Free, 2 Tbsp, 1 oz | 25 | 0 | 4 |
| **Dried:** Whole, ¼ cup, 1 oz | 160 | 9 | 12 |
| Skim/Non-Fat, ⅓ cup | 80 | 0 | 12 |
| Made-up, 1 cup, 8 fl.oz | 80 | 0 | 12 |
| Buttermilk (sweet cream): 1 oz | 110 | 2 | 14 |
| Non-Fat, 1 Tbsp | 25 | 0 | 3 |
| Malted (*Carnation*), dry, 1 Tbsp | 30 | 0.5 | 6 |

## Soy/Non-Dairy Drinks ~ *See Page 49*

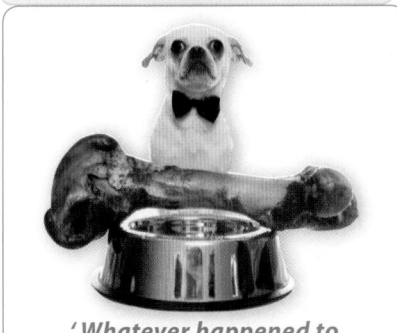

*'Whatever happened to sensible portion size?!'*

### Quick Guide | C | F | Cb

**Chocolate Milk:**
Average All Brands: Per 8 fl.oz Cup

| | C | F | Cb |
|---|---|---|---|
| **Whole Milk** (3.3%): 1 cup | 210 | 8 | 26 |
| 1 Pint, 16 fl.oz | 415 | 17 | 52 |
| **Reduced-Fat** (2%): 1 cup | 190 | 5 | 30 |
| 1 Pint, 16 fl.oz | 380 | 10 | 60 |
| **Low-Fat** (1%): 1 cup | 160 | 2.5 | 26 |
| 1 Pint, 16 fl.oz | 315 | 5 | 52 |

### Brands ~ Flavored Milk

Ready-To-Drink: Per 8 fl.oz Cup Unless Indicated

| | C | F | Cb |
|---|---|---|---|
| **Albertson's,** Choc Milk | 200 | 2.5 | 34 |
| **Alta Dena:** Chocolate: 8 fl.oz | 260 | 9 | 37 |
| 16 fl.oz | 520 | 18 | 74 |
| Low-Fat Chocolate: 8 fl.oz | 200 | 3 | 32 |
| 16 fl.oz | 400 | 6 | 64 |
| **Chug:** Per 12 fl.oz Bottle | | | |
| Chocolate; Cookies 'n' Cream | 420 | 12 | 68 |
| Vanilla | 440 | 11 | 75 |
| **Hood:** Chocolate | 230 | 9 | 31 |
| Low-Fat (1%), Chocolate | 170 | 3 | 28 |
| **Horizon Organic:** Low-Fat Choc. | 150 | 2.5 | 22 |
| Low-Fat Vanilla | 150 | 2.5 | 22 |
| **Kroger,** Choc Milk, Low-Fat, 1% | 180 | 2.5 | 33 |
| **Land O Lakes:** | | | |
| **Grip 'n Go:** Choc. (2% red-fat), 12 fl.oz | 285 | 8 | 39 |
| Strawberry (whole milk), 12 fl.oz | 285 | 12 | 33 |
| **Muscle Milk** (Cytosport ~ Hi Protein): | | | |
| **17 fl.oz Box:** Chocolate | 340 | 16 | 17 |
| Average other flavors | 310 | 12 | 16 |
| **11 fl.oz Box:** Choc./Choc Malt, av. | 230 | 11 | 11 |
| Average other flavors | 210 | 10 | 9 |
| **14 fl.oz Bottle:** Chocolate | 240 | 9 | 14 |
| Average other flavors | 220 | 9 | 11 |
| **Lite:** Chocolate | 170 | 4.5 | 12 |
| Cafe Late; Vanilla, average | 160 | 4.5 | 11 |
| **Nesquik:** Per 16 fl.oz Bottle | | | |
| Chocolate: Low Fat | 340 | 5 | 58 |
| Fat-Free | 300 | 0 | 58 |
| Strawberry, Low Fat | 360 | 5 | 62 |
| **Prairie Farms,** Choc., 16 fl.oz | 440 | 16 | 58 |
| **Quaker,** Milk Chillers, 14 fl.oz | 245 | 9 | 32 |
| **Ralphs,** Chocolate, Low-Fat, 8 fl.oz | 210 | 2.5 | 36 |
| **Skinny Cow,** Chocolate, Fat-Free | 150 | 0 | 26 |
| **TruMoo,** Choc.; Strawb., av, 1 cup | 145 | 0 | 26 |

### Flavored Milk (Cont) | C | F | Cb

Ready-To-Drink: Per 8 fl.oz Cup Unless Indicated

| | C | F | Cb |
|---|---|---|---|
| **Starbucks,** | | | |
| Vanilla Frappuccino, 9.5 fl.oz | 200 | 3 | 37 |
| **Yoo-Hoo,** | | | |
| Chocolate, 15.5 fl.oz bottle | 260 | 2 | 57 |

**Bottle Coffee Drinks ~ See Page 37**

### Shakes

| | C | F | Cb |
|---|---|---|---|
| **Arby's:** | | | |
| Chocolate; Jamocha, regular | 570 | 15 | 98 |
| Vanilla, regular | 480 | 15 | 74 |
| **Burger King:** | | | |
| Chocolate: | | | |
| Value, 12 fl.oz | 340 | 9 | 60 |
| Small, 16 fl.oz | 440 | 11 | 78 |
| Medium, 22 fl.oz | 650 | 16 | 119 |
| Large, 32 fl.oz | 960 | 23 | 176 |
| **Other flavors ~ See Page 186** | | | |
| **Denny's:** | | | |
| Chocolate; Strawberry, 12 fl.oz | 560 | 26 | 76 |
| Vanilla, 12 fl.oz | 560 | 26 | 76 |
| **Dreyers:** | | | |
| Slow Churned: Prep'd with ⅓ cup FF Milk | | | |
| Choc./Strawb./Vanilla, av, 8.1 oz | 220 | 5 | 38 |
| Cookies n' Cream | 270 | 6 | 45 |
| **Hardees,** av. all flav., 16 fl.oz | 700 | 33 | 86 |
| **McDonalds,** Triple Thick Shakes: | | | |
| Average all flavors: | | | |
| 12 fl.oz cup | 430 | 10 | 75 |
| 16 fl.oz cup | 570 | 13 | 101 |
| 21 fl.oz cup | 760 | 18 | 132 |
| 32 fl.oz cup | 1140 | 26 | 200 |

**Other Restaurants ~ See Fast-Foods Section**

### Smoothies

Made Up Ready-To-Drink
**(8 fl. oz Milk/Soy + Fruit):** Per 12 fl.oz
Average all types:

| | C | F | Cb |
|---|---|---|---|
| With Whole Milk | 300 | 8 | 50 |
| + Ice Cream, 1 scoop | 400 | 13 | 62 |
| With Non-Fat Milk | 240 | 0 | 50 |

**Fruit Smoothies ~ See Page 41**
**Freshens; Jamba Juice; TCBY ~ See Fast-Foods**

## Rice & Cereal Drinks

*Per 8 fl.oz Cup* **C F Cb**

| | C | F | Cb |
|---|---|---|---|
| **Almond Breeze** *(Blue Diamond)*: | | | |
| Original | 60 | 2.5 | 8 |
| Chocolate | 120 | 3 | 22 |
| Vanilla | 90 | 2.5 | 16 |
| **Unsweetened:** Orig.; Vanilla | 40 | 3 | 2 |
| Chocolate | 45 | 3.5 | 3 |
| **Almond Dream:** | | | |
| Enriched: Original | 50 | 2.5 | 6 |
| Unsweetened | 30 | 2.5 | 1 |
| **Amazake,** Oh So Original | 150 | 0 | 34 |
| **Better Than Milk:** | | | |
| **Rice Vegan Mix:** | | | |
| Original, 2 Tbsp powder, 0.67 oz | 100 | 2.5 | 16 |
| Vanilla, 2 Tbsp powder, 0.67 oz | 80 | 2 | 8 |
| **Cacique,** | | | |
| Horchata Rice Drink | 160 | 3.5 | 31 |
| **Don Jose:** | | | |
| Horchata Rice Drink | 140 | 4 | 25 |
| Cereal Match | 100 | 3 | 17 |
| **EdenBlend,** Rice & Soy | 120 | 3 | 18 |
| **Pacific:** | | | |
| **Rice Drinks,** | | | |
| Low-Fat Plain/Vanilla | 130 | 2 | 27 |
| **Organic Oat,** Original/Vanilla, av | 130 | 2.5 | 24 |
| **Nut Drinks:** Hazelnut, Orig. | 110 | 3.5 | 18 |
| Chocolate | 120 | 5 | 19 |
| **Almond:** Original, Low-Fat | 60 | 2.5 | 8 |
| Vanilla, Low-Fat | 70 | 2.5 | 11 |
| Organic: Original | 60 | 2.5 | 8 |
| Chocolate, Single Serve | 100 | 3 | 19 |
| Vanilla, Single Serve | 70 | 2.5 | 11 |
| **Rice Dream:** | | | |
| **Refrigerated,** Enriched, Original | 120 | 2.5 | 23 |
| **Shelf Stable:** Carob | 150 | 2.5 | 30 |
| Vanilla; Enriched Vanilla, average | 130 | 2.5 | 27 |
| **Heartwise,** Original; Vanilla, av | 135 | 2 | 29 |
| **Supreme:** Chocolate Chai | 160 | 3 | 35 |
| Vanilla Hazelnut | 140 | 2.5 | 29 |
| **Trader Joe's:** | | | |
| **Rice Drinks:** | | | |
| Original, Organic | 120 | 2.5 | 23 |
| Vanilla | 130 | 2.5 | 26 |
| **WestSoy,** Rice: Plain; Vanilla | 110 | 2.5 | 20 |

Note: Rice/Oat/Nut drinks are very low in protein. Unless enriched with protein (and calcium), they are not suitable for infants as a substitute for milk or calcium-enriched soy drinks.

## Soy Milk ~ Ready-To-Drink

*Per 8 fl.oz Cup* **C F Cb**

| | C | F | Cb |
|---|---|---|---|
| **365 Organic** *(Whole Foods)*: | | | |
| Original, unsweetened | 70 | 4 | 4 |
| Chocolate | 140 | 3.5 | 22 |
| Vanilla | 90 | 3.5 | 10 |
| Light: Original | 70 | 1.5 | 9 |
| Vanilla | 70 | 1.5 | 10 |
| **8th Continent:** | | | |
| Original | 80 | 2.5 | 7 |
| Complete Vanilla | 80 | 2.5 | 8 |
| Vanilla | 100 | 2.5 | 11 |
| Fat-Free: Original | 60 | 0 | 8 |
| Vanilla | 70 | 0 | 11 |
| Light: Original | 50 | 2 | 2 |
| Chocolate | 90 | 1.5 | 12 |
| **Bolthouse Farms:** | | | |
| Perfectly Protein: Mocha Cappuccino | 180 | 3 | 31 |
| Vanilla Chai Tea | 170 | 3.5 | 27 |
| **EdenBlend,** Organic | 120 | 3 | 18 |
| **Edensoy:** Original | 140 | 5 | 14 |
| Original, Unsweetened | 120 | 6 | 5 |
| Carob; Chocolate, average | 175 | 4 | 29 |
| Vanilla | 150 | 3 | 24 |
| Extra: Original | 130 | 4 | 13 |
| Vanilla | 150 | 3 | 23 |
| **Kidz Dream:** | | | |
| Smoothies: Berry Blast | 100 | 2 | 17 |
| Orange Cream | 120 | 2 | 21 |
| **O Organics** *(Safeway)*: | | | |
| Plain | 90 | 3.5 | 8 |
| Chocolate | 150 | 4 | 23 |
| Vanilla Soy | 90 | 3 | 9 |
| **Odwalla:** | | | |
| Super Protein: Original | 195 | 5.5 | 25 |
| Vanilla Al'Mondo | 195 | 5.5 | 25 |
| Protein Monster: Strawb. | 160 | 3.5 | 19 |
| Vanilla | 195 | 3.5 | 24 |
| **Pacific:** | | | |
| Select Soy: Plain, low fat | 70 | 2.5 | 9 |
| Vanilla, low fat | 80 | 2.5 | 11 |
| Organic, Original, Unsweetened | 90 | 4.5 | 4 |
| Ultra (Extra Protein/Calcium): Plain | 120 | 4 | 11 |
| Vanilla | 130 | 4 | 14 |

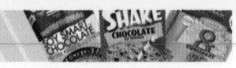

## Soy Milk ~ Ready-To-Drink

*Per 8 fl.oz Cup*

| | C | F | Cb |
|---|---|---|---|
| **Silk:** | | | |
| Refrigerated: Original | 100 | 4 | 8 |
| Chocolate | 140 | 3.5 | 23 |
| Vanilla | 100 | 3.5 | 10 |
| Shelf Stable: Heart Health | 80 | 1.5 | 10 |
| Plus DHA Omega-3 | 110 | 5 | 8 |
| Unsweetened | 80 | 4 | 4 |
| Very Vanilla | 130 | 4 | 19 |
| Light: Original | 60 | 1.5 | 6 |
| Chocolate | 90 | 1.5 | 15 |
| Vanilla | 70 | 1.5 | 7 |
| **Slim-Fast (Soy-Based)** ~ *See Page 40* | | | |
| **So Nice:** | | | |
| **Classic:** Original | 80 | 3 | 7 |
| Chocolate | 150 | 3 | 24 |
| Natural | 80 | 4 | 3 |
| Strawberry | 110 | 3 | 15 |
| **Omega 3,** Vanilla | 120 | 4 | 15 |
| **Prebiotic Fiber,** Original | 120 | 3 | 18 |
| **Soy Dream:** | | | |
| **Shelf Stable Enriched:** | | | |
| Original | 100 | 4 | 8 |
| Chocolate | 150 | 4 | 21 |
| Classic Vanilla | 140 | 4 | 18 |
| Vanilla | 120 | 4 | 14 |
| **Soy Slender:** Plain | 60 | 3 | 3 |
| Average other flavors | 70 | 3 | 4 |
| **Trader Joe's:** | | | |
| **Soy Milk:** Original | 110 | 2 | 13 |
| Chocolate | 130 | 2.5 | 23 |
| Vanilla | 100 | 2 | 16 |
| **Organic:** Original | 130 | 3 | 17 |
| Chocolate | 120 | 3 | 17 |
| Vanilla | 130 | 3 | 19 |
| Unsweetened | 70 | 3.5 | 3 |
| **WestSoy:** | | | |
| **Lite:** Plain | 60 | 2 | 6 |
| Vanilla | 70 | 2 | 8 |
| **Low-Fat:** Plain | 90 | 1.5 | 14 |
| Vanilla | 120 | 1.5 | 21 |
| **Non-Fat:** Plain | 70 | 0 | 10 |
| Vanilla | 80 | 0 | 12 |
| **Longevity,** Plain | 90 | 3.5 | 10 |
| **Plus** *(25% Less Sugar):* | | | |
| Plain | 90 | 3.5 | 7 |
| Vanilla | 100 | 3.5 | 10 |

## Soy Milk ~ Ready-To-Drink (Cont)

*Per 8 fl.oz Cup*

| | C | F | Cb |
|---|---|---|---|
| **WestSoy (Cont):** | | | |
| **Unsweetened:** Original | 90 | 4.5 | 5 |
| Chocolate; Vanilla, average | 100 | 4.5 | 6 |
| **Soy Shakes,** Chocolate; Vanilla, av. | 170 | 3.5 | 29 |

## Soy Powder Mix

*1 oz (¼ cup) mix makes 8 fl.oz Cup*

| | C | F | Cb |
|---|---|---|---|
| **Soy Protein Isolate,** 1 oz dry | 95 | 1 | 2 |
| **Better Than Milk:** | | | |
| Original, 2 Tbsp | 100 | 2.5 | 16 |
| Light, 2 Tbsp | 75 | 2.5 | 7 |
| Vanilla, 2¾ Tbsp | 80 | 2 | 8 |
| **Genisoy:** *Per 3 Rounded Tbsp* | | | |
| Natural, unflavored, 1 oz | 110 | 1.5 | 0 |
| Chocolate, 1.2 oz | 130 | 0.5 | 16 |
| Strawberry/Banana, 1.2 oz | 130 | 1 | 17 |
| Vanilla, 1.2 oz | 130 | 1 | 17 |
| Ultra Bone Health, Chocolate, 1.4 oz | 130 | 0.5 | 19 |
| Ultra-XT, Vanilla, 1.4 oz | 150 | 1 | 20 |
| **Now,** Soy, ¼ cup, 0.78 oz | 95 | 4.5 | 6.5 |
| **Revival Soy Shakes:** *Per Packet* | | | |
| Unsweetened: Plain | 90 | 1 | 1 |
| Vanilla Pleasure | 120 | 2 | 6 |
| Average other flavors | 115 | 2 | 4 |
| **Whole Foods:** | | | |
| Choc.with Spirulina, 1 oz | 100 | 1 | 10 |
| Vanilla with Spirulina, 1 oz | 100 | 0 | 11 |

## Coconut Milk Drink

| | C | F | Cb |
|---|---|---|---|
| **So Delicious:** *Per 8 fl.oz cup* | | | |
| Original | 80 | 5 | 7 |
| Unsweetened | 50 | 5 | 1 |
| Vanilla | 90 | 5 | 9 |
| **Trader Joes:** *Per 8 fl.oz cup* | | | |
| Light, ⅓ cup | 50 | 4 | 4 |
| Unsweetened | 60 | 5 | 1 |
| Vanilla | 90 | 5 | 9 |
| (Enriched with calcium + vitamins D & B12) | | | |

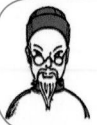

*Confucious say:*
{Man who eat with one chopstick never have problem with obesity⁹

### Quick Guide

**Cola Drinks:**
*Average All Brands*
*Includes Coca-Cola and Pepsi*

| | C | F | Cb |
|---|---|---|---|
| 8 fl.oz Cup/Can | 100 | 0 | 26 |
| 12 fl.oz Can | 150 | 0 | 39 |
| 16 fl.oz Bottle | 200 | 0 | 52 |
| 20 fl.oz Bottle | 250 | 0 | 65 |
| 24 fl.oz (Pepsi) | 300 | 0 | 84 |
| 1-Liter Bottle (34 fl.oz) | 400 | 0 | 100 |
| 2-Liter Bottle (68 fl.oz) | 800 | 0 | 200 |

**Other Soda Drinks:** *Av. All Brands, Per 12 fl.oz*

| | C | F | Cb |
|---|---|---|---|
| Club Soda | 0 | 0 | 0 |
| Cream Soda | 190 | 0 | 48 |
| Diet/Low Cal Drinks | 5 | 0 | 1 |
| Dr Pepper Type | 150 | 0 | 38 |
| Ginger Ale | 125 | 0 | 31 |
| Grape | 160 | 0 | 42 |
| Lemon Lime | 150 | 0 | 37 |
| Orange | 180 | 0 | 45 |
| Root Beer | 150 | 0 | 39 |
| Tonic Water | 125 | 0 | 2 |
| **Mineral Water:** Plain | 0 | 0 | 0 |
| Sweetened/flavored | 150 | 0 | 37 |
| With Fruit Juice | 120 | 0 | 30 |
| **Soda Water/Seltzer:** Plain/Diet | 0 | 0 | 0 |
| Sweetened/flavored | 155 | 0 | 39 |
| With Fruit Juice | 160 | 0 | 40 |

### Fountain, Movie Theater & Take-Out

*Average All Flavors*

| | C | F | Cb |
|---|---|---|---|
| Small Cup, 12 fl.oz: No Ice | 160 | 0 | 40 |
| With ⅓ Ice | 120 | 0 | 30 |
| Regular, 16 fl.oz: No Ice | 215 | 0 | 53 |
| With ⅓ Ice | 160 | 0 | 40 |
| Medium, 22 fl.oz: No Ice | 295 | 0 | 73 |
| With ⅓ Ice | 220 | 0 | 55 |
| Large, 32 fl.oz: No Ice | 430 | 0 | 105 |
| With ⅓ Ice | 320 | 0 | 80 |

*(Note: ⅓ Cup of Ice = ¼ Cup Liquid)*

### Soft Drinks Brands

*Per 12 fl.oz Unless Indicated*

| **A&W:** | C | F | Cb |
|---|---|---|---|
| Root Beer | 180 | 0 | 46 |
| Diet Cream Soda/Root Beer | 0 | 0 | 0 |
| **Albertson's:** | | | |
| Super Chill: Cola | 160 | 0 | 43 |
| Root Beer | 180 | 0 | 48 |

### Soft Drink Brands (Cont)

*Per 12 fl.oz Unless Indicated*

| | C | F | Cb |
|---|---|---|---|
| Barq's, Root Beer | 160 | 0 | 45 |
| Big Red, Soda, 20 fl.oz | 250 | 0 | 63 |
| **Blue Sky:** | | | |
| Natural Soda: Black Cherry | 140 | 0 | 37 |
| Cola; Orange Creme, av. | 160 | 0 | 43 |
| Bubble Up, Soda, 8 fl.oz | 110 | 0 | 28 |
| Cactus Cooler, 12 fl.oz | 150 | 0 | 40 |
| **Canada Dry:** *Per 8 fl.oz* | | | |
| Club Sod; Diet Ginger Ale | 0 | 0 | 0 |
| Ginger Ale | 90 | 0 | 25 |
| Tonic Water | 90 | 0 | 24 |
| **Capri Sun,** | | | |
| Juice Drinks, all flavors, 6 fl.oz | 60 | 0 | 16 |
| Cheerwine, 12 fl.oz | 150 | 0 | 42 |
| **Coca-Cola:** | | | |
| Classic/Caffeine Free | 140 | 0 | 39 |
| Diet Coke, all flavors | 0 | 0 | 0 |
| Cherry Coke/Vanilla Coke | 155 | 0 | 42 |
| Coca-Cola Zero | 0 | 0 | 0 |
| **Country Time** *(Kraft),* | | | |
| Lemonade, 11.25 fl.oz | 180 | 0 | 47 |
| **Crush:** | | | |
| Orange/Grape: 12 fl.oz | 195 | 0 | 53 |
| 20 fl.oz bottle | 325 | 0 | 88 |
| Diet Orange, 20 fl.oz | 35 | 0 | 10 |
| Strawberry, 20 fl.oz | 300 | 0 | 78 |
| **Dad's:** Orange Cream Soda | 180 | 0 | 46 |
| Root Beer | 165 | 0 | 41 |
| **Diet Rite,** Pure Zero | 0 | 0 | 0 |
| **Dr Pepper:** Regular | 150 | 0 | 40 |
| Cherry | 165 | 0 | 44 |
| Diet, all flavors | 0 | 0 | 0 |
| Fanta, all flavors, av. | 175 | 0 | 48 |
| **Fresca:** Original Citrus | 0 | 0 | 0 |
| Blackcherry Citrus | 0 | 0 | 0 |
| Peach Citrus | 0 | 0 | 0 |
| GuS, average all flavors | 95 | 0 | 23 |
| **Hansen's:** Diet Soda | 0 | 0 | 0 |
| Natural Cane Sugar: | | | |
| Creamy Root Beer | 160 | 0 | 43 |
| Pomegranate | 130 | 0 | 35 |
| **Hawaiian Punch,** Fruit Juicy Red | 105 | 0 | 26 |
| **Henry Weinhard's:** Root Beer | 170 | 0 | 43 |
| Cream flavor, average | 175 | 0 | 42 |
| Hires, Root Beer | 170 | 0 | 45 |
| **IBC:** Root Beer | 160 | 0 | 43 |
| Cream Soda; Black Cherry | 180 | 0 | 48 |
| **Icee:** Coca-Cola | 100 | 0 | 27 |
| Fanta, Lime | 105 | 0 | 27 |
| Minute Maid, Raspb. | 100 | 0 | 27 |

| Per 12 fl.oz Unless Indicated | C | F | Cb |
|---|---|---|---|
| **Jarritos**, all flavors, 12.5 fl.oz | 170 | 0 | 43 |
| **Jelly Belly**, all flavors | 180 | 0 | 28 |
| **Jolt:** Power Cola, 16 fl.oz | 200 | 0 | 52 |
| Blue Raspberry, 16 fl.oz | 240 | 0 | 60 |
| Or. Burst; Wired Grape, 16 fl.oz | 210 | 0 | 52 |
| **Jones Soda:** Cola | 160 | 0 | 40 |
| Whoopass, 16 fl.oz | 200 | 0 | 52 |
| Average other flavors | 185 | 0 | 46 |
| **Mello Yello**, Regular | 170 | 0 | 47 |
| **Minute Maid:** Fruit Punch | 160 | 0 | 44 |
| Lemonade, Regular: | | | |
| 12 fl.oz | 150 | 0 | 42 |
| 20 fl.oz | 250 | 0 | 70 |
| Orangeade | 160 | 0 | 43 |
| **Mountain Dew:** | | | |
| Live Wire; Code Red | 170 | 0 | 46 |
| Diet flavors | 0 | 0 | 0 |
| **Mug**, Root Beer | 160 | 0 | 43 |
| **Natural Brew:** Draft Root Beer | 180 | 0 | 44 |
| Outrageous Ginger Ale | 170 | 0 | 42 |
| Vanilla Cream | 170 | 0 | 42 |
| **Nehi**, Royal Crown Peach | 190 | 0 | 51 |
| **Orangina** | 160 | 0 | 39 |
| **Pepsi:** Regular; Caffeine Free | 150 | 0 | 41 |
| Diet Pepsi; Jazz; Pepsi One | 0 | 0 | 0 |
| Pepsi Next | 60 | 0 | 15 |
| Wild Cherry; Vanilla | 150 | 0 | 42 |
| **Perrier**, Carbonated Water | 0 | 0 | 0 |
| **Pibb**, Xtra | 150 | 0 | 39 |
| **RC Cola**, Regular | 160 | 0 | 43 |
| **Reed's**, Ginger Brew, | | | |
| average all varieties | 145 | 0 | 38 |
| **7•UP:** Regular; Cherry | 150 | 0 | 39 |
| Diet varieties | 0 | 0 | 0 |
| **Safeway:** Per 8 fl.oz | | | |
| Refreshe: Cola | 110 | 0 | 29 |
| Grape | 140 | 0 | 36 |
| Lemon Lime | 110 | 0 | 27 |
| Mountain Breeze | 120 | 0 | 32 |
| Strawberry | 120 | 0 | 29 |
| **Santa Cruz**, Sparkling, av., 10.5 fl.oz | 135 | 0 | 33 |
| **Schweppes:** Seltzer | 0 | 0 | 0 |
| Tonic Water; Ginger Ale, average | 130 | 0 | 35 |
| **Shasta:** Cream Soda | 190 | 0 | 47 |
| Cherry Cola | 180 | 0 | 45 |
| Dr. Shasta | 150 | 0 | 38 |
| Club Soda; Diet, all flavors | 0 | 0 | 0 |
| Tiki Punch; Pineapple; Or. | 200 | 0 | 50 |
| Ginger Ale | 130 | 0 | 33 |
| Other flavors, average | 170 | 0 | 41 |

| Per 12 fl.oz Unless Indicated | C | F | Cb |
|---|---|---|---|
| **Sierra Mist**, Lemon Lime | 150 | 0 | 39 |
| **Sprite:** Regular | 145 | 0 | 40 |
| Zero | 0 | 0 | 0 |
| **Squirt**, Ruby Red | 170 | 0 | 45 |
| **Stewarts:** Root Beer | 160 | 0 | 40 |
| Grape; Orange 'n Cream | 190 | 0 | 48 |
| **Sun Drop:** Citrus Soda, 20 fl.oz | 290 | 0 | 76 |
| Cherry Lemon | 180 | 0 | 46 |
| Diet Citrus Soda | 10 | 0 | 1 |
| **Sunkist:** Orange | 190 | 0 | 52 |
| Diet Sunkist | 0 | 0 | 0 |
| **TAB** | 0 | 0 | 0 |
| **Thomas Kemper:** Root Beer | 160 | 0 | 40 |
| Average other flavors | 160 | 0 | 40 |
| **Trader Joe's:** | | | |
| Sparkling: | | | |
| French Berry Lemonade, | | | |
| 1 cup, 8 fl.oz | 130 | 0 | 31 |
| 1 Bottle, 33.8 fl.oz | 520 | 0 | 124 |
| Lime Ade, 1 cup, 8 fl.oz | 110 | 0 | 28 |
| 1 Bottle, 33.8 fl.oz | 440 | 0 | 108 |
| Pink Lemonade, 1 cup, 8 fl.oz | 130 | 0 | 31 |
| 1 Bottle, 33.8 fl.oz | 520 | 0 | 124 |
| **Vernor's**, Ginger Soda | 150 | 0 | 39 |
| **Virgil's**, Root Beer | 160 | 0 | 42 |
| **Walgreens:** | | | |
| Orchard Grape Soda, 20 fl.oz | 300 | 0 | 84 |
| Cola; Zesty Lem. Lime, av., 20 fl.oz | 225 | 0 | 65 |
| Root Beer, 20 fl.oz | 225 | 0 | 75 |
| **Welch's**, | | | |
| Sparkling Grape Juice C'tail | 240 | 0 | 60 |
| **365 Organic** (Whole Foods), | | | |
| Spritzers, all flavors | 110 | 0 | 28 |

**Powdered Soft Drink Mix**

| Per 8 fl.oz Prepared, Unless Indicated | C | F | Cb |
|---|---|---|---|
| **Country Time:** | | | |
| Lemonade; Pink Lemonade | 60 | 0 | 16 |
| Average other flavors | 80 | 0 | 19 |
| Lite | 35 | 0 | 8 |
| **Crystal Light:** Orig., 8 fl.oz | 5 | 0 | 0 |
| Pure, av. all flav., 0.3 oz pkt | 15 | 0 | 4 |
| **Flavor Aid**, 1/8 package | 0 | 0 | 0 |
| **Kool-Aid:** All flavors | 60 | 0 | 16 |
| Unsweetened, 6 fl.oz | 0 | 0 | 0 |
| **Propel**, Fit, 3 grams | 10 | 0 | 3 |
| **Tang**, Regular, 2 Tbsp, 0.9oz | 105 | 0 | 28 |

## Quick Guide

### Teas

| | C | F | Cb |
|---|---|---|---|
| **Regular:** Bag, Loose or Instant Brewed, 1 cup, 8 fl.oz (Add extra for sugar/milk) | 2 | 0 | 0.5 |
| **Herbal:** Average all varieties, 1 cup | 2 | 0 | 0.5 |
| *Bigelow*, all flavors | 0 | 0 | 0 |
| *Celestial Seasonings*, all flavors | 0 | 0 | 0 |
| **Bubble Milk Tea,** w/ Pearls, 8 fl.oz | 175 | 0 | 41 |
| **Chai Tea** *(Cafe D' Vita)*, 2 Tbsp | 120 | 3.5 | 21 |
| **Starbucks ~** *See Fast-Foods Section* | | | |

### Iced Tea
*Average All Brands*

| | C | F | Cb |
|---|---|---|---|
| **Sweetened:** 8 fl.oz | 90 | 0 | 22 |
| 12 fl.oz | 140 | 0 | 34 |
| 16 fl.oz | 180 | 0 | 46 |
| **Unsweetened,** 8 fl.oz | 2 | 0 | 0.5 |

## Iced Tea Mixes

*Per 8 fl.oz Made-Up*

| | C | F | Cb |
|---|---|---|---|
| **4C Iced Teas:** | | | |
| Sweetened, average | 70 | 0 | 18 |
| Totally Light, all flavors | 0 | 0 | 0 |
| **Crystal Light,** sugar free | 5 | 0 | 0 |
| **Lipton:** Instant, unsweetened | 0 | 0 | 0 |
| Instant Raspberry | 80 | 0 | 19 |
| Lemon | 70 | 0 | 18 |
| Peach; Raspberry, Sugar Free | 5 | 0 | 1 |
| Iced Tea To Go | 0 | 0 | 0 |
| **Nestea:** | | | |
| Lemonade Tea, 1⅓ Tbsp | 60 | 0 | 15 |
| Lemon flavored Iced Tea, 1⅓ Tbsp | 60 | 0 | 15 |
| Sugar Free Lemon Iced Tea, 2 tsp | 5 | 0 | 2 |
| Unsweetened Tea, 2 tsp | 0 | 0 | 0 |

## Bottled & Canned Teas

**Arizona:** *Per 8 fl.oz*

| | C | F | Cb |
|---|---|---|---|
| **Black:** Cranberry | 80 | 0 | 22 |
| Sweet | 90 | 0 | 23 |
| With Ginseng | 60 | 0 | 15 |
| **Green Tea:** Flavored, average | 70 | 0 | 18 |
| Diet Blueberry | 5 | 0 | 2 |
| Lite, Half & Half Lemonade | 50 | 0 | 14 |
| **Fuze,** average all flavors, 16 fl.oz | 120 | 0 | 30 |
| **Gold Peak,** Lem.,16.9 fl.oz bottle | 170 | 0 | 44 |
| **Hansen's:** Green Tea: Reg., 16 fl.oz | 120 | 0 | 30 |
| Peach; Pomegranate, 16 fl.oz | 180 | 0 | 44 |

## Bottled & Canned Teas (Cont)

| | C | F | Cb |
|---|---|---|---|
| **Honest Tea,** Black Forest Berry/Peach, 16 fl.oz | 65 | 0 | 17 |
| **Lipton Brisk:** | | | |
| Av. all flavors: 12 fl.oz can | 130 | 0 | 33 |
| 20 fl.oz bottle | 215 | 0 | 55 |
| **Lipton Iced Tea:** | | | |
| Lemon; White w/ Raspb., 16.9 fl.oz | 120 | 0 | 32 |
| Green Tea with Citrus: | | | |
| 16.9 fl.oz bottle | 170 | 0 | 44 |
| 20 fl.oz bottle | 200 | 0 | 53 |
| Diet, all flavors | 0 | 0 | 0 |
| Sparkling, av. all flavors, 16 fl.oz | 120 | 0 | 32 |
| **Minute Maid,** Pomeg. Tea, 8 fl.oz | 40 | 0 | 9 |
| **Nantucket,** Lemon Tea 16 fl.oz | 160 | 0 | 44 |
| **Nestea Iced Tea:** | | | |
| With Lemon: 8 fl.oz | 80 | 0 | 22 |
| 16.9 oz bottle | 180 | 0 | 45 |
| 20 fl.oz bottle | 210 | 0 | 56 |
| Diet Green/Lemon | 0 | 0 | 0 |
| **POMx:** *Per 16 fl.oz* | | | |
| Pomegranate: Blackberry | 160 | 0 | 40 |
| Lychee | 140 | 0 | 36 |
| Peach Passion | 160 | 0 | 38 |
| Light flavors, average | 70 | 0 | 34 |

Note: Carbs figure for Light flavors includes Erythritol natural sweetener which has negligible calories.

| | C | F | Cb |
|---|---|---|---|
| **Snapple:** Diet/Unsweetened Teas | 0 | 0 | 0 |
| Iced Tea Blends, all flav., 16 fl.oz | 200 | 0 | 50 |
| Black Teas, average, 8 fl.oz | 40 | 0 | 10 |
| Green; White, 8 fl.oz | 60 | 0 | 10 |
| Red Tea, 8 fl.oz | 40 | 0 | 10 |
| **SoBe,** Green Tea, 20 fl.oz | 250 | 0 | 63 |
| **Ssips,** Lemon Iced, 6¾ fl.oz | 80 | 0 | 20 |
| **Steaz,** Green Tea, Peach/Mint, 16 fl.oz | 80 | 0 | 20 |
| **Tazo,** Sweet Organic Black, 13.8 fl oz | 60 | 0 | 15 |
| **TeaZazz:** Original; Peach, 20 fl.oz | 50 | 0 | 12 |
| Green Tea Lemon, 20 fl.oz | 60 | 0 | 15 |
| **Trader Joe's:** *Per 8 fl.oz* | | | |
| Organic Tea & Lemonade | 100 | 0 | 25 |
| Pomegranate Green Tea | 60 | 0 | 15 |
| Unsweetened *(Kettle/Green)* | 0 | 0 | 0 |
| **Turkey Hill:** Iced Tea, 16 fl.oz | 180 | 0 | 42 |
| Fruit flavors, average, 16 fl.oz | 205 | 0 | 50 |
| **365 Organic** *(Whole Foods):* | | | |
| Unsweetened: Black Tea | 0 | 0 | 0 |
| Green Tea | 0 | 0 | 0 |

Note: Most breads have similar calories on a weight basis. However, volume may vary.

For example, 1 oz of bread may equal 1 slice regular bread or 2 slices of a lighter bread.

It is best to weigh bread used and calculate using: 1 oz bread = 70 calories, 14g carb.

### Quick Guide

| Bread | C | F | Cb |
|---|---|---|---|
| **White or Wheat:** *Average Per Slice* | | | |
| **Thin or Light,** ¾ oz | 50 | 0.5 | 9 |
| **Sandwich slice,** 1 oz | 70 | 1 | 12 |
| **Thick or Large slice,** 1½ oz | 105 | 1.5 | 18 |
| **Thick,** 2 oz | 140 | 2 | 23 |
| **Extra Thick,** 3 oz | 210 | 3 | 35 |
| **Whole Loaf:** 16 oz | 1120 | 15 | 185 |
| 24 oz Loaf | 1680 | 24 | 280 |
| **Multi Grain/Whole Grain:** | | | |
| Sandwich slice, 1 oz | 75 | 1.5 | 12 |
| Thick Slice, 2 oz | 150 | 2.5 | 25 |

**Toast:** *Based on same counts as White/Wheat as shown above*

| 1 Slice (1 oz fresh): | C | F | Cb |
|---|---|---|---|
| With 1 tsp butter/margarine | 105 | 5 | 12 |
| With 1 tsp "light" butter/marg. | 90 | 3.5 | 12 |
| With 2 tsp butter/margarine | 140 | 9 | 12 |
| With 2 tsp "light" butter/marg. | 110 | 6 | 12 |

### Breads

*Per Slice Unless Indicated*

| | C | F | Cb |
|---|---|---|---|
| **12-Grain,** 1½ oz | 110 | 1.5 | 22 |
| **Bran style/Dark,** 1 oz | 70 | 1 | 14 |
| **Buttermilk,** average, 1½ oz | 110 | 1 | 22 |
| **Challah,** ¾ oz | 85 | 1.5 | 17 |
| **Chapati,** 1 oz | 110 | 3 | 18 |
| **Ciabatta,** 2 oz | 130 | 1 | 26 |
| **Cornbread,** average, 3 oz | 220 | 6 | 37 |
| **Cracked Wheat Sourdough,** 1½ oz | 130 | 0.5 | 27 |
| **Croissants** ~ *See Page 134* | | | |
| **Crustless Bread,** reg. slice, ¾ oz | 40 | 0.5 | 8.5 |
| **Crusts Only,** regular slice, ¼ oz | 30 | 0 | 7 |
| **English Toasting,** 2 oz | 140 | 1.5 | 27 |
| **Flax & Grain,** 1½ oz | 120 | 3 | 19 |
| **Foccacia:** Plain, 2 oz portion | 150 | 2.5 | 28 |
| Cheese & Garlic; Pesto, 2 oz | 160 | 6 | 21 |
| Tomato & Olive, 2 oz | 150 | 5 | 21 |

### Breads (Cont)

*Per Slice Unless Indicated*

| | C | F | Cb |
|---|---|---|---|
| **French Stick/Baguette,** 1 oz | 70 | 1 | 15 |
| **French Toast:** Slices, 1.6 oz | 140 | 2 | 26 |
| Sticks *(Aunt Jemima)*, av., 2 oz | 110 | 2 | 18 |
| **Garlic Bread/Toast:** | | | |
| Small slice + 1 tsp spread, ¾ oz | 80 | 5 | 7 |
| Medium slice + 2 tsp spread, 1½ oz | 160 | 10 | 14 |
| Thick slice + 3 tsp spread, 1.8 oz | 220 | 14 | 20 |
| *Pepperidge Farm*, 1 slice, 1.4 oz | 160 | 10 | 15 |
| **Hemp Bread,** 1.2 oz | 95 | 2 | 12 |
| **Italian Bread,** 2 oz | 140 | 1 | 28 |
| **Lower Carb** (higher protein/fiber), average all brands, 1 oz | 60 | 1.5 | 9 |
| **MultiGrain,** 1.5 oz | 100 | 2 | 21 |
| **Naan Flatbread,** 2 oz | 160 | 3.5 | 29 |
| **Nut/Health Nut,** 1.35 oz | 90 | 1.5 | 18 |
| **Oatmeal/Oatbran Bread,** 1½ oz | 90 | 0.5 | 19 |
| **Pita:** Average all types, | | | |
| Small (4" diam), 1.1 oz | 90 | 0 | 18 |
| Large (6½" diam), 2 oz | 140 | 1.5 | 27 |
| Extra Large (9" diam), 4 oz | 300 | 1.5 | 60 |
| **Popovers,** (1), without butter | 130 | 2 | 18 |
| **Pumpernickel:** | | | |
| Cocktail/Party size | 30 | 0.5 | 6 |
| Large slice, 1.35 oz | 80 | 0 | 15 |
| **Raisin Bread,** 1 oz | 80 | 1 | 15 |
| **Rye:** Average, 1 thin slice, 1 oz | 80 | 1 | 14 |
| 1 thick slice, 2 oz | 150 | 2 | 25 |
| Cocktail size, 0.4 oz | 25 | 0.5 | 4 |
| **Sandwich Pockets,** 2 oz | 140 | 1.5 | 27 |
| **Sourdough,** 1½ oz | 120 | 1 | 25 |
| **Sourdough French,** 1 oz | 75 | 0 | 14 |
| **Spelt,** 1.6 oz | 130 | 1 | 26 |
| **Sprouted 7-Grain,** 1.5 oz | 110 | 0.5 | 18 |
| **Squaw,** 1.1 oz | 85 | 0.5 | 13 |
| **Sweet Hawaiian Bread,** 1.3 oz | 110 | 2 | 19 |
| **Tacos/Tortillas** ~ *See Page 172* | | | |
| **Turkish/Middle Eastern,** 1 oz | 80 | 1.5 | 16 |
| **Wheat-Free Breads:** Spelt, 1.6 oz | 130 | 1 | 26 |
| Rice w/ Fruit Juice, 1½ oz | 110 | 2 | 21 |
| Healthseed Rye, 1.6 oz | 90 | 1 | 20 |
| Millet, 1.5 oz | 100 | 1 | 20 |

### Bread Brands

| | C | F | Cb |
|---|---|---|---|

*Per Slice Unless Indicated*

**Ener-G:** Gluten-Free Breads:

| | C | F | Cb |
|---|---|---|---|
| Brown Rice Loaf: Regular, 1.3 oz | 100 | 3 | 16 |
| Light, 0.67 oz | 50 | 2 | 7 |
| Corn Loaf, 0.67 oz | 40 | 2 | 7 |
| Light Tapioca, 0.67 oz | 45 | 1.5 | 7 |

**Ezekiel:**

| | C | F | Cb |
|---|---|---|---|
| **Sprouted Grain:** Low Sodium | 80 | 0.5 | 15 |
| Sesame, 1.2 oz | 80 | 0.5 | 14 |

**French Meadow:** *Per 1.2 oz Slice*

| | C | F | Cb |
|---|---|---|---|
| Flax & Sunflower | 90 | 1.5 | 15 |
| Hemp | 100 | 2.5 | 12 |
| Men's Bread | 100 | 4 | 10 |
| Spelt | 85 | 0.5 | 17 |

**Francisco International,**

| | C | F | Cb |
|---|---|---|---|
| Sourdough, Round Loaf, 1.6 oz | 110 | 0.5 | 22 |

**Nature's Path:**

| | C | F | Cb |
|---|---|---|---|
| **Manna:** Carrot Raisin; Millet Rice | 130 | 0 | 27 |
| Cinnamon Date | 150 | 0 | 29 |
| Fig Fennel Flax | 120 | 1.5 | 26 |
| Sunseed | 160 | 2 | 29 |
| **Oroweat:** 9 Grain DHA, 1.35 oz | 90 | 1 | 17 |
| 100% Whole Wheat, 1.35 oz | 90 | 1 | 17 |
| Country Buttermilk, 1.35 oz | 100 | 1.5 | 19 |
| Honey Wheat Berry, 1.2 oz | 80 | 1 | 17 |

**Pepperidge Farm:**

| | C | F | Cb |
|---|---|---|---|
| 100% Whole Wheat, Very Thin | 110 | 2 | 20 |
| 15 Grain, Small Slice | 70 | 1.5 | 13 |
| Farmhouse Soft Hearty White | 120 | 1.5 | 22 |
| Light Style, average | 130 | 1 | 26 |

**Frozen Breads:**

| | C | F | Cb |
|---|---|---|---|
| Garlic Bread: Parmesan, 2½" | 160 | 6 | 23 |
| Prem. Roasted Toast | 150 | 7 | 18 |
| Texas Toast | 150 | 7 | 18 |
| **Roman Meal:** Orig. Multigrain (2) | 130 | 1.5 | 25 |
| Honey Wheatberry, 1.5 oz | 100 | 1.5 | 19 |
| **Sara Lee:** Honey Wheat, 1 oz | 75 | 1 | 15 |

Hearty & Delicious,

| | C | F | Cb |
|---|---|---|---|
| 100% Multigrain, 1½ oz | 120 | 1.5 | 21 |
| 45 Cals & Delightful Wheat | 45 | 0.5 | 9 |

**Schwan's,** Frozen:

| | C | F | Cb |
|---|---|---|---|
| Cheese Stuffed Breadsticks, 2 oz | 160 | 7 | 18 |
| French Baguette Bread, ¼ loaf, 1.7 oz | 130 | 0 | 25 |
| **Trader Joe's:** Gourm. White, 1½ oz | 120 | 3.5 | 19 |
| Fat-Free Multi-Grain, 1.1 oz | 70 | 0 | 15 |
| Soft 10 Grain, 1½ oz | 90 | 1.5 | 16 |
| Sprouted Rye, 1.2 oz | 90 | 1 | 15 |
| **Wonder:** Classic White Sandwich, 1 oz | 70 | 1.5 | 14 |
| Light White, ¾ oz | 40 | 0 | 9 |
| Smartwhite, 1 slice, 0.92 oz | 50 | 1.5 | 11 |

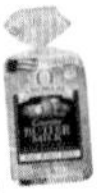

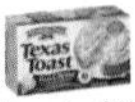

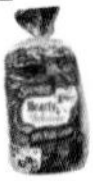

### Biscuits, Bread Rolls & Buns

| | C | F | Cb |
|---|---|---|---|
| **6" Roll,** Plain, average 2½ oz | 200 | 1 | 38 |

**Biscuits, Plain/B'Milk:** *Average, 2½" diameter*

| | C | F | Cb |
|---|---|---|---|
| Prepared from Recipe | 210 | 10 | 27 |
| Refrig. Dough, Baked | 95 | 4 | 13 |
| **Brown 'n Serve,** av., 1 oz | 70 | 1 | 13 |
| **Ciabatta Roll,** 3½ oz | 230 | 4 | 41 |

**Dinner Rolls:**

| | C | F | Cb |
|---|---|---|---|
| 1 small, 1 oz | 90 | 1.5 | 17 |
| 1 medium (3" diam),1½ oz | 110 | 1 | 23 |
| **Frankfurter/Hot Dog:** 1¼ oz | 110 | 1.5 | 21 |
| 1½ oz size | 130 | 2 | 25 |
| **French:** 1 med, 1.3 oz | 110 | 1.5 | 22 |
| 1 large, 3 oz | 230 | 2.5 | 42 |
| **Hamburger:** Regular, 1½ oz | 110 | 1.5 | 22 |
| Large, 3 oz | 210 | 3 | 40 |
| **Hoagie/Submarine,** Plain, 2⅓ oz | 200 | 1 | 38 |

**Kaiser Rolls:**

| | C | F | Cb |
|---|---|---|---|
| Small, 2 oz | 200 | 2.5 | 35 |
| Large, 3½ oz | 350 | 4 | 61 |

**Refrigerated Dough, Baked** *(Pillsbury):*

| | C | F | Cb |
|---|---|---|---|
| Buttermilk Biscuit (3), 2¼ oz | 150 | 2 | 30 |
| Crescent Roll, Original, 1 oz | 100 | 6 | 11 |
| Traditional Dinner Roll, 1.4 oz | 100 | 1.5 | 20 |
| **Sourdough Roll,** 1¼ oz | 110 | 1 | 21 |
| **Wheat Rolls:** Small, 1.2 oz | 100 | 1 | 17 |
| Medium, 1¾ oz | 130 | 1.5 | 23 |
| Large, 3½ oz | 260 | 3 | 46 |

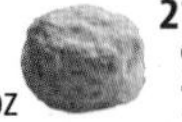

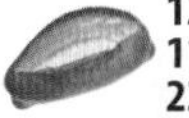

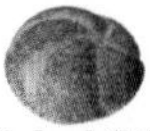

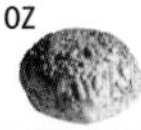

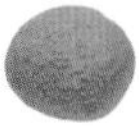

### Breadsticks, Croutons

**Breadsticks:**

| | C | F | Cb |
|---|---|---|---|
| Salt Sticks, plain, 1 oz | 110 | 1 | 20 |
| Fresh baked (1), 2 oz | 180 | 2.5 | 34 |
| *Stella D'oro:* Sesame (1) | 50 | 2 | 7 |
| Original (1) | 45 | 1 | 7 |
| **Croutons:** Seasoned, 2 Tbsp, ¼ oz | 35 | 1.5 | 4 |
| Zesty Italian *(Pepp. Farm)*, 6 croutons | 30 | 1 | 5 |

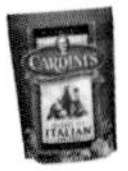

### Bread Products

**Bread Crumbs,** dry:

| | C | F | Cb |
|---|---|---|---|
| Plain or seasoned: 1 oz | 110 | 1.5 | 20 |
| 1 cup, 3½ oz | 385 | 5 | 70 |
| **Corn Flake Crumbs,** 1.1 oz | 120 | 0 | 29 |
| *Keebler*, Graham Cracker Crumbs:1 oz | 110 | 2.5 | 20 |
| 3 Tbsp, 0.65 oz | 70 | 1.5 | 13 |
| **Bread Dough:** Frozen, 1 sl., 2 oz | 140 | 2 | 26 |
| Refrigerated: French, 1" slice | 60 | 1 | 13 |
| Wheat; White, 1" slice | 80 | 2 | 14 |
| **Coating Mixes,** av., 2 Tbsp., 1 oz | 100 | 0.5 | 20 |
| **Stuffing:** Average, dry mix, 1 oz | 110 | 1 | 10 |
| Prepared, ½ cup, 4 oz | 180 | 9 | 11 |

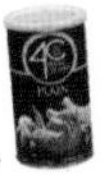

## Quick Guide

### Bagels — C F Cb

*Average All Brands*

**Plain/Onion:**

| | C | F | Cb |
|---|---|---|---|
| 1 mini/bagelette, 1 oz | 65 | 0.5 | 13 |
| 1 small bagel, 2 oz | 145 | 1 | 29 |
| 1 medium bagel, 3 oz | 220 | 1.5 | 43 |
| 1 large bagel, 4 oz | 290 | 2 | 57 |
| **Bagel Chips,** 1 oz | 130 | 4.5 | 19 |
| **Pizza Bagel Bites** (Bagel Bites), average all ,4 pieces, 3 oz | 190 | 5.5 | 27 |
| **Bagel Crisps** (New York Style), average all, 6 crisps, 1 oz | 130 | 5 | 17 |
| **Bagel Thins** (Thomas'), 1, 1.6 oz | 110 | 1 | 25 |

### Bagel Brands

*Per Bagel*

| | C | F | Cb |
|---|---|---|---|
| **Bubba's:** Plain; Onion, average | 220 | 1.5 | 46 |
| Blueberry | 230 | 2 | 49 |
| Cinnamon Raisin | 230 | 1.5 | 48 |
| **Costco Bakery:** Plain | 330 | 1.5 | 70 |
| Cinnamon Raisin | 340 | 1.5 | 73 |
| Honeywheat | 320 | 1.5 | 69 |
| **Enjoy Life,** all types, 3.2 oz | 275 | 6 | 50 |
| **Lenders:** Fresh, NY Style: Plain, 3.3 oz | 240 | 2 | 46 |
| Average other flavors, 3.3 oz | 250 | 1.5 | 51 |
| Mini, Plain, 2 oz | 140 | 0.5 | 29 |
| Whole Grain, 3.3 oz | 250 | 1.5 | 49 |
| Whole Wheat, 3.3 oz | 210 | 1.5 | 41 |
| **Panera Bread:** Blueberry, 4.25 oz | 330 | 1.5 | 68 |
| Cinnamon & Raisin, 3.75 oz | 320 | 2.5 | 64 |
| Everything, 4 oz | 300 | 2.5 | 59 |
| Whole Grain, 4.25 oz | 340 | 2.5 | 67 |
| **Sara Lee:** Mini, average, 1.3 oz | 100 | 0.5 | 20 |
| Plain, 3.35 oz | 260 | 1 | 50 |
| Blueberry, 3.7 oz | 280 | 1 | 54 |
| Cinnamon Raisin, 3.7 oz | 270 | 1 | 54 |
| Everything, 3.7 oz | 280 | 3.5 | 50 |
| Onion, 3 oz | 270 | 1 | 52 |
| **Western,** The Alternatives, av., 2 oz | 110 | 0 | 25 |

### Bagel Spreads

**Cream Cheese:**

| | C | F | Cb |
|---|---|---|---|
| Plain: 2 Tbsp, 1 oz | 100 | 9 | 1 |
| 2 oz mini-tub | 200 | 18 | 2 |
| Reduced Fat: 2 Tbsp, 1 oz | 60 | 5 | 2 |
| 2 oz mini-tub | 120 | 10 | 4 |
| **Flavors:** Lox, 1 oz | 90 | 8 | 2 |
| Honey Nut, 1 oz | 80 | 7 | 4 |
| Strawberry, 1 oz | 90 | 7 | 5 |
| Sundried Tomato, 1 oz | 80 | 7 | 2 |
| Vegetable, 1 oz | 90 | 8 | 2 |

### English Muffins — C F Cb

*Average All Brands*

**Plain/Whole Wheat:**

| | C | F | Cb |
|---|---|---|---|
| Regular, 2 oz | 135 | 1.5 | 26 |
| Heavier, 2½ oz | 155 | 2 | 31 |
| Super Size, 3.2 oz | 190 | 2 | 38 |
| **Raisin-Cinnamon,** 2.2 oz | 150 | 1 | 30 |

**Note:** *Actual weight of packaged muffins can be 10-15% heavier than stated net weight.*

### Rice Cakes

| | C | F | Cb |
|---|---|---|---|
| Reg. size, av.1 cake, 0.32 oz | 35 | 0.5 | 7.5 |
| *Hain,* Mini, plain, 10 pcs | 70 | 2 | 12 |
| *Lundberg,* all types, 0.65 oz | 70 | 0.5 | 14 |
| *Quaker,* Apple Cinnamon, 0.45 oz | 50 | 0 | 11 |

### Tortillas & Shells

**Corn Tortilla:** *Per Single Tortilla*

| | C | F | Cb |
|---|---|---|---|
| White/Yellow: 6", 1 oz | 55 | 1 | 11 |
| 7", 1.2 oz av. | 75 | 1 | 11 |

**Flour Tortilla:** *Per Single Tortilla*

| | C | F | Cb |
|---|---|---|---|
| 6", 1.2 oz | 100 | 3 | 16 |
| 8", 1.4 oz | 130 | 4 | 20 |
| 10", 2.3 oz | 200 | 6 | 31 |
| 12", 3.3 oz | 300 | 9 | 46 |

**Shells:** *Per Single Shell, Without Fillings*

**Taco Shells:**

| | C | F | Cb |
|---|---|---|---|
| Mini, 3", 0.2 oz | 25 | 1 | 3 |
| Medium, 5", 0.5 oz | 60 | 2.5 | 8 |
| Large, 6½", 0.7 oz | 100 | 4.5 | 13 |
| Extra Large, Salad Shell/Bowl (Taco Bell), Fried, 10", 2.4 oz | 360 | 21 | 40 |

**Tostada Shells:**

| | C | F | Cb |
|---|---|---|---|
| White Corn, 5½" diam. 0.4 oz | 55 | 2.5 | 8 |
| Yellow Corn, 5½" diam. 0.5 oz | 80 | 3.5 | 11 |
| **Sopes,** 1 shell, 4", 2 oz, av. | 110 | 1.5 | 23 |

**La Tortilla Factory,**

| | C | F | Cb |
|---|---|---|---|
| **Hand Made Style,** Corn, av., 1.45 oz | 90 | 1 | 14 |
| **Smart & Delicious:** | | | |
| Low Carb: Orig, 1.27 oz | 50 | 2 | 10 |
| Large, 2.19 oz | 80 | 3 | 18 |
| Soft Taco, Flour, 8", 1.5 oz | 130 | 3.5 | 18 |
| **Sonoma Wraps,** av., 2.3 oz | 180 | 6 | 29 |
| **Mission Foods:** | | | |
| **Soft Flour:** Carb Bal. (1), med.,1.48 oz | 120 | 3 | 19 |
| Life Balance (1), medium, 1.44 oz | 120 | 3.5 | 19 |
| Multi-Grain (1), medium, 1.8 oz | 170 | 6 | 24 |
| **White Corn Tortillas:** 2, 1.48 oz | 90 | 1 | 18 |
| Super Sized (1), 1.16 oz | 70 | 1 | 14 |
| **Yellow Corn,** Tortillas, (2), 1.3 oz | 80 | 1 | 16 |

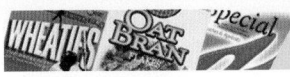

## Quick Guide

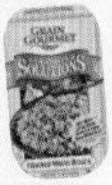

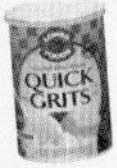

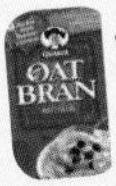

### Cooked Cereals

| | C | F | Cb |
|---|---|---|---|
| **Barley,** pearled, cooked, 1 cup | 195 | 0.5 | 44 |
| **Buckwheat Groats,** roasted: | | | |
| Dry, ½ cup, 3 oz | 285 | 2 | 61 |
| Cooked, 1 cup, 6 oz | 155 | 1 | 34 |
| **Bulgur:** Dry, ½ cup, 2½ oz | 240 | 1 | 53 |
| Cooked, 1 cup, 6½ oz | 150 | 0.5 | 34 |
| **Corn/Hominy Grits:** | | | |
| Dry, ¼ cup, 1.4 oz | 140 | 0.5 | 32 |
| Cooked, ¾ cup, 6½ oz | 110 | 0.5 | 23 |
| Instant: Dry, 0.8 oz packet | 75 | 0 | 18 |
| With Imitation Bacon Bits, 1 oz | 100 | 0.5 | 22 |
| **Cream of Rice,** cooked, ¾ cup, 6½ oz | 95 | 0 | 21 |
| **Cream of Wheat:** | | | |
| Regular, cooked, ¾ cup, 6½ oz | 95 | 0.5 | 20 |
| Quick, cooked, ¾ cup, 6½ oz | 100 | 0.5 | 22 |
| Instant, cooked, ¾ cup, 6½ oz | 105 | 0.5 | 21 |
| **Farina,** cooked, ¾ cup, 6 oz | 95 | 0.5 | 19 |
| **Millet,** dry, ¼ cup, 1¾ oz | 190 | 2 | 36 |
| **Oat Bran:** Raw, ⅓ cup, 1 oz | 70 | 2 | 19 |
| Cooked, ½ cup, 3¾ oz | 45 | 1 | 13 |
| **Oatmeal:** Dry, ⅓ cup, 1 oz | 100 | 1.5 | 18 |
| Regular: Cooked, ¾ cup, 6 oz | 125 | 2.5 | 21 |
| 1 cup, 8 oz | 165 | 3.5 | 28 |
| Instant: Regular, dry, average, 1 oz | 105 | 1.5 | 18 |
| Flavored, dry, average, 1½ oz | 165 | 2 | 34 |
| **Whole Wheat,** cooked, ¾ cup, 6.4 oz | 115 | 0.5 | 25 |

## Brans, Wheat Germ, Add-Ons

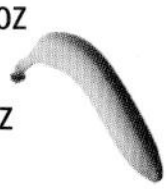

| | C | F | Cb |
|---|---|---|---|
| **Bran:** | | | |
| **Oat Bran:** Raw, 1 Tbsp, 0.18 oz | 10 | 0.5 | 4 |
| ⅓ cup, 1 oz | 70 | 2 | 19 |
| **Rice Bran:** Raw, 1 Tbsp, 0.18 oz | 15 | 1 | 2.5 |
| ¼ cup, 1 oz | 95 | 6 | 15 |
| **Wheat,** unprocessed, | | | |
| 1 Tbsp, 0.10 oz | 5 | 0 | 2 |
| **Wheat Germ:** Raw, 1 Tbsp, ¼ oz | 25 | 0.5 | 4 |
| ¼ cup, 1 oz | 105 | 3 | 15 |
| **Bee Pollen Granules,** 1 Tbsp, 0.28 oz | 25 | 1 | 2 |
| **Fruit:** Dried, average, 1 oz | 70 | 0 | 18 |
| Banana, ½ medium | 55 | 0 | 14 |
| Prunes in Syrup (5), 3 oz | 90 | 0 | 23 |
| **Honey,** 1 Tbsp, ¾ oz | 65 | 0 | 17 |
| **Lecithin Granules,** 1 Tbsp, 0.35 oz | 55 | 4 | 0.5 |
| **Nuts,** Almonds (6), ¼ oz | 40 | 4 | 1.5 |
| **Psyllium Husks,** 1 Tbsp, 0.18 oz | 15 | 0 | 4 |

## Hot/Cooked Cereals ~ Brands

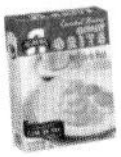

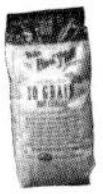

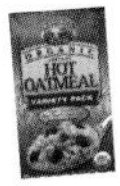

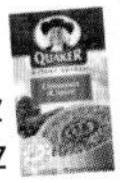

*Per Serving, Dry Mix only*

| | C | F | Cb |
|---|---|---|---|
| **Albers Grits,** | | | |
| ¼ cup, 1.4 oz | 140 | 0.5 | 31 |
| **B&G,** | | | |
| Cream of Wheat, Original, 1 oz | 150 | 1 | 30 |
| **Bobs Red Mill,** | | | |
| 10 Grain, ¼ cup, 1.6 oz | 140 | 1 | 28 |
| **Country Choice,** | | | |
| Quick Oats, ½ cup, 1.4 oz | 150 | 3 | 27 |
| **Dr McDougall's:** | | | |
| **Big Cup Organic Oatmeal:** *Per Cup* | | | |
| Grains: With Cranb. Muesli, 3.1 oz | 320 | 4 | 62 |
| With Peach Raspberry 3 oz | 300 | 4 | 62 |
| 4 Grain with Real Maple, 2.55 oz | 260 | 3 | 52 |
| Organic Instant Oatmeal: Per Packet | | | |
| Original, 1 oz | 120 | 2 | 21 |
| Light Apple Cinnamon, 1.95 oz | 120 | 1.5 | 24 |
| Light Maple Brown Sugar, 1.34 oz | 150 | 2 | 28 |
| **Great Value** *(Walmart),* Inst. Oatmeal: | | | |
| Orig.; Maple & Brown Sugar, av., 1 oz | 100 | 2 | 19 |
| Apple & Cinn.; Peaches & Crm, 1.23 oz | 130 | 1.5 | 27 |
| **McCann's:** | | | |
| **Instant Irish Oatmeal:** | | | |
| Original, 1 oz package | 100 | 2 | 19 |
| Apple & Cinnamon, 1.23 oz | 130 | 1.5 | 27 |
| Maple & Brown Sugar, 1.5 oz | 160 | 2 | 32 |
| **Malt-O-Meal:** Orig., 3Tbsp, 1.2 oz | 130 | 0.5 | 27 |
| Maple Brown Sugar, ¼ cup | 170 | 0 | 37 |
| **Natures Path:** | | | |
| **Oatmeal:** | | | |
| Apple Cinnamon, 1.7 oz | 210 | 2.5 | 40 |
| HempPlus, 1 pkt, 1.4 oz | 160 | 2.5 | 30 |
| Maple Nut, 1.7 oz | 210 | 4 | 38 |
| **NutriSystem,** | | | |
| Oatmeal, Apple Cinnamon, 1 pkt | 130 | 1.5 | 26 |
| **Ocean Spray,** | | | |
| Oatmeal, all flavors, 1.5 oz | 160 | 2 | 33 |
| **Quaker:** | | | |
| **Instant Oatmeal:** *Per Packet Unless Indicated* | | | |
| Regular, Organic 1 oz | 100 | 2 | 19 |
| Cinn. & Spice, 1.5 oz | 160 | 2.5 | 32 |
| Hearty Medley, av.,1.25 oz | 135 | 2.5 | 27 |
| Maple Brown Sugar, 1.5 oz | 160 | 2.5 | 32 |
| Peaches & Cream, 1.23 oz | 130 | 2 | 27 |
| Old Fash'nd/Quick Oats, ½ c., 1.4 oz | 150 | 3 | 27 |
| **Grits:** | | | |
| Instant, av. all types, 1 oz | 100 | 2 | 22 |
| Quick,Original, ¼ cup, 1.3 oz | 130 | 0.5 | 29 |
| **Silver Palate,** Oatmeal, 1.4 oz | 160 | 3 | 26 |

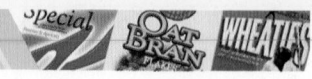

## Quick Guide

### Cold Cereals
*Average All Brands*

| | C | F | Cb |
|---|---|---|---|
| Bran Flakes, ¾ cup, 1 oz | 95 | 0.5 | 24 |
| Corn Flakes, 1 cup, 1 oz | 100 | 0 | 22 |
| Frosted Flakes, ¾ cup, 1 oz | 110 | 0 | 27 |
| Granola, 100% Nat., ½ cup, 1.7 oz | 205 | 6 | 35 |
| Oat Bran Cereal, ½ cup, 1½ oz | 145 | 3 | 25 |
| Puffed Rice, 1 cup, ½ oz | 55 | 0 | 13 |
| Puffed Wheat, 1 cup, ½ oz | 45 | 0 | 10 |
| Raisin Bran, ½ cup, 1 oz | 90 | 0.5 | 22 |
| Rice Crisps, 1 cup, 1 oz | 105 | 0.5 | 24 |
| Shredded Wheat, 1 biscuit, 1 oz | 85 | 0.5 | 20 |
| Wheat Flakes, ¾ cup, 1 oz | 105 | 1 | 24 |

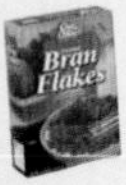

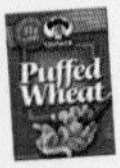

**Breakfast/Cereal Bars/Pop Tarts ~** *See Page 31*

### Ready-To-Eat Cereal

| | C | F | Cb |
|---|---|---|---|
| **Arrowhead Mills:** *Per Cup* | | | |
| **Flakes:** Amaranth, 1.2 oz | 140 | 2 | 26 |
| Kamut, 1.1 oz | 120 | 1 | 25 |
| Maple Buckwheat, 1.5 oz | 170 | 1 | 35 |
| Oat Bran, 1.2 oz | 140 | 2.5 | 24 |
| Rice, sweetened, 1.7 oz | 180 | 1 | 40 |
| Spelt, 1.1 oz | 120 | 1 | 24 |
| **Breadshop Granola:** | | | |
| Crunchy Oat Bran, w/ Almonds, 1.7 oz | 210 | 8 | 33 |
| Triple Berry Crunch, ½ cup, 1.75 oz | 210 | 8 | 34 |
| **Puffed:** Corn, ½ oz | 60 | 1 | 12 |
| Kamut, ½ oz | 50 | 0 | 11 |
| Millet, ½ oz | 60 | 0.5 | 11 |
| Rice, ½ oz | 60 | 0 | 14 |
| Wheat, ½ oz | 60 | 1 | 12 |
| **Shredded Wheat:** Original, 1.7 oz | 190 | 1 | 38 |
| Sweetened, 1.8 oz | 200 | 1 | 42 |
| **Back to Nature:** *Per ½ Cup, Unless Indicated* | | | |
| **Granola:** Apple Blueberry, 1.7 oz | 200 | 2.5 | 39 |
| Chocolate Delight, 1.8 oz | 220 | 6 | 37 |
| Classic, 1.7 oz | 200 | 3 | 39 |
| Cranberry Pecan, 1.65 oz | 180 | 4.5 | 36 |
| Honey Almond, 1.5 oz | 190 | 7 | 29 |
| Organic Cherry Vanilla, 1.75 oz | 200 | 4 | 38 |
| Sunflower & Pumpkin Seed, 1.75 oz | 210 | 7 | 30 |
| Wild Blueberry Walnut, 1.5 oz | 190 | 6 | 30 |

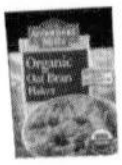

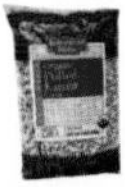

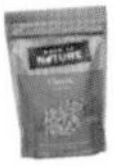

| | C | F | Cb |
|---|---|---|---|
| **Barbara's Bakery:** | | | |
| **Classics, Organic & Sweetened:** | | | |
| Brown Rice Crisps, 1.1 oz | 120 | 1 | 25 |
| Corn Flakes, 1 cup, 1.1 oz | 110 | 1 | 25 |
| Hole n' Oats, Honey Nut, 1.1 oz | 120 | 2 | 24 |
| **High Fiber:** | | | |
| Original, 1.95 oz | 180 | 1.5 | 42 |
| Cranberry, 2 oz | 190 | 1.5 | 42 |
| Flax & Granola, 1 cup, 2 oz | 200 | 3 | 42 |
| **Puffins:** Original, ¾ cup, 0.95 oz | 90 | 1 | 23 |
| Cinnamon, ⅔ cup, 1 oz | 90 | 1 | 26 |
| Multigrain, ¾ cup, 1 oz | 110 | 0 | 25 |
| Peanut Butter, ¾ cup, 1 oz | 110 | 2 | 23 |
| Peanut Butter & Choc., ¾ cup, 1 oz | 110 | 1 | 24 |
| Puffs: Crunchy Cocoa, ¾ c, 1 oz | 120 | 1 | 24 |
| Fruit Medley, ¾ cup, 1.1 oz | 120 | 1 | 26 |
| **Shredded Oats:** Orig., 1½ c, 2 oz | 220 | 2.5 | 46 |
| Cinnamon Crunch, 1 cup, 2 oz | 230 | 3 | 43 |
| Multigrain, ¾ cup, 1 oz | 120 | 1.5 | 24 |
| Vanilla Almond, 1 cup, 2 oz | 220 | 3 | 42 |
| **Cascadian Farm:** | | | |
| French Van. Almond Granola, 1.76 oz | 210 | 5 | 38 |
| Hearty Morning, ¾ cup, 1.9 oz | 200 | 3 | 43 |
| Honey Nut O's, 1 cup, 1 oz | 110 | 1 | 25 |
| Multi Grain Squares, ¾ cup, 1 oz | 110 | 1 | 25 |
| Oats & Honey Granola, ⅔ cup, 2 oz | 230 | 6 | 42 |
| Purely O's, 1 cup, 1.1oz | 110 | 1 | 24 |
| Raisin Bran, 1 cup, 1.9 oz | 180 | 1 | 43 |
| **Crapola,** ½ cup, 2 oz | 230 | 7 | 35 |
| **Emerald:** | | | |
| **Breakfast on the Go:** | | | |
| Breakfast Nut Blend, 1.5 oz | 180 | 7 | 27 |
| Berry Nut Blend, 1.5 oz | 180 | 9 | 24 |
| S'mores Nut Blend, 1.5 oz | 200 | 10 | 24 |
| **Ener-G,** Rice Bran, ½ cup, 2.4 oz | 220 | 14 | 34 |
| **EnviroKidz:** *Per 1 oz* | | | |
| Amazon Frosted Flakes, ⅔ cup | 120 | 0 | 26 |
| Gorilla Munch, ¾ cup | 120 | 0 | 27 |
| Koala Crisp, ¾ cup | 110 | 1 | 25 |
| Leapin Lemur, ¾ cup | 110 | 1 | 25 |
| Panda Puffs, ¾ cup | 130 | 2.5 | 24 |
| **Erewhon:** | | | |
| Corn Flakes, 1 cup, 2 oz | 130 | 0 | 30 |
| Crispy Brown Rice: Original, 1 oz | 110 | 0.5 | 25 |
| Gluten Free, 1 cup, 1 oz | 110 | 0.5 | 25 |
| With Mixed Berries, 1 cup, 1 oz | 120 | 0.5 | 27 |
| Raisin Bran, 1 cup, 1.8 oz | 180 | 1 | 40 |
| Rice Twice, ¾ cup, 1 oz | 120 | 0 | 26 |

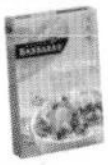

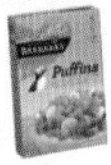

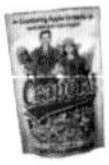

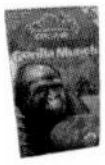

## Ready-To-Eat (Cont)

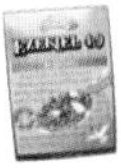
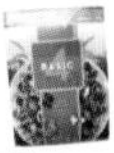
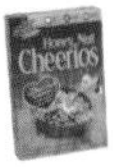
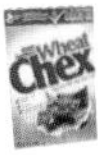
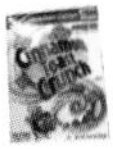
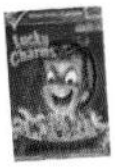
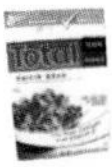

| | C | F | Cb |
|---|---|---|---|
| **Ezekiel 4.9:** | | | |
| **Flourless Cereals:** | | | |
| Original, ½ cup, 2 oz | 190 | 1 | 40 |
| Almond, ½ cup, 2 oz | 200 | 3 | 38 |
| Cinnamon Raisin, 2 oz | 190 | 1 | 41 |
| Golden Flax, ½ cup, 2 oz | 180 | 2.5 | 37 |
| **F-Factor,** Skinnys 'n Fruit, ½ cup | 70 | 1 | 27 |
| **General Mills:** | | | |
| **Basic 4,** 1 cup, 1.9 oz | 200 | 2 | 44 |
| **Cheerios:** *Per ¾ Cup Unless Indicated* | | | |
| Original, 1 oz | 100 | 2 | 20 |
| Apple Cinnamon, 1 oz | 120 | 1.5 | 24 |
| Banana Nut, 1 oz | 100 | 1 | 24 |
| Cinnamon Burst, 1 cup, 1.2 oz | 120 | 2 | 28 |
| Chocolate, 1 oz | 100 | 1.5 | 22 |
| Frosted, 1 oz | 110 | 1 | 23 |
| Fruity, 1 oz | 100 | 1 | 23 |
| Honey Nut, 1 oz | 110 | 1.5 | 22 |
| Multi Grain, 1 oz | 110 | 1 | 23 |
| Oat Cluster Crunch, 1.1 oz | 100 | 1 | 22 |
| Yogurt Burst, all flavors, 1 oz | 120 | 1.5 | 24 |
| **Chex:** Corn, 1 cup, 1 oz | 120 | 0.5 | 26 |
| Chocolate, ¾ cup, 1.1 oz | 130 | 2.5 | 26 |
| Honey Nut, ¾ cup, 1.1 oz | 120 | 1 | 28 |
| Multi-Bran, ¾ cup, 1.6 oz | 160 | 1.5 | 39 |
| Rice, 1 cup, 1 oz | 100 | 0 | 23 |
| Wheat, ¾ cup, 1.6 oz | 160 | 1 | 39 |
| **Cinnamon Toast Crunch,** ¾ cup, 1.2 oz | 130 | 3 | 25 |
| **Cocoa Puffs,** ¾ cup, 1 oz | 100 | 1.5 | 23 |
| **Count Chocula,** ¾ cup, 1 oz | 100 | 1.5 | 23 |
| **Fiber One:** Original, 1/2 cup, 1 oz | 60 | 1 | 25 |
| Honey Clusters, 1 cup | 160 | 1.5 | 44 |
| 80 Calorie Honey Squares, ¾ cup | 80 | 1 | 25 |
| **Golden Grahams,** 3/4 cup, 1 oz | 120 | 1 | 26 |
| **Honey Nut Clusters,** 1 cup, 2 oz | 210 | 1 | 48 |
| **Kix,** 1¼ cups, 1 oz | 110 | 1 | 25 |
| **Lucky Charms,** average, ¾ cup, 1 oz | 110 | 1 | 22 |
| **Oatmeal Crisp,** Almond, 1 cup, 2 oz | 240 | 4 | 47 |
| **Raisin Nut Bran,** 3/4 cup, 1¾ oz | 180 | 3 | 39 |
| **Reese's Puffs,** 3/4 cup, 1 oz | 120 | 3 | 22 |
| **Total:** Cinn. Crunch, 1 cup | 190 | 2.5 | 40 |
| Plus Omega-3s, 1.8 oz | 200 | 3.5 | 39 |
| Raisin Bran, 1 cup, 1.9 oz | 160 | 1 | 40 |
| **Wheaties,** ¾ cup, 1 oz | 100 | 0.5 | 22 |

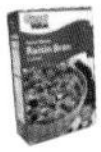
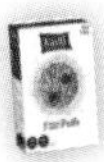

| | C | F | Cb |
|---|---|---|---|
| **Great Value** *(Walmart):* | | | |
| Apple Blasts, 1 c., 1.16 oz | 120 | 0 | 29 |
| Frosted Shredded Wheat, 1.83 oz | 180 | 11 | 42 |
| Fruit Spins, 1 cup, 1 oz | 110 | 1 | 25 |
| Honey Crunch, ¾ cup, 1 oz | 100 | 0 | 24 |
| Raisin Bran, 1 cup, 2 oz | 200 | 1 | 43 |
| Vanilla Alm. Awake, ¾ cup, 1.1 oz | 120 | 1 | 25 |
| **Health Valley:** | | | |
| **Organic Flakes:** | | | |
| Amaranth Flakes, 1¼ cups, 1.8 oz | 210 | 2 | 43 |
| Cranberry Crunch, ¾ cup, 1.8 oz | 190 | 4 | 38 |
| Fiber 7, Multigrain Flakes, 1 c., 1.7 oz | 160 | 1 | 37 |
| Golden Flax, 1 cup, 1¾ oz | 190 | 3.5 | 37 |
| Oat Bran Flakes: 1 cup, 1¾ oz | 190 | 1.5 | 39 |
| With Raisins, 1 cup, 1.9 oz | 200 | 1.5 | 43 |
| **Crunch-Ems!,** Rice; Corn, 1 cup, 1 oz | 110 | 0 | 27 |
| **Heart Wise,** 1 cup, 1.9 oz | 200 | 3 | 37 |
| **Heartland:** | | | |
| **Granola:** Original, ½ cup, 2¼ oz | 240 | 6 | 40 |
| Balanced Blend, ⅔ cup, 1.8 oz | 210 | 3 | 41 |
| Low-Fat Raisin, ½ cup, 2 oz | 200 | 3 | 40 |
| **Kashi:** | | | |
| **7 Whole Grain:** Flakes, 1 c., 1.8 oz | 180 | 1 | 41 |
| Honey Puffs, 1 cup, 1.1 oz | 120 | 1 | 25 |
| Nuggets, 1/2 cup, 2 oz | 210 | 1.5 | 47 |
| Puffs, 1 cup, 0.67 oz | 70 | 0.5 | 15 |
| **GoLEAN:** Original, 1 cup, 1.8 oz | 140 | 1 | 30 |
| Crunch!: Original, 1 cup, 1.9 oz | 190 | 3 | 37 |
| Honey Almond Flax, 1 cup, 1.9 oz | 200 | 4.5 | 36 |
| **Good Friends:** Orig., 1 cup, 1.9 oz | 160 | 1.5 | 42 |
| Cinna-Raisin Crunch, 1 cup, 1.8 oz | 160 | 1.5 | 40 |
| **Granola:** Cocoa Beach, ½ cup, 1.9 oz | 230 | 9 | 36 |
| Mountain Medley, ½ cup, 1.9 oz | 220 | 7 | 38 |
| Summer Berry, ½ cup, 1.9 oz | 220 | 6 | 39 |
| **Heart to Heart:** | | | |
| Honey Toasted Oat, ¾ cup, 1.2 oz | 120 | 1.5 | 26 |
| Oat Flakes & Blueb. Clusters, 1 c. | 200 | 2 | 44 |
| Warm Cinnamon Oat, ¾ cup, 1.2 oz | 120 | 1.5 | 25 |
| **Kashi U,** Blackcurrant & Walnuts, 1 c. | 200 | 3.5 | 42 |
| **Whole Wheat Biscuit:** | | | |
| Autumn Wheat, 1 cup, 1.9 oz | 180 | 1 | 43 |
| Cinnamon Harvest, 1 cup, 1.9 oz | 180 | 1 | 43 |
| Island Vanilla, 1 cup, 1.9 oz | 190 | 1 | 44 |

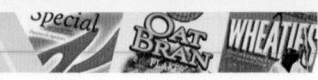

| Ready-To-Eat (Cont) | C | F | Cb |
|---|---|---|---|
| **Kellogg's:** | | | |
| **All-Bran:** Original, ½ cup, 1.1 oz | 80 | 1 | 23 |
| Bran Buds, ⅓ cup, 1.1 oz | 70 | 1 | 24 |
| Complete Wheat Flakes, ¾ cup, 1.1 oz | 90 | 0.5 | 23 |
| **Apple Jacks,** 1 cup, 1 oz | 100 | 0.5 | 25 |
| **Cinnabon,** 1 cup, 1.1 oz | 120 | 2 | 25 |
| **Cocoa Krispies,** ¾ cup, 1.1 oz | 120 | 1 | 27 |
| **Corn Flakes:** Original, 1 cup, 1 oz | 100 | 0 | 24 |
| Simply Cinnamon, 1 cup, 1.1oz | 120 | 0 | 27 |
| **Corn Pops,** 1 cup, 1.1 oz | 120 | 0 | 29 |
| **Cracklin' Oat Bran,** | | | |
| ¾ cup, 1.8 oz | 200 | 7 | 35 |
| **Crispix,** Original, 1 cup, 1 oz | 110 | 0 | 25 |
| **Crunchy Nut:** Flakes, ¾ cup, 1.1 oz | 120 | 1 | 27 |
| Roasted Nut & Honey, ¾ cup, 1oz | 100 | 1 | 23 |
| **Fiber Plus,** | | | |
| Caramel Pecan, ¾ cup, 1.7 oz | 170 | 1.5 | 43 |
| **Fruit Loops:** Original, 1 cup, 1 oz | 110 | 1 | 25 |
| Marshmallow, 1 cup, 1.1 oz | 110 | 1 | 25 |
| **Frosted Flakes:** Orig., ¾ cup, 1.1 oz | 110 | 1 | 27 |
| With Fiber, Less Sugar, | | | |
| 1 cup, 1.1 oz | 110 | 0 | 26 |
| **Granola,** Low-Fat: | | | |
| With Raisins, ⅔ cup, 2.1 oz | 230 | 3 | 48 |
| Without Raisins, ½ cup, 1.7 oz | 190 | 2.5 | 40 |
| **Honey Smacks,** ¾ cup, 1 oz | 100 | 0.5 | 24 |
| **Mini-Wheats:** Frosted Big Bite (5) | 180 | 1 | 41 |
| Frosted: Bite Size (24), 2.1 oz | 200 | 1 | 48 |
| Blueberry Muffin (24) | 180 | 1 | 43 |
| Fruit In Middle (21) | 190 | 1 | 45 |
| Little Bites: Original (51) | 190 | 1 | 46 |
| Chocolate (52) | 200 | 2 | 45 |
| Unfrosted (30), 2.1 oz | 200 | 1.5 | 46 |
| **Mueslix,** ⅔ cup, 2 oz | 200 | 3 | 40 |
| **Nutri-Grain Bars** ~ *See Page 31* | | | |
| **Product 19,** 1 cup, 1.1 oz | 100 | 0 | 25 |
| **Raisin Bran:** Regular, 1 cup, 2.1 oz | 190 | 1 | 46 |
| Extra, 1 cup, 1.7 oz | 170 | 2.5 | 38 |
| **Rice Krispies:** Original, 1¼ cups | 130 | 0 | 29 |
| Cocoa, ¾ cup, 1.1 oz | 120 | 1 | 27 |
| Frosted, ¾ cup, 1.1 oz | 110 | 0 | 27 |
| Gluten Free, 1.1 oz | 110 | 1 | 25 |
| Treats, ¾ cup, 1.1 oz | 120 | 1 | 26 |
| **Smart Start,** | | | |
| Antioxidants, 1 cup, 1.8 oz | 190 | 0.5 | 43 |

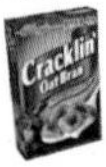

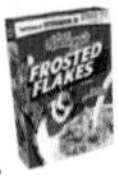

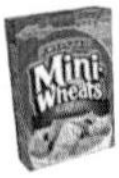

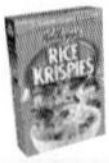

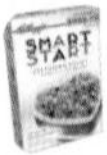

| Kellogg's (Cont) | C | F | Cb |
|---|---|---|---|
| **Special K:** Original 1 cup, 1.1 oz | 120 | 0.5 | 23 |
| Blueberry, ¾ cup, 1.1 oz | 110 | 0 | 26 |
| Fruit & Yogurt, ¾ cup, 1.1 oz | 120 | 1 | 27 |
| Red Berries, 1 cup, 1.1 oz | 110 | 0 | 27 |
| Vanilla Almond, ¾ cup | 110 | 1.5 | 25 |
| Low Fat Granola, | | | |
| ½ cup, 1.8 oz | 190 | 3 | 39 |
| **Kozy Shack:** | | | |
| **Ready Grains:** *Per 7 oz Pkg* | | | |
| Original | 180 | 2.5 | 29 |
| Apple & Cinnamon | 210 | 2 | 38 |
| Maple Brown Sugar | 180 | 2 | 31 |
| Strawberry | 210 | 2 | 37 |
| **Malt-O-Meal:** | | | |
| Apple Zings, 1 cup, 1.1 oz | 130 | 1 | 30 |
| Blueb. Muffin Tops, ¾ cup | 130 | 3.5 | 24 |
| Cocoa Dyno-Bites, ¾ cup | 120 | 1 | 26 |
| Coco Roos, ¾ cup, 1 oz | 120 | 1.5 | 26 |
| Colossal/Berry Crunch, ¾ cup, 1.1 oz | 120 | 1.5 | 26 |
| Frosted Flakes, ¾ cup, 1 oz | 120 | 0 | 28 |
| Frosted Mini Spooners, 1 c. | 190 | 1 | 45 |
| Golden Puffs, ¾ cup, 1 oz | 110 | 0 | 24 |
| Honey Nut Scooters, 1 cup, 1 oz | 110 | 1.5 | 24 |
| Raisin Bran, 1 cup, 1.7 oz | 220 | 1.5 | 49 |
| **Natural Ovens,** | | | |
| Great Granola, ½ cup, 2 oz | 250 | 9 | 36 |
| **Nature's Path:** | | | |
| Heritage, average, ¾ cup, 1 oz | 120 | 1 | 24 |
| Honey'd Cornflakes, ¾ cup, 1 oz | 120 | 0 | 26 |
| Multigr. Oatbran Flakes, ¾ cup, 1 oz | 110 | 1 | 24 |
| **Flax Plus:** Maple Pecan Cr., ¾ cup | 220 | 7 | 38 |
| Pumpkin Raisin Crunch, ¾ cup | 210 | 4.5 | 40 |
| Raisin Bran Flakes, ¾ cup, 2 oz | 190 | 2.5 | 41 |
| Kamut Puffs, 1 cup, ½ oz | 50 | 0 | 11 |
| **Optimum:** Banana Almond, 1.9 oz | 190 | 6 | 35 |
| Blueberry Cinnamon, 1 cup 2 oz | 200 | 3 | 38 |
| **New England Natural Bakers:** | | | |
| **Granola Pouches:** | | | |
| Organic Crispy Fruity, ⅔ cup, 1.9 oz | 250 | 9 | 39 |
| All Natural: | | | |
| Banana Walnut, ½ cup, 1.95 oz | 260 | 12 | 34 |
| Honey Nut Cinn., ½ cup, 2.1 oz | 270 | 12 | 35 |
| **Organic Muesli,** ½ cup, 2.1 oz | 220 | 5 | 40 |

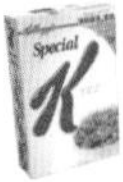

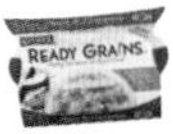

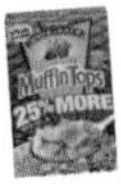

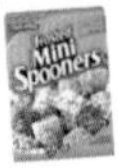

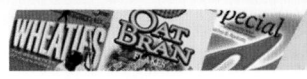

### Ready-To-Eat (Cont)

| | C | F | Cb |
|---|---|---|---|
| **New Morning:** | | | |
| Fruit-e-O's, Organic, 1 cup, 1 oz | 120 | 1.5 | 25 |
| Grahams: Cinnamon (2), 1.1 oz | 130 | 2.5 | 24 |
| Honey (2), 1.1 oz | 130 | 3 | 24 |
| Oatios, Original, 1 cup, 1 oz | 110 | 2 | 22 |
| **NutriSystem:** *Per Packet* | | | |
| Granola, Low-Fat | 160 | 2.5 | 31 |
| NutriCinnamon Squares | 120 | 0.5 | 23 |
| NutriFlakes (40% Bran Flakes) | 110 | 1 | 23 |
| NutriFrosted Crunch | 120 | 0.5 | 24 |
| **Peace:** | | | |
| Clusters & Flakes, av. all flav., 1.95 oz | 225 | 2.5 | 46 |
| Crispy Rice & Flakes, | | | |
| Blueberry Pomegranate, 1.95 oz | 240 | 6 | 41 |
| Hearty Raisin Bran, 1.95 oz | 190 | 2 | 44 |
| Granola, average all varieties, ⅔ cup | 240 | 6 | 41 |
| **Post:** | | | |
| Alpha Bits, 1 cup, 1 oz | 110 | 1 | 23 |
| Bran Flakes, ¾ cup, 1 oz | 100 | 0.5 | 24 |
| Grape-Nuts: Original, ½ cup | 200 | 1 | 48 |
| Flakes, ¾ cup, 1 oz | 110 | 1 | 24 |
| Great Grains, ¾ cup, 2 oz, average | 205 | 4 | 38 |
| **Honey Bunches of Oats:** | | | |
| With Almonds, ¾ cup | 130 | 2.5 | 25 |
| With Van. Bunches, 1 cup | 220 | 3 | 46 |
| Raisin Medley, 1 cup | 200 | 2 | 42 |
| Average other varieties, ¾ cup | 120 | 1.5 | 25 |
| Just Bunches, | | | |
| Cinnamon; Honey, av., ⅔ cup | 250 | 7 | 43 |
| Honeycomb, Cinna Graham, 1½ cups | 130 | 1.5 | 27 |
| Pebbles, all flavors, ¾ cup | 120 | 1 | 26 |
| Raisin Bran, 1 cup | 190 | 1 | 46 |
| Selects: Banana Nut Crunch, 1 cup | 240 | 6 | 44 |
| Maple Pecan Crunch, ¾ cup | 220 | 5 | 40 |
| Waffle Crisp, 1 cup, 1 oz | 120 | 2.5 | 25 |
| **Quaker:** | | | |
| **100% Natural Granola:** | | | |
| Oats & Honey, ½ cup, 1.7 oz | 200 | 6 | 35 |
| Oats & Honey & Raisins, 1.8 oz | 210 | 5 | 38 |
| Low-Fat, ⅔ cup, 1.95 oz | 210 | 3 | 45 |
| **Cap 'n Crunch:** Original, ¾ cup, 1 oz | 110 | 1.5 | 23 |
| Crunch Berries, ¾ cup, 1 oz | 100 | 1.5 | 22 |
| Peanut Butter, ¾ cup, 1 oz | 110 | 2.5 | 21 |
| Oat Bran, 1¼ cups, 2 oz | 210 | 3 | 43 |
| Oatmeal Squares, Brown Sugar, 1 c. | 210 | 2.5 | 44 |

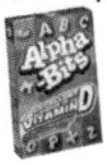

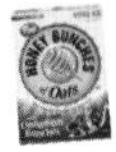

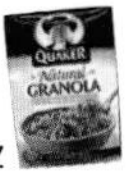

| **Quaker (Cont):** | C | F | Cb |
|---|---|---|---|
| Crunchy Corn Bran, ¾ cup, 1 oz | 90 | 1 | 23 |
| Honey Graham Oh's, ¾ cup | 110 | 2 | 23 |
| King Vitaman, 1½ c., 1.1 oz | 120 | 1 | 26 |
| Life, all types, ¾ cup, 1.1 oz | 120 | 1.5 | 26 |
| **Sweet Home Farm:** | | | |
| Honey Nut Granola, ½ cup, 1.9 oz | 250 | 10 | 37 |
| Low-Fat Granola, ½ cup, 1.9 oz | 210 | 3 | 44 |
| **Trader Joe's:** | | | |
| **Clusters:** Raisin Bran, 1 cup, 2 oz | 190 | 3 | 41 |
| Super Nutty Toffee, ¾ cup, 2 oz | 250 | 9 | 38 |
| Average all other flavors | | | |
| ⅔ cup, 1.3 oz | 145 | 3.5 | 26 |
| 1 cup, 2 oz | 220 | 5 | 39 |
| Cornflakes, 1 cup, 1.1 oz | 110 | 0 | 26 |
| Golden Flax Cereal, ¾ cup, 1.7 oz | 200 | 3.5 | 37 |
| Granola: Mango Passion, 2 oz | 240 | 8 | 37 |
| Pecan Praline, ½ cup, 1.65 oz | 210 | 7 | 31 |
| Trek Mix, ⅔ cup, 2 oz | 240 | 8 | 37 |
| High Fiber, ⅔ cup, 1 oz | 80 | 0.5 | 23 |
| Honey Nut O's, ¾ cup, 1 oz | 120 | 1.5 | 24 |
| Joe's O's, 1 cup, 1 oz | 110 | 1.5 | 22 |
| Morning Lite, 1 cup, 1.85 oz | 170 | 2.5 | 40 |
| Shredded Wheats, Bite Size, 1 c., 1.7 oz | 180 | 1 | 38 |
| Triple Berry O's, ¾ cup, 1 oz | 110 | 1 | 25 |
| Toasted Oatmeal Flakes, ¾ cup, 1.1 oz | 110 | 1 | 23 |
| Wheats, average, 1 cup, 2 oz | 200 | 1 | 42 |
| **Twigs,** Flakes & Clusters, 1 c., 1.9 oz | 170 | 1.5 | 41 |
| **Udi's,** Granola, Au Naturel, ½ cup, 2 oz | 240 | 8 | 38 |
| **Uncle Sam:** | | | |
| Original, ¾ cup, 1.95 oz | 190 | 5 | 38 |
| Strawberry, ¾ cup, 2.1 oz | 240 | 5 | 40 |
| **Weetabix:** | | | |
| 2 biscuits, 1.3 oz | 130 | 0.5 | 29 |
| Crispy Flakes: Original, ¾ cup, 1.1 oz | 110 | 0.5 | 24 |
| and Fiber, 1¼ cup, 2 oz | 170 | 1.5 | 44 |
| **Whole Foods (365):** | | | |
| Corn Flakes, 1 cup, 1 oz | 110 | 0 | 26 |
| Honey Puffed Wheat, 1 oz | 110 | 0 | 24 |
| Frosted Flakes, ¾ cup, 1 oz | 110 | 0 | 27 |
| Oat Bran Flakes, 1 cup, 2 oz | 220 | 2.5 | 44 |
| Raisin Bran, 1 cup, 2 oz | 200 | 0.5 | 44 |
| Shredded Wheat: Reg., 1 cup, 1.7 oz | 180 | 1 | 38 |
| Frosted, 1 cup, 2 oz | 210 | 1 | 45 |

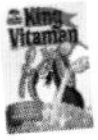

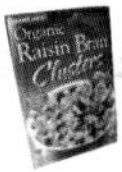

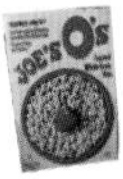

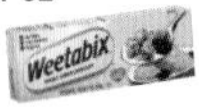

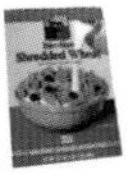

## Ready-to-Eat

| | C | F | Cb |
|---|---|---|---|
| **Angel Food:** Plain: W/out oil, 2 oz | 145 | 0 | 33 |
| With oil, 2 oz | 145 | 1 | 27 |
| With Cream Frosting | 255 | 7 | 45 |
| **Almond Croissant,** 5 oz | 620 | 35 | 67 |
| **Apple Danish,** 5 oz | 450 | 18 | 67 |
| **Apple Pie** ~ *See Pies/Tarts Page 134* | | | |
| **Baklava,** 1½" square, 1.75 oz | 200 | 10 | 27 |
| **Banana,** with Butter Cream, 2 oz | 230 | 9 | 37 |
| **Banana Walnut,** 3 oz | 270 | 11 | 40 |
| **Bear Claw,** 4.5 oz | 540 | 24 | 71 |
| **Black Forest,** 3 oz slice, (½ cake) | 345 | 11 | 59 |
| **Brownie:** Small, 2" Square, 1 oz | 130 | 8 | 14 |
| Large, 3 oz | 390 | 24 | 42 |
| **Bundt:** Average all types, | | | |
| 3 oz slice, (⅒ cake) | 300 | 13 | 42 |
| Mini-Bundt, 5 oz | 500 | 22 | 70 |
| **Cannoli** | 375 | 17 | 44 |
| **Carrot Cake:** Plain, 3 oz | 300 | 16 | 37 |
| With Cream Cheese Frosting | 400 | 22 | 48 |
| **Cheesecake:** Small serving, 3 oz | 235 | 13 | 26 |
| Large serving, 5 oz | 395 | 21 | 44 |
| With Low-Fat Cheese/Fruit, 3 oz | 170 | 4 | 28 |
| *Denny's,* NY Style, 5oz slice | 510 | 34 | 43 |
| **Chocolate Cake:** | | | |
| Plain: With chocolate frosting, 4 oz | 415 | 18 | 62 |
| Without frosting, ½₂ of 9", 3.5 oz | 340 | 14 | 51 |
| **Chocolate Croissant,** 4.25 oz | 470 | 26 | 46 |
| **Chocolate Eclair,** w/ Custard, 3.5 oz | 260 | 16 | 24 |
| **Chocolate Fudge Cake,** 3 oz | 270 | 12 | 40 |
| **Chocolate Meringue,** ⅙ pie | 320 | 13 | 48 |
| **Churros,** 1 stick, 1.5 oz | 165 | 8 | 21 |
| **Cinnamon Crumb Cake,** 2.5 oz | 260 | 9 | 40 |
| **Cinnamon Roll:** Small, 2 oz | 220 | 8 | 34 |
| Regular, 4 oz | 440 | 16 | 68 |
| Large, 6 oz | 660 | 24 | 102 |
| **Brands** ~ *See Page 67* | | | |
| **Coffee Cake,** 2 oz | 180 | 6 | 30 |
| **Concha:** Small, 2 oz | 240 | 9 | 33 |
| Large (5" diameter), 5.5 oz | 615 | 23 | 85 |
| **Cream Puff,** (custard fill), 4.6 oz | 335 | 20 | 30 |
| **Cream Horn,** (1), 3 oz | 210 | 5 | 36 |
| **Crumble Coffee Cake,** 4.5 oz | 500 | 25 | 65 |
| **Danish Pastry:** | | | |
| Small, 2.5 oz | 250 | 14 | 25 |
| Large, 5 oz | 500 | 28 | 50 |
| **Donuts** ~ *See Page 66* | | | |
| **Eclair,** Chocolate, Custard fill, 3.5 oz | 260 | 16 | 24 |
| **Fig Bar,** (1), average | 160 | 3 | 31 |

## Ready-to-Eat (Cont)

| | C | F | Cb |
|---|---|---|---|
| **Fruit Cake,** Dark/Light, 2 oz | 185 | 5 | 34 |
| **Fudge Nut Brownie,** (1), 3.5 oz | 380 | 18 | 54 |
| **Gingerbread,** from mix, 3" square | 210 | 4 | 41 |
| **Honey Bun,** (1), 2.7 oz | 310 | 15 | 39 |
| **Jelly Roll,** ½₂ roll, 1.8 oz | 150 | 2 | 32 |
| **Key Lime Pie,** 4.3 oz | 400 | 25 | 41 |
| **Lady Fingers,** 3 oz | 310 | 4.5 | 59 |
| **Lemon Cake,** 4 oz | 440 | 24 | 49 |
| **Lemon Poppy Seed Creme,** 1.6 oz | 180 | 9 | 23 |
| **Marble Cake,** 1 slice, 4 oz | 430 | 23 | 50 |
| **Mississippi Mud Pie,** 4 oz | 480 | 22 | 67 |
| **Mud Cake,** 1 slice, 4.5 oz | 380 | 20 | 44 |
| **Muffins** ~ *See Page 67* | | | |
| **Palmier Cookie,** large, 4.5 oz | 490 | 25 | 62 |
| **Pineapple Upside Down,** 2.5 oz | 230 | 9 | 36 |
| **Peach Melba,** 3.5 oz | 300 | 8 | 52 |
| **Pecan Sticky Roll,** 6.5 oz | 690 | 22 | 91 |
| **Pecan Twirls,** 1 piece, 1.3 oz | 170 | 7 | 26 |
| **Pies & Tarts** ~ *See Page 134* | | | |
| **Pound Cakes:** Iced Lemon, 3.5 oz | 360 | 17 | 50 |
| Marble, 3.75 oz | 350 | 13 | 53 |
| **Raspberry Rugulah,** | | | |
| 1 piece, 1.2 oz | 110 | 9 | 7 |
| **Scone,** fruit, 2 oz | 200 | 9 | 30 |
| **Sponge:** Plain, 2.5 oz | 220 | 10 | 33 |
| With Chocolate Frosting | 290 | 12 | 45 |
| With Cream & Strawberry Jam | 390 | 12 | 69 |
| **Starbucks Cakes** ~ *Page 244* | | | |
| **Strawberry Creme,** 4.7 oz | 400 | 27 | 33 |
| **Strudel Bites,** ¾ oz | 60 | 2.5 | 9 |
| **Strudel,** fruit, av., 4.4 oz | 300 | 17 | 32 |
| **Swiss Rolls,** (2) | 270 | 12 | 38 |
| **Tiramisu,** 4.4 oz | 440 | 22 | 34 |
| **Turnovers,** fruit, average, 3 oz | 290 | 15 | 35 |

## Cupcakes

| | C | F | Cb |
|---|---|---|---|
| *Average all Varieties* | | | |
| **Regular:** | | | |
| Cake only, 1.5 oz | 140 | 5.5 | 20 |
| Cake + Icing, 2.5 oz | 260 | 13 | 34 |
| Large (Muffin Size): | | | |
| Cake only, 2.5 oz | 235 | 9 | 34 |
| Cake + Icing, 5 oz | 520 | 27 | 67 |
| **Mini,** (2-Bite): | | | |
| Cake only, 0.4 oz | 40 | 1.5 | 5.5 |
| Cake + Icing, 1 oz | 110 | 5.5 | 13 |
| **Icing Only:** Per 1 oz | 115 | 7 | 13 |
| Thick/Tall amount, 2.5 oz | 290 | 17 | 32 |
| Very Berry | 350 | 10 | 58 |

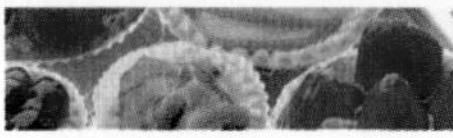

## Cakes ~ Brands

| | C | F | Cb |
|---|---|---|---|
| **Albertson's Bakery:** | | | |
| **Ring Cakes:** *Per ⅛ Cake* | | | |
| Angle Food, 2 oz | **160** | 0 | 36 |
| Butter, 3 oz | **310** | 16 | 39 |
| Chocolate, 3 oz | **300** | 14 | 38 |
| **Cake Slices:** | | | |
| Banana Nut Loaf | **330** | 17 | 39 |
| Butter Creme | **110** | 6 | 20 |
| Creme Cake (2), 3.17 oz | **300** | 12 | 43 |
| Cinnamon Streusel (2), 3.17 oz | **350** | 18 | 43 |
| **Bimbo:** | | | |
| Concha, Vanilla, 2.1 oz | **260** | 11 | 35 |
| Mini Pound Cake, 1.76 oz | **170** | 4.5 | 29 |
| Pecan Pound Cake, 2.25 oz | **260** | 11 | 36 |
| Raisin Pound Cake, 2.25 oz | **240** | 9 | 38 |
| **Bon Appetit:** | | | |
| Banana Bread | **440** | 25 | 49 |
| Cream Cheese Cake, 4 oz | **430** | 24 | 49 |
| Walnut Brownie, 3.5 oz | **380** | 18 | 54 |
| Sliced: Cheesecake, 4 oz | **430** | 24 | 49 |
| Lemon Cake, 4 oz | **430** | 24 | 49 |
| Marble Cake, 4 oz | **430** | 24 | 50 |
| **Danish:** Apple (1), 5 oz | **420** | 22 | 50 |
| Bear Claw (1), 5 oz | **480** | 26 | 54 |
| Cheese & Berries (1), 5 oz | **500** | 28 | 52 |
| Vienna Cream (1), 5 oz | **480** | 28 | 54 |
| **Cheesecake Factory** ~ *See Fast-Foods Section* | | | |
| **Entenmann's:** | | | |
| **Crumb Cakes:** All Butter French, 1.75 oz | **210** | 10 | 29 |
| Average other vrieties, ⅒, 2 oz | **255** | 13 | 34 |
| **Danish:** Pecan Danish Ring, ⅛, 2 oz | **240** | 15 | 24 |
| Cheese-Filled Crumb Coffee, ⅑, 1.9 oz | **200** | 10 | 25 |
| Raspberry Danish Twist, ⅛, 2 oz | **220** | 11 | 29 |
| **Dessert Cakes:** Ban. Crunch, ⅛, 2 oz | **230** | 10 | 33 |
| Carrot, Iced, ⅛ cake | **280** | 13 | 39 |
| Chocolate Fudge, ⅛, 2.5 oz | **270** | 11 | 40 |
| **Muffins/Sweet Rolls** ~ *See Page 67* | | | |
| **Glenny's:** | | | |
| **100 Calorie Brownies:** *Per Brownie* | | | |
| Original, Chocolate Chip, 1.45 oz | **100** | 4 | 12 |
| Blondie, 1.45 oz | **100** | 4 | 15 |
| Peanut Butter, 1.45 oz | **100** | 4 | 15 |

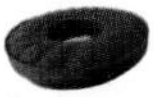
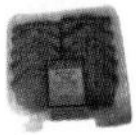
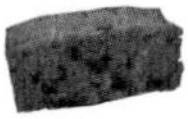
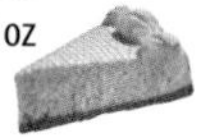
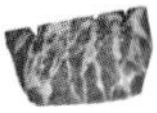

**Updated Nutrition Data ~ www.CalorieKing.com**
**Persons with Diabetes ~ See Disclaimer (Page 22)**

| | C | F | Cb |
|---|---|---|---|
| **Great American Cookies:** | | | |
| **Cookie Cakes:** *Per Slice* | | | |
| By the Slice, 4.6 oz | **580** | 27 | 83 |
| Heart Shaped, 3.5 oz | **440** | 21 | 64 |
| M&M, 1 slice, 4 oz | **500** | 24 | 73 |
| **Great Value** *(Walmart):* | | | |
| Choc. Cup Cake (1) | **170** | 5 | 31 |
| Devil's Food Cake (1) | **160** | 7 | 23 |
| Swiss Rolls (2), 2.2 oz | **240** | 10 | 35 |
| **Hostess:** | | | |
| 100 Calorie Packs, | | | |
| Coffee Cakes, Cinn. Streusel (3) | **100** | 3 | 21 |
| Cinnamon Streusel Cake (1) | **150** | 5 | 26 |
| Chocodiles | **240** | 11 | 33 |
| Cupcakes: Chocolate (1), 1.76 oz | **180** | 7 | 29 |
| Orange (2), 3.74 oz | **410** | 14 | 68 |
| Ding Dongs (2), 2.82 oz | **360** | 19 | 47 |
| Ho Ho's (3), 3 oz | **370** | 17 | 54 |
| Sno Balls (2) | **360** | 11 | 61 |
| Suzy Q, (2), 4 oz | **440** | 18 | 68 |
| **Pies,** Apple/Cherry, av.,4.5 oz | **475** | 20 | 70 |
| **Twinkies,** 1 cake, 1.5 oz | **150** | 4.5 | 27 |
| Fried Twinkie | **360** | 28 | 26 |
| **Zingers:** | | | |
| Chocolate (1) | **150** | 5 | 25 |
| Devils Food (3) | **440** | 15 | 74 |
| Raspberry (3) | **480** | 20 | 71 |
| Vanilla (3) | **470** | 16 | 81 |
| **Kroger:** | | | |
| Cinnamon Rolls: With Icing | **150** | 5 | 23 |
| Reduced Fat | **140** | 3.5 | 24 |
| **Little Debbie:** | | | |
| 100 Calories: Choc. Cake (1), 1 oz | **100** | 3 | 17 |
| Yellow Cake with Icing (1), 1 oz | **100** | 3 | 18 |
| Brownie: Choc Chip (1), 2.2 oz | **270** | 11 | 41 |
| Fudge (1), 2.15 oz | **280** | 12 | 40 |
| Choc. Cup Cake (1) | **210** | 8 | 33 |
| Coffee Cake (1) | **190** | 5 | 35 |
| Devil Creme (1), 1.65 oz | **200** | 9 | 29 |
| Devil Squares (2), 2.2 oz | **260** | 11 | 38 |
| Fancy Cake (2) | **300** | 13 | 44 |
| Frosted Fudge Cake, 1.5 oz | **190** | 9 | 27 |
| Star Crunch (1) | **150** | 6 | 22 |
| S'mores (1) | **190** | 7 | 30 |
| Strawberry Shortcake Roll, 2.1 oz | **240** | 9 | 40 |
| Swiss Cake Roll (2), 2.15 oz | **270** | 12 | 38 |
| Zebra Cake (2), 2.6 oz | **320** | 14 | 48 |
| **Nemo's:** | | | |
| **Cake Squares:** Banana, 3 oz | **300** | 12 | 45 |
| Carrot, 3.6 oz | **390** | 21 | 47 |
| Chocolate, 3 oz | **300** | 12 | 44 |
| **Crumble Cake:** Blueberry (1), 3.9 oz | **390** | 17 | 54 |
| Cinnamon Streusel (1), 3.9 oz | **420** | 18 | 59 |
| Lemon Raspberry (1), 3.9 oz | **400** | 19 | 55 |

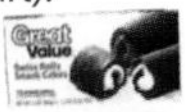

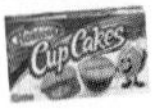

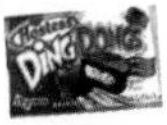

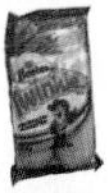
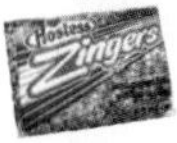

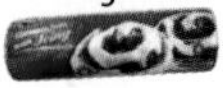
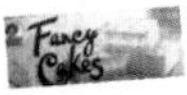

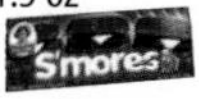

## Cakes ~ Brands (Cont)

| | C | F | Cb |
|---|---|---|---|
| **Oreo:** | | | |
| **Brownie,** | | | |
| Creme Filled, 1.5 oz | 190 | 9 | 25 |
| **Soft Cakesters:** | | | |
| Chocolate (2), 2 oz | 250 | 12 | 36 |
| Double Stuf (2), 2.65 oz pkt | 350 | 18 | 48 |
| Golden (2), 1.76 oz | 220 | 10 | 32 |
| **Pillsbury:** | | | |
| **Sweet Moments Brownies (Frozen),** | | | |
| average all varieties, 3 pcs, 1.48 oz | 185 | 9 | 24 |
| **Pepperidge Farm:** | | | |
| **3-Layer Cakes:** *Per ⅛ cake* | | | |
| Chocolate Fudge | 250 | 13 | 32 |
| Coconut | 240 | 10 | 35 |
| Devil's Food | 220 | 9 | 34 |
| Fudge Stripe; German Chocolate | 240 | 10 | 34 |
| Peppermint | 230 | 11 | 31 |
| Vanilla Bean | 230 | 9 | 35 |
| Dumplings: Apple (1) | 230 | 11 | 29 |
| Peach (1) | 250 | 11 | 34 |
| **Turnovers (Frozen):** *Each* | | | |
| Apple; Cherry | 260 | 13 | 31 |
| Peach; Raspberry | 270 | 13 | 34 |
| **Safeway Select,** | | | |
| Molten Choc. Lava Cake, 4.5 oz | 440 | 26 | 50 |
| **Sara Lee:** | | | |
| **Cheesecake:** *Per Slice* | | | |
| French Strawberry, ⅙ | 320 | 18 | 37 |
| New York Style Classic, ⅙ cake | 480 | 30 | 47 |
| Original Cream Cherry, ¼ cake | 320 | 11 | 50 |
| Original Cream, ¼ cake | 320 | 17 | 36 |
| **Coffee Cakes:** | | | |
| Banana, ⅕ cake | 280 | 10 | 46 |
| Carrot, ⅙ cake | 340 | 18 | 41 |
| Deluxe Cinnamon Rolls, | | | |
| with Icing (1) | 260 | 12 | 33 |
| Pecan Cake, ⅙ cake | 190 | 10 | 22 |
| **Layer Cakes:** *Per ⅛ Whole* | | | |
| Chocolate Gold, ⅛ cake | 320 | 14 | 46 |
| Layer Coconut, ⅛ cake, 2.7 oz | 290 | 12 | 44 |
| Layer Double Chocolate, ⅛ cake | 290 | 9 | 49 |
| Layer Vanilla, ⅛ cake | 260 | 14 | 32 |
| **Pound Cakes:** *Per ¼ of Cake* | | | |
| All Butter | 300 | 16 | 35 |
| Free & Light | 220 | 4 | 41 |
| Strawberry Swirl | 225 | 7.5 | 38 |
| **Bites:** *Per Serving* | | | |
| Original: (1) | 20 | 1 | 3 |
| (25) | 440 | 27 | 44 |
| Strawberry: (1) | 20 | 1 | 2 |
| (25) | 430 | 25 | 45 |

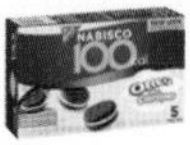

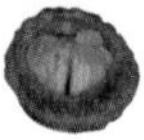

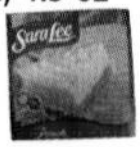

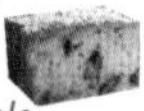

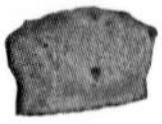

| | C | F | Cb |
|---|---|---|---|
| **Smart Ones** *(Weight Watchers)*: | | | |
| Brownie à la Mode, 3.13 oz | 200 | 4 | 36 |
| Chocolate Eclair, 2 oz | 140 | 4 | 24 |
| Choc. Chip Cookie Dough S'dae, 2.64 oz | 170 | 3 | 32 |
| Double Fudge Cake, 2.1 oz | 170 | 4 | 31 |
| Key Lime Pie, 2.78 oz | 190 | 4.5 | 33 |
| Mint Choc Chip Sundae, 2.5 oz | 150 | 3 | 28 |
| Mocha Fudge Sundae, 2.5 oz | 160 | 4 | 27 |
| Peanut Butter Cup Sundae, 2.5 oz | 170 | 5 | 28 |
| Strawberry Shortcake, 3.3 oz | 170 | 6 | 26 |
| **Starbucks** ~ *See Page 244* | | | |
| **Tastykake:** | | | |
| **Creme Filled Cupcakes:** | | | |
| Chocolate: (3), 3.5 oz | 390 | 15 | 59 |
| W/ Van. Icing (3), 3.5 oz | 390 | 15 | 60 |
| Crumb Topped Koffee (3), 3.5 oz | 370 | 17 | 52 |
| Kandy Kake (3), 2 oz | 270 | 16 | 30 |
| Krimpets, Butterscotch (3), 3 oz | 350 | 10 | 60 |
| **Trader Joe's:** | | | |
| **Bakery:** | | | |
| Apricot Almond Tart, ⅙, 4 oz | 450 | 24 | 56 |
| Cheesecake Brownie Bites (1) | 110 | 7 | 9 |
| Chocolate Ganache Cake, ⅛, 3 oz | 390 | 22 | 44 |
| Cranberry Walnut Tart, ¼ | 390 | 23 | 42 |
| Flourless Chocolate Cake, | | | |
| 1 piece, 2 oz | 260 | 17 | 23 |
| Lemon Cake, ⅛, 3.25 oz | 350 | 19 | 43 |
| Mini Bundt, Triple Choc., ½ cake | 340 | 21 | 41 |
| Mini Carrot Cake, 5 oz | 450 | 19 | 68 |
| Pear, Blueberry Galette Pie, | | | |
| ⅙, 3.4 oz | 240 | 13 | 34 |
| Whoopie Pie (1), 2.5 oz | 350 | 14 | 54 |
| **Bread Cake:** | | | |
| Banana Bonanza, ⅙, 2.65 oz | 250 | 9 | 39 |
| Walnut Streusel Coffee, ¹⁄₁₂, 2 oz | 180 | 8 | 25 |
| Zucchini Carrot, ⅛, 2 oz | 200 | 7 | 32 |
| Pumpkin Nut, ⅐, 2.65 oz | 270 | 10 | 43 |
| Walnut Streusel Coffee, ¹⁄₁₂, 2 oz | 180 | 8 | 25 |
| **Loaf Cakes:** | | | |
| Cranberrry Pumpkin, ⅛, 2 oz | 140 | 2 | 30 |
| Pumpkin Nut, ⅐, 2.65 oz | 270 | 10 | 43 |
| **Frozen Dessert:** | | | |
| Apple Raspb. Turnovers, 3.17 oz | 280 | 14 | 34 |
| Chocolate Dilema Cheesecake: | | | |
| Plain, 3.5 oz | 320 | 19 | 30 |
| Choc. Chip, 3.5 oz | 350 | 20 | 34 |
| Triple Choc, 3.5 oz | 340 | 19 | 34 |
| Tuxedo, 3.5 oz | 320 | 17 | 34 |
| Choc Lava Cake (1), 3.8 oz | 360 | 23 | 40 |
| Karat Cake, ⅛, 2.9 oz | 320 | 19 | 37 |
| N.Y. Style Cheesecake, ⅐, 4.5 oz | 400 | 28 | 32 |
| Tiramisu Torte, ⅐, 3.2 oz | 230 | 12 | 24 |
| Tarts: Pear, ⅙, 3.5 oz | 250 | 9 | 39 |
| Raspberry, ¼, 4.83 oz | 290 | 10 | 51 |
| Wild Blueberry, ⅙, 3.5 oz | 260 | 6 | 52 |

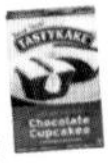

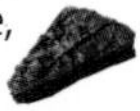

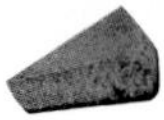

## Cakes ~ Mixes

| *Prepared as Directed* | C | F | Cb |
|---|---|---|---|
| **Arrowhead Mills:** | | | |
| **Brownie Mix:** Choc Chip, 1/20 pkg | 150 | 7 | 21 |
| Gluten Free, 1/20 pkg | 160 | 9 | 21 |
| **Cake Mix:** Chocolate, org., 1/12, 1.55 oz | 260 | 11 | 39 |
| Vanilla, 1/12, 1.73 oz | 270 | 10 | 41 |
| **Betty Crocker:** | | | |
| **Bars:** Caramelita, 1/16 pkg | 190 | 8 | 28 |
| Reese's, 1/15 pkg | 180 | 10 | 20 |
| Sunkist Lemon, 1/16 pkg | 140 | 4 | 24 |
| **Decadent Supreme Cake Mix:** | | | |
| Chocolate Molten Lava, 1/8 pkg | 290 | 14 | 38 |
| Chocolate Mousse, 1/12 pkg | 290 | 13 | 42 |
| Cinnamon Swirl, 1/12 pkg | 240 | 9 | 39 |

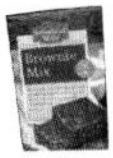

| **Cakes (SuperMoist):** *Per 1/12 Pkg Unless Indicated* | C | F | Cb |
|---|---|---|---|
| Butter Recipe Yellow | 240 | 9 | 36 |
| Carrot | 310 | 18 | 35 |
| Cherry Chip | 240 | 14 | 36 |
| Devil's Food | 280 | 14 | 35 |
| Milk Chocolate, 1/10 pkg | 250 | 10 | 35 |
| Average other Choc. varieties | 280 | 14 | 35 |
| White | 240 | 9 | 39 |

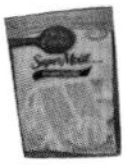

If using No-Cholesterol Recipe, deduct 40 cals and 4g fat.

| **FUN da-Middles:** *Per 1/12 Package* | C | F | Cb |
|---|---|---|---|
| Choc/Yellow Cake, Vanilla Middle | 200 | 9 | 27 |
| Yellow Cake, Choc Middle | 190 | 9 | 25 |
| **Brownie Mix:** *Per 1/20 Pkg* | | | |
| Dark Chocolate Fudge | 160 | 7 | 24 |
| Fudge | 170 | 8 | 23 |
| Low-Fat Fudge, 1/18 pkg | 140 | 3 | 28 |
| Premium: Chocolate Chunk | 170 | 7 | 27 |
| Original Supreme | 160 | 6 | 27 |
| Peanut Butter; Walnut, av., | 160 | 6 | 25 |
| Triple Chunk | 170 | 6 | 28 |

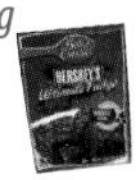

| **Duncan Hines:** | C | F | Cb |
|---|---|---|---|
| **Brownie Mix:** *Per 1 oz Brownie* | | | |
| Decadent, Caramel Turtle | 150 | 7 | 23 |
| Premium: Chewy Fudge | 170 | 8 | 24 |
| Milk Chocolate | 170 | 9 | 22 |
| **Cake Mix:** *Per 1/12 Pkg.* | | | |
| Decadent: Apple Caramel | 280 | 12 | 39 |
| Classic Carrot; Triple Choc, av | 265 | 11 | 39 |
| Moist Deluxe: | | | |
| Banana Supreme; Classic Yellow | 270 | 12 | 36 |
| Coconut Supreme | 250 | 11 | 34 |
| Dark Choc. Fudge; Devil's Food | 290 | 15 | 35 |
| French Vanilla | 270 | 12 | 34 |

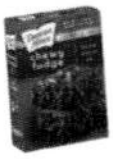

| *Prepared as Directed* | C | F | Cb |
|---|---|---|---|
| **Jell-O No Bake Cheesecakes:** | | | |
| Cherry, 1/9 pkg | 290 | 11 | 48 |
| Homestyle, 1/6 | 360 | 15 | 51 |
| Real, 1/8 pkg | 360 | 21 | 42 |
| Strawberry, 1/9 pkg | 290 | 10 | 48 |
| **Krusteaz:** Cinn. Crumb Cake, 2" | 220 | 5 | 40 |
| Lemon; Key Lime Bar, 2½x2" bar | 160 | 4.5 | 29 |
| **Pillsbury:** | | | |
| **Moist Supreme:** *Per 1/12 Pkg, Dry Mix Only* | | | |
| Classic White; Classic Yellow | 170 | 3.5 | 34 |
| Devils Food | 160 | 2.5 | 34 |
| **Premium Brownie Mix:** *Dry Mix Only* | | | |
| Caramel Swirl, 1/12 pkt, 1.2 oz | 130 | 3 | 26 |
| Cheesecake Swirl, 1/18 pkt, 0.85 oz | 100 | 2.5 | 19 |
| Chocolate Extreme, 1/16 pkt, 1 oz | 120 | 3 | 22 |

## Cookie ~ Mixes

| *Prepared as Directed* | C | F | Cb |
|---|---|---|---|
| **Betty Crocker:** | | | |
| **Pouch Mix:** *Per 2 Cookies* | | | |
| Chocolate Chip | 150 | 6.5 | 23 |
| Double Chocolate Chunk | 140 | 6 | 21 |
| Oatmeal | 150 | 6 | 22 |
| Oatmeal Chocolate Chip | 160 | 8 | 22 |
| Peanut Butter | 140 | 6.5 | 19 |
| Rainbow Chocolate Candy | 160 | 7 | 22 |
| Sugar Cookie | 160 | 8 | 22 |
| Walnut Chocolate Chip | 170 | 9 | 20 |

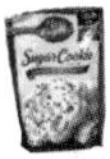

## Cake Frostings

| | C | F | Cb |
|---|---|---|---|
| **Betty Crocker:** | | | |
| Rich & Creamy, av., 2 T. | 140 | 5 | 23 |
| Whipped, all flavors, 2 T. | 100 | 4.5 | 15 |
| **Duncan Hines:** | | | |
| Creamy Homestyle, av. all flav., 2T. | 140 | 6 | 23 |
| Whipped, average 2 Tbsp | 100 | 4.5 | 15 |
| **Pillsbury:** *Per 2 Tbsp (approx. 1/12 Tub)* | | | |
| Creamy Supreme: Choc Fudge | 130 | 6 | 20 |
| Classic White | 140 | 5 | 22 |
| Milk Choc | 130 | 6 | 20 |
| Vanilla; Vanilla Funfetti | 140 | 5 | 22 |
| Sugar Free: Choc. Fudge, 2 Tbsp | 100 | 6 | 16 |
| Vanilla, 2 Tbsp | 100 | 6 | 17 |
| Whipped Supreme, av. all flavors | 100 | 5 | 14 |

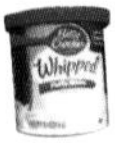

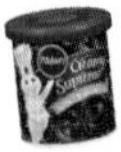


Persons with Diabetes ~ See Disclaimer (Page 22)

### Quick Guide

| | C | F | Cb |
|---|---|---|---|
| **Donuts** | | | |
| *Average All Brands* | | | |
| **Plain,** cake, 1¾ oz | 205 | 12 | 23 |
| **Sugared,** cake, 1¾ oz | 205 | 10 | 29 |
| **Glazed,** non-cake, 2 oz | 225 | 11 | 29 |
| **Chocolate Iced,** cake, 2 oz | 255 | 14 | 29 |

### Donuts ~ Brands

| | C | F | Cb |
|---|---|---|---|
| **Albertson's:** | | | |
| Donut Holes: | | | |
| Glazed Old Fashioned (4) | 240 | 12 | 31 |
| Powdered Sugar (4,) 1.7 oz | 210 | 12 | 24 |
| Gem Donuts: Plain Cake (3), 1.6 oz | 190 | 12 | 20 |
| Cinnamon Sugar (3), 1.83 oz | 240 | 15 | 23 |
| Glazed (1), 1.6 oz | 140 | 6 | 21 |
| **Bon Appetit:** | | | |
| Mini Donuts: Chocolate (4) | 270 | 16 | 29 |
| Powdered; Crumb (4), average | 245 | 12 | 33 |
| **Dolly Madison:** | | | |
| Regular, 1¾ oz | 270 | 12 | 40 |
| Donut Gems, | | | |
| Powdered Mini's (4), 2 oz | 230 | 11 | 31 |
| **Dunkin' Donuts:** | | | |
| Apple N' Spice | 270 | 14 | 32 |
| Blueberry Cake | 340 | 17 | 44 |
| Boston Kreme | 310 | 16 | 39 |
| Chocolate Frosted Cake | 370 | 23 | 45 |
| Chocolate Glazed Cake | 370 | 24 | 35 |
| Cinnamon Cake | 340 | 22 | 38 |
| Glazed Cake | 360 | 22 | 44 |
| Jelly Filled | 290 | 14 | 36 |
| Old Fashioned Cake | 320 | 22 | 33 |
| Powdered Cake | 340 | 22 | 38 |
| Sugar Raised | 230 | 14 | 22 |
| Vanilla Kreme Filled | 380 | 23 | 42 |
| **Entenmann's:** | | | |
| Crumb, 2 oz | 350 | 12 | 36 |
| Frosted Devil's, 2.36 oz | 310 | 18 | 36 |
| Glazed Buttermilk, 2.25 oz | 260 | 16 | 27 |
| Plain, 1½ oz | 190 | 11 | 21 |
| Rich Frosted, 2 oz | 300 | 20 | 30 |

### Donuts ~ Brands (Cont)

| | C | F | Cb |
|---|---|---|---|
| **Entenmann's (Cont):** | | | |
| **Pop'ems (bite size):** *Per 3 pieces* | | | |
| Frosted, 1.7 oz | 230 | 15 | 23 |
| Glazed, 1.83 oz | 220 | 10 | 30 |
| **Popettes:** Cinnamon (4), 2 oz | 250 | 13 | 31 |
| Glazed Krullers (2), 1.62 oz | 210 | 12 | 25 |
| **Great Value** *(Walmart)*: | | | |
| **Minis:** Chocolate Frosted (4) | 280 | 16 | 32 |
| Powdered (4) | 210 | 10 | 30 |
| **Hostess:** | | | |
| Donut Bites: (5) | 250 | 13 | 32 |
| Mini Crullers (3), 2.25 oz | 270 | 14 | 34 |
| Regular: Plain, 1.4 oz | 160 | 9 | 18 |
| Choc. Frosted, 2 oz | 230 | 13 | 26 |
| Powdered, 1.7 oz | 190 | 9 | 25 |
| Old Fashioned Glazed, 2.1 oz | 260 | 13 | 33 |
| Donettes, Mini: Choc Frosted: (4), 2 oz | 270 | 17 | 29 |
| (6), 3 oz | 405 | 26 | 44 |
| Crumb (6), 4 oz | 360 | 16 | 62 |
| Powdered: (4), 2 oz | 230 | 12 | 28 |
| (6), 3 oz | 340 | 18 | 42 |
| **Krispy Kreme:** | | | |
| Chocolate Iced Glazed Cruller | 260 | 12 | 38 |
| Chocolate Iced Glazed | 240 | 11 | 33 |
| Chocolate Iced Kreme Filled | 360 | 21 | 40 |
| Chocolate Iced Glazed w/ Sprinkles | 270 | 11 | 41 |
| Cinnamon Twist | 240 | 15 | 23 |
| Glazed Cruller | 220 | 12 | 27 |
| Glazed Kreme Filled | 340 | 20 | 38 |
| Maple Iced Glazed | 230 | 11 | 32 |
| New York Cheesecake | 350 | 21 | 36 |
| Original Glazed | 190 | 11 | 21 |
| Powdered Cake | 220 | 11 | 27 |
| Traditional Cake Doughnut | 190 | 12 | 19 |
| Glazed Doughnut Holes, Orig., (4) | 200 | 11 | 26 |
| **Little Debbie,** | | | |
| Donut Sticks (2), 1.65 oz | 230 | 14 | 25 |
| **Tastykake:** | | | |
| Cinnamon, 1.8 oz | 210 | 11 | 26 |
| Mini: Coated, 3 oz | 380 | 22 | 42 |
| Powdered Sugar (6), 2.5 oz | 280 | 13 | 37 |

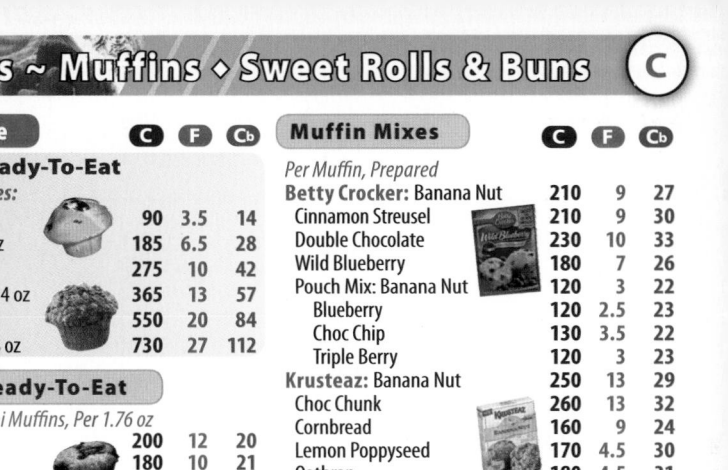

## Quick Guide
| | C | F | Cb |
|---|---|---|---|
| **Muffins: Ready-To-Eat** | | | |
| *Average All Types:* | | | |
| **Small,** 1 oz | 90 | 3.5 | 14 |
| **Medium,** 2 oz | 185 | 6.5 | 28 |
| **Large,** 3 oz | 275 | 10 | 42 |
| **Extra Large,** 4 oz | 365 | 13 | 57 |
| **Giant,** 6 oz | 550 | 20 | 84 |
| **Super Size,** 8 oz | 730 | 27 | 112 |

## Brands ~ Ready-To-Eat
| | C | F | Cb |
|---|---|---|---|
| **Albertsons:** *Mini Muffins, Per 1.76 oz* | | | |
| Banana Nut (2) | 200 | 12 | 20 |
| Blueberry (2) | 180 | 10 | 21 |
| Honey Raisin Bran (2) | 170 | 7 | 24 |
| **Entenmann's:** *Per Muffin* | | | |
| Individually wrapped, all varieties | 190 | 9 | 26 |
| Little Bites, all varieties, 1.65 oz | 180 | 8 | 25 |
| **Hostess:** Mini, 1 pouch, average | 260 | 15 | 30 |
| Regular, av. all varieties, 1.76 oz | 150 | 3 | 28 |
| **Fiber One** *(General Mills):* | | | |
| 4-Pack, av., 1 muffin, 2.3 oz | 175 | 4.5 | 35 |
| 3-Pack, av., 1 muffin, 2.3 oz | 195 | 4 | 36 |
| **Great Value** *(Walmart),* | | | |
| Double Blueberry (1), 4 oz | 430 | 16 | 65 |
| **Little Debbie:** Banana Nut (1), 1.9 oz | 210 | 9 | 30 |
| Blueberry (1), 1.9 oz | 190 | 8 | 27 |
| Chocolate Chip (1), 1.9 oz | 210 | 9 | 28 |
| **My Favorite Muffin:** *Per 6 oz* | | | |
| Banana Nut | 585 | 33 | 63 |
| Blueberry | 505 | 24 | 66 |
| Boston Cream Pie | 530 | 21 | 78 |
| Chocolate Chip | 635 | 33 | 81 |
| Lemon Poppyseed | 605 | 30 | 75 |
| Fat-Free, Blueberry; Cherry Pie, av. | 325 | 0 | 78 |
| **Otis Spunkmeyer:** *Per Whole 4 oz Muffin* | | | |
| Banana Nut | 440 | 22 | 58 |
| Chocolate Chip | 420 | 24 | 54 |
| Wild Blueberry | 400 | 16 | 56 |
| **Starbucks** ~ *See Fast-Foods Section* | | | |
| **Trader Joe's:** | | | |
| Apple Cranberry, 4.8 oz | 220 | 5 | 38 |
| Banana Chocolate Chip, 4 oz | 400 | 18 | 57 |
| Carrot, 4 oz | 320 | 11 | 52 |
| Triple Berry (1), 4 oz | 310 | 11 | 49 |
| **VitaMuffins:** Av. all flavors, 2 oz | 100 | 1 | 24 |
| Large, average all flavors, 4 oz | 200 | 2 | 50 |
| Sugar-Free, Banana Nut, 2 oz | 90 | 2.5 | 21 |
| **VitaTops:** Average all flavors, 2 oz | 100 | 1.5 | 24 |
| Sugar free, av. all flavors, 2 oz | 90 | 2.5 | 22 |
| **Weight Watchers:** Blueb., 2.5 oz | 190 | 2.5 | 42 |
| Double Chocolate, 2.5 oz | 180 | 3 | 41 |

## Muffin Mixes
| | C | F | Cb |
|---|---|---|---|
| *Per Muffin, Prepared* | | | |
| **Betty Crocker:** Banana Nut | 210 | 9 | 27 |
| Cinnamon Streusel | 210 | 9 | 30 |
| Double Chocolate | 230 | 10 | 33 |
| Wild Blueberry | 180 | 7 | 26 |
| Pouch Mix: Banana Nut | 120 | 3 | 22 |
| Blueberry | 120 | 2.5 | 23 |
| Choc Chip | 130 | 3.5 | 22 |
| Triple Berry | 120 | 3 | 23 |
| **Krusteaz:** Banana Nut | 250 | 13 | 29 |
| Choc Chunk | 260 | 13 | 32 |
| Cornbread | 160 | 9 | 24 |
| Lemon Poppyseed | 170 | 4.5 | 30 |
| Oatbran | 180 | 4.5 | 31 |
| **Sunmaid,** English, Honey Raisin | 170 | 0.5 | 36 |
| **Trader Joe's,** Triple Berry | 150 | 2 | 28 |

## Sweet Rolls & Buns
| | C | F | Cb |
|---|---|---|---|
| *Note: It is best to weigh for accuracy as actual weight can be 10-50% higher than label weight* | | | |
| **Bimbo,** Bimbolete (1), 2.2 oz | 240 | 9 | 36 |
| **Bon Appetit,** Cinnamon Roll, 5 oz | 620 | 42 | 50 |
| **Cinnabon:** Classic | 880 | 36 | 127 |
| Caramel | 1080 | 50 | 147 |
| **Cloverhill Bakery,** | | | |
| Jumbo Honey Bun, 4.75 oz | 600 | 35 | 64 |
| **Entenmann's,** Cinn. Swirl Bun (1), 3 oz | 320 | 14 | 44 |
| **Hostess:** Cinn. Sweet Roll (1) | 200 | 6 | 34 |
| Honey Bun, Glazed: | | | |
| Net weight, 3.75 oz | 410 | 22 | 50 |
| Actual weight, 4.65 oz | 510 | 27 | 62 |
| Iced/Frosted, 3.5 oz | 410 | 24 | 42 |
| **Little Debbie:** Honey Buns, 1.76 oz | 230 | 13 | 26 |
| Pecan Spinwheels, 1 oz | 100 | 4 | 16 |
| **McDonald's,** | | | |
| Cinnamon Melts, 4 oz | 460 | 19 | 66 |
| **Pillsbury:** | | | |
| **Sweet Rolls, Refrigerated:** | | | |
| Caramel Roll (1), 1.72 oz | 160 | 6 | 25 |
| Cinnamon Rolls with Icing, all var. (1) | 140 | 5 | 23 |
| Reduced Fat (1) | 130 | 3.5 | 24 |
| Cinnamon Mini-Bites with Icing (3) | 160 | 4.5 | 27 |
| Flaky Cinnamon Twists with Icing (1) | 160 | 7 | 23 |
| Orange Flavored Sweet Roll (1), 1.7 oz | 160 | 6 | 26 |
| **Grands:** Cinnabon w/ Crm Chse (1) | 360 | 17 | 48 |
| Other Varieties (1), 3.49 oz | 300 | 8 | 54 |
| Flaky Supreme Cinnabon, all varieties (1), 3.49 oz | 360 | 17 | 48 |
| **7-Eleven,** Iced Honey Bun, 4.75 oz | 520 | 24 | 71 |

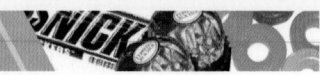

## Quick Guide

### Chocolate
*Average All Brands*

| | **C** | **F** | **Cb** |
|---|---|---|---|
| **Milk Chocolate,** regular: | | | |
| **Plain/Nuts/Fruit,** average, 1 oz | **150** | 9 | 17 |
| 1½ oz Bar | **230** | 13 | 25 |
| 2 oz Bar | **305** | 17 | 34 |
| 4 oz Block | **610** | 34 | 68 |
| 8 oz Block | **1220** | 68 | 136 |
| 1 Pound, 16 oz | **2440** | 136 | 272 |
| Dark/White Chocolate, 1 oz | **155** | 9 | 17 |
| Sugar Free *(Hershey's)*,1 piece, 0.3 oz | **40** | 2 | 5 |
| **Milk Chocolate-Coated:** | | | |
| Almonds, 5-6, 1 oz | **150** | 10 | 15 |
| Clusters, Nut, 3 pieces, 1.2 oz | **210** | 14 | 20 |
| Coffee Beans, 1.4 oz | **220** | 13 | 22 |
| Cherry Cordial Centers, 2 pcs, 1 oz | **145** | 6 | 21 |
| Macadamias, 10 pieces, 1.4 oz | **220** | 16 | 21 |
| Mints, 1 medium, ½ oz | **55** | 1 | 11 |
| Nougat & Caramel, 1 oz | **150** | 9 | 15 |
| Peanuts, 12 medium, 1 oz | **145** | 10 | 14 |
| Raisins, 28 medium, 1 oz | **110** | 4 | 19 |
| **Baking Chocolate:** | | | |
| Bittersweet *(Baker's)*, 1 oz | **140** | 12 | 14 |
| Semi-sweet *(Baker's)*, 1 oz | **140** | 9 | 16 |
| Chips *(Nestle)*: Dark, 1 T., ½ oz | **70** | 5 | 3 |
| Semi-Sweet, 1 Tbsp, ½ oz | **70** | 4 | 9 |
| Unsweetened, 1 oz | **140** | 14 | 8 |
| **Carob,** Plain, 1 oz | **155** | 9 | 16 |

## Brands & Generic

| | **C** | **F** | **Cb** |
|---|---|---|---|
| *Per Piece/Serving* | | | |
| **3 Musketeers:** Orig., 1 bar, 2.13 oz | **260** | 8 | 46 |
| 2 To Go, 1.65 oz Bar | **200** | 6 | 35 |
| Fun Size (3), 1.58 oz | **190** | 6 | 34 |
| Minis, 7 pieces, 1.4 oz | **170** | 5 | 32 |
| **100 Calorie Crisp Bars** *(Hershey's)*, 0.6 oz | **100** | 5 | 12 |
| **100 Grand:** 1.5 oz bar | **190** | 8 | 30 |
| Super Size, 2.8 oz | **360** | 14 | 58 |
| Snack Size (1), ¾ oz | **95** | 4 | 15 |
| **Abba Zabba,** 2 oz bar | **250** | 5 | 48 |
| **After Dinner Mints,** 1 small | **25** | 1.5 | 3 |
| **After Eight Mint** *(Nestlé)*, each | **35** | 1.5 | 4 |
| **Air Head,** 1 bar, ½ oz | **60** | 1 | 14 |
| **Almond Joy:** 2 bars, 1.58 oz | **220** | 13 | 26 |
| King Size, 4 bars, 3.25 oz | **460** | 26 | 54 |
| Snack, 0.6 oz bar | **80** | 4.5 | 10 |
| Pieces (46), 1.4 oz | **200** | 10 | 27 |

## Brands & Generic (Cont)

| | **C** | **F** | **Cb** |
|---|---|---|---|
| *Per Piece/Serving* | | | |
| **Almond Roca,** 3 pieces, 1.27 oz | **200** | 15 | 17 |
| **Almonds,** sugar-coated (15), 1.4 oz | **190** | 7 | 27 |
| **Almond Clusters:** | | | |
| 1 oz *(True North)* | **170** | 12 | 9 |
| 1.2 oz *(Trader Joe's)* | **190** | 14 | 13 |
| **Altoids,** (C & B), 3 pieces | **10** | 0 | 2 |
| **Andes,** Thins, av., all flav. (8), 1.4 oz | **205** | 13 | 22 |
| **Anthon Berg:** | | | |
| Creamy Mint (4), 1.4 oz | **180** | 6 | 31 |
| Marzipan with Plum, in Madeira | **120** | 6 | 14 |
| **Atomic Fireball,** 1 piece, 0.3 oz | **35** | 0 | 9 |
| **Baby Ruth:** King Size, 3.7 oz bar | **500** | 24 | 66 |
| 2.1 oz bar | **280** | 14 | 39 |
| Fun size, 2 bars | **170** | 8 | 24 |
| Minis, 4 bars | **210** | 9 | 30 |
| **Baci** *(Perugina)*: | | | |
| 1 piece, ½ oz | **75** | 6 | 7 |
| **Baskin-Robbins:** Sugar Candy, 3 pcs | **60** | 1 | 12 |
| Sugar Free, 4 pieces, 0.6 oz av | **40** | 1 | 15 |
| **Big Hunk,** 2 oz Bar | **230** | 3 | 47 |
| **Bit-O-Honey:** 1.7 oz | **180** | 3.5 | 39 |
| Chews, 6 pieces, 1.4 oz | **150** | 3 | 32 |
| **Bliss** *(Hershey's)*: | | | |
| Milk/Dark Choc., 6 pieces | **210** | 14 | 25 |
| Meltaway Centers: | | | |
| Milk Choc, 6 pieces | **220** | 15 | 24 |
| Raspberry, 6 pieces | **220** | 14 | 24 |
| **Blow Pops,** each, 0.6 oz | **60** | 0 | 17 |
| **Bon Bons,** 3 pieces | **65** | 0 | 15 |
| **Boston Baked Beans,** (11), ½ oz | **70** | 2 | 11 |
| **Brach's:** Almond Supremes (10) | **200** | 14 | 20 |
| Bridge Mix (15), 1.4 oz | **190** | 10 | 26 |
| Double Dippers (15), 1.4 oz | **210** | 14 | 22 |
| Gummi Bears (14), 1.4 oz | **130** | 0 | 30 |
| Lemon Drops, (Sugar Free), 4 pieces, 0.6 oz | **35** | 0 | 17 |
| (Note: Carbs include 16g Sugar Alcohols) | | | |
| Mandarin/Orange Slices (3), 1.6 oz | **150** | 0 | 37 |
| Maple Nut Goodies (8), 1.5 oz | **190** | 9 | 27 |
| Milk Maid Caramel (4), 1.4 oz | **150** | 4 | 25 |
| Peanut Butter Poppins (25), 1.5 oz | **200** | 11 | 24 |
| Peanut Cluster (3) | **210** | 15 | 20 |
| **Breath Savers,** all types, each | **5** | 0 | 2 |
| **Bubble Gum** ~ *See 'Gum' Page 75* | | | |
| **Bulls Eyes,** 3 pieces, 1.2 oz | **130** | 3 | 23 |
| **Buncha Crunch:** ⅓ cup, 1.4 oz | **180** | 9 | 25 |
| Movie Box, 3.2 oz | **450** | 20 | 65 |
| **Burnt Peanuts,** (31), 1.4 oz | **170** | 6 | 29 |

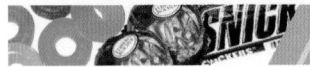
## Brands & Generic (Cont)

*Per Piece/Serving* | **C** | **F** | **Cb**
---|---|---|---
**Butterfinger:** 2.1 oz bar | 270 | 11 | 43
King Size (3 bars), 3.7 oz | 480 | 18 | 75
Fun Size, (1), 0.75 | 100 | 4 | 15
Giant, (Pieces in Chocolate), | | |
  ¼ bar, 1.1 oz | 150 | 8 | 21
Miniatures: | | |
  1 piece, 0.35 oz | 45 | 2 | 7.5
  4 pieces, 1.4 oz | 180 | 8 | 29
  Snack Pack 4 pcs, 1.4 oz | 180 | 7 | 29
Crisp Bar: Original, 2.1 oz | 270 | 11 | 43
  King Size, 2 oz | 310 | 17 | 38
  Minis, 2 bars, 1.4 oz | 210 | 11 | 25
Snackerz: | | |
  Single, 1 pouch, 1.25 oz | 170 | 8 | 23
  Fun Size, 2 pches, 1.2 oz | 150 | 7 | 21
  King Size, 10 pcs, 1.4 oz | 190 | 8 | 25
**Butter Mints,** 7 pieces, 0.46 oz | 50 | 0 | 12
**Butterscotch:** 3 pieces | 60 | 0 | 15
Discs (Walgreens), 3 pcs, 0.63 oz | 70 | 0 | 17
**Cadbury:** Caramello Bar, 1.6 oz | 220 | 10 | 29
Caramel Egg, 1.2 oz | 170 | 8 | 22
Dairy Milk Bar, 7 pieces,1.4 oz | 200 | 11 | 23
Mini Eggs (Candy), 12 pcs,1.4 oz | 190 | 8 | 28
**Candy Apple,** medium, 6.5 oz | 280 | 0 | 60
**Candy Cane,** medium, 5", ½ oz | 40 | 0 | 14
**Candy Corn,** 20 pieces | 150 | 0 | 38
**Candy Jar Mix** (Jewel) (3), 0.6 oz | 60 | 0 | 14
**Candy Necklaces,** each, 0.7 oz | 80 | 0 | 20
**Caramels:** Each, 0.35 oz | 40 | 1 | 8
Chocolate, each, 0.23 oz | 25 | 0.3 | 6
Creams (3), 1.25 oz | 130 | 3 | 23
**Caramel Popcorn,** ⅔ cup | 150 | 6 | 23
**Cella's Cherries,** 3 pieces, 1.52 oz | 160 | 6 | 27
**Certs,** Breath Mints, 1 piece | 5 | 0 | 2
**Charleston Chew:** | | |
Chocolate Bar (1), 1.4 oz | 160 | 4.5 | 30
Mini, 1.5 oz | 190 | 6 | 34
**Charms:** Blow Pop | 60 | 0 | 17
Flat Pop, ½ oz | 50 | 0 | 14
**Chew-ets Peanut Chews,** | | |
Original (4), 1.65 oz | 230 | 12 | 29
**Chewz,** 1 roll, 1 oz | 120 | 1 | 28
**Chick O Stick,** 2 oz | 240 | 9 | 42
**Chocolate Parfait Nips,** 2 pieces | 60 | 2 | 11

*Per Piece/Serving* | **C** | **F** | **Cb**
---|---|---|---
**Chunky Bar** (Nestlé), | | |
King Size, 2.5 oz | 340 | 19 | 44
**Chupa Chups,** 1 Pop | 50 | 0 | 12
**Cinn. Buttons** (Walgreens), 3 pcs | 60 | 0 | 18
**Cinnamon Disks** (Walmart), 3 pcs | 70 | 0 | 18
**Circus Peanuts** (Spangler), | | |
6 pieces, 1.35 oz | 165 | 0 | 41
**CocoaVia,** Original, 0.8 oz | 100 | 6 | 12
**Coconut Stacks,** (8) | 320 | 16 | 46
**Coffee Go,** Candy, (4) | 60 | 1 | 12
**Coffee Rio-Gold,** Sugar Free, (4) | 45 | 1.5 | 10
**Conversation Hearts** (Necco), 1 lge | 10 | 0 | 3
**Cookie Dough Bites,** 1.4 oz | 200 | 10 | 27
**Cote d'Or:** Dark 86% Coca, 3.5 oz | 605 | 55 | 19
Dark 70%, Orange, 3.5 oz | 575 | 46 | 34
Dark Raspberry, 3.5 oz | 580 | 46 | 34
Milk Intense, 3.5 oz | 575 | 40 | 45
**Cotton Candy,** 1 oz | 110 | 0 | 28
**Cough Drops** ~ See Page 75 | | |
**Cracker Jack,** ½ cup, 1 oz | 120 | 2 | 23
**Creme Savers** ~ See Lifesavers | | |
**Crisped Rice,** Choc Chip, 1 bar, 1 oz | 115 | 4 | 20
**Crows,** 11 pieces, 1.4 oz | 130 | 0 | 33
**Crunch:** Original, 1.55 oz bar | 220 | 11 | 30
Fun Size, 3 bars, 1.34 oz | 180 | 9 | 26
Miniatures, 4 bars, 1.4 oz | 200 | 10 | 27
Buncha Crunch, ⅓ cup, 1.2 oz | 180 | 9 | 25
Crunch Crisp, 1.72 oz | 190 | 11 | 24
**Dots,** 11 dots, 1.4 oz | 130 | 0 | 33
**Double Dip Stick,** 1 stick | 16 | 0.5 | 3
**Dove:** | | |
Milk Choc: Singles Bar, 1.4 oz | 220 | 13 | 24
Large Tablet Bar, 9 pcs, 1.48 oz | 230 | 13 | 25
Choc. Covered Almonds, 13 pcs, 1.4 oz | 220 | 15 | 19
Promises: Milk Choc., 1 pce, 0.3 oz | 45 | 2.5 | 5
  With Caramel, 1 piece, 0.3 oz | 40 | 2 | 5
  W/ Peanut Butter, 1 pce, 0.3 oz | 45 | 3 | 4
Swirls, all varieties, 9 pieces 1.48 oz | 230 | 14 | 25
Dark Choc: Singles Bar, 1.3 oz | 220 | 13 | 24
  Large Tablet Bar, 9 pcs, 1.48 oz | 220 | 14 | 25
  Choc. Covered. Almds, 13 pcs, 1.4 oz | 210 | 15 | 19
  Promises, Almond, 1 piece, 0.3 oz | 40 | 3 | 4
  Swirls, Raspberry, 9 pieces, 1.4 oz | 220 | 14 | 24
**Sugar Free,** all flav., 5 pcs, 1.4 oz | 195 | 15 | 21
**Dum Dum Pops** (Spangler), 1 pop | 25 | 0 | 7
**Drops** (Hershey's): | | |
Milk Chocolate, 15 pieces, 1.4 oz | 200 | 12 | 25
Cookies 'n' Creme, 14 pieces, 1.45 oz | 210 | 11 | 26

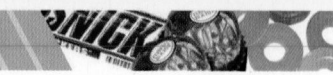

## Brands & Generic (Cont)

| *Per Piece/Serving* | **C** | **F** | **Cb** |
|---|---|---|---|
| **English Toffee,** 1 piece, 0.42 oz | 70 | 4 | 6 |
| **5th Avenue:** 2 oz bar | 260 | 12 | 38 |
| King Size, 3.4 oz | 440 | 20 | 64 |
| **Fannie May:** | | | |
| Mint Meltaway (1), 1.51 oz | 230 | 15 | 24 |
| Pixie (1), 1.51 oz | 210 | 12 | 24 |
| Trinidad (1), 1.5 oz | 200 | 12 | 23 |
| **Fast Break** *(Reese's):* 2 oz bar | 260 | 12 | 35 |
| 3.5 oz bar | 460 | 22 | 62 |
| **Ferrero Rocher:** Each | | | |
| (3), 1.3 oz | 75 | 5 | 5 |
| | 220 | 16 | 16 |
| Rondnoir (4), 1.4 oz | 220 | 14 | 21 |
| **Fifty 50 Snack Bars:** | | | |
| Almond, 7 pieces, 1.4 oz | 200 | 17 | 18 |
| Crunch Bar, 7 pieces, 1.1 oz | 140 | 12 | 16 |
| Dark Chocolate, 7 pieces, 1.4 oz | 170 | 14 | 21 |
| Milk Chocolate, 7 pieces, 1.4 oz | 190 | 16 | 19 |
| Peanut Butter, 2 bars, 1.2 oz | 200 | 14 | 21 |
| **Fluffy Stuff** *(Charms),*1.4 oz | 150 | 0 | 40 |
| **Fondant:** Choc-coated, 1.2 oz | 125 | 3 | 27 |
| Mint, 1 oz | 105 | 0 | 25 |
| **Fran's:** Gold Bar, Almond, 1.6 oz | 250 | 14 | 27 |
| GoldBite, Almond, 0.8 oz | 120 | 7 | 13 |
| **Frooties,** 12 pieces, 1.4 oz | 160 | 3.5 | 32 |
| **Fruit Drops,** (1), ¼ oz | 20 | 0 | 4 |
| **Fruit Gems** *(Sunkist),* (4), 1.4 oz | 130 | 0 | 33 |
| **Fruit Leathers,** average, 0.5 oz | 50 | 0.5 | 12 |
| **Fruit Pastilles** *(Rowntree),* 1 roll | 185 | 0 | 45 |
| **Fruit Rolls,** 1 roll | 80 | 1 | 17 |
| **Fruit Roll-Ups** *(Betty Crocker/Sunkist),* | | | |
| 1 roll, ½ oz | 50 | 1 | 12 |
| **Fruit Runts** *(Walgreens),* | | | |
| 12 pieces | 60 | 0 | 14 |
| **Fruit Flavored Shapes** *(Betty Crocker):* | | | |
| Scooby Doo, 1 pouch, 0.8 oz | 80 | 0 | 19 |
| All Other Character Shapes, 0.8 oz | 80 | 0 | 19 |
| Mixed Fruit *(Sunkist),* 1 pouch, 0.8 oz | 80 | 0 | 19 |
| **Fudge:** Chocolate/Vanilla: (1), 1 oz | 120 | 4 | 20 |
| With Nuts (1), 1 oz | 145 | 9 | 15 |
| Chocolate Marshmallow: (1), 1 oz | 130 | 5 | 20 |
| With Nuts (1), 1 oz | 135 | 6 | 19 |
| Peanut Butter, 1 oz | 115 | 3 | 19 |
| **Ghirardelli:** | | | |
| Squares: Dark Chocolate (4), 1.5 oz | 210 | 16 | 23 |
| Milk & Caramel (3), 1.6 oz | 220 | 12 | 27 |
| 3 oz Bars: Dark Chocolate, 4 squares | 220 | 17 | 23 |
| Filled, Peanut Butter, 4 squares | 250 | 17 | 22 |
| Intense Dark: Evening Dream, 3 pcs | 190 | 15 | 20 |
| Twilight Delight, 3 pieces | 200 | 17 | 17 |

| *Per Piece/Serving* | **C** | **F** | **Cb** |
|---|---|---|---|
| **Godiva:** | | | |
| Bars: Milk/Dark, average, 1.5 oz | 230 | 14 | 26 |
| Extra Dark: 75%, 1.5 oz | 230 | 17 | 18 |
| 85%, 1.4 oz | 260 | 21 | 14 |
| Chocoiste: | | | |
| Dark Chocolate Cherries (12) | 190 | 7 | 30 |
| Milk Chocolate Cashews (14) | 230 | 15 | 19 |
| Hearts: Dark Ganache (4) | 200 | 12 | 23 |
| Milk Praline (4) | 220 | 13 | 23 |
| **Go Lightly:** | | | |
| Bags: Assorted Taffy, 5 pieces | 130 | 3 | 36 |
| Vanilla Caramels, 5 pieces | 150 | 6 | 32 |
| Hard Candy (4), ½ oz | 45 | 0 | 15 |
| **Goobers Peanuts,** 1 pkg, 1.4 oz | 200 | 13 | 21 |
| **Good & Plenty** *(Hershey's),* 1.4 oz | 140 | 0 | 35 |
| **GooGoo Clusters,** 1 piece, 1.75 oz | 240 | 12 | 30 |
| **Gum Drops:** 1 small, 0.1 oz | 15 | 0 | 3 |
| 5 pieces, 0.63 oz | 75 | 0 | 15 |
| **Gummi:** Bears (22 ) 1.4 oz | 150 | 0 | 34 |
| Chewy Sweet Tarts (4), 1.5 oz | 160 | 0 | 36 |
| Novelties (Walgreens), 7 | 140 | 0 | 34 |
| Worms (5), 1.25 oz | 130 | 0 | 31 |
| **Guylian:** | | | |
| Bars: Dark Chocolate, 0.3 oz | 55 | 4 | 3 |
| Milk Choc. w/ Hazelnuts, 0.3 oz | 55 | 4 | 3 |
| White Choc. w/ Hazelnuts, 0.3 oz | 60 | 4 | 6 |
| No Sugar Added Bars: | | | |
| Milk Chocolate, 3 squares | 150 | 11 | 16 |
| 54% Cocoa, Dark Choc., 3 squares | 140 | 11 | 16 |
| Seashell: Bar, 1.4 oz | 210 | 13 | 21 |
| Boxed, Originals (1), 0.35 oz | 60 | 4 | 6 |
| Truffles (1), 0.4 oz | 70 | 5.5 | 5 |
| **Heath:** Original (1), 1.38 oz | 210 | 13 | 24 |
| King Size, 2.8 oz | 410 | 22 | 49 |
| Snack Size, 3 pieces, 1.5 oz | 230 | 14 | 27 |
| **Hershey's:** | | | |
| **Cookies 'N' Creme,** 1.5 oz Bar | 220 | 12 | 26 |
| **Milk Chocolate:** 1.55 oz Bar | 210 | 13 | 26 |
| With Almonds, 1 bar, 1.4 oz | 210 | 14 | 21 |
| King Size, 1 Bar, 2.6 oz | 370 | 22 | 44 |
| Air Delight, 1 bar, 1.4 oz | 200 | 12 | 24 |
| Kisses, 11 pieces, 1.4 oz | 200 | 12 | 24 |
| Nuggets: 4 pieces, 1.35 oz | 180 | 12 | 20 |
| W/ Toffee & Alm., 4 pcs, 1.3 oz | 200 | 12 | 25 |
| Sugar Free Choc.,,, 5 pieces, 1.4 oz | 160 | 13 | 24 |
| **Pot of Gold Chocolate Asstd:** | | | |
| Carmel (4), 1.4 oz | 190 | 10 | 26 |
| Average other varieties (4), 1.4 oz | 210 | 12 | 24 |

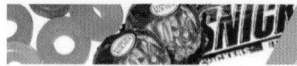 

## Brands & Generic (Cont)

*Per Piece/Serving* **C** **F** **Cb**

**Hershey's (Cont):**

| | C | F | Cb |
|---|---|---|---|
| **Extra Dark Choc.,** 4 pieces, 1.4 oz | **180** | 14 | 21 |
| **Special Dark Choc.:** 1.45 oz bar | **180** | 12 | 25 |
| Sugar Free, 5 pieces, 1.4 oz | **190** | 15 | 23 |
| Nuggets, with Almonds, 4 pcs | **200** | 13 | 20 |
| **Candy-Coated Eggs:** | | | |
| Milk Choc (8), 1.2 oz | **170** | 8 | 27 |
| With Almonds (8), 1.2 oz | **200** | 12 | 18 |
| **Honeycomb:** Plain, 1 oz | **115** | 0 | 27 |
| Choc-coated, 2 pieces | **180** | 7 | 31 |
| **Hot Tamales,** 20 pieces, 1.4 oz | **150** | 0 | 36 |
| **Hugs ~ See Kisses** | | | |
| **Jawbreakers** *(Sathers)*, (15), 0.6 oz | **60** | 0 | 16 |
| **Jellies,** 3 medium, 1 oz | **130** | 0 | 33 |
| **Jells,** *(Joyva),* Raspb., 3 pcs, 1.55 oz | **160** | 0 | 38 |
| **Jelly Beans:** Small, 37 beans, 1.4 oz | **120** | 0 | 35 |
| Regular, 13 beans, 1.4 oz | **150** | 0 | 37 |
| 1 bean | **15** | 0 | 3 |
| Sugar Free, 35 beans | **80** | 0 | 37 |
| (Carbs include 25g sugar alcohol) | | | |
| Jumbo, 1 bean | **20** | 0 | 5 |
| *Jewel,* 13 beans, 1.4 oz | **140** | 0 | 36 |
| *Sathers/Walgreens,* 13 beans | **150** | 0 | 37 |
| Wonderbeans, 33 beans | **100** | 0 | 24 |
| **Jelly Bellys:** Each | **5** | 0 | 1 |
| 35 beans, 1.4 oz | **175** | 0 | 37 |
| Sugar Free Beans/Sours (35), 1.4 oz | **80** | 0 | 37 |
| Dips (Choc Covered), av. all, 40 pcs | **150** | 3.5 | 32 |
| **Jelly Rings** *(Jewel),* 5 pcs, 1.4 oz | **110** | 0 | 26 |
| **Jolly Rancher:** | | | |
| Gummies, 9 pieces | **120** | 0 | 28 |
| Hard Candy, 3 pieces | **70** | 0 | 17 |
| Jelly Beans, 30 pieces, 1.4 oz | **140** | 0 | 36 |
| Lollipops (1), 0.55 oz | **60** | 0 | 15 |
| Sours, 16 pieces, 1.4 oz | **140** | 0 | 36 |
| **Jujubees,** all types, (52), 1.4 oz | **110** | 0 | 28 |
| **Juju Bears,** 5 pieces | **130** | 0 | 34 |
| **Juju Mix** *(Sathers),* 11 pieces, 1.5 oz | **150** | 0 | 36 |
| **Jujyfruits,** 16 pieces, 1.4 oz | **120** | 0 | 32 |
| **Junior Caramels:** 13 pieces, 1.48 oz | **190** | 6 | 33 |
| Mini, 2 boxes, 1 oz | **130** | 4 | 23 |

*Per Piece/Serving* **C** **F** **Cb**

| | C | F | Cb |
|---|---|---|---|
| **Junior Mints,** 1.83 oz | **220** | 4 | 45 |
| 16 pieces, 1.4 oz | **170** | 3 | 35 |
| **Justin's Peanut Butter Cups:** | | | |
| Milk Choc, 2 cups, 1.4 oz pkg | **210** | 14 | 18 |
| Dark Choc, 2 cups, 1.4 oz pkg | **235** | 16 | 20 |
| **Kissables,** 39 pcs, 1.4 oz | **180** | 9 | 28 |
| **Kisses:** | | | |
| Milk Choc.: 1 pce, 0.16 oz | **25** | 1.5 | 3 |
| 9 pieces, 1.4oz | **200** | 12 | 25 |
| With Almonds (9), 1.4 oz | **200** | 13 | 22 |
| Air Delights, 11 pieces, 1.4 oz | **200** | 12 | 24 |
| Caramel Filled 9 pieces, 1.5 oz | **190** | 9 | 27 |
| Special Dark, 9 pieces, 1.4 oz | **180** | 12 | 25 |
| **Kit Kat:** | | | |
| **Milk Chocolate:** | | | |
| 4 piece bar, 1.5 oz | **210** | 11 | 28 |
| King Size, 8 pieces, 3 oz bar | **420** | 22 | 56 |
| Snack Size, 6 pieces, 1.48 oz | **210** | 11 | 27 |
| Extra Crispy, 1.58 oz bar | **220** | 12 | 29 |
| **White Chocolate,** 4 pieces, 1.5 oz | **220** | 12 | 26 |
| **Kraft,** Caramels (5), 1.4 oz | **160** | 3.5 | 30 |
| **Kudos ~ See Page 33** | | | |
| **Lance,** Peanut Bar, 2.2 oz package | **340** | 19 | 29 |
| **Lemon Drops:** (4), 0.6 oz | **60** | 0 | 16 |
| Sugar Free *(Walgreens),* (3), 0.6 oz | **50** | 0 | 17 |
| **Lemonhead,** (26), 1.4 oz | **140** | 0 | 36 |
| **Licorice:** Average all types, 1oz | **100** | 0 | 25 |
| Bites *(Switzer),* (1) | **10** | 0 | 3 |
| Chews *(Panda),* (1) | **10** | 0 | 3 |
| Tid Bits (1) | **10** | 0 | 1.5 |
| Twists: Black/Red, av., 1 pce | **35** | 0 | 8 |
| Sugar Free, 1 piece | **13** | 0 | 2.5 |
| *American Licorice Co.:* Extinguisher (1) | **160** | 1.5 | 37 |
| Natural Vines: Black, 9 pcs, 1.4 oz | **140** | 1 | 33 |
| Red, 9 pcs, 1.4 oz | **150** | 1 | 34 |
| Red Vines, 7 pieces, 1.4 oz | **140** | 0 | 33 |
| Sip-n-Chew, 1 package 1 oz | **100** | 1 | 23 |
| Snaps, 31 pieces, 1.4 oz | **140** | 0.5 | 33 |
| Sour Punch, 6 pieces, 1.4 oz | **150** | 0.5 | 34 |
| Super Ropes, 1 piece, 2 oz | **200** | 0 | 46 |
| *Young & Smiley:* Strawberry, 11 pcs | **150** | 1.5 | 33 |
| Traditional Black, 11 pcs, 1.48 oz | **140** | 1.5 | 32 |
| **Lifesavers:** Large size, 1 candy | **15** | 0 | 3 |
| Regular: All flavors, 1 candy | **10** | 0 | 2.5 |
| 1 Roll (14 candies), 1.14 oz | **140** | 0 | 35 |
| Creme Savers: 3 pieces, ½ oz | **60** | 1 | 11 |
| Sugar Free, 4 pieces | **45** | 1.5 | 13 |
| Pep-o-mint (3), 0.2 oz | **20** | 0 | 5 |
| Fruit Splosion (10), 1.4 oz | **130** | 0 | 31 |
| **Sugar-Free Delites:** *Per Candy* | | | |
| Orchard Fruits; Summer Blend | **7** | 0 | 2.5 |
| Butter Toffee; European Collect. | **10** | 1 | 2.5 |

### Brands & Generic (Cont)

*Per Piece/Serving*

| | C | F | Cb |
|---|---|---|---|
| **Lik-m-aid** (*Wonka*), Fun Dip, 1 pkg | 50 | 0 | 13 |
| **Lindt:** Lindor Truffles, average, (1) | 75 | 6 | 5 |
| **Swiss Milk Chocolate Bars:** | | | |
| 70% Cocoa, 4 pieces | 220 | 17 | 13 |
| Classic, with Hazelnuts, 10 pieces | 230 | 16 | 20 |
| Raspberry filled, 7 pieces | 200 | 10 | 25 |
| **Dark Choc. Truffles,** | | | |
| w/ filling, 7 pieces | 240 | 18 | 18 |
| **Lollipops:** Mini, ¼ oz | 25 | 0 | 6 |
| Small, ½ oz | 50 | 0 | 12 |
| Medium, 1 oz | 100 | 0 | 25 |
| Giant (4″ diam), 7 oz | 790 | 0 | 198 |
| **Look Bar,** 1.5 oz | 190 | 6 | 49 |
| **M & M's:** | | | |
| Milk Chocolate: 1 pce | 5 | 0.1 | 0.5 |
| 20 pieces, 0.6 oz | 70 | 3 | 10 |
| 1.7 oz package | 240 | 10 | 34 |
| 13 pieces, 1.5 oz | 210 | 9 | 30 |
| Almond Choc., 1.5 oz | 220 | 12 | 25 |
| Minis, 1 tube, 1.08 oz | 150 | 7 | 21 |
| Peanut, 1.74 oz pkg | 250 | 13 | 30 |
| Peanut Butter, 1.63 oz package | 240 | 14 | 26 |
| Dark Chocolate: 1.5 oz pkg | 210 | 10 | 29 |
| Peanuts, 1.5 oz | 220 | 12 | 25 |
| Premiums: Chocolate Trio, 1.5 oz | 230 | 14 | 25 |
| Mint Thrills, 1.5 oz | 240 | 14 | 25 |
| Pretzels, 1.14 oz | 150 | 5 | 24 |
| **Mamba,** 6 pieces, 0.88 oz | 170 | 2.5 | 36 |
| **Marshmallow Egg,** 1 egg, 1 oz | 120 | 3 | 22 |
| **Mary Jane,** (*Necco*), 5 pcs, 1.4 oz | 160 | 3.5 | 32 |
| **Marshmallows:** Firm/Soft, 1 oz | 90 | 0 | 23 |
| Regular size, 4 pieces, 1 oz | 100 | 0 | 24 |
| Mini-Marshmallow, ⅔ cup, 1 oz | 95 | 0 | 24 |
| Choc-coat. Twists (*Joyva*), each | 95 | 2 | 10 |
| *Fluff,* 2 Tbsp, 0.63 oz | 60 | 0 | 15 |
| *Kraft:* Mini, 1 oz | 90 | 0 | 23 |
| Creme, ½ oz | 45 | 0 | 11 |
| Jet-Puffed, 5 pieces, 1 oz | 100 | 0 | 24 |
| Funmallows, ⅔ cup, 1 oz | 100 | 0 | 24 |
| **Marzipan,** 2 Tbsp, 1.4 oz | 160 | 4 | 29 |
| **Mauna Loa,** Mountains, 4 pcs | 230 | 17 | 21 |
| **Mexican Hats,** (7), 1.34 oz | 120 | 0 | 30 |
| **Mentos:** Regular (1) | 10 | 0 | 3 |
| Sugar Free (1) | 5 | 0 | 2.5 |
| **Mike & Ike:** | | | |
| Original: 1 pkg, 2.1 oz | 220 | 0 | 55 |
| 23 pieces, 1.4 oz | 140 | 0 | 36 |
| **Milk Duds,** 1 box, 1.83 oz | 230 | 8 | 38 |

*Per Piece/Serving*

| | C | F | Cb |
|---|---|---|---|
| **Milky Way:** | | | |
| Bars: Single, 2.1 oz | 260 | 10 | 41 |
| Fun Size, 2 bars, 1.2 oz | 150 | 6 | 24 |
| To Go, 1.8 oz | 230 | 9 | 36 |
| Minis, 5 pieces, 1.52 oz | 190 | 7 | 30 |
| Midnight Bar: (1), 1.76 oz | 220 | 8 | 36 |
| Minis, 5 pieces, 1.4 oz | 190 | 7 | 30 |
| More Caramel, 2.05 oz | 260 | 10 | 41 |
| Simply Caramel, 1.9 oz | 250 | 11 | 37 |
| **Mints:** Uncoated, 3 pieces | 70 | 0 | 17 |
| 1 mint | 7 | 0 | 1 |
| 1 large mint | 15 | 0 | 3 |
| **Mon Cheri** (*Ferrero*), 4 pcs, 1.59 oz | 260 | 18 | 20 |
| **Mounds:** 1.73 oz bar | 230 | 13 | 29 |
| Snack Size, 1 piece, 0.6 oz | 80 | 4.5 | 10 |
| King Size, 4 pcs, 3.5 oz | 460 | 26 | 58 |
| **Mr Goodbar:** 1.73 oz bar | 250 | 17 | 26 |
| King Size, 2.6 oz bar | 380 | 26 | 38 |
| **Munch Bar,** 1.42 oz | 220 | 15 | 18 |
| **Necco,** Candy Wafers (40) 2 oz | 220 | 0 | 56 |
| **Newman's Own:** | | | |
| Milk Chocolate: Caramel Cups (3) | 160 | 8 | 21 |
| Peanut Butter Cups (3) | 180 | 12 | 17 |
| Dark Chocolate: Caramel Cups (3) | 160 | 9 | 20 |
| Peanut Butter Cups (3) | 180 | 13 | 16 |
| **Nips,** all flavors, 2 pieces, ½ oz | 60 | 2 | 11 |
| **Nougat:** 3 pcs, 1.48 oz | 170 | 1 | 39 |
| Choc. Covered, 1 oz | 125 | 4 | 22 |
| **Nuggets:** Milk Chocolate, 4 pieces | 200 | 12 | 25 |
| W/ Toffee & Almonds, 4 pieces, 1.3 oz | 200 | 12 | 25 |
| Special Dark w/ Almonds, 4 pieces | 200 | 13 | 20 |
| **Nutrageous Bar** (*Reese's*), 1.8 oz | 260 | 16 | 28 |
| **Oh Henry!,** 2.2 oz bar | 300 | 17 | 26 |
| **Orange Slices:** | | | |
| *Jewel,* 3, 1.5 oz | 140 | 0 | 35 |
| *Walgreens,* 4 pieces, 1.6 oz | 160 | 0 | 39 |
| **Pastel Mints** (*Walgreens*), 20 pcs | 60 | 0 | 14 |
| **PayDay Bar:** 1.8 oz bar | 240 | 13 | 27 |
| King Size, 3.4 oz bar | 440 | 24 | 50 |
| Snack Size, 0.7 oz | 90 | 5 | 10 |
| Avalanche, 1.8 oz bar | 250 | 13 | 29 |
| **Peanut Bar,** 1.6 oz bar | 235 | 15 | 21 |
| **Peanut Butter Cups** ~ *See Reese's; Newman's Own* | | | |
| **Peanut Brittle:** 1 piece, 1.5 oz | 190 | 5 | 32 |
| Sugar Free (*Russell Stover*) | | | |
| 4 pcs, 1.3 oz | 140 | 10 | 24 |
| **Peanuts,** choc-covered, 14 pieces | 230 | 14 | 23 |
| **Pearson's Mint Patties,** (5), 1.34 oz | 150 | 2.5 | 31 |
| **Peppermints:** 7 small, 0.5 oz | 60 | 0 | 15 |
| *Brach's,* 3 pieces | 60 | 0 | 16 |

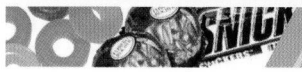 
### Brands & Generic (Cont)

*Per Piece/Serving* **C** **F** **Cb**

| | C | F | Cb |
|---|---|---|---|
| **Pez,** 1 roll | 35 | 0 | 9 |
| **Planters:** Choc. Peanuts , 1.4 oz | 210 | 15 | 18 |
| Double Peanut Bar, 1.6 oz | 220 | 13 | 21 |
| **Pops ~** *See Lollipops* | | | |
| **Pop Rocks,** 0.34 oz package | 35 | 0 | 9 |
| **Pot of Gold:** | | | |
| Assortment: Caramel, 4 pieces | 190 | 10 | 25 |
| Nut, 4 pieces | 210 | 13 | 23 |
| **Pretzels:** Choc-covered, Mini (6) | 200 | 9 | 25 |
| White Choc Bites (23), 1.4 oz | 200 | 9 | 25 |
| **Pretzel Flipz** *(Nestlé)*, 8 pcs, 1 oz | 130 | 5 | 20 |
| **Raisinets:** Milk Choc: 1 pkg, 1.6 oz | 190 | 8 | 30 |
| King Size, 2.8 oz | 330 | 13 | 56 |
| Movie Pack, 3.5 oz | 380 | 16 | 64 |
| Dark Choc., ¼ cup, 1.6 oz | 180 | 8 | 32 |
| **Reese's:** | | | |
| Clusters, 3 pieces, 1.5 oz | 220 | 12 | 24 |
| Crispy Crunchy Bar: 1.7 oz | 260 | 18 | 22 |
| 2 pieces, 1.2 oz | 170 | 10 | 19 |
| King Size, 3.1 oz | 480 | 32 | 40 |
| Fast Break, 2 oz bar | 260 | 12 | 35 |
| Peanut Butter Chips, 1 Tbsp, ½ oz | 80 | 4 | 8 |
| Peanut Butter Cups: 2 cups, 1.48 oz | 210 | 13 | 24 |
| Mini, 5 pieces, 1.55 oz | 220 | 13 | 26 |
| 8-Pack, 1 piece, ½ oz | 80 | 4.5 | 9 |
| Snack Size, 1 piece, 0.74 oz | 110 | 6.5 | 12 |
| Sugar Free: 5 pieces, av., 1.38 oz | 180 | 13 | 27 |
| Caramel Filled (2),1.4 oz | 150 | 11 | 27 |
| Big Cup: Regular, 1.38 oz | 200 | 12 | 22 |
| Dark Chocolate (2), 1.5 oz | 210 | 14 | 23 |
| White Chocolate (2), 1.5 oz | 220 | 13 | 22 |
| Pieces: Regular (51), 1.4 oz | 190 | 9 | 25 |
| Special Dark (50), 1.4 oz | 180 | 8 | 29 |
| Sticks: 1.5 oz | 220 | 13 | 23 |
| King Size (1), 3 oz | 440 | 26 | 46 |
| Snack Size (1), 0.6 oz | 90 | 5 | 9 |
| Snacksters, 1 package, ¾ oz | 100 | 4 | 14 |
| Whipps, (40% less fat), 1½ oz | 230 | 9 | 37 |
| **Rice Krispies Treats** *(Kellogg's)*, | | | |
| 1 bar, av. all varieties, 0.8 oz | 95 | 2.5 | 17 |
| **Riesen,** Choc. Chew, 4 pieces, 1.26 oz | 170 | 6 | 28 |
| **Rocky Road,** Milk/Dark 1.8 oz bar | 240 | 11 | 34 |
| **Roca Thins,** all flavors, 3 pieces | 200 | 15 | 17 |
| **Rolo,** all types, per roll, 1.7 oz | 220 | 10 | 33 |
| **Root Beer Barrels,** (3) 0.63 oz | 60 | 0 | 17 |

*Per Piece/Serving* **C** **F** **Cb**

**Russell Stover Candy:**

| | C | F | Cb |
|---|---|---|---|
| Boxed Chocolates: Chocolate Coated | | | |
| Assorted (2),1.13 oz | 150 | 7 | 23 |
| Cherry Cordials (3), .34 oz | 150 | 5 | 25 |
| Dairy Cream Caramels (2), 1.16 oz | 150 | 7 | 22 |
| Elegant Collection (3), 1.59 oz | 210 | 10 | 29 |
| French Choc. Mints (4), 1.34 oz | 220 | 13 | 22 |
| Nut, Chewy & Crisp Centers (2) | 160 | 8 | 21 |
| Sugar Free: Assort. Candies (3), 1.55 oz | 180 | 12 | 26 |
| Pecan Delights (2), 1.7 oz | 220 | 17 | 26 |
| Bags: Caramel (3), 1.3 oz | 180 | 8 | 25 |
| Coconut (3), 1.5 oz | 200 | 10 | 26 |
| Mint Patty (3), 1.5 oz | 180 | 7 | 30 |
| Pecan Delight (2), 1.2 oz | 180 | 11 | 20 |
| **Salt Water Taffy** *(Brach's)*, (5) | 170 | 2.5 | 36 |
| **Seashells** *(Guylian)*, 4 shells, 1.6 oz | 260 | 17 | 24 |
| **See's Candies:** | | | |
| Almond Royal (5), 1.3 oz | 190 | 13 | 18 |
| Butterscotch Chews (5), 1.5 oz | 210 | 12 | 27 |
| Krispy's: Caffe Latte (5),1.3 oz | 180 | 8 | 27 |
| Mint (5), 1.3 oz | 170 | 8 | 27 |
| Little Pops: | | | |
| Butterscotch (4), 0.5 oz | 60 | 2 | 12 |
| Chocolate (4), 0.5 oz | 60 | 3 | 10 |
| Vanilla (4), 0.5 oz | 50 | 2 | 9 |
| Lollypops, average, 0.7 oz | 90 | 3 | 17 |
| Milk Molasses Chips, 6 pcs, 1.4 oz | 180 | 8 | 27 |
| Milk Peppermints, 2 pieces, 1.23 oz | 150 | 4 | 28 |
| Peanut Brittle Bar, 1 oz | 150 | 10 | 15 |
| Peanut Butter Patties, 1.2 oz | 170 | 10 | 16 |
| Peppermint Twists (3), 0.53 oz | 60 | 0 | 15 |
| Toffee-ettes, 3 pieces, 1.6 oz | 270 | 21 | 18 |
| Sugar Free: Dark Bar, 1.5 oz | 180 | 16 | 24 |
| Dark Walnut Clusters, 1.5 oz | 230 | 21 | 17 |
| Peanut Brittle, 1.5 oz | 170 | 14 | 17 |
| **Skinny Cow:** | | | |
| Dreamy Clusters, all varieties, 1 pouch | 120 | 6 | 20 |
| Heavenly Crips, all varieties, 1 bar | 110 | 6 | 14 |
| **Skittles:** | | | |
| Original, 2.17 oz | 250 | 2.5 | 56 |
| Sour, 1.8 oz | 200 | 2 | 44 |
| Tropical; Wild Berry, 2.17 oz | 250 | 2.5 | 56 |
| Fun Size, 1 bag, 0.5 oz | 60 | 1 | 14 |
| Tear & Share, 4 oz bag | 420 | 4.5 | 93 |
| **Skor,** Toffee Bar (1), 1.4 oz | 200 | 12 | 25 |
| **Smarties:** Candy Rolls (1), ¼ oz | 25 | 0 | 6 |
| Giant, 1 roll, 1 oz | 100 | 0 | 25 |

## Brands & Generic (Cont)

*Per Piece/Serving*

| | C | F | Cb |
|---|---|---|---|
| **Snickers:** 2.07 oz bar | 280 | 14 | 35 |
| King Size, 3.29 oz | 440 | 22 | 56 |
| Amond Bar, 1.76 oz | 230 | 11 | 32 |
| P'nut Butter Squared, 2 bars, 1.78 oz | 250 | 13 | 30 |
| To Go Bar, 1.66 oz | 220 | 11 | 28 |
| Dark Chocolate Bar (1), 1.83 oz | 250 | 12 | 31 |
| Miniatures: 4 pieces, 1.27 oz | 170 | 9 | 22 |
| Sugar Free, 5 pieces | 180 | 13 | 27 |
| **Sno Caps,** ¼ cup, 1.4 oz | 180 | 8 | 30 |
| **Soft 'N Chewy,** Butter Toffee, each | 30 | 0.5 | 5 |
| **Sorbee,** | | | |
| Crystal Light Hard Candy, 4 pieces | 25 | 0 | 13 |
| (Note: Carb figures include Isomalt which has fewer calories than sugar.) | | | |
| **Sour Patch:** All types, 1.5 oz | 150 | 0 | 37 |
| 1 straw | 20 | 0 | 5 |
| **Spearmint Leaves**: *Jewel*, (5), 1.4 oz | 140 | 0 | 35 |
| *Walgreens*, 4 pieces, 1.62 oz | 160 | 0 | 39 |
| **Spree Candies:** Original, 15 pieces | 50 | 0 | 13 |
| Chewy Spree, 8 pieces | 60 | 0 | 13 |
| **Starburst:** Candy Canes, 0.5 oz | 70 | 0 | 18 |
| Fruit Chews: Each | 20 | 0.4 | 4 |
| 8 pieces, 1.4 oz | 160 | 3.5 | 33 |
| Gummibursts, 9 pieces, 1.4 oz | 130 | 0 | 31 |
| Jellybeans, 1.5 oz | 150 | 0 | 37 |
| Jellybean Egg, 2 oz | 200 | 0 | 51 |
| Tropical Fruit (8), 1.4 oz pack | 160 | 3.5 | 34 |
| **Starlight Mints,** 3 pieces, 0.56 oz | 60 | 0 | 15 |
| **Suckers** (*Walgreens*), (1), 0.39 oz | 45 | 0 | 11 |
| **Sugar Babies,** Original, 1.4 oz | 160 | 1.5 | 37 |
| **Sugar Coated Peanuts,** 1 oz | 120 | 8 | 10 |
| **Sunbursts Sunflowers** (*Kimmie*): | | | |
| Choco Rocks Milk, 1.4 oz | 210 | 10 | 27 |
| Kettle Corn Nuggets, 1.41 oz | 200 | 9 | 29 |
| Sunburst Milk, 1.4 oz | 210 | 11 | 23 |
| **Swedish Fish,** (7), 1.48 oz | 150 | 0 | 38 |
| **Sweet 'N Low:** Chews (1) | 20 | 0.5 | 5 |
| Coffee Cremes (1) | 40 | 3 | 6 |
| Wafer Bars, average, 3 pieces | 140 | 7 | 23 |
| Mint Cremes, 3½ pieces | 120 | 9 | 22 |
| **Symphony:** | | | |
| Milk Choc.  1.5 oz bar | 220 | 14 | 23 |
| Large Block: 5 pieces, 1.34 oz | 200 | 12 | 22 |
| W/ Alm. & Toffee, 5 pieces, 1.3 oz | 200 | 13 | 21 |

*Per Piece/Serving*

| | C | F | Cb |
|---|---|---|---|
| **Taffy,** 1 piece, 1 oz | 60 | 0 | 17 |
| **Take 5** (*Hershey's*): Orig., 1.48 oz | 200 | 11 | 25 |
| King Size, 2.25 oz | 300 | 16 | 37 |
| Snack Size, 2 pcs | 210 | 11 | 26 |
| **3 Musketeers:** Original, 2.13 oz | 260 | 8 | 46 |
| 2 To Go, 1 bar, 1.06 oz | 200 | 6 | 35 |
| Fun Size, 3 bars, 1.6 oz | 190 | 6 | 34 |
| Minis, 7 pcs, 1.4 oz | 170 | 5 | 32 |
| **Tang-a-Roos,** 1 roll | 25 | 0 | 6 |
| **Terry's:** Choc. Orange (5), 1.5 oz | 230 | 12 | 27 |
| Dark Choc. Orange (5), 1.5 oz | 240 | 13 | 28 |
| **Tic Tac,** all varieties, each | 2 | 0 | 0 |
| **Toblerone:** 1.23 oz bar | 180 | 9 | 23 |
| 1.4 oz bar | 210 | 11 | 26 |
| 1.8 oz bar | 260 | 13 | 32 |
| Truffle Peaks (1), 1.45 oz | 240 | 15 | 23 |
| **Toffees,** Regular, 1 oz | 160 | 9 | 18 |
| **Tootsie Pops,** (1), 0.6 oz | 60 | 0 | 15 |
| **Tootsie Roll:** 2.25 oz roll | 245 | 2 | 55 |
| Mini Chews, 1.4 oz | 140 | 3 | 28 |
| **Trader Joes:** | | | |
| Peanut Butter Cups: | | | |
| Milk/Dark Choolate (3), average | 190 | 12 | 21 |
| Mini Milk Choc., (27) | 210 | 13 | 24 |
| **Truffles:** Regular, 1 piece, 0.42 oz | 60 | 4 | 6 |
| Large (*Godiva*), ¾ oz | 110 | 6.5 | 12 |
| Extra Large (*J.Schmidt*), 1.5 oz | 220 | 13 | 24 |
| **Turtles** (*Nestlé*): Average, each | 80 | 4.5 | 10 |
| Sugar Free, 1 pieces, 0.42 oz | 60 | 3.5 | 7 |
| **Twists,** Sugar Free: Licorice; Strawb., | | | |
| 7 pieces, 1.4 oz | 90 | 0 | 25 |
| **Twix:** | | | |
| Caramel: 2 cookies, 1.8 oz | 250 | 12 | 33 |
| Family Size, 1 cooki, 0.88 oz | 130 | 6 | 17 |
| King Sixe, 1 cookie, 0.78 oz | 110 | 4 | 14 |
| Minis, 3 pcs, 1 oz | 150 | 8 | 20 |
| Peanut Butter: Single, | | | |
| 2 cookies, 1.69 oz | 250 | 15 | 26 |
| King Size, 1 cookie, 0.71 oz | 100 | 6 | 11 |
| **Twizzlers:** Cherry Bites (17), 1.4 oz | 140 | 0.5 | 32 |
| Cherry Nibs, 29 pieces, 1.4 oz | 140 | 1 | 32 |
| Pull 'n' Peel, Cherry, 1 pc, 1.16 oz | 110 | 0.5 | 24 |
| Twists Strawb., 1.6 oz | 160 | 0.5 | 36 |
| **U-No Bar,** 1.5 oz | 250 | 17 | 22 |
| **Weight Watchers** (*Whitman's*): | | | |
| Butter Cream Caramel (3) | 150 | 8 | 23 |
| Caramel Medallions (3) | 160 | 9 | 24 |
| Coconut (3) | 150 | 9 | 23 |
| English Toffee Squares (3) | 150 | 9 | 21 |
| Mint Patties (3) | 150 | 9 | 23 |
| Peanut Butter Cups (4) | 180 | 8 | 31 |
| Pecan Crowns (3) | 160 | 10 | 24 |

## Brands & Generic (Cont)

| Per Piece/Serving | C | F | Cb |
|---|---|---|---|
| **Werther's:** Original (3), 0.56 oz | 70 | 1.5 | 14 |
| Sugar-Free Original (5 ) | 40 | 1 | 15 |
| Caramelts (7), 1.4 oz | 190 | 7 | 28 |
| Chewy Caramel (6), 1.31 oz | 170 | 6 | 28 |
| **Whatchamacallit:** 1.6 oz Bar | 230 | 12 | 28 |
| King Size Bar, 2.6 oz | 370 | 20 | 45 |
| **Whitman's,** Boxed Chocolates: | | | |
| Sampler (4), 1.75 oz | 240 | 11 | 34 |
| 12 oz Box, 4 pieces, 1.59 oz | 230 | 12 | 27 |
| Sugar Free, 10 oz Box, 3 pcs, 1.42 oz | 180 | 13 | 25 |
| Reserve, 7 oz Box, 2 pieces, 1.16 oz | 160 | 9 | 21 |
| **Whoppers,** av. all flav., 18 pieces | 190 | 8 | 31 |
| **Wonka:** Bar (1), 2.6 oz | 360 | 19 | 49 |
| Exceptional Bars, average all, 4 pcs | 200 | 13 | 23 |
| Gobstopper, 0.5 oz | 60 | 0 | 14 |
| Laffy Taffy: Original, 5 bars, 1.5 oz | 160 | 2 | 36 |
| Stretchy & Tangy, all flav., 1.5 oz | 150 | 3.5 | 29 |
| Nerds, Giant, Chewy, 1.8 oz | 170 | 0 | 44 |
| **Yogurt Candy,** | | | |
| Coated Raisins, 27 pieces, 1.4 oz | 180 | 8 | 28 |
| **York Peppermint Pattie,** | | | |
| Regular, 1.4 oz | 140 | 2.5 | 31 |
| **York Mints,** (3) | 10 | 0 | 3 |
| **Zachary,** Choc. Peanuts, 1.48 oz | 240 | 15 | 21 |
| **Zagnut,** 1.73 oz bar | 220 | 9 | 35 |
| **Zero Bar:** 1.8 oz bar | 230 | 8 | 37 |
| King Size, 3.4 oz | 400 | 14 | 68 |
| **Zingos,** 3 pieces, 0.07 oz | 5 | 0 | 2 |

## Gum

| Per Piece | C | F | Cb |
|---|---|---|---|
| **Bazooka,** each | 15 | 0 | 4 |
| **Beechies** | 6 | 0 | 2 |
| **Big League Chews** | 10 | 0 | 2 |
| **Bubble Yum,** | 25 | 0 | 6 |
| Sugarless | 10 | 0 | 3 |
| Candilicious | 30 | 0 | 2 |
| **Carefree,** Sugarless/Regular | 5 | 0 | 2 |
| **Chiclets,** 1 piece | 5 | 0 | 1 |
| **Dentyne** | 5 | 0 | 0.5 |
| **Double Bubble Ball** | 20 | 0 | 5 |
| **Estee,** bubble/regular | 5 | 0 | 2 |
| **Extra** (Wrigley's), Sugar-Free | 5 | 0 | 2 |
| **Freshen-Up** | 10 | 0 | 3 |
| **Hubba Bubba:** Regular | 25 | 0 | 6 |
| Sugar-free, average | 14 | 0 | 0.5 |
| **Ice Breakers** | 5 | 0 | 2 |
| **Jolt Gum,** 2 pieces | 10 | 0 | 3 |
| **Super Bubble** | 15 | 0 | 4 |
| **Trident,** Orig.; White | 5 | 0 | 1 |
| **Wrigley's,** all flavors | 10 | 0 | 2 |

## Carob Candy

| Per Piece/Serving | C | F | Cb |
|---|---|---|---|
| **Carob,** Plain/Natural, 1 oz | 155 | 9 | 15 |
| **Carob Coated:** Raisins, 1 oz | 130 | 8 | 15 |
| Almonds/Peanuts, 1 oz | 150 | 10 | 14 |
| Malt Balls, 1 oz | 135 | 8 | 15 |
| Caramels, 1 oz | 110 | 4 | 18 |
| Dates, 1 oz | 125 | 5 | 20 |
| Soybeans | 145 | 9 | 16 |
| Trail/Party Mix, 1 oz | 150 | 9 | 15 |
| **Carob Chips,** unsweetened, 1 oz | 155 | 9 | 15 |

## Cough Drops

| | C | F | Cb |
|---|---|---|---|
| **Beech Nut,** 1 drop | 10 | 0 | 2 |
| **CVS,** Sour Lemon Throat Drops | | | |
| **Diabetic Tussin,** 1 drop | 0 | 0 | 0 |
| **Halls:** Defense Vit. C, 1 drop | 15 | 0 | 4 |
| Sugar Free, 1 drop | 5 | 0 | 3 |
| Fruit Breezers, 1 drop | 15 | 0 | 4 |
| Menthol Drops, 1 drop | 15 | 0 | 4 |
| Sugar Free, 1 drop | 5 | 0 | 4 |
| Plus, 1 drop | 20 | 0 | 5 |
| **Listerine,** Lozenge (Amer. Chicle) | 10 | 0 | 2 |
| **Luden's,** Throat Drops, all flavors, 1 | 10 | 0 | 2 |
| Sugar Free, 1 drop | 0 | 0 | 0 |
| **Pine Bros,** 1 cough drop | 10 | 0 | 2 |
| **Ricola:** Cough Drops (1) | 10 | 0 | 3 |
| Sugar-Free Lemon Mint (2) | 0 | 0 | 1 |
| **Robitussin:** Regular, 1 drop | 15 | 0 | 3 |
| Honey Cough, 1 drop | 40 | 0 | 10 |
| Sugar Free Throat, 1 drop | 10 | 0 | 3 |
| Sunny Orange Vit. C, 1 drop | 10 | 0 | 3 |
| **Rolaids,** Sodium Free, 1 | 5 | 0 | 1 |
| **Sathers,** Peppermint Lozenges, 1 | 15 | 0 | 3 |
| **Squibb,** Cough/Throat Loz.'s, 1 | 15 | 0 | 4 |
| **Sucrets** (Beecham), Lozenges, 1 | 10 | 0 | 2 |
| **Wintergreen Loz.** (Walgreens), 1 | 15 | 0 | 3 |

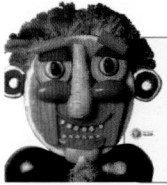

*Eat at least 5 servings of fruit and vegetables every day . . . and Enjoy Better Health!*

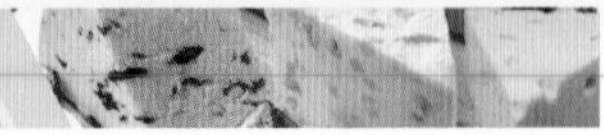

## Quick Guide | C | F | Cb

### Firm/Hard Cheeses
(American, Cheddar, Jack, Swiss, av. all Unless Indicated))

**Regular Cheese:**

| | C | F | Cb |
|---|---|---|---|
| Thin Deli slice, ¾ oz | 80 | 6 | 0.5 |
| 1 oz slice/piece | 110 | 9 | 0.5 |
| American/Cheddar/Jack: 8 oz | 870 | 72 | 2.5 |
| 16 oz (1lb) package, average | 1740 | 143 | 5.5 |
| Swiss: 8 oz package | 860 | 63 | 12 |
| 16 oz package | 1725 | 126 | 24 |
| **Cubes:** 1" cube, ¾ oz | 65 | 5 | 0.5 |
| 1¼" cube, 1 oz slice | 115 | 9 | 0.5 |
| **Diced,** 1 cup, 4.5 oz | 510 | 41 | 3 |

**Melted:** *Per ¼ cup, 2.1 oz*

| | C | F | Cb |
|---|---|---|---|
| Cheddar | 245 | 20 | 1 |
| Swiss | 230 | 17 | 3 |
| **Shredded:** ¼ cup, 1 oz | 110 | 9 | 0.5 |
| 1 cup, 4 oz | 440 | 36 | 2 |
| **Low-Fat: Jack,** 1 oz | 90 | 6 | 0 |
| American/Cheddar/Swiss, av., 1 oz | 50 | 2 | 1 |
| **Reduced Fat,** Cheddar, 1 oz | 80 | 5 | 0.5 |
| **Imitation,** American/Cheddar, 1.oz | 110 | 9 | 0 |

**Mozzarella:**

| | C | F | Cb |
|---|---|---|---|
| Whole Milk, ¼ cup, 1 oz | 85 | 6.5 | 0.5 |
| Part-Skim, ¼ cup, 1 oz | 70 | 4.5 | 1 |
| Nonfat, ¼ cup, 1 oz | 40 | 0 | 1 |

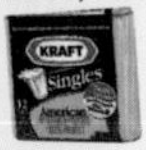

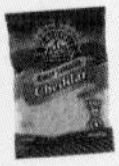

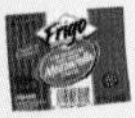

## Cheese | C | F | Cb

*Per 2 Tbsp, 1 oz Unless Indicated*

**American:**

| | C | F | Cb |
|---|---|---|---|
| Regular: 1 slice, 1 oz | 95 | 7 | 2 |
| *Alpine Lace,* | | | |
| Deli, 25% Red. Fat, 0.8 oz | 90 | 6 | 1 |
| *Kraft,* 0.67 oz slice | 60 | 4.5 | 1 |
| *Land O'Lakes,* 0.8 oz slice | 80 | 7 | 1 |
| Light (2% Milk), *Kraft,* 0.67 oz | 45 | 2.5 | 2 |
| Fat-Free: *Kraft,* 0.67 oz sl. | 25 | 0 | 2 |
| *Borden,* 1 slice, 0.7 oz | 30 | 0 | 3 |

**Babybel** *(Laughing Cow),* Mini

| | C | F | Cb |
|---|---|---|---|
| Original (1), ¾ oz | 70 | 6 | 0 |
| Bonbel (1), ¾ oz | 70 | 6 | 0 |
| Light Original (1), ¾ oz | 50 | 3 | 0 |
| Gouda (1), ¾ oz | 80 | 6 | 0 |

**Blue/Bleu**

| | C | F | Cb |
|---|---|---|---|
| *Alouette,* Crumbled, ¼ c. 1 oz | 100 | 8 | 0 |
| Light, 0.75 oz | 35 | 1.5 | 2 |
| **Brie** *(Alouette):* Creme di Brie, 2T. | 90 | 8 | 0 |
| *Alouette,* Baby Brie, 1 oz | 110 | 10 | 1 |
| **Camembert** | 85 | 7 | 0 |
| **Caraway** | 105 | 8 | 1 |
| **Castello** | 120 | 12 | 0 |

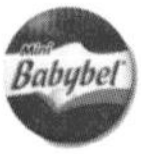

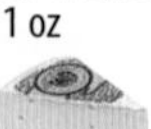

## Cheese (Cont) | C | F | Cb

*Per 2 Tbsp, 1 oz Unless Indicated*

**Cheddar:** (Also see 'Quick Guide')

| | C | F | Cb |
|---|---|---|---|
| Regular | 115 | 9 | 0.5 |
| Reduced Fat: | | | |
| *Kraft,* 25% Reduced Fat, | 90 | 7 | 0 |
| *Borden,* Shredded, ¼ cup, 1 oz | 80 | 6 | 1 |
| *Cabot,* 50% Light, 1 oz | 70 | 4.5 | 0.5 |
| Fat-Free *(Kraft),* 0.67 oz slice | 25 | 0 | 2 |
| **Cheese Balls** *(Kaukauna),* average | 100 | 7 | 4 |
| **Cheese Curds:** Fresh, ¼ cup, 1 oz | 110 | 9 | 0 |
| **Breaded & Fried** ~ *See Page 78* | | | |
| **Cheese Logs** *(Kaukauna),* average | 90 | 6 | 4 |
| **Cheshire** | 110 | 9 | 1.5 |
| **Colby:** Regular | 110 | 8 | 1 |
| Reduced-Fat *(Kraft)* | 80 | 6 | 0 |
| **Colby-Jack,** regular | 110 | 9 | 1 |

**Cottage Cheese:** *Average All Brands*

| | C | F | Cb |
|---|---|---|---|
| Creamed (4% milk fat): 2 Tbsp, 1 oz | 30 | 1 | 1.5 |
| ½ cup, 4 oz | 120 | 5 | 6 |
| With fruit, ½ cup, 4 oz | 130 | 4 | 15 |
| Reduced-Fat (2%): 2 Tbsp, 1 oz | 25 | 0.5 | 1 |
| ½ cup, 4 oz | 100 | 2 | 4 |
| Low-Fat (1%): 2 Tbsp, 1 oz | 20 | .5 | 1 |
| ½ cup, 4 oz | 80 | 1 | 3 |
| Fat-Free/Non-Fat: 2 Tbsp, 1 oz | 20 | 0 | 1 |
| *(Jewel),* ½ cup, 4 oz | 80 | 0 | 5 |
| *Fiber One,* 1% Fat, ½ cup, 4 oz | 80 | 2 | 8 |
| *Friendship:* 1% Low-Fat Pineapple, 4 oz | 120 | 1 | 16 |
| Nonfat with P'apple, ½ cup, 4 oz | 110 | 0 | 17 |
| Pot Style, 2%, ½ cup, 4 oz | 90 | 2.5 | 3 |
| *Hood,* with Chive/Onion, 4 oz | 90 | 1 | 5 |
| *Knudsen/Breakstone's:* | | | |
| Free, Non-Fat, ½ cup, 4.oz | 70 | 0 | 7 |
| 2% Milk Fat, ½ cup, 4 oz | 100 | 2.5 | 6 |
| On the Go!: Free, 4 oz ctn | 70 | 0 | 7 |
| Low-Fat, 4 oz carton | 90 | 2.5 | 6 |
| *Lactaid,* Low-Fat, ½ cup, 4 oz | 80 | 1 | 7 |
| *Light N' Lively:* Fat-Free, 4.4 oz | 80 | 0 | 8 |
| Low-Fat, ½ cup, 4.4 oz | 80 | 1.5 | 6 |

**Cream Cheese** ~ *See Page 79*

| | C | F | Cb |
|---|---|---|---|
| **Edam,** Regular | 100 | 8 | 0.5 |
| **Farmer,** Low-Fat | 40 | 2.5 | 0 |
| **Feta:** Regular | 75 | 6 | 1 |
| Crumbled, ½ cup, 2.5 oz | 190 | 15 | 3 |
| Reduced-Fat *(Athenos)* | 60 | 4 | 1 |
| **Fontina,** 2 Tbsp | 110 | 9 | 0.5 |

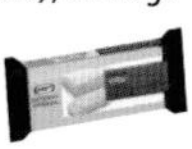

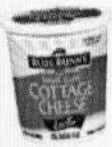

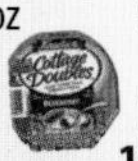

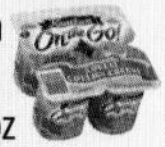

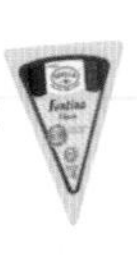

## Cheese (Cont)

*Per 2 Tbsp, 1 oz Unless Indicated*

| | C | F | Cb |
|---|---|---|---|
| **Goat's Milk Cheese:** | | | |
| *Chevre*, Soft | 80 | 6 | 1 |
| *Chavril:* Regular | 60 | 4.5 | 0.5 |
| Semi-Soft | 100 | 8.5 | 1 |
| Hard | 130 | 10 | 0.5 |
| Gjetost, fresh | 130 | 8 | 12 |
| Myzithra, grated | 80 | 4 | 2 |
| **Gorgonzola** | 100 | 8 | 0.5 |
| **Galbani Dolcelatte** | 95 | 8 | 1 |
| **Gouda** | 100 | 8 | 0.5 |
| **Gruyere** | 115 | 9 | 1 |
| **Havarti** (Land O'Lakes), 0.75 oz | 80 | 7 | 0 |
| **Italian Pasta Blend** (Sargento), 1 oz | 90 | 6 | 2 |
| **Jarlsberg** (Wegman's), | 100 | 8 | 0 |
| Reduced Fat, shredded | 70 | 3.5 | 0 |
| **Labneh,** (Lebanese Cream Chse), 1.8 oz | 70 | 4 | 4 |
| **Limburger** | 95 | 8 | 0 |
| **Mascarpone:** | 125 | 13 | 0.5 |
| (BelGioioso), 1 oz | 120 | 12 | 0 |
| (Trader Joe's), 1 oz | 150 | 13 | 5 |
| **Mexican:** | | | |
| *Cacique:* Cotija | 100 | 8 | 0 |
| Enchilado; Manchego | 90 | 7 | 0 |
| Panela | 80 | 6 | 0 |
| Queso Fresco | 80 | 6 | 0 |
| Queso Quesadilla | 90 | 7 | 0 |
| Ranchero | 80 | 6 | 0 |
| *Chi-Chi's*, Salsa Con Quéso, Mild | 45 | 3 | 4 |
| *Kraft*, 4 Cheese; Taco, shredded | 100 | 8 | 1 |
| *Sargento,* Shredded | 110 | 9 | 1 |
| *Supremo Chihuahua:* Quéso Bianco | 100 | 8 | 0 |
| Quéso Oaxaca; Queso Del Caribe | 85 | 6.5 | 1 |
| **Monterey Jack:** Regular, shredded | 100 | 8 | 1 |
| *Alpine Lace,* Co-Jack | 70 | 5 | 0 |
| **Mozzarella:** | | | |
| **Regular:** | 85 | 6.5 | 0.5 |
| Land O'Lakes/Polly-O: | | | |
| Slice (1), average, 1 oz | 90 | 6 | 1 |
| Shredded, 1 oz | 90 | 6 | 1 |
| **Light:** Polly-O Lite, Shredded | 60 | 2.5 | 1 |
| *Kraft,* 2% Milk Fat, Reduced Fat | 70 | 4 | 1 |
| **Part Skim:** *Alpine Lace*, 25% Red. | 60 | 4 | 1 |
| *Borden/Kraft,* Shredded | 80 | 5 | 1 |
| *Kraft Polly-O,* | | | |
| String (2% milk) | 70 | 5 | 1 |
| **Fat-Free,** Kraft Polly-O | 35 | 0 | 1 |
| **Muenster:** Regular | 105 | 9 | 0.5 |
| Low-Fat | 85 | 5 | 1 |

## Cheese (Cont)

*Per 2 Tbsp, 1 oz Unless Indicated*

| | C | F | Cb |
|---|---|---|---|
| **Parmesan:** Fresh/Block, Dry | 110 | 7.5 | 1 |
| Grated (Packaged): 1 Tbsp | 20 | 1.5 | 0 |
| 1 oz | 120 | 8 | 1 |
| ½ cup, 1.75 oz | 215 | 14 | 2 |
| With Romano (*Frigo*), grated | 110 | 7 | 0 |
| *Kraft,* Reduced-Fat Topping, 1 T. | 20 | 1 | 2 |
| **Pizza Cheese,** shredded, | | | |
| Regular (*Kraft*), ¼ cup, 1 oz | 90 | 7 | 1 |
| **Port de Salut** | 100 | 8 | 0 |
| **Port Wine** (*Kaukauna*), 1 oz | 90 | 6 | 4 |
| **Provolone:** Regular | 100 | 7.5 | 0.5 |
| Reduced-Fat: *Alpine Lace* , 0.8 | 60 | 4.5 | 0 |
| *Sargento,* 1 slice, 0.67 oz | 70 | 5 | 0 |
| **Pub** (*Rondele*), average | 95 | 7 | 1 |
| **Quark:** 40% fat | 47 | 3 | 1 |
| 20% fat | 32 | 1.5 | 1 |
| Skim/Non-Fat | 22 | 0 | 1.5 |
| **Queso:** Anejo/Asadero/Blanco | 105 | 9 | 1 |
| Chichuahua/De Papa | 110 | 9 | 2 |
| **Ricotta Cheese:** | | | |
| Whole Milk | 50 | 3.5 | 1 |
| ½ cup, 4.5 oz | 215 | 16 | 4 |
| Part Skim, | 40 | 2 | 1.5 |
| ½ cup, 4.5 oz | 170 | 10 | 6 |
| Light/Low-Fat | 25 | 1 | 1.5 |
| ½ cup, 4.5 oz | 125 | 5 | 6 |
| Fat-Free, ½ cup, 4.5 oz | 100 | 0 | 10 |
| Baked Ricotta, 2 oz portion | 130 | 9 | 3 |
| **Romano:** Block/Loaf | 110 | 8 | 1 |
| Grated (Package), | 120 | 9 | 1 |
| 1 Tbsp, 0.2 oz | 20 | 1.5 | 0 |
| **Roquefort** | 105 | 9 | 0.5 |
| **Sheep's Milk** | 45 | 3 | 1 |
| **Smoked Cheddar:** | | | |
| *Wegman's,* 1 oz | 110 | 10 | 0 |
| *Tillamook,* Smoked Cheddar | 110 | 9 | 0 |
| Stilton (*Wegman's*) | 110 | 10 | 0 |
| String (*Frigo/Kraft/Sargento*) | 80 | 6 | 0.5 |
| Light String-Ums (*Kraft*) | 80 | 4.5 | 1 |
| String Lite (*Frigo*) | 60 | 2.5 | 0.5 |
| Light (*Sargento*), 0.75 oz | 50 | 2.5 | 1 |
| **Swiss:** Regular | 110 | 8 | 1.5 |
| Reduced-Fat: Alpine Lace, 0.8 oz | 70 | 4.5 | 1 |
| *Kraft,* 2% Milk, 0.67 oz slice | 45 | 2.5 | 2 |
| **Tilsit** | 100 | 7.5 | 0.5 |
| **Tybo** | 100 | 7 | 0.5 |
| **Vermont** (*Cabot*), Cheddar | 120 | 10 | 0 |
| **Wensleydale** | 100 | 8 | 0.5 |
| **Whey Cheese** | 125 | 8 | 9 |

### Cheese Products | C | F | Cb

| | C | F | Cb |
|---|---|---|---|
| **Cheese Food:** | | | |
| Average all flavors: ¾ oz slice | 70 | 5 | 2 |
| 1 oz slice | 95 | 7 | 2.5 |
| **Alouette:** | | | |
| **Soft Spreadable:** *Per 2 Tbsp., 0.8 oz* | | | |
| Garlic & Herb | 80 | 8 | 1 |
| Light Garlic & Herb | 50 | 4 | 2 |
| Spinach Artichoke | 70 | 7 | 1 |
| **Cabot**, 50% Red-Fat Ched., av., 1 oz | 70 | 4.5 | 0.5 |
| **Cracker Barrel,** | | | |
| Extra Sharp Cheddar, 1 oz | 120 | 10 | 0 |
| **Handi-Snacks** *(Kraft)*: | | | |
| Breadsticks 'n Cheez Single, 1.1 oz | 110 | 4.5 | 14 |
| Ritz Crackers 'n Cheez Single, 0.95oz | 100 | 6 | 11 |
| **Kraft:** | | | |
| **American:** Singles, 2% Milk, | | | |
| 1 slice, 0.67 oz | 45 | 2.5 | 2 |
| Fat-Free, 1 slice, 0.67 oz | 25 | 0 | 2 |
| **Easy Cheese,** | | | |
| American, 2 Tbsp, 1.2 oz | 90 | 6 | 2 |
| **Kraft Natural:** Cheddar, all var, 1 oz | 120 | 10 | 0 |
| Colby; Monterey Jack, 1 oz | 100 | 9 | 0 |
| Mozzarella, part skim, 1 oz | 90 | 6 | 1 |
| **String-ums,** Mozzarella, 1 stick, 1 oz | 80 | 6 | 1 |
| **Laughing Cow:** | | | |
| **Wedges:** | | | |
| Orig. Creamy Swiss (1) | 50 | 4 | 1 |
| Light Varieties, av., 1 wedge | 35 | 2 | 2 |
| **Mini Babybel** ~ *See Page 76* | | | |
| **Lifetime,** Cholesterol Reducing, | | | |
| Low Fat, all varieties, 1 Slice, 1 oz | 45 | 1.5 | 1 |
| **Precious,** Sticksters, Cheddar, 1 oz | 110 | 9 | 1 |
| **Rondele:** | | | |
| **Spreadable:** All Flav., 2 Tbsp., 1 oz | 70 | 7 | 1 |
| Light, Garlic & Herb, 2 Tbsp., 1 oz | 50 | 3 | 1 |
| **Sargento:** | | | |
| **Artisan Blends:** Dble Cheddar,1 oz | 110 | 9 | 0 |
| Authentic Mexican, 1 oz | 100 | 8 | 1 |
| Mozzarella & Provolone, 1 oz | 90 | 7 | 1 |
| Snack Bars, Mild Cheddar, (1) | 90 | 7 | 1 |
| Sticks, Pepper Jack, (1), 0.74 oz | 80 | 7 | 0 |
| **Velveeta** *(Kraft)*: | | | |
| Original, shredded, ¼ cup, 1.3 oz | 60 | 4 | 2 |
| Extra Thick, 1.2 oz | 100 | 7 | 3 |
| Regular, 1 oz | 80 | 6 | 3 |
| **WisPride:** | | | |
| Port Wine: Ball/Cup, 0.8 oz | 80 | 6 | 2 |
| Cup, Lite, 2 Tbsp, 0.8 oz | 50 | 2.5 | 4 |

### Cheez Whiz | C | F | Cb

| | C | F | Cb |
|---|---|---|---|
| Original, 2 Tbsp, 1.1 oz | 90 | 7 | 4 |
| Light, 2 Tbsp, 1.1 oz | 80 | 3.5 | 6 |
| Salsa Con Queso, 2 Tbsp, 1.1 oz | 90 | 7 | 4 |

### Cheese Curds

| | C | F | Cb |
|---|---|---|---|
| **Fresh:** ¼ cup, 1 oz | 110 | 9 | 0 |
| 1 cup, 4 oz | 440 | 36 | 0 |
| **Breaded & Fried:** | | | |
| *A&W*, 5 oz | 570 | 40 | 27 |
| *Culver's*, 6.7 oz | 670 | 38 | 54 |

### Cheese Substitutes

| | C | F | Cb |
|---|---|---|---|
| **Galaxy:** | | | |
| Grated Parmesan Flavor, 2 tsp, 0.18 oz | 15 | 0 | 0 |
| Rice, Mozzarella flavor, 1 sl., 0.6 oz | 40 | 2.5 | 0.5 |
| Veggy, all varieties, 1 slice, ½ oz | 40 | 2.5 | 0.5 |
| **Lifetime,** Swiss Rice Chunk, 1" cube | 95 | 7 | 2 |
| **Lisanatti:** Almond Chse Chunks, av. | 50 | 1 | 3 |
| Rice Cheese Chunks, average, 1 oz | 60 | 3 | 2 |
| **Soya Kaas:** | | | |
| American, 1 slice, 0.67 oz | 45 | 2 | 3 |
| Cheddar, Mild, 1 oz | 50 | 2 | 8 |
| Fat-Free, all varieties, 1 oz | 35 | 0 | 1 |
| Parmesan, grated, 1 tsp, 0.18 oz | 20 | 1.5 | 1 |
| **Soy Sation**, Chunks, all varieties, 1 oz | 60 | 3 | 2 |
| **Tofutti,** Better Than Cream Cheese, | | | |
| all varieties, 1 oz | 85 | 5 | 9 |
| **Trader Joe's:** *Per Slice* | | | |
| Soy Cheese, Cheddar flavor, 0.7 oz | 45 | 2 | 3 |
| Yogurt Cheese: Regular, 1 oz | 100 | 8 | 0 |
| Jalapeno, 1 oz | 100 | 8 | 0 |

**New Diet Aid
- The Refrigerator Air Bag!**

POOF!

## Cream Cheese

| | C | F | Cb |
|---|---|---|---|
| **Regular/Soft:** *Average all brands:* | | | |
| 2 Tbsp, 1 oz | 90 | 9 | 2 |
| 8 oz package | 720 | 72 | 13 |
| with Chives; Herbs; Pimento, 1 oz | 75 | 2.5 | 10 |
| with Strawberry; Pineapple, 1 oz | 90 | 8 | 4 |
| **Philadelphia:** *Per 2 Tbsp* | | | |
| **Cooking Creme,** av. all flav., ¼ c. | 110 | 9 | 4 |
| **Cream Cheese:** Original, 1 oz | 100 | 9 | 1 |
| 3 oz package | 300 | 27 | 3 |
| **Flavored:** | | | |
| Blueberry, 1 oz | 90 | 7 | 5 |
| Honey Nut; Strawberry, av., 1 oz | 80 | 7 | 5 |
| Garden Vegetable, 1 oz | 80 | 7 | 2 |
| Salmon, 1.1 oz | 70 | 7 | 1 |
| **Light,** Plain, 1.1 oz | 70 | 5 | 2 |
| ⅓ **Less Fat:** Plain, 1.1 oz | 70 | 6 | 2 |
| Garden Vege.; Chive & Onion, 1.1 oz | 70 | 5 | 2 |
| Neufchatel, 1 oz | 70 | 6 | 1 |
| **Fat-Free,** Plain, 1 oz | 30 | 0 | 2 |
| **Whipped:** Reg., 0.7 oz | 60 | 6 | 1 |
| Mixed Berry, 0.7 oz | 70 | 5 | 3 |

## Dips/Spreads

*Per 2 Tbsp, 1 oz, Unless Indicated*

| ***Average All Brands*** | C | F | Cb |
|---|---|---|---|
| Avocado/Guacamole | 45 | 4 | 2 |
| Baba Ghanoush (Eggplant/Sesame) | 70 | 6 | 2 |
| Cheese Fondue, ½ cup, 4 oz | 260 | 15 | 4 |
| French Onion Dip | 60 | 4.5 | 3 |
| Hummus: 2 Tbsp | 50 | 1 | 5 |
| ½ cup, 4.5 oz | 220 | 4.5 | 23 |
| Tzatziki (Cucumber/Yogurt) | 30 | 2.5 | 2 |
| **Clearman's,** Original Spread | 150 | 15 | 2 |
| **De La Casa,** 5 Layer Party Dip | 45 | 2.5 | 4 |
| **Fritos:** | | | |
| Dips: | | | |
| Chili Cheese | 45 | 3 | 3 |
| Bean; Hot Bean w/ Jalap. | 35 | 1 | 5 |
| Jalapeno Cheddar Cheese | 50 | 3.5 | 3 |
| **Guiltless Gourmet,** | | | |
| Spicy Black Bean Dip | 40 | 0 | 7 |
| **Heluva Good Cheese:** | | | |
| Dips: Fiesta Salsa; French Onion, av. | 60 | 5 | 3 |
| French Onion, Fat-Free | 25 | 0 | 3 |
| **Kaukauna** *(Wisconsin)* | | | |
| Spreadable Cheddar: | | | |
| Sharp/Smokey Cheddar | 90 | 7 | 3 |

## Dips/Spreads (Cont)

*Per 2 Tbsp, 1 oz, Unless Indicated*

| **Kemps:** | C | F | Cb |
|---|---|---|---|
| Dips: Bacon & Onion; French Onion | 60 | 5 | 2 |
| Ranch Style | 60 | 5 | 2 |
| Top The Tater, | | | |
| Chive, Onion & Sour Cream | 60 | 6 | 2 |
| **Kroger,** Dips, all flavors | 60 | 5 | 2 |
| **Kraft:** | | | |
| Dips: Average all flavors | 60 | 5 | 4 |
| Cheez Whiz: Original | 90 | 7 | 4 |
| Light | 80 | 3.5 | 6 |
| Salsa Con Queso | 90 | 7 | 4 |
| Spreads: Olive & Pimento, 1.13 oz | 70 | 6 | 3 |
| Old English Sharp; Roka Blue, av. | 85 | 8 | 2 |
| **Marie's:** *Per 2 Tbsp* | | | |
| Dips: Buttermilk Ranch | 100 | 9 | 2 |
| Creamy Dill | 100 | 10 | 2 |
| Guacamole | 40 | 3 | 3 |
| **Marzetti:** | | | |
| Dips: Choc Fruit, 1.34 oz | 110 | 2 | 23 |
| Caramel Apple, fat free, 1.4 oz | 100 | 0 | 25 |
| Veggie: Dill, Light, 1.1 oz | 60 | 5 | 2 |
| Ranch, Singles, 1.5 oz | 180 | 18 | 2.5 |
| Ranch, Fat-Free | 30 | 0 | 6 |
| **Nalley's,** Dip, Ranch Chip | 100 | 10 | 2 |
| **Naturally Fresh:** | | | |
| Dips: Chocolate | 70 | 0 | 12 |
| Cream Cheese Strawberry | 90 | 3.5 | 14 |
| Caramel | 100 | 4 | 16 |
| **Old Dutch,** French Onion | 50 | 3 | 5 |
| **Old El Paso:** | | | |
| Dips: Cheese & Red Pepper | 35 | 2 | 3.5 |
| Thick N' Chunky | 10 | 0 | 2.5 |
| **Price's:** | | | |
| Dips: Pimiento Cheese | 85 | 7 | 3 |
| Light Pimiento | 55 | 3 | 3 |
| **Stop & Shop:** | | | |
| Dips: Veggie | 100 | 10 | 3 |
| Sour Cream French Onion | 60 | 4.5 | 2 |
| **TGI Fridays,** | | | |
| Spinach, Cheese & Artichoke Dip | 35 | 2 | 2 |
| **Toby's:** Tofu Pate | 80 | 7 | 2 |
| Average other spreads | 40 | 2.5 | 2 |
| **Tostitos:** | | | |
| Dips: Creamy Spinach, 1.1 oz | 50 | 4 | 2 |
| Salsa Con Quéso | 40 | 2.5 | 5 |
| Smooth & Cheesy, 1.1 oz | 50 | 3.5 | 4 |
| **Wise:** French Onion, 1.15 oz | 60 | 5 | 3 |
| Ranch, 1.15 oz | 50 | 4 | 3 |

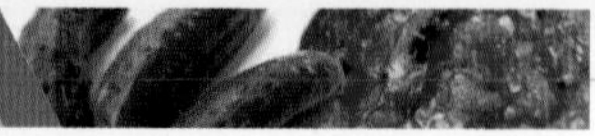

### Condiments, Sauces — C F Cb

*Average of Brands & Homemade*

| Food | C | F | Cb |
|---|---|---|---|
| **Apple Sauce** ~ *Also See Page 102* | | | |
| Sweetened, ¼ cup, 2.5 oz | 55 | 0 | 13 |
| Unsweetened, ¼ cup, 2 oz | 25 | 0 | 7 |
| **Barbecue Sauce:** | | | |
| Av., 2 Tbsp, 1 oz | 40 | 0 | 10 |
| *Bull's Eye,* Original, 1 oz | 60 | 0 | 14 |
| **Bearnaise Sauce,** ¼ cup, 2.5 oz | 190 | 19 | 5 |
| **Buffalo Wing Sce:** Hon. Mustard, 1 T. | 40 | 3 | 3 |
| Average other varieties, 1 Tbsp | 25 | 2 | 2 |
| **Cheese,** h/made, ¼ cup, 2.5 oz | 150 | 10 | 12 |
| **Chef-Mate,** Hot Dog, ¼ cup | 70 | 2.5 | 9 |
| **Chili Sauce:** *Heinz,* 1 T., 0.5 oz | 20 | 0 | 5 |
| *Del Monte,* 1 Tbsp, 0.5 oz | 20 | 0 | 5 |
| **Cocktail Sauce,** ¼ cup | 110 | 0 | 15 |
| Fat-Free *(Walden Farms)* 1 Tbsp | 0 | 0 | 0 |
| **Cranberry Sce:** Av all types, 2 T., 1 oz | 45 | 0 | 11 |
| ¼ cup, 2.5 oz | 110 | 0 | 27 |
| **Demi Glaze Gold,** 2 tsp | 30 | 0.5 | 3 |
| **Honey Mustard** *(French's),* 2 Tbsp | 60 | 0.5 | 12 |
| **Horseradish:** 1 tsp | 2 | 0 | 0 |
| Kraft, 1 tsp | 15 | 1.5 | 1 |
| **Ketchup:** Regular, 1 T., 0.5 oz | 15 | 0 | 4 |
| *Heinz,* One-Carb, 1 Tbsp | 5 | 0 | 1 |
| *Simply Heinz,* 1 Tbsp | 20 | 0 | 5 |
| **Mole:** *Dona Maria,* 2 Tbsp, 1 oz | 200 | 13 | 10 |
| *Rogelio Bueno,* 2 Tbsp, 1 oz | 160 | 11 | 12 |
| **Mushroom Sce,** ½ cup, 2 oz | 50 | 2 | 5 |
| **Mustard,** average, 1 tsp | 5 | 0 | 0.5 |
| **Pesto Sauce,** ¼ cup, 2 oz | 270 | 28 | 2 |
| **Pizza Sauce,** cnd., ¼ cup, 2 oz | 30 | 0 | 6 |
| **Seafood Cocktail Sce,** ¼ cup | 60 | 0 | 15 |
| **Soy Sauce:** Av., 1 Tbsp | 10 | 0 | 1 |
| *Kikkoman,* Lite Soy, 1 Tbsp | 10 | 0 | 1 |
| **Sour Cream Sce,** ½ cup | 250 | 15 | 22 |
| **Spaghetti Sce,** ½ cup, 4.5 oz | 135 | 6 | 19 |
| **Steak Sauce:** A1, 1 Tbsp, 0.5oz | 15 | 0 | 3 |
| *Lea & Perrins,* 1 Tbsp, 0.5 oz | 20 | 0 | 5 |
| **Strawb. Puree Sce,** Unsweet., 2 T. | 10 | 0 | 2 |
| **Sweet & Sour Sauce:** | | | |
| *Contadina,* 1 Tbsp | 40 | 1 | 8 |
| *Kraft,* 1 Tbsp | 60 | 0 | 13 |
| *La Choy,* 2 Tbsp, 1.2 oz | 60 | 0 | 14 |
| **Tabasco Sauce,** 1 tsp | 2 | 0 | 0 |
| **Taco Sauce,** average, 2 Tbsp, 1 oz | 10 | 0 | 1 |
| **Tartar Sauce:** Heinz, 2 Tbsp, 1 oz | 120 | 11 | 4 |
| *Hellmann's,* Regular, 2 Tbsp, 1 oz | 80 | 7 | 4 |
| *McCormick,* Fat-Free, 2 Tbsp, 1 oz | 30 | 0 | 7 |
| **Teriyaki Sauce** *(Kikkoman),* 1 T., 0.5 oz | 15 | 0 | 2 |
| **Vinegar,** White or Wine, 2 Tbsp | 4 | 0 | 1 |
| **White Sauce,** ½ cup, 5 oz | 130 | 7 | 10 |
| **Worcestershire Sauce,** 1 tsp | 5 | 0 | 1 |

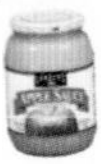

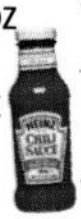

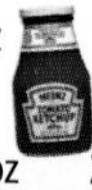

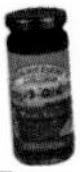

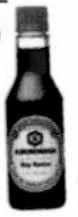

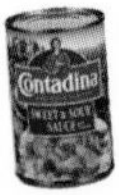

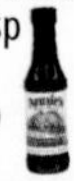

### Pickles & Relish — C F Cb

*Average All Brands*

| Food | C | F | Cb |
|---|---|---|---|
| **Bread & Butter Pickles,** 4 sl., 1 oz | 25 | 0 | 6 |
| **Chutney,** 2 Tbsp, 1.25 oz | 50 | 0 | 11 |
| **Dill Pickle:** | | | |
| Slices, 4 slices, 1 oz | 4 | 0 | 1 |
| 1 large, (3¾"x 1¼" diam.), 2.25 oz | 12 | 0 | 3 |
| Extra lrg (4"x 1¾" diam.), 5 oz | 30 | 0 | 6 |
| Halves: Small, 1 oz | 3 | 0 | 0.5 |
| Large, 2.5 oz | 8 | 0 | 2 |
| **Gherkins,** sweet, 1 medium, 1 oz | 30 | 0 | 7 |
| **Green Chiles,** chopped, 2 Tbsp | 5 | 0 | 1 |
| **Horseradish,** 1 Tbsp | 10 | 0 | 2 |
| **Jalapenos,** pickled (2), 2 oz | 10 | 0.5 | 2 |
| **Jalapeno Relish,** 1 Tbsp, 0.5oz | 5 | 0 | 1 |
| **Mustard,** avg. all brands, 1 tsp | 5 | 0 | 0.5 |
| **Peppers,** Hot/Mild (1), 1.6 oz | 20 | 0 | 4 |
| **Pickled:** Beets, ½ cup, 4 oz | 75 | 0 | 19 |
| Onions, 1 medium, 0.75 oz | 10 | 0 | 2 |
| Cocktail Onion, 1 onion | 2 | 0 | 0 |
| Red Cabbage, ½ cup, 3 oz | 65 | 0 | 15 |
| **Pickles:** Sweet, 2 Tbsp, 1 oz | 35 | 0 | 8 |
| Large (3"x ¾ diam.),1.25 oz | 40 | 0 | 10 |
| Pickle in a Pouch, 1 large | 12 | 0 | 3 |
| **Relishes:** S'wich Spread, 1 tsp | 20 | 1 | 5 |
| Cranberry-Orange, 1 Tbsp | 30 | 0 | 7 |
| Hot Dog *(Heinz),* 1 Tbsp, 0.5 oz | 17 | 0 | 3 |
| Sweet Pickle, 1 Tbsp, 0.5 oz | 20 | 0 | 5 |
| Sweet Cauliflower, 1 oz | 35 | 0 | 8 |
| Sugar Free Relish, 1 tsp | 5 | 0 | 1 |
| Sweet Gherkins (2), 1 oz | 5 | 0 | 1 |
| **Sauerkraut,** Drained, 1 cup, 5 oz | 25 | 0 | 6 |

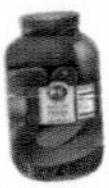

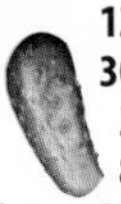

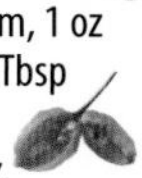

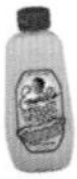

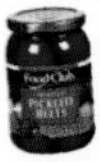

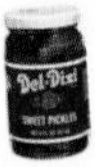

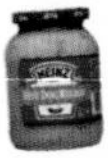

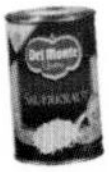

### Salsa

*Average all Types:*

| Food | C | F | Cb |
|---|---|---|---|
| Reg., w/out oil, 2 Tbsp, 1 oz | 15 | 0 | 3.5 |
| Made with oil, 2 Tbsp, 1 oz | 40 | 3 | 8 |
| *La Victoria,* 2 Tbsp, 1 oz | 10 | 0 | 2 |
| *Old El Paso,* 1 Tbsp, 1 oz | 10 | 0 | 3 |
| *TGI Friday's,* 1.2 oz | 15 | 0 | 4 |

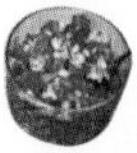

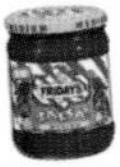

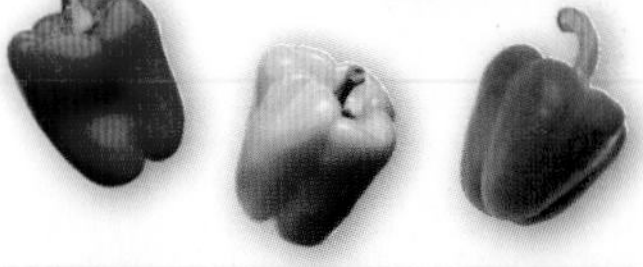

## Quick Guide | C | F | Cb |

### Cookies
**Average All Brands:** *Per Cookie*

| | C | F | Cb |
|---|---|---|---|
| **Biscotti:** Small, 0.5 oz | 70 | 3 | 10 |
| Regular, 1 oz | 140 | 6.5 | 18 |
| **Chocolate Chip Cookies:** | | | |
| Small/Thin 0.5 oz | 70 | 3.5 | 9 |
| Regular, 1 oz | 140 | 7 | 18 |
| Large, 2.93 oz (Mrs Fields) | 350 | 17 | 45 |
| Extra Large, 4 oz | 555 | 28 | 73 |
| **Oatmeal/Oatmeal Raisin:** | | | |
| Small/Thin 0.5 oz | 65 | 2.5 | 10 |
| Regular, 1 oz | 130 | 5 | 20 |
| Large, 2.5 oz *(Mrs Fields)* | 330 | 14 | 44 |
| Extra Large, 4 oz | 510 | 20 | 78 |
| **Peanut Butter:** | | | |
| Small/Thin 0.5 oz | 70 | 3.5 | 9 |
| Regular, 1 oz | 135 | 7 | 17 |
| Large, 2.5 oz *(Mrs Fields)* | 330 | 17 | 41 |
| Extra Large, 4 oz | 540 | 27 | 67 |
| **Low-Fat Cookies:** | | | |
| Choc Chip (Low-Fat), (1), 0.5 oz | 65 | 2 | 10 |
| Oatmeal Raisin (Fat-Free), (1),1 oz | 95 | 0.5 | 22 |
| Peanut Butter (Low-Fat), (1),1 oz | 105 | 5 | 15 |

## Quick Guide | C | F | Cb |

### Crackers
**Average All Brands:** *Per Cracker Unless Indicated*

| | C | F | Cb |
|---|---|---|---|
| **Cheese Crackers:** Plain, 1" square | 5 | 0 | 0.5 |
| Bag, single serving, 1 oz | 140 | 7 | 16 |
| Sandwich: | | | |
| Cheese/P'nut Butter filled | 30 | 1.5 | 4 |
| **Crispbread,** Rye | 35 | 0 | 8 |
| **Graham,** 2½" square | 30 | 0.5 | 5 |
| **Melba Toast,** plain, 1 piece | 20 | 0 | 4 |
| **Matzo,** Plain, 1 oz | 110 | 0.5 | 23 |
| **Oyster/Soup,** ½ cup | 95 | 2 | 17 |
| **Rice Crackers:** 1 small | 10 | 0 | 1.5 |
| Rice Snacks, Oriental-Style, 1 oz | 130 | 2.5 | 23 |
| **Saltines,** 5 crackers | 65 | 2 | 11 |
| **Snack-type,** 1 round cracker | 15 | 1 | 2 |
| **Soda Crackers** *(Saltine),* 2 | 25 | 1 | 4.5 |
| **Water Cracker** *(Carr's),* Original | 14 | 0.5 | 2.5 |
| **Wheat:** Wheat Thin | 10 | 0.5 | 1.5 |
| Sandwich, Cheese/P'nut Butter filled | 35 | 2 | 4 |

## Brands | C | F | Cb |

*Per Cookie/Cracker, Unless indicated*

**Albertsons:**

| | C | F | Cb |
|---|---|---|---|
| Animal Crackers (6), 1 oz | 130 | 3.5 | 22 |
| Chocolate Chip: | | | |
| Original (3), 1 oz | 150 | 7 | 20 |
| Chewy (2), 1 oz | 130 | 6 | 18 |
| Chunky, 0.6 oz | 80 | 3.5 | 10 |
| Chocolate Sandwich Cremes (3) 1.1oz | 150 | 6 | 25 |
| Double Filled (2) 1 oz | 140 | 6 | 21 |
| Fudge Graham (3), 1 oz | 140 | 7 | 19 |
| Fudge Wafer (3), 1 oz | 140 | 8 | 18 |
| Graham Crackers: Cinnamon (2) | 130 | 3 | 25 |
| Honey (2), 1 oz | 140 | 3 | 24 |
| Low-Fat Honey (2), 1 oz | 110 | 1 | 22 |
| Marshmallow Ring (1) | 120 | 5 | 19 |
| Pinwheels, Choc. Marshmallow (1) | 120 | 5 | 20 |
| Vanilla Wafers (9), 1.1 oz | 140 | 4 | 25 |

**Annie's:**

| | C | F | Cb |
|---|---|---|---|
| **Cheddar Bunnies:** | | | |
| Regular: 1 oz Snack Pack | 140 | 6 | 19 |
| 7½ oz Box | 1050 | 45 | 145 |
| Sour Cream & Onion, 1 oz | 150 | 7 | 19 |
| White Cheddar, 1 oz | 150 | 7 | 19 |
| Whole Wheat, 1 oz | 140 | 6 | 18 |
| **Bunny Grahams:** | | | |
| Chocolate; Choc Chip, 1 oz | 130 | 4.5 | 21 |
| Friends, 1 oz | 130 | 4.5 | 22 |
| Honey, 1 oz | 140 | 4.5 | 22 |
| **Organic Bunny Classics:** | | | |
| Buttery Rich, 1 oz | 140 | 7 | 18 |
| Cheddar, 1 oz | 140 | 7 | 18 |
| Saltine, 1 oz | 140 | 3 | 22 |

**Austin:**

| | C | F | Cb |
|---|---|---|---|
| **Sandwich Cookies:** *Per Package* | | | |
| Choco Cremes, 1.8 oz | 240 | 10 | 37 |
| Lemon OHs!; Vanilla Cremes, 1.8 oz | 250 | 11 | 37 |
| **Sandwich Crackers:** *Per Package* | | | |
| Cheese: With Cheddar Cheese | 190 | 10 | 23 |
| With Peanut Butter | 190 | 10 | 23 |
| Chocolatey Peanut Butter Flavored | 190 | 8 | 26 |
| Grilled Cheese Flavored, 1.38 oz | 190 | 9 | 24 |
| PB & J Flavored, 1.38 oz | 190 | 8 | 26 |
| Toasty Crackers w/ P'nut Butter, 1.3 oz | 190 | 9 | 23 |
| **Zoo Animal Crackers,** 1 oz | 120 | 1.5 | 25 |

*Per Cookie/Cracker, Unless Indicated*

| Barbara's Bakery: | C | F | Cb |
|---|---|---|---|
| **Cookies:** Fig Bars, av., 1.35 oz | 120 | 0 | 27 |
| Blueberry, low fat, 1.35 oz | 120 | 1 | 27 |
| Snackimals: Double Choc., 1 oz | 140 | 4.5 | 23 |
| Peanut Butter, 1 oz | 150 | 7 | 20 |

| Bear Naked: | | | |
|---|---|---|---|
| **Soft Baked Cookies:** | | | |
| Double Chocolate | 130 | 5 | 20 |
| Fruit & Nut | 130 | 6 | 18 |

| Blue Diamond: | | | |
|---|---|---|---|
| **Nut Chips:** | | | |
| Average all flavors: 14 chips, 1.1 oz | 130 | 4 | 21 |
| ½ package, 28 chips, 2.2 oz | 260 | 8 | 42 |
| **Nut Thins Crackers:** | | | |
| Av. all flavors: 17 crackers, 1.1 oz | 130 | 3 | 23 |
| ½ Package, 2.2 oz | 260 | 6 | 46 |

| Brent & Sam's: | | | |
|---|---|---|---|
| Chocolate Chip Pecan | 140 | 8 | 15 |
| Key Lime White Choc. | 130 | 7 | 16 |
| Oatmeal Raisin with Pecans | 130 | 7 | 16 |
| Triple Chocolate Bliss (2), 1 oz | 110 | 5 | 14 |
| White Chocolate Macadamia (2), 1 oz | 130 | 7 | 14 |

| Carr's: | | | |
|---|---|---|---|
| **Cookies,** Ginger Lem. Cremes (2) | 130 | 5 | 20 |
| **Crackers:** Poppy & Sesame (4) | 80 | 5 | 9 |
| Table Water (5) | 70 | 1.5 | 13 |
| Whole Wheat (2) | 80 | 4 | 10 |

**Cheez·It** ~ *See Sunshine, Page 87*
**Chips Ahoy!** ~ *See Nabisco, Page 85*

| Country Choice: | | | |
|---|---|---|---|
| Sandwich Cremes (2), all varieties | 130 | 5 | 19 |
| Snacking: Ginger Snaps (5) | 140 | 5 | 22 |
| Vanilla Wafers (7) | 140 | 5 | 22 |
| Soft Baked, average all flavors | 95 | 4 | 16 |

| Dr. Kracker: | | | |
|---|---|---|---|
| **Crackers:** Flatbread,  av. all flav. | 100 | 4 | 11 |
| Snacker Krackers (8), av all flav. | 120 | 5 | 13 |

| Erin Baker's: | | | |
|---|---|---|---|
| **Original Breakfast Cookies:** *Per 3 oz* | | | |
| Banana Walnut | 300 | 8 | 52 |
| Peanut Butter | 320 | 11 | 47 |
| Vegan Peanut Butter Choc. Chunk | 320 | 10 | 48 |
| **Minis:** *Per 1 oz Cookie* | | | |
| Peanut Butter | 110 | 3.5 | 16 |
| Average other varieties | 100 | 2 | 18 |
| **Organic Brownie Bites,** average | 95 | 2 | 18 |

*Per Cookie/Cracker, Unless Indicated*

| Famous Amos: | C | F | Cb |
|---|---|---|---|
| **Bite Size Cookies:** | | | |
| Chocolate Chip: | | | |
| 4 Cookies, 1 oz | 150 | 7 | 20 |
| 15 oz box | 2250 | 105 | 300 |
| Chocolate Chip & Pecans (4) | 150 | 8 | 18 |
| Sandwich, Creme Filled: | | | |
| Chocolate (3), 1 oz | 160 | 7 | 25 |
| Vanilla (3), 1 oz | 170 | 7 | 25 |

**Fig Newtons** ~ *See Nabisco, Page 85*

| Fresh & Easy: | | | |
|---|---|---|---|
| Chocolate Cookie Cremes (3), 1.3 oz | 180 | 7 | 26 |
| Iced Oatmeal (3), 1 oz | 120 | 3 | 21 |
| Peanut Sensation (1) | 170 | 9 | 20 |
| Pecan Shortbread (2) | 150 | 9 | 20 |

| Girl Scouts: | | | |
|---|---|---|---|
| **Cookies:** Caramel DeLites/Samoas (2) | 140 | 7 | 19 |
| Do-si-dos (2) | 110 | 5 | 16 |
| Peanut Butter Sandwich (3) | 160 | 6 | 26 |
| Shortbreads (4) | 120 | 4.5 | 19 |
| Thanks-A-Lot (9) | 150 | 6 | 22 |
| Thin Mints (4) | 160 | 8 | 21 |

**Goldfish** ~ *See Pepperidge Farm, Page 86*

| Grandma's: *Per Package* | | | |
|---|---|---|---|
| **Cookies:** | | | |
| Homestyle: | | | |
| Chocolate Chip | 170 | 9 | 22 |
| Oatmeal Raisin | 150 | 6 | 23 |
| Peanut Butter | 170 | 9 | 19 |
| Rich 'N Chewy, Choc Chip (6) | 240 | 12 | 32 |
| Sandwich Cremes: P'nut Butter (5) | 200 | 9 | 25 |
| Vanilla (5) | 190 | 9 | 27 |
| Mini S'wich Cremes, Van./Choc (9) | 150 | 7 | 22 |

| Great American Cookies: | | | |
|---|---|---|---|
| **Cookies:** | | | |
| Chewy Chocolate Supreme | 180 | 7 | 27 |
| Chewy Pecan Supreme | 230 | 12 | 31 |
| Double Fudge with Reese's | 230 | 12 | 32 |
| Original, with Reese's  M&M's | 240 | 12 | 32 |
| Peanut Butter with M&M's | 250 | 14 | 30 |
| Snickerdoodles | 240 | 11 | 33 |
| White Chunk Macadamia | 250 | 14 | 30 |
| **Double Doozies:** Original | 690 | 34 | 94 |
| M&M Big Bite | 340 | 17 | 46 |
| **Cookie Cakes:** 16", 3.63 oz slice | 460 | 22 | 67 |
| 16" M&M, 3.95 oz slice | 500 | 24 | 73 |
| Heart Shaped, 3.49 oz slice | 440 | 21 | 64 |

*Per Cookie/Cracker, Unless Indicated*

| Great Value *(Walmart)*: | C | F | Cb |
|---|---|---|---|
| **Cookies:** Choc Chip (3) | 150 | 7 | 21 |
| Switch-A-Roos (2) | 140 | 6 | 21 |
| Twist & Shout (3) | 170 | 6 | 26 |
| **Crackers:** Buttery Rounds, Baked (5) | 80 | 4.5 | 10 |
| Reduced Fat (5) | 70 | 2 | 11 |
| Saltines (1) | 60 | 1 | 12 |
| Woven Squares (6) | 120 | 4.5 | 19 |

**Health Valley:**
**Cookies:**

| | C | F | Cb |
|---|---|---|---|
| Cookie Cremes Sandwich (2), average | 130 | 5 | 19 |
| Oatmeal Raisin Cookie | 90 | 3.5 | 14 |
| Mini: Chocolate Chip (4) | 140 | 6 | 18 |
| Chocolate Chocolate Chip (4) | 140 | 7 | 18 |

**Crackers:**

| | C | F | Cb |
|---|---|---|---|
| Grahams: Amaranth (6) | 120 | 3 | 22 |
| Oat/Rice Bran (6) | 120 | 3 | 22 |
| Organic (4), average all varieties | 70 | 3 | 10 |

**Joseph's Lite Cookies:**

| **Crispy Bite Size:** *Sugar Free, Per 4 Cookies* | | | |
|---|---|---|---|
| Almond; Chocolate Peanut Butter | 95 | 5 | 13 |
| Chocolate Mint | 95 | 5 | 14 |
| Choc. Walnut; Pecan Chocolate Chip | 95 | 5 | 13 |
| Chocolate Chip | 95 | 5 | 13 |
| Average other varieties | 95 | 4 | 15 |
| Each cookie contains 6 grams Malitol | | | |

**Kashi:**

| **TLC Cookies:** *Per Cookie* | | | |
|---|---|---|---|
| Happy Trail Mix, Chewy | 140 | 5 | 21 |
| Oatmeal: Dark Choc. | 130 | 5 | 20 |
| Raisin Flax | 130 | 4.5 | 20 |

**Crackers:**

| Heart To Heart Whole Grain: | | | |
|---|---|---|---|
| Original (7) | 120 | 3.5 | 22 |
| Roasted Garlic (7) | 120 | 3.5 | 22 |
| TLC Crackers: | | | |
| Country Cheddar (18) | 130 | 4.5 | 20 |
| Fire Roasted Vegetables (15) | 120 | 3.5 | 19 |
| Honey Sesame (15) | 120 | 3 | 22 |
| Original 7 Grain (15) | 120 | 3.5 | 19 |
| Toasted Asiago (15) | 130 | 4 | 21 |
| TLC Pita Crisps: | | | |
| Original 7 Grain with Salt (11) | 120 | 3 | 22 |
| Zesty Salsa (11) | 120 | 3 | 22 |

*Per Cookie/Cracker Unless indicated*

| Keebler: | C | F | Cb |
|---|---|---|---|
| **Cookies:** *Per 2 Cookies Unless Indicated* | | | |
| **Chips Deluxe:** Original | 160 | 8 | 19 |
| Chocolate Lovers | 160 | 9 | 20 |
| Coconut | 160 | 9 | 18 |
| Rainbow Choc Chip | 160 | 8 | 20 |
| Minis, 1.4 oz package | 200 | 10 | 27 |
| Soft & Chewy | 140 | 6 | 21 |
| Country Style Oatmeal with Raisins | 130 | 6 | 19 |
| Danish Wedding (4) | 130 | 6 | 18 |
| **E.L. Fudge:** Original | 170 | 7 | 25 |
| Double Stuffed | 180 | 9 | 24 |
| **Fudge Shoppe:** | | | |
| Deluxe Grahams (3) | 140 | 7 | 18 |
| Fudge Sticks (3) | 150 | 8 | 20 |
| Fudge Stripes (3) | 150 | 7 | 21 |
| Mini's, 1 package | 200 | 9 | 27 |
| Grasshopper (4) | 140 | 7 | 20 |
| Peanut Butter Filled | 160 | 9 | 17 |
| 100 Calorie Rite Bites: | | | |
| Mini Fudge Stripes, 1 pouch | 100 | 3.5 | 16 |
| Variety Pack, average, 1 pouch | 100 | 3 | 16 |
| **Gripz,** Graham Cinn, 1 pouch | 100 | 3 | 19 |
| **Iced Animal,** (6) | 140 | 4.5 | 22 |
| **Sandies Cookies:** | | | |
| Choc Chip Pecan | 170 | 10 | 18 |
| Pecan Shortbread | 170 | 10 | 18 |
| 100 Calorie Rite Bites, 1 pouch | 100 | 3.5 | 16 |
| **Vienna Fingers:** Regular | 150 | 6 | 23 |
| Reduced Fat | 140 | 4.5 | 24 |
| **Wafers:** Vanilla (8) | 140 | 5 | 22 |
| Mini Vanilla (18) | 140 | 5 | 22 |
| **Crackers:** | | | |
| **Club:** Original (4) | 70 | 3 | 9 |
| Reduced Fat (5) | 70 | 2 | 12 |
| **Grahams:** | | | |
| Original (8) | 120 | 3.5 | 22 |
| Cinnamon (8) | 130 | 3.5 | 23 |
| Honey (8) | 140 | 4.5 | 23 |
| **Town House:** | | | |
| Original (5) | 80 | 4.5 | 10 |
| Reduced Fat (6) | 60 | 1.5 | 11 |
| **Wheatables:** | | | |
| Original Gldn. Wheat (17) | 140 | 6 | 20 |
| Toasted Honey Wheat (17) | 140 | 6 | 20 |
| Nut Crisps, all flavors, (16), av | 140 | 6.5 | 20 |

*Per Cookie/Cracker, Unless Indicated*

| Kroger: | C | F | Cb |
|---|---|---|---|
| **Cookies:** Chip Mates | | | |
| Original (3), 1.5 oz | 160 | 8 | 22 |
| Chewy (2), 1 oz | 130 | 6 | 20 |
| Chunky (2), 1 oz | 130 | 6 | 18 |
| Olde Sthrn Pecan Shortbread (2),1 oz | 150 | 9 | 15 |
| Sugar Wafers (4), 1.1 oz | 160 | 7 | 24 |
| Vanilla Wafers (7), 1.1 oz | 130 | 3.5 | 24 |
| **Crackers:** | | | |
| Grahams, Original; Honey (4) | 120 | 3 | 20 |
| Saltines, Original, (5), 0.5 oz | 60 | 1.5 | 10 |
| **Kid-O's:** | | | |
| Mint (2) 1 oz | 140 | 6 | 22 |
| Chocolate Lovers (2), 1 oz | 140 | 6 | 21 |
| Double Filled Sandwich (2) 1 oz | 140 | 6 | 21 |
| Chocolate Sandwich (3) 1.15 oz | 150 | 6 | 25 |
| **Lance:** *Per Package of 6* | | | |
| **Cookies:** | | | |
| Nekot, Peanut Butter | 240 | 11 | 32 |
| Choc-O-Lunch, Vanilla Cream | 230 | 10 | 32 |
| Strawberry | 230 | 10 | 33 |
| **Crackers:** | | | |
| Creations (2), av. all flav. , 1 oz | 150 | 8 | 14 |
| Sandwich: | | | |
| Malt | 190 | 10 | 19 |
| Nip Chee, Chedd. Chse | 190 | 9 | 23 |
| Toastchee: | | | |
| Peanut Butter | 220 | 12 | 23 |
| Peanut Butter Red. Fat | 190 | 8 | 23 |
| Toasty, Peanut Butter | 180 | 9 | 19 |
| Wholegrain, av. all varieties | 185 | 9 | 24 |
| **Little Debbie:** | | | |
| Fig Bar | 160 | 3 | 32 |
| Marshmallow Pie, average | 180 | 7 | 28 |
| Marshmallow Treat | 160 | 4 | 31 |
| Oatmeal Creme Pie , 1.34 oz | 170 | 7 | 26 |
| Nutty Bar (2), 2 oz | 310 | 18 | 33 |
| **Lu:** | | | |
| Le Petit Beurre (4) | 140 | 4 | 24 |
| Le Petit Ecolier, average (2) | 130 | 7 | 15 |
| Pim's, Orange (2) | 100 | 3 | 17 |
| **Macaroni & Cheese,** *(Nabisco),* | | | |
| average all flavors | 150 | 7 | 18 |
| **Manischewitz** | | | |
| Chocolate Macaroon | 45 | 2 | 8 |
| Matzo Cracker, Miniatures (10) | 110 | 0 | 24 |
| Tam Tam Snack Crackers: | | | |
| Everything (10) | 140 | 5 | 19 |
| Onion (10) | 140 | 5 | 21 |

*Per Cookie/Cracker, Unless Indicated*

| Mary's Gone Crackers: | C | F | Cb |
|---|---|---|---|
| **Cookies:** Choc. Chip ; Dble Choc (2) | 130 | 6 | 19 |
| Ginger Snaps (3) | 140 | 5 | 23 |
| "N'Oatmeal" Raisin w/out Oats (2) | 120 | 4 | 20 |
| **Crackers,** all varieties (13) | 140 | 5 | 21 |
| **Miss Meringue:** | | | |
| Chocolettes (10), average | 130 | 3.5 | 24 |
| **Macaroons,** Traditional, 1.3 oz | 180 | 10 | 20 |
| **Madeleines:** | | | |
| Traditional & Dipped (2), 1.2 oz | 160 | 9 | 18 |
| Traditional Recipe (2), 1.2 oz | 160 | 9 | 19 |
| **Meringue Classiques:** | | | |
| Cappuccino (4), 1.1 oz | 110 | 0 | 26 |
| Mint Chocolate Chip (4), 1.1 oz | 120 | 1.5 | 25 |
| Triple Chocolate (4), 1.1 oz | 120 | 1.5 | 25 |
| Vanilla Rainbow/Van. (4), 1.1 oz | 110 | 0 | 27 |
| **Meringue Minis:** | | | |
| Chocolate (13), 1.1 oz | 110 | 0 | 26 |
| Chocolate Chip (12), 1.1 oz | 130 | 1.5 | 27 |
| Mint Chocolate Chip (12), 1.1 oz | 120 | 1.5 | 26 |
| Vanilla; Rainbow Van. (13), 1.1 oz | 110 | 0 | 27 |
| Sugar-Free: Chocolate (13), 0.5 oz | 40 | 0 | 8 |
| Vanilla (13), 0.5 oz | 35 | 0 | 9 |
| Mother's: | | | |
| Chocolate Chip (4), 1 oz | 150 | 7 | 20 |
| Circus Animal (6), 1 oz | 150 | 7 | 20 |
| Coconut Cocadas (5), 1.2 oz | 160 | 8 | 21 |
| Double Fudge (2), 1.3 oz | 170 | 7 | 27 |
| English Tea (2), 1.3 oz | 180 | 7 | 27 |
| Macaroons (2), 1 oz | 170 | 11 | 17 |
| Oatmeal (2), 1 oz | 130 | 5 | 19 |
| Taffy (2), 1.3 oz | 180 | 8 | 27 |
| Vanilla Creme (2), 1.3 oz | 180 | 7 | 26 |
| Iced: Lemonade (4), 1 oz | 150 | 7 | 19 |
| Oatmeal (4), 1.13 oz | 150 | 6 | 23 |
| **Mrs Fields Cookies** ~ *Fast-Foods Section, Page 219* | | | |
| **Murray Sugar Free Cookies:** | | | |
| Fudge-Dipped: Grahams (4) | 140 | 8 | 19 |
| Mint Cookies (4) | 130 | 7 | 17 |
| Vanilla Wafers (4) | 150 | 10 | 19 |
| Sandwiches, | | | |
| Chocolate; Lemon, average | 130 | 6 | 20 |
| Oatmeal (3) | 140 | 7 | 21 |
| Peanut Butter (3) | 150 | 9 | 16 |
| Shortbread (8) | 130 | 5 | 21 |
| Shortbread Pecan (3) | 160 | 11 | 18 |
| Vanilla Wafers (9) | 130 | 5 | 24 |
| Vanilla Creme Wafers (4) | 130 | 8 | 19 |

*Per Cookie/Cracker Unless Indicated*

**Nabisco:**    **C**   **F**   **Cb**

**Cookies:**

**Chips Ahoy!:**

| | C | F | Cb |
|---|---|---|---|
| Chewy, 1 oz | 120 | 5 | 18 |
| Chewy Gooey, all varieties, 1.1 oz | 150 | 7 | 21 |
| Chocolate Chip, 1.16 oz | 160 | 8 | 21 |
| Chunky, Chocolate Chunk, 0.6 oz | 80 | 4 | 10 |
| Mini Choc. Chips Bite-Size (14) | 150 | 7 | 21 |
| Snak Saks (5) | 150 | 7 | 21 |
| **Ginger Snaps,** (4) | 120 | 2.5 | 23 |
| **Lorna Doone,** (4) | 140 | 7 | 20 |
| Mallomars | 120 | 5 | 18 |

**Newtons:**

| | C | F | Cb |
|---|---|---|---|
| Fig: 1 oz | 110 | 2 | 22 |
| 2 oz | 200 | 4 | 39 |
| Mini, 1.34 oz pkg | 130 | 3 | 26 |
| Fat-Free, 1 oz | 90 | 0 | 22 |
| 100% Whole Grain, 1 oz | 110 | 2 | 22 |
| Raspberry; Strawberry: 1 oz | 100 | 1.5 | 21 |
| Mini Strawberry, 1.34 oz pkg | 130 | 3 | 26 |
| Fruit Crisps (1), av. all varieties, 1 oz | 100 | 2 | 20 |
| Fruit Thins (1), av. all varieties, 1 oz | 140 | 5 | 21 |

**Nilla Wafers:** (8), 1 oz    140   6   21
Reduced-Fat (8), 1 oz    120   2   24

**Nutter Butter:**

| | C | F | Cb |
|---|---|---|---|
| Sandwich Cookies, 1 oz | 130 | 5 | 20 |
| Bites: 1.25 oz | 170 | 7 | 24 |
| Go-Paks (10), 1 oz | 140 | 6 | 21 |
| Creme Patties, Peanut Butter (5) | 160 | 9 | 19 |

**Oreo,** Sandwich Cookies:

| | C | F | Cb |
|---|---|---|---|
| Original, White Creme Filling: 1.2 oz | 160 | 7 | 25 |
| Reduced-Fat, 1.2 oz | 150 | 4.5 | 27 |
| Snak-Sak, Mini Bite Size, 1 oz | 130 | 6 | 21 |
| Chocolate Creme Filling, 1.2 oz | 160 | 7 | 28 |
| Chocolate Fudge Covered, 0.7 oz | 100 | 5 | 13 |
| Dble Delight, Choc Mint'n Crm, 1 oz | 140 | 7 | 20 |
| Golden: Original, 1.2 oz | 170 | 7 | 25 |
| Double Stuff, 1 oz | 150 | 7 | 21 |
| Uh-Oh with Choc. Cream, 1.2 oz | 170 | 7 | 25 |

**Teddy Grahams:**

| | C | F | Cb |
|---|---|---|---|
| Snacks: Honey; Cinn. (24) | 130 | 4 | 23 |
| Chocolate (24), av. | 130 | 4.5 | 22 |
| Snak Saks, Mini Honey (47) | 130 | 4 | 22 |

*Per Cookie/Cracker Unless Indicated*

**Nabisco Cookies (Cont):**    **C**   **F**   **Cb**

**100 Calorie Packs:** *Per Pack*

Thin Crisps/Cookie Crisps:

| | C | F | Cb |
|---|---|---|---|
| Chips A'hoy, 0.74 oz | 100 | 3 | 18 |
| Variety Pack, 0.74 oz | 100 | 3 | 16 |
| Cookie Crisps: Lorna Doone, 0.74 oz | 100 | 3 | 16 |
| Lorna Doone Shortbreads, 0.7 oz | 100 | 3 | 16 |
| Planters, Peanut Butter, 0.85 oz | 100 | 3 | 17 |

**Snackwells ~** *See Page 87*

**Crackers:**

**Barnum's:** 1 oz    120   3.5   22
Snack Saks, 1.1 oz    140   4   24

**Flavor Originals:**

| | C | F | Cb |
|---|---|---|---|
| Baked: Better Cheddars, 1.1 oz | 160 | 8 | 18 |
| Sociables, Savory, 0.5 oz | 70 | 3.5 | 9 |
| Vegetable Thins, 1.1 oz | 150 | 7 | 20 |
| Chicken In A Biscit, 1.1 oz | 160 | 8 | 19 |

**Honey Maid:**

| | C | F | Cb |
|---|---|---|---|
| Grahams: Orig.; Honey, 1.1 oz | 130 | 3 | 24 |
| Chocolate, 1.23 oz | 140 | 3.5 | 27 |
| Low-Fat, av., 1.23 oz | 140 | 2 | 28 |
| Mini S'Mores, 1 oz | 140 | 6 | 21 |

**Premium Crackers:** Original, 0.5 oz   70   1.5   12

| | C | F | Cb |
|---|---|---|---|
| Minis, 0.5 oz | 70 | 2 | 11 |
| Saltine: Original, 0.5 oz | 70 | 1.5 | 12 |
| Minis (21), 0.5 oz | 70 | 2.5 | 10 |
| Fat-Free, 0.5 oz | 60 | 0 | 13 |
| Hint of Salt, 0.5 oz | 70 | 1.5 | 11 |
| Multigrain, 0.5 oz | 70 | 2 | 12 |
| Unsalted Tops, 0.5 oz | 70 | 1.5 | 13 |

**Wheat Thins:**

| | C | F | Cb |
|---|---|---|---|
| Crackers: Original (9), 1.1 oz | 140 | 5 | 22 |
| Baked, Reduced-Fat (9), 1 oz | 130 | 3.5 | 22 |
| Av. other varieties, 1 oz | 140 | 5 | 22 |
| Fiber Selects, av. all var,, 1.oz | 120 | 4 | 22 |
| Flatbread, av. all var., 0.5 oz | 60 | 1.5 | 12 |
| Multigrain, 1.1 oz | 140 | 4.5 | 22 |
| 100 Calorie Packs, | | | |
| Minis, Multi-Grain, 0.75 oz | 100 | 3 | 16 |

**Wheatsworth,**
Stone Ground Wheat (5)    80   3.5   10

**Zwieback,** 1 piece, 0.3 oz    35   1   6

Per Cookie/Cracker, Unless Indicated **C** **F** **Cb**

**Newman's Own Organics**

| | C | F | Cb |
|---|---|---|---|
| Alphabet Cookies, 10, av. | 120 | 3 | 21 |
| Fig Newman's: Fat-Free, 2 bars | 120 | 0 | 28 |
| Low-Fat, 2 bars | 140 | 2 | 28 |
| Wheat/Dairy-Free, 2 bars | 120 | 1.5 | 26 |
| Newman-O's: Original (2) | 110 | 4.5 | 18 |
| Choc. Creme (2); Mint Creme (2) | 110 | 5 | 18 |
| Ginger-O's (2) | 120 | 4 | 19 |

**Nonni's Biscotti:**

| | C | F | Cb |
|---|---|---|---|
| Original (1), 0.7 oz | 90 | 3 | 14 |
| Decadence (1), 0.85 oz | 100 | 4 | 16 |
| Average other varieties (1), 0.85 oz | 110 | 4 | 17 |

**Oreo Cookies** ~ See Nabisco, Page 85

**Peek Freans:**

| | C | F | Cb |
|---|---|---|---|
| Assorted Creme (3) | 140 | 6 | 19 |
| Nice Biscuits (1) | 160 | 6 | 25 |
| Shortcake (2) | 140 | 7 | 18 |

**Pepperidge Farm:**

**American Collection:**

| | C | F | Cb |
|---|---|---|---|
| Chesapeake, Dark Chocolate Pecan | 130 | 6 | 17 |
| Montauk, Milk Chocolate | 130 | 6 | 18 |
| Nantucket: Dark Chocolate | 130 | 6 | 18 |
| Double | 140 | 7 | 19 |
| Sausalito, Milk Chocolate | 130 | 6 | 17 |
| Tahoe, White Choc. Macadamia | 130 | 6 | 17 |
| Brussels, (3) | 150 | 7 | 20 |
| Chessmen, (3) | 120 | 5 | 18 |
| Favorites, Chocolate (2) | 130 | 7 | 17 |
| Geneva, (3) | 160 | 9 | 19 |

**Homestyle:**

| | C | F | Cb |
|---|---|---|---|
| gingerman (4) | 130 | 3.5 | 22 |
| Shortbread (2) | 130 | 6 | 17 |
| Sugar (3) | 150 | 7 | 21 |
| Milano: Original; Milk Choc (3), av. | 175 | 10 | 21 |
| Double Chocolate | 140 | 8 | 17 |
| Orange; Raspberry; Strawberry (2) | 130 | 7 | 16 |
| Melts, all varieties, (2) | 140 | 7 | 18 |
| Pirouettes, (2), average all var. | 120 | 5 | 19 |
| Tahiti, Coconut (2) | 170 | 10 | 17 |
| Tim Tams: Caramel (2) | 190 | 9 | 29 |
| Chocolate Creme (2) | 190 | 10 | 24 |
| Verona, Strawberry; Raspberry (3) | 140 | 5 | 22 |

**100 Calorie Pouches,**

| | C | F | Cb |
|---|---|---|---|
| average all varieties, 1 pouch | 100 | 4.5 | 12 |

Per Cookie/Cracker, Unless Indicated **C** **F** **Cb**

**Pepperidge Farm (Cont):**

**Crackers:**

| | C | F | Cb |
|---|---|---|---|
| Baked Naturals: Cheese Crisps, (20), all varieties | 140 | 6 | 19 |
| Crackers (2), av. all varieties | 135 | 4.5 | 23 |
| Entertaining Quartet (4) | 70 | 2.5 | 10 |
| Golden Butter (4) | 70 | 2.5 | 11 |
| Harvest Wheat (4) | 100 | 4 | 14 |
| Wheat Crisps (17) | 140 | 5 | 21 |

**Goldfish:**

| | C | F | Cb |
|---|---|---|---|
| Average all flavors: (55), 1 oz | 140 | 5 | 23 |
| 1.5 oz pouch | 210 | 8 | 37 |
| 2 oz carton | 280 | 10 | 46 |

**Pretzel Thins,**

| | C | F | Cb |
|---|---|---|---|
| Baked Naturals (11) | 110 | 0 | 21 |

**Snack Sticks,**

| | C | F | Cb |
|---|---|---|---|
| Toasted Sesame (12) | 140 | 5 | 20 |

**Ritz:**

| | C | F | Cb |
|---|---|---|---|
| Crackers: Original, 0.5oz | 80 | 4.5 | 10 |
| Reduced-Fat, 0.5 oz | 70 | 2 | 11 |
| Hint of Salt, 0.5 oz | 80 | 4 | 10 |
| Honey Butter (5), 0.6 oz | 80 | 4 | 10 |
| Roasted Vegetable, 0.6 oz | 80 | 3.5 | 10 |
| With Peanut Butter, 1.4 oz pkg | 190 | 9 | 24 |
| With Real Cheese, 1.4 oz package | 200 | 12 | 22 |
| Whole Wheat, 0.5 oz | 70 | 2.5 | 11 |
| 100 Calorie Toasted Chips, Snack Mix, 0.78 oz | 100 | 3 | 16 |
| Crackerfuls, all varieties, 1 oz | 130 | 7 | 17 |

**Ritz Bits Cracker Sandwiches:**

| | C | F | Cb |
|---|---|---|---|
| Cheese: Single Serve, 1.5 oz | 220 | 13 | 24 |
| 3 oz Pack | 450 | 25 | 50 |
| Go-Pak (13), 1 oz | 150 | 9 | 17 |
| Cheddar Cheese, 1 oz pack | 130 | 7 | 17 |
| Four Cheese, 1 oz pack | 130 | 7 | 17 |
| P'nut Butter: Single Serve, 1.25 oz | 170 | 10 | 20 |
| Big Bag: (12), 1 oz | 140 | 8 | 16 |
| Whole Bag (36), 3 oz | 420 | 23 | 48 |

**Ritz Toasted Chips:**

| | C | F | Cb |
|---|---|---|---|
| Main Street Originals 1 oz | 130 | 4.5 | 21 |
| All other Varieties, 1 oz | 130 | 6 | 19 |

**Safeway Select:**

| | C | F | Cb |
|---|---|---|---|
| Homestyle, Oatmeal Raisin, 1 oz | 130 | 6 | 18 |
| Indulgent: Dble Choc Chunk, 1 oz | 130 | 7 | 18 |
| Milk Choc. Macadamia Nut, 1 oz | 140 | 8 | 17 |

**Gourmet Sandwich Cremes:**

| | C | F | Cb |
|---|---|---|---|
| Maple Creme (2), 1.1 oz | 170 | 7 | 25 |
| Raspberry Swirl (2), 1.1 oz | 130 | 5 | 20 |
| Strawberry Swirl (2), 1. oz | 130 | 6 | 19 |

| | C | F | Cb |
|---|---|---|---|
| **Shar:** *Gluten Free* | | | |
| **Cookies:** Chocolate O's (3) | 150 | 7 | 19 |
| Lady Fingers (3) | 110 | 2 | 22 |
| S'wich Cremes: Choc.; Vanilla (2) | 130 | 6 | 16 |
| Wafers, Cocoa; Vanilla (4), average | 160 | 8 | 19 |
| **Crackers:** Snack (8) | 240 | 11 | 29 |
| Table (5) | 130 | 3 | 24 |
| **Snackwell's:** | | | |
| Creme S'wich (2) 1 oz | 110 | 3 | 20 |
| Devil's Food Cake, Fat-Free, 0.5 oz | 50 | 0 | 12 |
| 100 Calorie Packs, all flavors, 0.74 oz | 100 | 4.5 | 17 |
| **Stella D'Oro:** | | | |
| **Cookies:** | | | |
| Biscotti, average, 0.75 oz | 100 | 4.5 | 13 |
| Breakfast Treats: Choc. Cookie | 90 | 2.5 | 15 |
| Original (1), 0.75 oz | 90 | 3 | 14 |
| Viennese Cinnamon | 90 | 2.5 | 16 |
| Margherite (2) | 130 | 5 | 20 |
| Roman Egg Biscuits, 1.1 oz | 130 | 4 | 21 |
| Swiss Fudge (2) 1.1 oz | 170 | 9 | 22 |
| **Toast & Sponge:** | | | |
| Almond Toast (2) | 100 | 2 | 20 |
| Anisette Sponge (2) | 90 | 1 | 18 |
| Anisette Toast, 1.1 oz | 130 | 1 | 27 |
| **Streit's:** | | | |
| **Wafers:** Chocolate (3) | 160 | 9 | 19 |
| Lemon (3) | 170 | 10 | 19 |
| Rolls, Chocolate (3) | 105 | 6 | 12 |
| **Sunshine:** | | | |
| **Crackers:** | | | |
| Krispy: Original; Whole Wheat (5) | 60 | 1.5 | 11 |
| Soup & Oyster, 16 crackers | 60 | 1.5 | 11 |
| Cheez-It: Original (27), 1 oz | 150 | 8 | 17 |
| Reduced-Fat (29), 1 oz | 130 | 4.5 | 20 |
| **Trader Joe's:** | | | |
| **Cookies:** | | | |
| 100 Calorie Packs, average | 100 | 2.5 | 18 |
| Almond Windmill (2), 1 oz | 140 | 6 | 18 |
| Charmingly Chewy Choc Chip (2), 1 oz | 130 | 5 | 20 |
| Cherry Granola (2), 1 oz | 110 | 4 | 18 |
| Chocolate Almond Lacey's (1) | 120 | 8 | 12 |
| Chocolate Chip: Small (4), 1.1 oz | 140 | 7 | 18 |
| Large, Singles , 1.7 oz | 280 | 14 | 35 |
| Vegan (1), 1 oz | 130 | 6 | 18 |
| Caramel Cashew (3), 1 oz | 140 | 7 | 16 |
| Dark Choc Chunks w/ Almonds (3) | 140 | 7 | 17 |
| *Also See Snacks ~ Page 150* | | | |

| | C | F | Cb |
|---|---|---|---|
| *Per Cookie/Cracker, Unless Indicated* | | | |
| **Trader Joe's (Cont):** | | | |
| Dunkers: Choc. Chip (2), 1.2 oz | 160 | 7 | 21 |
| Choc. Coated Choc. Chip (2), 1.3 oz | 190 | 9 | 25 |
| Ginger Snaps, Gluten Free, (5), 1 oz | 140 | 6 | 21 |
| Highbrow Chocolate (2) | 140 | 7 | 17 |
| Joe Joe's S'wich Cremes, | | | |
| Choc./ Vanilla (2), 1 oz | 130 | 5 | 20 |
| Lemon Crisps (5) | 120 | 4 | 19 |
| Macarons A La Parisienne, | | | |
| 2 cookies, ¾ oz | 90 | 3 | 10 |
| Meringues, Fat-Free, | | | |
| Vanilla (4) | 110 | 0 | 27 |
| Oatmeal Raisin, 1.8 oz | 270 | 12 | 35 |
| Pecan Southern Style (4), 1 oz | 150 | 9 | 15 |
| Petite Cocoa Batons (17), 1 oz | 140 | 5 | 22 |
| Thins: Meyer Lemon (9), 1 oz | 160 | 5 | 25 |
| Triple Ginger (9), 1 oz | 140 | 4.5 | 24 |
| Triple Choc Chunk, 1 oz | 140 | 7 | 20 |
| Ultimate Vanilla Wafers (5), 1 oz | 120 | 6 | 15 |
| **Crackers,** Water (4) | 60 | 1 | 12 |
| **Triscuit:** *Per Serving* | | | |
| **Whole Grain Wheat Crackers:** | | | |
| Original (15), 1 oz | 120 | 4.5 | 19 |
| Roasted Garlic (8), 1 oz | 120 | 4.5 | 20 |
| Thin Crisps, all var., 1.1 oz | 140 | 5 | 22 |
| **Voortman:** | | | |
| **Classic:** Almond Krunch (2), 1 oz | 140 | 6 | 20 |
| Chunky Chip (1), 0.74 oz | 100 | 4.5 | 14 |
| Sugar Free, Choc. Chip (1), 0.7 oz | 80 | 5 | 13 |
| **Wafers:** All varieties (3), 1 oz | 140 | 6 | 20 |
| Sugar Free, Peanut Butter (4), 1 oz | 150 | 7 | 17 |
| **365** *(Whole Foods):* | | | |
| Choc Chip (5), 1 oz | 130 | 6 | 19 |
| Classic Fig Bars (2), 1.3 oz | 140 | 2.5 | 27 |
| Lemon Wafers (5), 0.9 oz | 120 | 5 | 17 |
| Oatmeal (6), 1 oz | 130 | 4.5 | 20 |
| Sandwich Cremes (2), average | 130 | 5 | 20 |
| Sugar (5), 1.1 oz | 130 | 4 | 22 |

## Thaw, Bake & Serve  | C | F | Cb |

**Pillsbury Cookies:** *Per Cookie Unless Indicated*

### Refrigerated Cookie Dough:

| | C | F | Cb |
|---|---|---|---|
| Chocolate Chip Cookies | 130 | 6 | 18 |
| Gingerbread (2) | 130 | 6 | 18 |
| Peanut Butter | 120 | 5 | 17 |
| Sugar | 120 | 5 | 18 |

### Ready To Bake:

| | C | F | Cb |
|---|---|---|---|
| Chocolate Chip (2) | 170 | 8 | 23 |
| Chocolate Chunk & Chip (2) | 170 | 8 | 23 |
| Holiday Cookies, Sugar, (2), av all | 120 | 6 | 15 |
| Sugar Cookie (2) | 170 | 8 | 22 |

#### Big Deluxe Classics:

| | C | F | Cb |
|---|---|---|---|
| Chocolate Chip | 170 | 8 | 23 |
| Oatmeal Raisin | 150 | 6 | 24 |
| Peanut Butter Cup | 170 | 8 | 22 |
| White Chunk Macadamia Nut | 170 | 9 | 22 |
| **Simply Cookies:** Chocolate Chip | 150 | 7 | 20 |
| Peanut Butter | 140 | 6 | 19 |

**Refrigerated Sweet Buns/Rolls~** *See Page 67*

**Toll House (Nestle):** *Per Cookie Unless Indicated*

### Refrigerated Dough:

| | C | F | Cb |
|---|---|---|---|
| Chocolate Chunk (2) | 200 | 10 | 26 |
| Jumbo Chocolate Chip (1) | 170 | 9 | 23 |
| Mini Brownie Bites (3) | 160 | 8 | 20 |
| Mini Chocolate Chip (3) | 160 | 8 | 21 |
| Peanut Butter Chocolate Chip (1) | 80 | 4.5 | 10 |
| Walnut Chocolate Chip (2) | 180 | 9 | 22 |

### Ultimates Refrigerated Dough:

| | C | F | Cb |
|---|---|---|---|
| Chocolate Chip Lovers | 180 | 9 | 23 |
| Choc. Chips & Chunks with Pecans | 190 | 10 | 22 |
| Peanut Butter Chips & Choc Chunks | 180 | 9 | 23 |
| Ultimate Filled, Turtle | 160 | 7 | 23 |
| White Chocolate Macadamia Nut | 190 | 10 | 22 |

## Crispbreads  | C | F | Cb |

*Per Crispbread Unless Indicated*

**Finn Crisp:**

| | C | F | Cb |
|---|---|---|---|
| Classic: Traditional, Rye | 40 | 0.5 | 7 |
| Hi-Fibre | 40 | 0 | 6.5 |
| Round: Original | 45 | 0.5 | 7.5 |
| Sesame | 50 | 1 | 8 |

**Kavli Norwegian:**

| | C | F | Cb |
|---|---|---|---|
| Crispy Thin (3) | 50 | 0 | 11 |
| Hearty Thick (2) | 60 | 0 | 12 |
| **Malsovit,** Meal Wafers | 75 | 4 | 7 |

**New York Flatbread Crisps,**

| | C | F | Cb |
|---|---|---|---|
| Everything, 0.4 oz | 50 | 1.5 | 7 |
| **Ry-Krisp:** Natural (2) | 50 | 0 | 11 |
| Seasoned (2) | 60 | 1 | 11 |
| Sesame (2) | 60 | 1.5 | 10 |

**Ryvita:**

| | C | F | Cb |
|---|---|---|---|
| **Crackerbreads:** Orig.; Wholegrain | 20 | 0 | 4 |
| **Crispbreads:** Original; Dark | 70 | 0 | 13 |
| **WASA:** Crisp'n Light 7 Grain (3) | 60 | 0 | 13 |
| Fiber, 0.35 oz | 35 | 0.5 | 8 |
| Hearty, 0.5 oz | 45 | 0 | 11 |
| Light Rye (2), 0.5 oz | 60 | 0 | 14 |
| Multi Grain, 0.5 oz | 45 | 0 | 10 |
| Whole Wheat, 0.5 oz | 50 | 1 | 10 |

## Matzos

**Manischewitz:**

| | C | F | Cb |
|---|---|---|---|
| **Matzos:** Passover Egg, 1.1 oz | 100 | 0 | 20 |
| Egg 'n Onion, 1 oz | 80 | 0.5 | 17 |
| Thin Salted; Thin Tea,av., 0.9 oz | 95 | 0 | 20 |
| Unsalted, 1 oz | 110 | 0 | 24 |
| Whole Wheat, 1 oz | 110 | 1 | 21 |

**Crackers:**

| | C | F | Cb |
|---|---|---|---|
| **Tam Tam:** Original (10), 1 oz | 110 | 4 | 16 |
| Everything; Onion (10), 1 oz | 140 | 5 | 19 |
| Sesame (10), 1 oz | 140 | 6 | 19 |

**Streit's:**

| | C | F | Cb |
|---|---|---|---|
| Mediterranean Matzos, 1 Matzo, 1 oz | 90 | 0.5 | 18 |
| Unsalted Matzos, 1 Matzo, 1 oz | 100 | 0 | 23 |

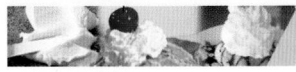

## Quick Guide | C | F | Cb |

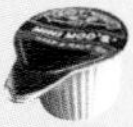

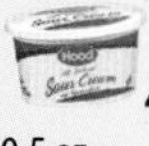

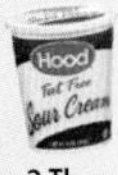

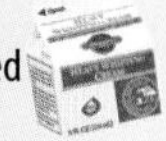

### Cream
*Average All Brands*
**Half & Half Cream:**

| | C | F | Cb |
|---|---|---|---|
| 1 Tbsp, 0.5 oz | 20 | 1.5 | 0.5 |
| 2 Tbsp, 1 oz | 40 | 3 | 1 |
| ¼ cup, 2 oz | 80 | 6 | 2 |
| Single Serve Cup, ⅜ fl.oz | 15 | 1.5 | 0.5 |
| **Light:** Coffee/table (20% fat): 1 Tbsp | 30 | 3 | 0.5 |
| 2 Tbsp, 1 oz | 60 | 6 | 0.5 |

**Sour Cream:**

| | C | F | Cb |
|---|---|---|---|
| **Regular:** 1 Tbsp, 0.5 oz | 25 | 2.5 | 1 |
| 1 cup, 8 oz | 445 | 45 | 7 |
| **Low-Fat/Light:** 1 Tbsp, 0.5 oz | 20 | 1.5 | 1 |
| 2 Tbsp, 1 oz | 40 | 3 | 2 |
| **Fat-Free:** Av., 2 Tbsp, 1 oz | 20 | 0 | 4.5 |
| *Hood,* 2 Tbsp, 1 oz | 25 | 0 | 4 |
| *Kroger,* 2 Tbsp, 1 oz | 20 | 0 | 3 |
| *Naturally Yours; Oak Farm,* 2 Tbsp | 20 | 0 | 3 |
| *Knudsen,* 2 Tbsp, 1 oz | 30 | 0 | 5 |

**Sour Cream Substitute:**

| | C | F | Cb |
|---|---|---|---|
| *Albertson's,* 2 Tbsp, 1 oz | 60 | 5 | 2 |
| *Tofutti Sour Supreme,* 2 Tbsp, 1 oz | 85 | 5 | 9 |

**Whipping Cream:**
**Heavy:** (37% fat):

| | C | F | Cb |
|---|---|---|---|
| 1 T. fluid/2 T. whipped | 50 | 5.5 | 0.5 |
| ¼ cup whipped | 105 | 11 | 1 |
| ½ cup fluid/1 cup whipped | 410 | 44 | 3.5 |

**Light:** (30% fat):

| | C | F | Cb |
|---|---|---|---|
| 1 Tbsp fluid/2 Tbsp whipped | 45 | 4.5 | 0.5 |
| ½ cup fluid/1 cup whipped | 350 | 37 | 3.5 |

### Coconut Cream/Milk

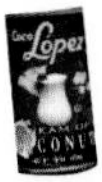

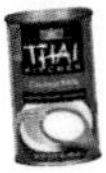

| | C | F | Cb |
|---|---|---|---|
| **Coconut Cream:** (Canned), | | | |
| Plain/unsweetened: 2 Tbsp, 1 oz | 75 | 6.5 | 3 |
| ½ cup, 4 oz | 285 | 26 | 12 |
| Sweetened: | | | |
| Coco Lopez: 1 oz | 130 | 5 | 21 |
| ½ cup, 4 oz | 520 | 20 | 84 |
| **Coconut Milk:** (Canned): | | | |
| **Thai Kitchen:** | | | |
| Lite, ¼ cup, 2 fl.oz | 50 | 4.5 | 1 |
| Premium, 2 fl.oz | 140 | 14 | 3 |
| **Coconut Water,** (Center), 1 cup | 45 | 0.5 | 9 |

### Whipped Toppings | C | F | Cb |

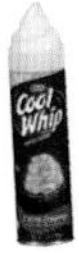

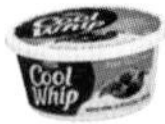

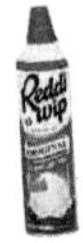

*Average All Brands*

| | C | F | Cb |
|---|---|---|---|
| **Cream (Pressurized):** 2 Tbsp | 20 | 1.5 | 1 |
| ¼ cup | 40 | 3.5 | 2 |
| ½ cup | 75 | 6.5 | 4 |
| **Cream Topping,** Lite, 2 Tbsp | 20 | 1 | 3 |
| **Cool Whip:** Original, ⅓ oz | 25 | 1.5 | 2 |
| Extra Creamy, 2 Tbsp | 25 | 2 | 2 |
| Lite, 2 Tbsp, ¼ oz | 20 | 1 | 3 |
| Free, 2 Tbsp, 0.32 oz | 15 | 0 | 3 |
| **Kraft,** Dream Whip, 2 Tbsp | 10 | 0 | 2 |
| **Reddi-Wip:** | | | |
| Original, 2 T., 0.28 oz | 15 | 1 | 1 |
| Chocolate, 2 Tbsp, 0.28 oz | 15 | 1 | 1 |
| Extra Creamy, 2 Tbsp, 0.28 oz | 15 | 1 | 1 |
| Fat-Free, 2 Tbsp, 0.28 oz | 5 | 0 | 1 |

### Creamers (Non-Dairy)
**Powder:**
**Coffee-Mate/Cremora/N-Rich:**

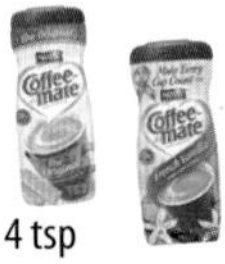

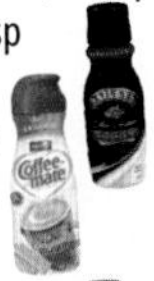

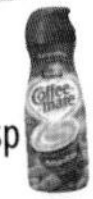

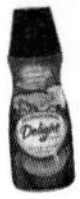

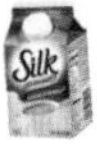

| | C | F | Cb |
|---|---|---|---|
| Original: 1 tsp | 10 | 0.5 | 1 |
| 1 heaping tsp | 25 | 2 | 2 |
| Lite, 1 tsp | 10 | 0 | 2 |
| Flavors: 4 tsp | 60 | 3 | 8 |
| Fat-Free, Average, 4 tsp | 50 | 0 | 11 |

**Liquid/Refrigerated:** *Per Tablespoon*

| | C | F | Cb |
|---|---|---|---|
| **Bailey's:** Average all flavors, 1 Tbsp | 40 | 1.5 | 6 |
| Fat Free, all flavors, 1 Tbsp | 25 | 0 | 5 |
| **Coffee-Mate:** | | | |
| Unflavored: Original, 1 Tbsp | 20 | 1 | 2 |
| Fat-Free, 1 Tbsp | 10 | 0 | 1 |
| Low-Fat, 1 Tbsp | 10 | 0.5 | 2 |
| Flavors: Av. all flav., 1 Tbsp | 35 | 1.5 | 5 |
| Fat-Free, all flavors, 1 Tbsp | 25 | 0 | 5 |
| **Hood,** Country Creamer, 1 Tbsp | 20 | 1.5 | 2 |
| **International Delight:** | | | |
| Average all flavors, 1 Tbsp | 40 | 1.5 | 7 |
| Fat-Free French Vanilla, 1 Tbsp | 30 | 0 | 7 |
| **Kroger:** | | | |
| Coffee, Fat-Free & Lactose Free: | | | |
| Caramel Vanilla, 1 Tbsp | 25 | 1.5 | 6 |
| Hazelnut, 1 Tbsp | 35 | 1.5 | 6 |
| **Silk:** Original, 1Tbsp | 15 | 1 | 1 |
| French Van.; Hazelnut, 1 Tbsp | 20 | 1 | 3 |

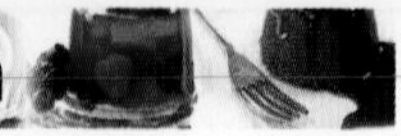

## Ready-To-Serve

**Hunt's Snack Pack:** *Per 3.5oz Cup*

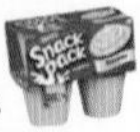

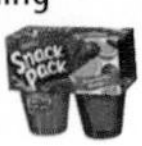

| | C | F | Cb |
|---|---|---|---|
| **Puddings:** Av. all flavors | 120 | 3.5 | 21 |
| Fat Free, av. all flavors | 80 | 0 | 19 |
| Sugar Free, av. all flavors | 65 | 3 | 13 |
| Dessert Twists, av. all flavors | 120 | 3 | 21 |
| Fruit Blasts: Lemon Pudding | 130 | 2.5 | 25 |
| Juicy Gels, av. all flav. | 100 | 0 | 25 |
| Sugar Free, av. all flav. | 10 | 0 | 1 |

**Jell-O** *(Kraft)*:

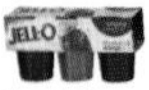

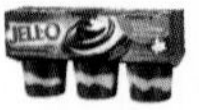

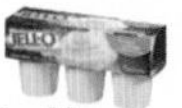

| | C | F | Cb |
|---|---|---|---|
| **Cheesecake Snacks (6 Pack),** Strawberry | 130 | 2 | 25 |
| **Gelatin Snacks (6 Pack),** all varieties, 3.5 oz Cup | 10 | 0 | 0 |
| **Gel Cups (6 Pack):** *Per 3.5 oz Cup* | | | |
| Xtreme: Cherry & Blue Raspberry | 70 | 0 | 17 |
| Watermelon & Green Apple | 100 | 0 | 24 |
| **Pudding Snacks (6 Pack):** *Per 4 oz Cup* | | | |
| Original: Chocolate | 120 | 1.5 | 25 |
| With Van. Swirls | 110 | 1.5 | 24 |
| Sundae Toppers | 110 | 1 | 23 |
| Tapioca, fat free | 100 | 0 | 23 |
| Vanilla | 110 | 1.5 | 23 |
| **Smoothie Snacks (6 Pack),** Mixed Berry; Strawb, Ban., 4 oz cup | 100 | 2.5 | 18 |

**Kozy Shack Puddings:**

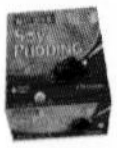

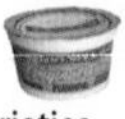

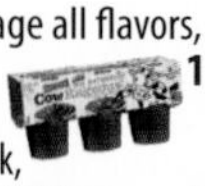

| | C | F | Cb |
|---|---|---|---|
| Chocolate, ½ cup, 4 oz | 140 | 3.5 | 24 |
| **Rice:** *Per 1 Cup, 4 oz* | | | |
| Original | 130 | 3 | 22 |
| Cinnamon Raisin | 140 | 3 | 24 |
| European Style | 130 | 3.5 | 21 |
| No Sugar Added, av. all varieties | 80 | 1 | 11 |
| **No Sugar Added:** | | | |
| Chocolate; Tapioca, average, 1 cup | 65 | 1 | 11 |
| Vanilla, ½ cup | 90 | 3 | 10 |
| **Bread Pudding,** average all flavors, ½ cup, 4 oz | 155 | 3.5 | 28 |
| **Cowrageous:** | | | |
| Low-Fat (1% Milk), 6-Pack, Av., 1 pudding cup, 3.75 oz | 100 | 1 | 20 |
| **Simplywell,** 4 oz, av. all flavors | 100 | 1 | 17 |
| **SmartGels,** 4 oz, average all flavors | 80 | 0 | 22 |
| **Flan,** Creme Caramel, 1 cup | 150 | 3.5 | 27 |

**Kraft:**

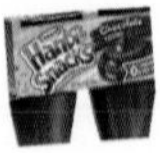

| | C | F | Cb |
|---|---|---|---|
| **Handi Snacks (4 Pack):** *Per cup, 3.5 oz* | | | |
| Banana | 90 | 1 | 20 |
| Butterscotch | 90 | 1 | 1 |
| Chocolate | 100 | 1 | 23 |
| Fat Free | 90 | 0 | 21 |
| Rice Pudding | 140 | 6 | 19 |
| Vanilla | 90 | 0 | 20 |

## Ready-To-Serve (Cont)

**Kroger:** *Per Container*

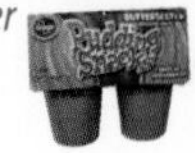

| | C | F | Cb |
|---|---|---|---|
| Butterscotch, 3.5 oz | 110 | 2 | 22 |
| Chocolate, 3.5 oz | 110 | 2.5 | 21 |

**Swiss Miss:**

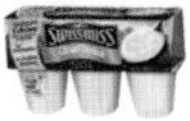

| | C | F | Cb |
|---|---|---|---|
| **Puddings:** *Per 4 oz Cup* | | | |
| Chocolate Dream | 160 | 4 | 27 |
| Classic Butterscotch | 10 | 3.5 | 22 |
| Creamy vanilla | 140 | 3.5 | 24 |
| **Pudding Snacks:** *Per 4 oz Cup* | | | |
| Banana Cream Pie; Blueberry Muffin | 110 | 3.5 | 18 |
| Caramel Cream; Vanilla, average | 120 | 3 | 21 |
| Chocolate | 130 | 3 | 22 |
| Fat Free | 80 | 0 | 20 |

## Homemade Puddings

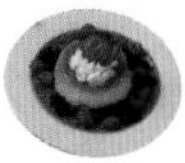

| | C | F | Cb |
|---|---|---|---|
| Apple Tapioca, ½ cup | 150 | 0 | 32 |
| Bread Pudding, ½ cup | 250 | 8 | 40 |
| Blancmange, ½ cup | 140 | 5 | 19 |
| Chocolate, ½ cup | 190 | 6 | 30 |
| Crème Brûlée, ½ cup | 400 | 35 | 16 |
| Plum Pudding, 2 oz | 170 | 3 | 32 |
| Rice with Raisins, ½ cup | 200 | 4 | 38 |
| Sponge Pudding, 3.5 oz | 340 | 16 | 45 |
| Tapioca Cream, ½ cup | 110 | 4 | 15 |
| Trifle, ½ cup | 180 | 7 | 26 |

## Custards

| | C | F | Cb |
|---|---|---|---|
| **Custard Mix:** Dry, ⅙ package | 85 | 1 | 17 |
| Prepared with 2% milk, ½ cup | 140 | 3.5 | 21 |
| Jello Flan, with 2% milk, ½ cup | 140 | 2.5 | 20 |
| *Royal-Flan,* Prep. w/ 2% milk, ½ cup | 130 | 2.5 | 24 |
| **Homemade Custard:** | | | |
| Baked: Plain, ½ cup, 4.5oz | 150 | 7 | 16 |
| With non fat milk, and sugar subsititute | 70 | 3 | 4 |
| Boiled, ½ cup | 165 | 7 | 18 |

## Gelatin • Parfait • Jell-O

| | C | F | Cb |
|---|---|---|---|
| **Gelatin Dessert Mix:** *Prepared* | | | |
| *Jell-O:* Regular, all flavors, ¼ pkg | 80 | 0 | 18 |
| Sugar Free/Low Calorie, ¼ pkg | 10 | 0 | 0 |
| **Creme Gelatin/Parfait:** *Per ½ Cup* | | | |
| *Ida Mae,* ½ cup | 60 | 2 | 10 |
| *Reser's,* Rasp. Parfait, 3.88 oz | 100 | 2 | 19 |

## Meringues

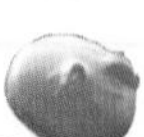

| | C | F | Cb |
|---|---|---|---|
| Meringue Swirl, ½ oz | 50 | 0 | 8 |
| Meringue Shell, 1 oz shell | 100 | 0 | 16 |

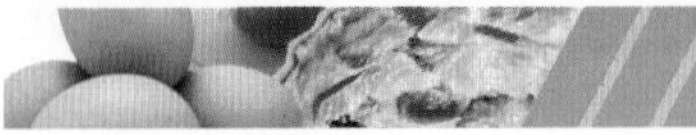

### Chicken Eggs  C  F  Cb

**Fresh Eggs:**
**Raw (weight with shell):**

| | C | F | Cb |
|---|---|---|---|
| Small, 1.4 oz | 65 | 4 | 0 |
| Medium, 1.55 oz | 70 | 4 | 0 |
| Large, 1.76 oz | 75 | 4.5 | 0 |
| Extra Large, 1.98 oz | 80 | 5 | 0 |
| Jumbo, 2.22 oz | 90 | 5.5 | 0 |
| **Egg Yolk,** 1 extra large | 63 | 5 | 0 |
| **Egg White,** 1 extra large | 16 | 0 | 0 |

**Dried Egg Powder:**

| | C | F | Cb |
|---|---|---|---|
| **Whole Egg:** ¼ **cup,** 1 oz | 170 | 12 | 0 |
| 1 Tbsp | 30 | 2 | 0 |
| **Egg White,** ¼ cup, 1 oz | 105 | 0 | 0 |
| **Egg Yolk,** ¼ cup, 1 oz | 195 | 18 | 0 |

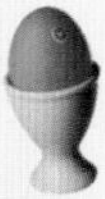

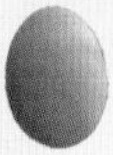

### Egg Substitutes

*¼ Cup (Equivalent to 1 Egg) ~ Zero Cholesterol*

| | C | F | Cb |
|---|---|---|---|
| **All Whites** (Crystal Farms), 1.62 oz | 25 | 0 | 0 |
| **Better 'n Eggs** (Crystal Farms): | | | |
| Regular, ¼ cup, 2 oz | 30 | 0 | 1 |
| Plus, ¼ cup, 2 oz | 35 | 0 | 1 |
| **Egg Beaters** (Conagra): | | | |
| Original, 3 Tbsp, 1.62 oz | 25 | 0 | 1 |
| Southwestern Style, 3 Tbsp, 1.62 oz | 20 | 0 | 1 |
| **Egg Replacer** (Ener-g), 1½ tsp, | 15 | 0 | 4 |
| **Eggs** (Second Nature), | | | |
| Fat-Free, ¼ cup, 2 fl.oz | 35 | 0 | 0.5 |
| **Egg Substitute** (Albertson's), ¼ cup | 30 | 0 | 1 |
| **Naturegg** (Burnbrae Farms), | | | |
| Simply Egg White, ¼ cup, 2 oz | 30 | 0 | 0 |

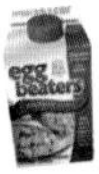

### Other Eggs

| | C | F | Cb |
|---|---|---|---|
| Duck, 1 large, 2.5 oz | 130 | 9.5 | 0 |
| Goose, 1 large, 5 oz | 280 | 19 | 0 |
| Quail, 3 eggs, 1 oz | 42 | 3 | 0 |
| Turkey, 1 large, 3 oz | 135 | 9.5 | 0 |
| Turtle, 1 egg, 1.75 oz | 75 | 5 | 0 |

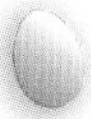

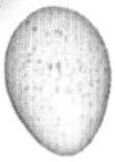

### Omega-3 Fat Enriched

| | C | F | Cb |
|---|---|---|---|
| **Eggland's Best,** 1 large | 70 | 4 | 0 |
| **Eggs Plus** (Pilgrim's Pride), 1 large | 70 | 4.5 | 1 |

**Note:** Cholesterol content same as regular eggs, but Omega-3 fats inhibit blood cholesterol increase.
**Extra Notes ~** *See Page 259*

### Cooked Eggs  C  F  Cb

| | C | F | Cb |
|---|---|---|---|
| **Boiled Egg:** *Same as raw egg* | | | |
| **Hard-Cooked** (Egg·Lands), Small, Peeled | 65 | 4 | 0 |
| **Fried Egg:** | | | |
| With fat: 1 large egg | 105 | 9 | 0.5 |
| 2 small eggs | 175 | 13 | 1 |
| No fat/nonstick pan, 1 large | 75 | 5 | 0.5 |
| **Deviled Egg,** 2 halves | 145 | 13 | 0.5 |
| **Eggs Benedict,** (2) | | | |
| on Toast or English Muffin | 860 | 56 | 25 |
| **Eggs Florentine,** (2) | | | |
| on Toast or English Muffin | 890 | 59 | 25 |
| **Pickled Egg,** 1 large | 80 | 5.5 | 0 |
| **Poached Egg,** 1 large | 65 | 4 | 0 |
| **Quiche** (Homemade): | | | |
| Egg & Bacon, 1 slice, 5.3 oz | 580 | 43 | 27 |
| Ham & Cheese, 1 slice, 5.3 oz | 475 | 33 | 29 |
| **Scotch Egg,** 1 egg | 300 | 21 | 16 |
| **Scrambled Eggs:** 1 large egg: | | | |
| With 1 Tbsp milk + 1 tsp fat | 120 | 9 | 1 |
| With 1 Tbsp skim milk/no fat | 85 | 5.5 | 1 |
| 2 large eggs: | | | |
| With 2 Tbsp milk + 2 tsp fat | 260 | 20 | 2 |
| With 2 Tbsp skim milk, w/o fat | 180 | 11 | 2 |

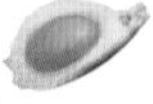

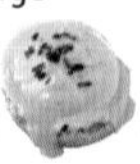

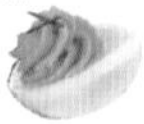

### Omelets

| | C | F | Cb |
|---|---|---|---|
| **1 Egg:** Plain (with 1 tsp fat) | 125 | 10 | 0.5 |
| With ½ oz cheese | 175 | 15 | 0.5 |
| W/ ½ oz cheese + ½ oz ham | 200 | 16 | 0.5 |
| **2 Eggs:** Plain (with 2 tsp fat) | 250 | 20 | 1 |
| With 1 oz cheese | 360 | 29 | 2 |
| With 1 oz cheese+1 oz ham | 410 | 32 | 2 |
| **3 Eggs:** Plain (with 1 Tbsp fat) | 360 | 29 | 1.5 |
| With 2 oz cheese | 580 | 47 | 2.5 |
| With 2 oz cheese+2 oz ham | 680 | 53 | 2.5 |
| **Extras:** Tomato/Onion/Veggies | 20 | 0 | 4.5 |
| **Egg Substitute** (EggBeaters): | | | |
| 2 eggs (½ cup) + 1 tsp fat | 100 | 4 | 2 |
| 3 eggs (¾ cup) + 2 tsp fat | 160 | 8 | 3 |
| Extras: 1 oz Cheese | 110 | 9 | 1 |
| 1 oz Ham | 50 | 3 | 1 |
| Tomato/Onion/veggies | 20 | 0 | 4.5 |

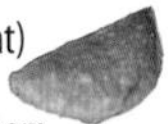

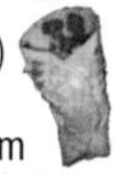

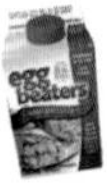

### Egg Nog

*Average all Brands*

| | C | F | Cb |
|---|---|---|---|
| ½ cup, 4 oz | 170 | 9.5 | 17 |
| **Regular** (Borden), ½ cup | 160 | 9 | 17 |
| **Golden** (Hood), ½ cup | 180 | 9 | 22 |
| **Light/Low-Fat,** (Horizon; Hood) | 140 | 4 | 22 |

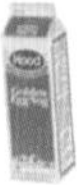

Updated Nutrition Data ~ www.CalorieKing.com
Persons with Diabetes ~ See Disclaimer (Page 22)

## Breakfast Sides

| | C | F | Cb |
|---|---|---|---|
| **Toast:** Plain, 1 thick slice | 85 | 1 | 13 |
| With 2 tsp butter/margarine | 155 | 9 | 13 |
| With 3 tsp/1 Tbsp fat | 190 | 13 | 13 |
| **English Muffin:** Plain, 2 oz | 130 | 1 | 26 |
| With 3 tsp fat | 230 | 12 | 26 |
| **Bacon,** 2 strips | 70 | 5 | 0 |
| **Ham,** Lean, 2 oz | 100 | 3 | 0 |
| **Hash Browns:** | | | |
| ½ cup, 3 oz | 125 | 6.5 | 14 |
| 1 cup serving, 6 oz | 250 | 13 | 28 |
| **Sausages,** 2 links (1 oz each) | 180 | 16 | 1.5 |

## Frozen Egg Breakfasts

| | C | F | Cb |
|---|---|---|---|
| **Aunt Jemima Breakfast Sandwiches:** *Per Package* | | | |
| Biscuit, Sausage, Egg & Cheese | 340 | 21 | 27 |
| Croissant, Sausage, Egg & Cheese | 350 | 23 | 23 |
| Griddlecake, Ham, Egg & Cheese | 240 | 8 | 33 |
| **Jimmy Dean Sandwiches:** | | | |
| Biscuit, Sausage, Egg & Cheese, (1) | 440 | 31 | 27 |
| Croissant, Sausage, Egg & Cheese, (1) | 430 | 29 | 30 |
| Muffin, Sausage, Egg & Cheese, (1) | 350 | 21 | 28 |
| Omelet: Three Cheese (1) | 290 | 23 | 4 |
| Ham & Cheese (1) | 250 | 19 | 4 |
| **Red Baron:** | | | |
| **Scrambles:** | | | |
| Bacon (1), 5 oz | 390 | 19 | 38 |
| Sausage (1), 5 oz | 360 | 17 | 38 |
| Western (1), 5 oz | 360 | 17 | 38 |
| **Frozen Pancake/Waffles ~** *See Page 132* | | | |

## Frozen Egg Rolls

| | C | F | Cb |
|---|---|---|---|
| **Kahiki:** | | | |
| Chicken (1), 3 oz | 90 | 3.5 | 12 |
| Pork (1), 3 oz | 110 | 6 | 11 |
| Vegetable (1), 3 oz | 80 | 3 | 12 |
| Sauce, 1 packet | 10 | 0 | 3 |
| **La Choy Mini,** | | | |
| Chicken (1), 3 oz | 140 | 4.5 | 18 |
| **Lotus:** Chicken, 3 oz | 160 | 7 | 25 |
| Pork (1), 3 oz | 160 | 7 | 25 |
| Vegetarian (1), 3 oz | 120 | 4.5 | 21 |
| **Minh,** | | | |
| Chicken (1), 3 oz | 160 | 5 | 20 |
| **Pagoda Express,** | | | |
| Vegetable (1), without sauce, 3 oz | 130 | 4.5 | 20 |
| **TGI Friday's,** | | | |
| Thai Style Chkn (1), 3 oz | 150 | 5 | 19 |
| **Trader Joes,** | | | |
| Vegetable (1), 3 oz | 110 | 4 | 16 |

## Fast-Foods/Restaurants

| | C | F | Cb |
|---|---|---|---|
| **Arby's,** | | | |
| Bacon, Egg & Cheese Croissant | 390 | 24 | 24 |
| **Au Bon Pain,** Egg on a Bagel | 430 | 12 | 58 |
| **Bob Evans:** | | | |
| Farmers Market Omelet | 640 | 45 | 14 |
| Ham & Cheddar Omelet | 515 | 36 | 4 |
| Western Omelet | 530 | 36 | 8 |
| **Bojangles:** Egg & Cheese Biscuit | 515 | 34 | 35 |
| Bacon, Egg & Cheese Biscuit | 555 | 37 | 35 |
| **Bruegger's Bagels:** | | | |
| Breakfast Sandwiches: | | | |
| Bagel: With Egg & Cheese, 6.8 oz | 410 | 6 | 63 |
| With Egg, Chse & Sausage, 8.8 oz | 630 | 14 | 64 |
| **Burger King:** Croissan'wich | | | |
| Bacon Egg & Cheese | 360 | 19 | 26 |
| Ham Egg & Cheese | 350 | 17 | 27 |
| Double, Sausage, Egg & Cheese | 700 | 49 | 29 |
| **Carl's Jr,** Bacon & Egg Burrito | 550 | 31 | 37 |
| **Chick-Fil-A,** | | | |
| Chkn, Egg & Chse on Multigr. Bagel | 490 | 20 | 49 |
| **Denny's:** T-Bone Steak & Eggs | 780 | 36 | 4 |
| Omelette: Fit Fare, without sides | 390 | 18 | 25 |
| Ultimate with Hash Browns | 830 | 60 | 34 |
| Veg.-Cheese with Hash Browns | 670 | 45 | 35 |
| **Del Taco,** Egg & Cheese Burrito | 400 | 17 | 22 |
| **Dunkin Donuts:** | | | |
| Bacon, Egg & Cheese Croissant | 530 | 33 | 38 |
| Ham, Egg & Cheese Bagel | 510 | 16 | 66 |
| **Eat 'N Park:** Cheese Omelette | 390 | 30 | 2.5 |
| Western Omelette | 345 | 21 | 6.5 |
| **Hardee's:** Loaded Omelet Biscuit | 610 | 42 | 36 |
| Smoked Sausage & Egg Biscuit | 750 | 56 | 38 |
| **IHOP:** T-Bone Steak & Eggs | 1250 | 68 | 74 |
| Colorado Omelette | 1120 | 82 | 24 |
| **Jack in the Box:** | | | |
| Bacon, Egg & Cheese Biscuit | 420 | 24 | 36 |
| Sausage, Egg & Cheese Biscuit | 570 | 39 | 37 |
| **McDonald's:** Egg McMuffin | 300 | 12 | 30 |
| Bacon, Egg & Cheese Biscuit, regular | 420 | 23 | 37 |
| **Whataburger,** | | | |
| Breakfast Platter with Bacon | 730 | 45 | 93 |

### Quick Guide    **C** **F** **Cb**

#### Butter
*Average All Brands*

| | C | F | Cb |
|---|---|---|---|
| **Regular:** 1 tsp, 0.18 oz | 35 | 4 | 0 |
| 1 Pat/Single Portion, 0.18 oz | 35 | 4 | 0 |
| 1 Tbsp, approximately 0.5 oz | 100 | 11 | 0 |
| 2 Tbsp, 1 oz | 205 | 23 | 0 |
| 1 Stick, ½ cup, 4 oz | 810 | 92 | 0 |
| 1 Pound, 2 cups, 16 oz | 3255 | 368 | 0 |
| **Light:** (Regular) 40% Fat: | | | |
| 1 tsp, 0.18 oz | 25 | 3 | 0 |
| 1 Tbsp, 0.5 oz | 75 | 8.5 | 0 |
| 2 Tbsp, 1 oz | 145 | 16 | 0 |
| **Whipped Butter:** (Regular): | | | |
| 1 tsp, 0.14 oz | 30 | 3 | 0 |
| 1 Tbsp, 0.35 oz | 65 | 7.5 | 0 |
| 1 Stick, ½ cup, 2 .66 oz | 545 | 62 | 0 |
| **Whipped Light Butter** (*Land O Lakes*): | | | |
| 1 tsp, 0.15 oz | 15 | 1.5 | 0 |
| 1 Tbsp, 0.4 oz | 45 | 5 | 0 |
| 2 Tbsp, 0.8 oz | 90 | 10 | 0 |

**Unsalted:** Same as Salted

### Flavored Butter/Spreads

*Average All Brands*

| | C | F | Cb |
|---|---|---|---|
| **Honey Butter:** (60% Fat): | | | |
| 1 Tbsp, ½ oz | 90 | 8 | 4 |
| *Downey's*, 1 Tbsp, 0.5 oz | 60 | 1 | 11 |
| **Garlic Butter:** (80% Fat): | | | |
| 1 Tbsp, ½ oz | 100 | 11 | 0 |
| **Sweet Cream Butter:** | | | |
| Regular, 1 Tbsp | 100 | 11 | 0 |
| **Stick** (*Parkay*), 60% Fat, 1 Tbsp | 80 | 9 | 0 |
| **Tub** (*Land O'Lakes*), 50% Fat, 1 Tbsp | 70 | 8 | 0 |

### Ghee (Clarified Butter)

(Example: *Purity Farms*)
Note: Ghee is 100% fat compared to regular butter (80% fat + 20% water)

| | C | F | Cb |
|---|---|---|---|
| 1 tsp, 0.18 oz | 45 | 5 | 0 |
| 1 Tbsp, 0.5 oz | 120 | 14 | 0 |
| 2¼ Tbsp, 1 oz | 250 | 28 | 0 |

### Light & Reduced Fat Spreads

*Per 1 Tablespoon, ½ oz*    **C** **F** **Cb**

| | C | F | Cb |
|---|---|---|---|
| **Albertson's:** Country Style (48%) | 60 | 7 | 0 |
| Butter Blend | 90 | 9 | 0 |
| **Best Life,** Buttery Spread | 60 | 6 | 0 |
| **Benecol:** Spread | 70 | 8 | 0 |
| Light Spread | 50 | 5 | 0 |
| **Blue Bonnet,** Light Marg. Stick | 60 | 7 | 0 |
| **Brummel & Brown,** Spread | 45 | 5 | 0 |
| **Country Crock** (*Shedd's*): | | | |
| Regular | 70 | 7 | 0 |
| Light; Calcium & Vitamins | 50 | 5 | 0 |
| Spreadable Butter | 80 | 8 | 0 |
| **Downey's,** Honey Butter | 60 | 1 | 11 |
| **Fleischmann's:** | | | |
| Original Stick | 80 | 9 | 0 |
| Original Whipped Tub | 60 | 7 | 0 |
| **'I Can't Believe It's Not Butter':** | | | |
| Regular | 70 | 8 | 0 |
| Light Soft Spread | 50 | 5 | 0 |
| **Imperial:** Stick | 80 | 9 | 0 |
| Tub | 50 | 5 | 0 |
| **Land O'Lakes:** Butter | 100 | 11 | 0 |
| Honey Butter | 90 | 8 | 4 |
| Light Butter | 50 | 6 | 0 |
| Light Butter, Whipped | 45 | 5 | 0 |
| **Parkay:** Squeeze | 70 | 8 | 0 |
| Original Spread | 70 | 7 | 0 |
| Original Stick | 80 | 9 | 0 |
| Light Stick | 45 | 5 | 0 |
| **Promise:** Buttery | 80 | 8 | 0 |
| Fat-Free | 5 | 0 | 0 |
| Light | 45 | 5 | 0 |
| **Smart Balance:** | | | |
| **Buttery Spread:** Original | 80 | 9 | 0 |
| Original, Light | 50 | 5 | 0 |
| HeartRight: Original | 80 | 8 | 0 |
| Light | 45 | 5 | 0 |
| Omega 3: Original | 80 | 8 | 0 |
| Light | 50 | 5 | 0 |
| Whipped, low sodium | 60 | 7 | 0 |
| **Smart Beat,** Unsalted, Light | 25 | 2.5 | 0 |

### Butter Substitutes

| | C | F | Cb |
|---|---|---|---|
| **Butter Buds:** | | | |
| 1 serving, ½ tsp | 5 | 0 | 2 |
| Sprinkles, 1 tsp | 5 | 0 | 0 |
| **Earth Balance,** Non GMO, 1 Tbsp | 100 | 11 | 0 |
| **Molly McButter,** ½ tsp | 5 | 0 | 1 |
| **Shedd's Willow Run,** Soy, 1 Tbsp | 100 | 11 | 0 |
| **Sunsweet,** (Butter/Oil Replacement) | | | |
| Lighter Bake, 1 Tbsp, 0.67 oz | 35 | 0 | 9 |

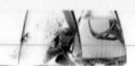

## Animal Fats/Lards    C   F   Cb

*Average All Types*

**Beef Tallow/Drippings, Lard (Pork),**
**Chicken, Duck, Goose, Turkey:**

| | C | F | Cb |
|---|---|---|---|
| 1 Tbsp, 13g | **115** | **13** | 0 |
| 2¼ Tbsp, 1 oz | **255** | **28** | 0 |
| 1 cup, 7.25 oz | **1850** | **205** | 0 |
| ½ pound, 8 oz | **2040** | **227** | 0 |

**Ghee/Butter/ Oil** ~ *See Page 93*

## Vegetable Shortening

*Average All Types*

| | C | F | Cb |
|---|---|---|---|
| 1 Tbsp, 13g | **115** | **13** | 0 |
| 2¼ Tbsp, 1 oz | **250** | **28** | 0 |
| 1 cup, 7.25 oz | **1810** | **205** | 0 |

## Vegetable Oils

Includes almond, avocado, canola, corn, coconut, flaxseed, grapeseed, linseed, mustard, olive, palm, peanut, rice bran, safflower, sesame, sunflower, soybean, wheat germ. Note: Oil is 100% fat.

| | C | F | Cb |
|---|---|---|---|
| 1 tsp, 5g | **45** | **5** | 0 |
| 1 Tbsp, 0.5 oz | **120** | **14** | 0 |
| 2 Tbsp, 1 oz | **240** | **28** | 0 |
| 1 cup, 7.25 oz | **1930** | **205** | 0 |

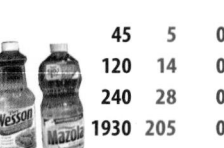

## Fish Oils

*Average All Types*

(Includes Cod Liver, Herring,
Salmon, Sardines): 1 Tbsp, 0.5 oz   **125**   **14**   0

## Cooking Sprays/Squeezes

**Cooking Sprays:** *(PAM, Mazola, I Can't Believe It's Not Butter, Weight Watchers, Wesson):*

| **Per serving** | **2** | **0** | **0** |
|---|---|---|---|
|    1-3 second spray | **6** | **1** | 0 |
| *I Can't Believe It's Not Butter* | **0** | **0** | **0** |
| *Parkay Buttery Spray* | **0** | **0** | **0** |
| Squeeze, *(Parkay)*, 1 Tbsp, 0.5 oz | **70** | **8** | 0 |

## Olestra (Olean)    C   F   Cb

**Olestra** *(Olean)*     **0**   **0**   **0**

Note: Olean is Proctor & Gamble's brand name for Olestra – a no-calorie cooking oil that gives snacks (like potato chips, tortilla chips and crackers) taste and texture without adding fat or calories.

**Examples:**
- *Frito-Lay,* Light Products
  *(Lays, Ruffles, Tostitos, Doritos)*
- *Pringles,* Fat-Free Potato Crisps

### Mayonnaise ~ Quick Guide

### Mayonnaise

**Regular:** *Per 1 Tbsp, 0.5 oz*

| | C | F | Cb |
|---|---|---|---|
|    Average All Brands | **90** | **10** | 0 |
| **Best Foods/Hellmans; Kraft:** | | | |
|    1 Tbsp | **90** | **10** | 0 |
|    ½ cup, 4 oz | **720** | **80** | 0 |
| **Hain,** Safflower Oil | **120** | **14** | 0 |
| **Spectrum,** Canola Mayo | **100** | **11** | 0 |

**Light/Reduced Fat:** *Per 1 Tbsp, 0.5 oz*

| | C | F | Cb |
|---|---|---|---|
| **Best Foods/Hellman's,** 1 Tbsp | **35** | **3.5** | 1 |
| **Kraft,** 1 Tbsp | **45** | **4** | 2 |
| **Smart Balance,** Omega Plus, 1 Tbsp | **50** | **4.5** | 2 |
| **Spectrum,** | | | |
|    **Light Canola Mayo Eggless,** 1 Tbsp | **35** | **3.5** | 0 |

**Fat Free:** *Per 1 Tbsp, 0.5 oz*

| | C | F | Cb |
|---|---|---|---|
| **Kraft:** 1 Tbsp | **10** | **0** | 2 |
|    ½ cup, 4 oz | **80** | **0** | 16 |
| **Sugar Free,** Dukes Mayo, 1 Tbsp | **100** | **12** | 0 |

### Mayonnaise Style Dressing

| | C | F | Cb |
|---|---|---|---|
| **Best Foods:** Sandwich Spread, 1 T. | **60** | **5** | 2 |
|    Light, 1 Tbsp, 0.5 oz | **35** | **3.5** | 1 |
| **Kraft:** | | | |
|    *Miracle Whip Salad Dressing:* | | | |
|     Original, 1 Tbsp, 0.5 oz | **40** | **3.5** | 2 |
|     Light, 1 Tbsp, 0.5 oz | **20** | **1.5** | 2 |
|     Free, 1 Tbsp, 0.5 oz | **15** | **0** | 3 |
|    *Sandwich Shop Mayo:* | | | |
|     Chipotle, 1 Tbsp, 0.5 oz | **40** | **4** | 2 |
|     Horseradish-Dijon, 1 Tbsp, 0.5 oz | **40** | **3.5** | 2 |
|     Hot & Spicy, 1 Tbsp, 0.5 oz | **100** | **11** | 0 |
| **Nasoya:** Tofu Base/Dairy Free/Eggless | | | |
|    Regular, 1 Tbsp, 0.5 oz | **35** | **3.5** | 1 |
|    Fat-Free, 1 Tbsp, 0.5 oz | **10** | **0** | 2 |

## Quick Guide

### Fresh Fish    C F Cb

**Low Oil (Less than 2.5% fat):**
**White/Lightly-colored flesh. Examples:**
Cod, Flounder, Haddock, Halibut, Mahi Mahi,
Perch, Pike, Pollock, Snapper, Sole, Whiting.

*Per 4 oz Edible Portion*

| | C | F | Cb |
|---|---|---|---|
| **Raw,** 4 oz (without bones) | 90 | 1 | 0 |
| **Steamed,** Broiled, Baked | 130 | 1 | 0 |
| **Fried:** Lightly Floured | 210 | 8 | 3.5 |
| Breaded | 260 | 12 | 8 |
| In Batter | 320 | 16 | 27 |

**Medium Oil (2.5-5% fat):**
**Lightly-colored flesh. Examples:** C F Cb
Bluefin Tuna, Catfish, Kingfish, Orange Roughy,
Salmon (Pink), Swordfish, Rainbow Trout, Yellowtail.

| | C | F | Cb |
|---|---|---|---|
| **Raw,** 4 oz (without bones) | 145 | 7 | 0 |
| **Baked,** Broiled, 4 oz | 195 | 8 | 0 |
| **Fried,** 4 oz | 230 | 11 | 8 |

**High Oil (Over 5% fat):** C F Cb
**Darker-colored flesh. Examples:**
Albacore Tuna, Mackerel, Salmon
(Atlantic/Chinook/Sockeye), Sardines, Trout.

| | C | F | Cb |
|---|---|---|---|
| **Raw,** 4 oz (without bones) | 220 | 14 | 0 |
| **Baked,** Broiled, 4 oz | 275 | 17 | 0 |
| **Fried,** 4 oz | 340 | 23 | 12 |

---

**Cooking Yields (Fin Fish):**
4 oz Raw wt. = 3.5 oz Cooked weight
4 oz Cooked wt. = 5 oz Raw weight

**Calorie & Fat Variations:**
The amount of fat/oil in fish varies with the species,
season and locality. Within the same fish, fat/oil
content is generally higher towards the head.

---

*Get Moving!*
*Take a computer*
*break every hour.*

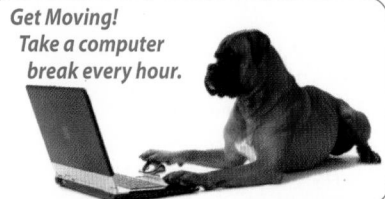

### Fish & Shellfish    C F Cb

*Edible Weights: (no bones/shell)*

| | C | F | Cb |
|---|---|---|---|
| **Abalone,** Raw, 3 oz | 90 | 0.5 | 5 |
| **Ahi Tuna,** grilled, 6 oz fillet (w/o fat) | 235 | 2 | 0 |
| **Anchovy:** Paste, 1 Tbsp, 0.5 oz | 45 | 3 | 0 |
| Canned in oil, drained, 5 only, 0.75 oz | 40 | 2 | 0 |
| Pickled, 1 oz | 50 | 3 | 0 |
| **Barracuda (Pacific),** raw, 4 oz | 130 | 3 | 0 |
| **Bass:** Sea, raw, 4.6 oz fillet | 125 | 2.5 | 0 |
| Striped: Raw, 1 fillet, 5.5 oz | 150 | 3.5 | 0 |
| Baked, 3 oz | 105 | 3 | 0 |
| **Blue Fish:** Raw, 1 fillet, 5.25 oz | 185 | 6.5 | 0 |
| Baked, 3 oz | 130 | 5 | 0 |
| **Butterfish,** raw, 3 oz | 125 | 7 | 0 |
| **Cajun & Creole Dishes** ~ *See Page 168* | | | |
| **Calamari,** breaded/fried, 7 oz | 350 | 15 | 16 |
| **Carp,** raw, 3 oz | 110 | 5 | 0 |
| **Catfish (Wild):** Raw, 1 fillet, 6 oz | 135 | 5 | 0 |
| Baked/Broiled (6 oz raw wt), 1 fillet, 5.25 oz | 160 | 4.5 | 0 |
| Fried, breaded (6 oz raw wt) 1 fillet, 5.87oz | 390 | 24 | 14 |
| **Caviar,** black/red, 1 Tbsp, 16g | 40 | 3 | 0.5 |
| **Clams:** Raw, 3 oz (4 large/9 small) | 65 | 1 | 2 |
| Fried, breaded, 6.6 oz (20 small) | 380 | 21 | 20 |
| Canned, drained, ½ cup, 2.5 oz | 120 | 1.5 | 4 |
| Minced, ¼ cup, 2 oz | 25 | 0 | 2 |
| **Clam Juice** *(Snow's)* 1 Tbsp | 0 | 0 | 0 |
| **Cod, Atlantic/Pacific:** Raw, 4 oz | 95 | 0.5 | 0 |
| Baked/Broiled, 1 fillet, 6.35 oz | 190 | 1.5 | 0 |
| Canned, 3 oz | 90 | 1 | 0 |
| Minced, ¼ cup, 2 oz | 25 | 0 | 0 |
| Smoked/Dry Heat, 3 oz | 90 | 1 | 0 |
| **Crab:** Alaska King, raw, 1 leg, 6 oz | 145 | 1 | 0 |
| 1 leg, cooked, 4.75 oz | 130 | 2 | 0 |
| Blue: Raw, 1 crab (⅓ lb whole crab, 0.75 oz flesh) | 20 | 0.2 | 0 |
| Steamed, 3 oz | 85 | 1 | 0 |
| Canned, drained, ½ cup, 2.5 oz | 65 | 1 | 0 |
| Dungeness, 1 crab, 5.75 oz edible (from 1.5 lb whole crab) | 180 | 2 | 2 |
| Imitation Crab Legs/Stix, 3oz | 80 | 0.5 | 13 |
| **Crab Cakes (Low-fat),** (1), 2 oz | 95 | 4.5 | 0.5 |
| Regular (1), 3 oz | 130 | 6.5 | 0.5 |
| **Crayfish,** raw, 4 oz (edible) | 90 | 1 | 0 |
| **Croaker,** raw, 3 oz | 90 | 3 | 0 |
| **Cuttlefish,** raw, 3 oz | 70 | 1 | 1 |
| **Dolphinfish,** raw, 1 fillet, 7 oz | 175 | 1.5 | 0 |
| **Eel:** Raw, 3 oz | 155 | 10 | 0 |
| Smoked/Dry Heat, 3 oz | 200 | 13 | 0 |
| **Fish & Chips** *(Arthur Treacher)*, 3 pieces fish & triple chips | 1420 | 63 | 183 |
| **Fish S'wich,** W/ Tartar Sauce, 5.5 oz | 430 | 23 | 41 |

## Fish & Shellfish (Cont)

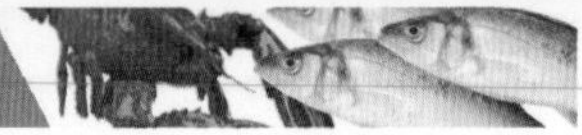

| *Edible Weights: (no bones/shell)* | C | F | Cb |
|---|---|---|---|
| **Fish Oil,** 1 Tbsp, 0.5 oz | 125 | 14 | 0 |
| **Flounder/Sole:** Raw, 4 oz | 105 | 1.5 | 0 |
| Baked, 1 fillet, 4.5 oz | 150 | 2 | 0 |
| **Frozen Fish** ~ *See Page 97* | | | |
| **Gefilte Fish** ~ *See Kosher/Deli Foods, Page 171* | | | |
| **Grouper,** raw, 4 oz | 105 | 1 | 0 |
| **Haddock:** Raw, 4 oz | 100 | 1 | 0 |
| Baked, 3 oz | 95 | 1 | 0 |
| Broiled, 1 fillet, 5.25 oz | 170 | 1.5 | 0 |
| Smoked, 3 oz | 100 | 1 | 0 |
| **Halibut:** Raw, 4 oz | 105 | 1.5 | 0 |
| Baked, ½ fillet, 5.6 oz | 175 | 2.5 | 0 |
| **Herring:** Atlantic, raw, 4 oz | 180 | 10 | 0 |
| Canned: Plain, drained, 3 oz | 130 | 8 | 0 |
| In Tomato Sauce, 3.5 oz | 140 | 8 | 2 |
| Party Snacks, ¼ cup, drained, 2 oz | 120 | 5 | 0 |
| Pickled: 2 pieces, 1 oz | 80 | 5 | 3 |
| In Sour Cream, 1 oz | 55 | 3 | 5 |
| Rollmops, 1½ oz | 110 | 8 | 6 |
| Smoked, kippered, 4 oz | 245 | 14 | 0 |
| **Jellyfish:** Raw, 4 oz | 30 | 0 | 0 |
| Dried, Salted, 1 cup, 2 oz | 20 | 1 | 0 |
| **King Fish,** raw, 4 oz | 120 | 2.5 | 0 |
| **Ling,** raw, 4 oz | 100 | 0.5 | 0 |
| **Lobster, Northern:** Raw, 4 oz | 105 | 1 | 0.5 |
| 1 Lobster, 6.25 oz | | | |
| (from 1.5 lb whole lobster) | 160 | 1.5 | 1 |
| Cooked, 1 cup, 5 oz | 140 | 1 | 2 |
| Lobster Newberg, av., ¾ cup | 360 | 20 | 9 |
| Lobster Thermidor, av., 1 serving | 370 | 22 | 15 |
| Lobster Salads, average, ½ cup | 220 | 13 | 5 |
| Lobster Tail, restaurant *(Red Lobster)* | 260 | 3 | 0 |
| **Lomi Salmon,** ¼ cup, 4 oz | 20 | 1 | 3 |
| **Lox,** Regular/Nova, 2 oz | 65 | 2.5 | 0 |
| **Mackerel:** Atlantic, raw, 4 oz | 230 | 16 | 0 |
| Broiled, 3 oz fillet | 230 | 16 | 0 |
| Jack, canned, ½ cup, 3.35 oz | 150 | 6 | 0 |
| King, raw, 4 oz | 120 | 2 | 0 |
| Pacific/Jack: Raw, 4 oz | 180 | 9 | 0 |
| Broiled, 3 oz | 170 | 9 | 0 |
| Spanish, raw, 4 oz | 160 | 7 | 0 |
| **Mahi-Mahi,** raw, 4 oz | 125 | 1 | 0 |
| **Milkfish,** raw, 4 oz | 170 | 7.5 | 0 |
| **Monkfish:** Raw, 4 oz | 85 | 1.5 | 0 |
| Baked, 3 oz | 80 | 2 | 0 |
| **Mullet,** striped, raw, 4 oz | 135 | 4.5 | 0 |
| **Mussels:** Raw, 4 oz (edible weight) | 100 | 2.5 | 4 |
| 1 cup, 5.25 oz (edible weight) | 130 | 3.5 | 5 |
| Cooked, moist heat, 3 oz | 150 | 4 | 6 |

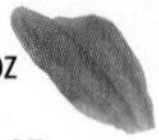

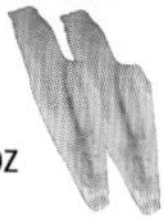

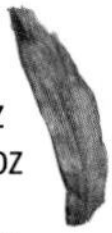

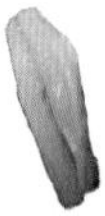

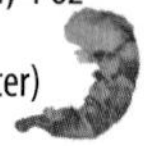

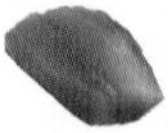

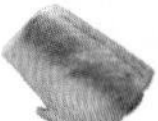

| | C | F | Cb |
|---|---|---|---|
| **Ocean Perch:** Raw, 4 oz | 105 | 2 | 0 |
| Baked, 3 oz | 105 | 2 | 0 |
| **Octopus,** common, raw, 4 oz | 95 | 1 | 2.5 |
| **Orange Roughy,** raw, 4 oz | 85 | 1 | 0 |
| **Oysters:** Common, raw, 3 oz | 70 | 2 | 4 |
| Eastern, raw: 6 medium, 3 oz | 50 | 1.5 | 4.5 |
| 1 cup, 8.75 oz | 150 | 4 | 14 |
| Fried/breaded, 6 medium, 3 oz | 170 | 11 | 10 |
| Pacific, raw, 1 medium, 1.75 oz | 40 | 1 | 2 |
| Oysters Rockerfeller, 3 oysters | 220 | 13 | 12 |
| **Perch,** average, raw, 4 oz | 105 | 1 | 0 |
| **Pike:** Northern, raw, 4 oz | 100 | 1 | 0 |
| Walleye, raw, 4 oz | 105 | 1.5 | 0 |
| **Pollock,** raw, 4 oz | 105 | 1 | 0 |
| **Pout (Ocean),** raw, 4 oz | 90 | 1 | 0 |
| **Pompano,** Florida, raw, 4 oz | 185 | 11 | 0 |
| **Porgy/Scup,** raw, 4 oz | 150 | 4 | 0 |
| **Red-Snapper,** raw, 4 oz | 115 | 1.5 | 0 |
| **Rockfish,** Pacific, raw, 4 oz | 110 | 2 | 0 |
| **Roe,** raw, 2 Tbsp, 1 oz | 40 | 2 | 0.5 |
| **Sablefish:** Raw, 4 oz | 220 | 17 | 0 |
| Smoked, 3 oz | 220 | 17 | 0 |
| **Salmon:** | | | |
| **Raw:** Chinook, 4 oz | 205 | 12 | 0 |
| Atlantic; Coho/Silver, 4 oz | 210 | 12 | 0 |
| Chum; Pink, 4 oz | 135 | 4 | 0 |
| Red/Sockeye, 4 oz | 190 | 10 | 0 |
| **Baked,** Atlantic/Coho, 3 oz | 160 | 5 | 0 |
| **Canned Salmon:** *Average All Brands* | | | |
| **Pink:** 1 oz | 40 | 2 | 0 |
| ¼ cup, 2.2 oz | 90 | 5 | 0 |
| 3¾ oz can, whole | 155 | 8.5 | 0 |
| 7½ oz can, whole | 300 | 17 | 0 |
| Skinless/boneless, ¼ cup, 2 oz | 70 | 2 | 0 |
| **Red Sockeye:** 1 oz | 50 | 3 | 0 |
| ¼ cup, 2.2 oz | 110 | 7 | 0 |
| 3¾ oz can, whole | 190 | 12 | 0 |
| Atlantic, ½ cup, 3.5 oz | 230 | 14 | 0 |
| Chinook/King, ½ cup | 210 | 14 | 0 |
| Chum, ½ cup, 3.5 oz | 140 | 5 | 0 |
| Coho/Silver, ½ cup | 155 | 5 | 0 |
| **Atlantic Steaks:** Small, 8 oz | 320 | 14 | 0 |
| Medium, 12 oz | 480 | 21 | 0 |
| Large, 16 oz | 640 | 28 | 0 |
| **Salmon:** Cake, take-out, 3 oz | 240 | 15 | 6 |
| Burger (Trident), 1 pce, 2.8 oz | 130 | 7 | 1 |
| **Smoked Salmon:** Chinook, 3 oz | 100 | 4 | 0 |
| Pacific Supreme, 2 oz | 100 | 4 | 0 |

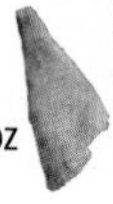

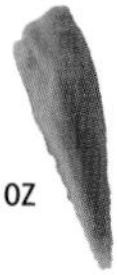

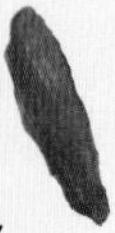

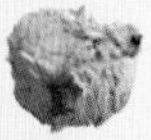

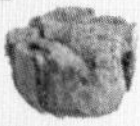

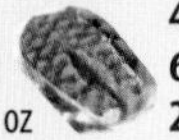

## Fish (Cont)

| | C | F | Cb |
|---|---|---|---|
| **Sardines (Canned):** *Average All Brands* | | | |
| In Oil, undrained, 1 oz | 85 | 7 | 0 |
| Drained of Oil: 1 oz | 60 | 3 | 0 |
| 3.25 oz | 190 | 11 | 0 |
| 1 large/2 med. ⅗" small, 0.8 oz | 50 | 3 | 0 |
| In Tomato/ Mustard Sauce: 1 oz | 55 | 3 | 0 |
| 3.75 oz can (3 sardines) | 210 | 12 | 1 |
| **Sashimi** ~ *See Japanese Foods, Page 171* | | | |
| **Scallop:** Raw, 6 large/15 small, 3 oz | 80 | 0.5 | 2 |
| Breaded/fried, 6 pieces, 3.5 oz | 200 | 10 | 10 |
| **Sea Bass,** raw, 4 oz | 110 | 2 | 0 |
| **Seafood Salad,** Deli Style, ½ cup, 3.5 oz | 250 | 21 | 11 |
| **Shark:** Raw, 4 oz | 150 | 5 | 0 |
| Baked, 4 oz | 185 | 7 | 0 |
| Batter-dipped, fried, 4 oz | 220 | 13 | 6 |
| Shark Fin, dried, 1 oz | 30 | 0 | 0 |
| **Shrimp:** Raw, in shell, 8 oz | 140 | 2 | 1.5 |
| Raw, shelled, 3 oz (12 large) | 90 | 1.5 | 0.5 |
| Breaded/fried, 3 oz (11 large) | 210 | 11 | 10 |
| Canned, 1 oz (10 shrimp) | 30 | 0.5 | 0 |
| Cocktail Shrimp, restaurant-style | 140 | 2 | 1 |
| Tiger: Cooked, 1 shrimp, 0.5 oz | 15 | 0.5 | 0 |
| Battered, fried, 1 shrimp | 60 | 4 | 3 |
| **Smelt,** Rainbow, raw, 4 oz | 110 | 3 | 0 |
| **Snapper:** Raw, 3 oz | 85 | 1 | 0 |
| Cooked, 1 fillet, 6 oz | 220 | 3 | 0 |
| **Sole,** Raw, 4 oz | 105 | 1.5 | 0 |
| **Squid:** Raw, 4 oz | 105 | 1.5 | 3.5 |
| Fried, 3 oz | 150 | 6 | 7 |
| **Surimi (Imitation Crab),** 4 oz | 110 | 0.5 | 17 |
| **Sweet & Sour Fish,** ½ dish, 10 oz | 580 | 29 | 53 |
| **Swordfish,** raw: | | | |
| Small Steak, 4 oz | 135 | 4.5 | 0 |
| Medium Steak, 6 oz | 205 | 7 | 0 |
| **Tilapia,** Rain Forest Fillets, 4 oz | 110 | 2 | 0 |
| **Trout,** Rainbow: Raw, 4 oz | 135 | 4 | 0 |
| Broiled, 3 oz | 125 | 5 | 0 |
| Smoked, 2 oz | 110 | 6 | 0 |
| **Tuna:** *Average All Brands* | | | |
| Raw: Albacore, 4 oz | 190 | 8 | 0 |
| Bluefin, 4 oz | 165 | 5.5 | 0 |
| Skipjack, Yellowfin, 4 oz | 125 | 1 | 0 |
| **Broiled,** 3 oz | 115 | 1 | 0 |
| **Canned:** | | | |
| In Water, drained: | | | |
| Chunk/Solid: 2 oz can | 75 | 1.5 | 0 |
| 3 oz can | 110 | 2.5 | 0 |
| 6 oz can | 220 | 5 | 0 |

| **Tuna (Cont):** | C | F | Cb |
|---|---|---|---|
| In Oil, drained: | | | |
| Chunk Light: 2 oz | 110 | 5 | 0 |
| 6 oz can, drained | 315 | 14 | 0 |
| Solid White, 2 oz | 105 | 4.5 | 0 |
| 6.3 oz can, drained | 330 | 14 | 0 |
| **Tuna Salad,** Deli Style, ½ cup, 4oz | 280 | 20 | 8 |
| **Whitefish:** Raw, 4 oz | 150 | 6.5 | 0 |
| Baked, 3 oz | 145 | 6.5 | 1 |
| Smoked, 3 oz | 90 | 1 | 0 |
| **Whiting:** Raw, 4 oz | 100 | 1.5 | 0 |
| Baked, 3 oz | 100 | 1.5 | 0 |
| **Yellowtail:** Raw, 4 oz | 165 | 6 | 0 |
| Grilled, 3 oz (from 4 oz raw) | 160 | 6 | 0 |

## Other Canned/Packaged Fish

| | C | F | Cb |
|---|---|---|---|
| **Bumble Bee:** | | | |
| **Tuna Salad Kits:** *With Crackers* | | | |
| Original: 3.5 oz pkg | 300 | 22 | 18 |
| With Mayonnaise | 420 | 22 | 24 |
| Fat-Free, 3.5 oz | 150 | 1.5 | 24 |
| **Lunch on the Run,** 8.2 oz | 510 | 28 | 50 |
| **Seafood Salad,** with Crackers, 3.3 oz pkg | 180 | 5.5 | 27 |
| **Sensations Bowls:** | | | |
| Lemon & Cracked Pepper Tuna, 3 oz | 110 | 3 | 2 |
| Spicy Thai Chili Tuna, 3 oz | 160 | 7 | 9 |
| **Chicken of the Sea:** | | | |
| Albacore Tuna in Water, 2.5 oz pouch | 100 | 1.5 | 0 |
| Pink Salmon, skinless/boneless, 2 oz | 60 | 2 | 0 |
| Shrimp, medium, 4 oz can | 90 | 1 | 2 |
| **Gorton's** *(Frozen)* ~ Page 119 | | | |
| **Kroger** *(Frozen)* ~ Page 119 | | | |
| **Starkist:** | | | |
| **Pouch:** *Per 2.6 oz Pouch* | | | |
| Albacore Tuna in water | 90 | 2 | 1 |
| Light Tuna Chunks in water | 80 | 0.5 | 1 |
| **Lunch-To-Go Kit:** Chunk Light Tuna With Mayo & Crackers, 4.5 oz | 240 | 9 | 20 |
| **SeaSations** ~ *Page 121* | | | |
| **Tuna Creations,** av. all varieties, 2 oz | 70 | 1 | 2 |
| **Van De Kamp's** *(Frozen)* ~ Page 122 | | | |

## Restaurant Chains

Captain D's Seafood ~ *Page 187*
Long John Silver's ~ *Page 213*
Shoney's ~ *Page 239*
Southern Tsunami ~ *Page 242*
Wahoo's Fish Taco ~ *Page 254*

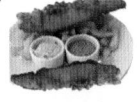

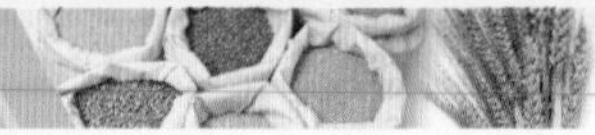

F

# Flours & Grains

| Flours & Grains | C | F | Cb |
|---|---|---|---|
| **Amaranth Flour,** ½ cup, 3.5 oz | 365 | 6.5 | 65 |
| **Arrowroot Flour,** ½ cup, 2.25 oz | 230 | 0 | 56 |
| **Barley:** Grain, reg., ½ cup, 2.6 oz | 255 | 1 | 55 |
| Pearled, raw, 3½ oz | 350 | 1 | 78 |
| **Buckwheat:** Grain, ½ cup, 3 oz | 290 | 3 | 61 |
| Flour, whole-groat, ½ cup, 2 oz | 200 | 2 | 42 |
| Groats: Roasted, dry, ½ cup, 2.9 oz | 285 | 2 | 62 |
| Roasted, cooked, 3.5 oz | 80 | 0.5 | 17 |
| **Bulgur:** Dry, ½ cup, 2.5 oz | 240 | 1 | 53 |
| Cooked, ½ cup, 3.2 oz | 75 | 0.5 | 17 |
| **Carob Flour,** ½ cup, 1.8 oz | 115 | 0.5 | 46 |
| **Corn Kernels,** av., ckd, ½ cup | 80 | 0.5 | 18 |
| **Corn Bran,** ½ cup, 1.3 oz | 85 | 0.5 | 33 |
| **Corn Flour/Masa,** ½ cup, 2 oz | 215 | 2.5 | 43 |
| **Corn Grits:** Dry, ½ cup, 2.75 oz | 290 | 1 | 62 |
| Cooked, ½ cup, 4¼ oz | 70 | 0.5 | 15 |
| **Corn Germ,** toasted, ½ cup, 4 oz | 100 | 1.5 | 22 |
| **Cornmeal:** Average all Types, | | | |
| 3 Tbsp, 1 oz | 105 | 0.5 | 22 |
| ½ cup, 2½ oz | 255 | 1 | 54 |
| Mixes: same as above | 230 | 1 | 48 |
| **Cornstarch:** 1 Tbsp, 0.3 oz | 30 | 0 | 8 |
| ½ cup, 2¼ oz | 245 | 0 | 58 |
| **Couscous:** Dry, 1 oz (3 oz cooked) | 110 | 0 | 22 |
| 1 cup cooked, 5.5 oz | 175 | 0.5 | 37 |
| **Farina:** Dry, ½ cup, 3.1 oz | 325 | 0.5 | 69 |
| Cooked, ½ cup, 4.1 oz | 55 | 0 | 12 |
| **Flaxseed:** Whole, 1 Tbsp, 0.3 oz | 45 | 3.5 | 2 |
| Ground, 2 Tbsp, 0.3 oz | 60 | 4.5 | 4 |
| **Garbanzo** (Chick Pea), ½ cup, 1.6 oz | 180 | 3 | 27 |
| **Gluten Free** (King Arthur), 3 Tbsp | 110 | 0 | 24 |
| **Matzo Meal,** ½ cup, 2.2 oz | 230 | 0.5 | 48 |
| **Millet:** Raw, ½ cup, 3.5 oz | 380 | 4 | 73 |
| Cooked, ½ cup, 3 oz | 105 | 1 | 21 |
| **Oat Bran:** Raw, ⅓ cup, 1.1 oz | 75 | 2 | 21 |
| Cooked, ½ cup, 3.75 oz | 45 | 1 | 13 |
| **Oats,** rolled/oatmeal: | | | |
| Dry/Groats, ½ cup, 1.5 oz | 160 | 3 | 28 |
| Cooked, ½ cup, 4.2 oz | 75 | 1 | 13 |
| **Polenta ~** *See Cornmeal* | | | |
| **Potato Flour,** ½ cup, 2.8 oz | 285 | 0.5 | 66 |
| **Psyllium Husks,** 1 Tbsp, 0.15 oz | 20 | 0 | 4 |
| **Quinoa:** Dry ½ cup, 3 oz | 320 | 5 | 59 |
| Cooked, ½ cup, 3¾ oz | 130 | 2 | 24 |
| **Rice Bran,** ½ cup, 2 oz | 180 | 12 | 28 |
| **Rice Flour,** ½ cup, 2.75 oz | 290 | 1 | 63 |

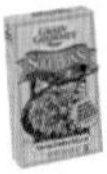

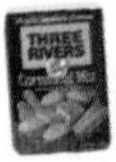

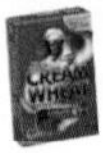

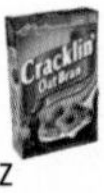

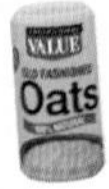

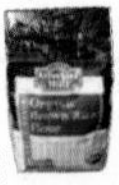

| Flours & Grains (Cont) | C | F | Cb |
|---|---|---|---|
| **Rice Polish,** ½ cup, 3.5 oz | 360 | 0.5 | 80 |
| **Rye Flour:** Dark, ½ cup, 2.3 oz | 210 | 2 | 44 |
| Medium, ½ cup, 1.8 oz | 180 | 1 | 40 |
| Light, ½ cup, 1.8 oz | 190 | 1 | 41 |
| **Rye Grain:** ½ cup, 3 oz | 280 | 2 | 59 |
| Flakes, ¼ cup, 1 oz | 100 | 0.5 | 21 |
| **Semolina,** ½ cup, 3 oz | 300 | 1 | 61 |
| **Sorghum,** ½ cup, 3.4 oz | 325 | 3 | 72 |
| **Soy Flour:** | | | |
| Defatted, 1 cup, 3.5 oz | 330 | 1 | 38 |
| Low-Fat, 1 cup, 3 oz | 325 | 6 | 33 |
| Full-Fat, 1 cup, 3 oz | 365 | 17 | 29 |
| **Soy Meal,** defatted, 1 cup, 4.3 oz | 415 | 3 | 49 |
| **Spelt Flour,** ½ cup, 2 oz | 190 | 1 | 41 |
| **Tapioca, Pearl:** | | | |
| Dry, ½ cup, 2.7 oz | 270 | 0 | 67 |
| 3 Tbsp, 1 oz | 100 | 0 | 25 |
| **Teff (Seed) Flour,** 2 oz | 215 | 2 | 42 |
| **Tortilla Flour Mix,** ½ cup, 2 oz | 220 | 6 | 37 |
| **Triticale:** ½ cup, 3.4 oz | 325 | 2 | 70 |
| Flour, wholegrain, ½ cup, 2.3 oz | 220 | 1 | 48 |
| **Wheat Bran,** unproc., ½ cup, 1 oz | 65 | 1 | 19 |
| **Wheat Flakes,** ½ cup, 1.5 oz | 160 | 1 | 35 |
| **Wheat Germ:** | | | |
| Raw, ¼ cup, 1 oz | 105 | 3 | 15 |
| Toasted, ¼ cup, 1 oz | 110 | 3 | 14 |
| **Wheat Flour:** | | | |
| White, All Purpose/Self-Rising, | | | |
| 1 level Tbsp, 0.28 oz | 30 | 0 | 6 |
| ½ cup, 2.2 oz | 230 | 0.5 | 48 |
| 1 cup, 4.4 oz | 455 | 1.5 | 95 |
| Whole Wheat, 1 cup, 4.2 oz | 405 | 2 | 87 |

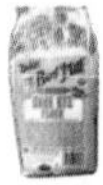

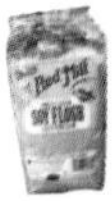

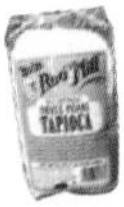

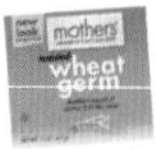

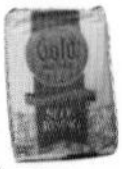

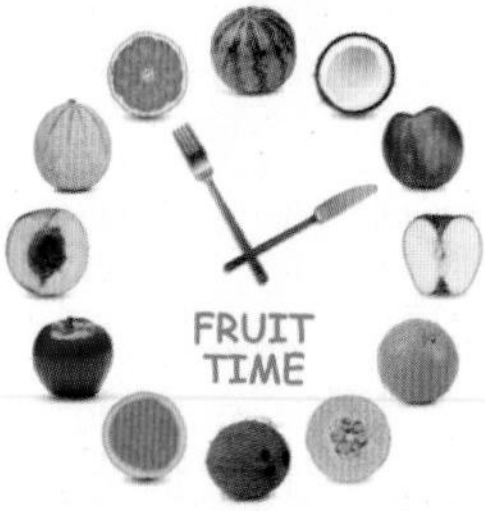

FRUIT TIME

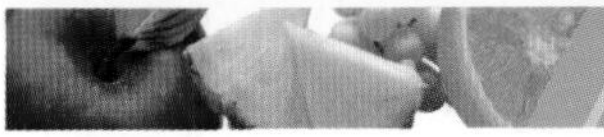

# Fruit ~ Fresh (F)

| Weights As Purchased | C | F | Cb |
|---|---|---|---|
| **Apples:** Average all varieties, Whole (with skin): | | | |
| 1 small (4 per lb), 4 oz | 55 | 0 | 14 |
| 1 med., (3 per lb), 5.5 oz | 75 | 0 | 19 |
| 1 large (2 per lb), 8 oz | 110 | 0 | 28 |
| 1 extra large, 11 oz | 145 | 0 | 36 |
| Flesh only (no skin or core): 1 oz | 15 | 0 | 3.5 |
| 1 cup slices, 4 oz | 55 | 0 | 14 |
| Candy/Caramel Apple, 1 med., 6.5 oz | 245 | 4 | 54 |
| *Chiquita Apple Bites*, 10 slices, 3.5 oz | 50 | 0 | 12 |
| **Apricots:** 1 small (12 per lb) | 17 | 0 | 4 |
| 1 medium (8 per lb), 2 oz | 25 | 0 | 6 |
| 1 large (5-6 per lb), 3 oz | 40 | 0 | 10 |
| **Asian Pear,** (Nashi Fruit), 1 med., 7 oz | 85 | 0 | 21 |
| **Avocado,** (without seed/skin): | | | |
| Average, ½ medium, 3.5 oz | 160 | 15 | 8 |
| 1 salad slice, 0.5 oz | 25 | 2 | 1 |
| Mashed/Puree, 2 Tbsp, 1 oz | 50 | 4.5 | 2 |
| ¼ cup, 2 oz | 90 | 9 | 5 |
| Californian, ½ medium, 3 oz | 160 | 14 | 8 |
| Mashed/Puree, ½ cup, 4 oz | 190 | 18 | 10 |
| Florida, ½ medium, 5.5 oz | 180 | 15 | 12 |
| Mashed/Puree, ½ cup, 4 oz | 140 | 11 | 9 |
| ½ cup cubed, 3 oz | 105 | 8 | 7 |
| **Banana,** (weight with skin): | | | |
| 1 small (6", 4 per lb), 4 oz | 90 | 0 | 23 |
| 1 medium (7", 3 per lb), 5 oz | 105 | 0 | 27 |
| 1 large (8"), 7 oz | 120 | 0 | 30 |
| 1 extra large (9"), 9 oz | 135 | 0 | 35 |
| without skin, 1 oz | 25 | 0 | 6 |
| **Black Raspberries,** 1 cup, 5 oz | 70 | 0 | 15 |
| **Blackberries,** 1 cup, 5 oz | 60 | 0.5 | 14 |
| **Blueberries:** ¼ cup, 1 oz | 15 | 0 | 4 |
| 1 cup, (½ pint) | 80 | 0.5 | 20 |
| **Boysenberries,** 1 cup, 4.5 oz | 60 | 4.5 | 14 |
| **Breadfruit,** ½ cup, 4 oz | 115 | 0 | 30 |
| **Cactus Pear,** 1 fruit, 3.5 oz | 40 | 0 | 9 |
| **Cantaloupe:** Flesh (without rind), 1 oz | 10 | 0 | 2 |
| 1 cup pieces/balls, 5.5 oz | 55 | 0 | 13 |
| Slices, ½ Circle (no rind): | | | |
| 1 thin (buffet), (⅛"), 0.5 oz | 5 | 0 | 1 |
| 1 medium (¼"), 1 oz | 10 | 0 | 2 |
| 1 thick (½"), 2 oz | 20 | 0 | 5 |
| Wedges, (Length cut, w/o rind): | | | |
| 1 thin, 1/16 medium, 2 oz | 20 | 0 | 5 |
| 1 thick, ⅛ medium, 4 oz | 40 | 0 | 9 |
| Whole, (Weights with seeds and rind): | | | |
| ½ small, 20 oz | 195 | 1 | 46 |
| ½ medium, 28 oz | 270 | 1.5 | 65 |
| ½ large, 2.5 lb | 370 | 2 | 90 |
| **Carambola,** (Starfruit), 1 med., 3 oz | 30 | 0 | 6 |

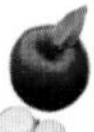

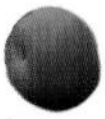

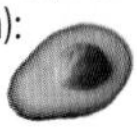

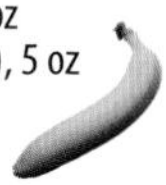

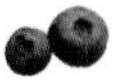

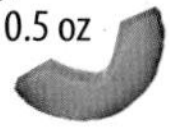

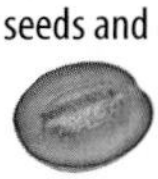

| Weights As Purchased | C | F | Cb |
|---|---|---|---|
| **Cassava,** ⅓ cup, 2.5 oz | 115 | 0 | 27 |
| **Cherimoya,** 1 fruit, 11 oz, 8¼ oz edible | 175 | 1.5 | 41 |
| **Cherries:** Sweet (Red/White), raw, 8 cherries, 2 oz | 30 | 0 | 8 |
| 1 cup, 4.5 oz | 75 | 0 | 19 |
| ½ lb (30 cherries) | 130 | 0.5 | 32 |
| Sour, red, raw, 1 cup, 4 oz | 50 | 0 | 12 |
| **Clementine,** 1 medium, 2.6 oz | 35 | 0 | 9 |
| **Coconut:** Fresh, 1 piece, 2"x2"x ½", 1 oz | 100 | 10 | 4.5 |
| Shredded, fresh, ½ cup, 1.4 oz | 140 | 13 | 6 |
| Sweetened, dried, ½ cup, 1.6 oz | 235 | 16 | 22 |
| **Crabapples,** ½ cup slices, 2 oz | 40 | 0 | 11 |
| **Cranberries,** ¼ cup, 1 oz | 25 | 0 | 6.5 |
| **Currants,** raw, ½ cup, 2 oz | 35 | 0 | 8 |
| **Custard Apple ~** *See Cherimoya* | | | |
| **Dragon Fruit,** (Pitahaya), 1 medium, 12 oz | 145 | 0.5 | 39 |
| **Durian,** flesh, 2 oz | 165 | 6 | 31 |
| **Elderberries,** ½ cup, 2.5 oz | 55 | 0.5 | 13 |
| **Feijoa,** (Pineapple Guava), 1 medium, 2 oz | 30 | 0.5 | 5.5 |
| **Figs,** green/black: 1 medium, 2 oz | 40 | 0 | 10 |
| 1 large, 3 oz | 60 | 0 | 15 |
| **Gooseberries,** raw, ½ cup, 2.5 oz | 35 | 0 | 7 |
| **Grapefruit:** Average all types, ½ fruit, 10 oz (6 oz flesh) | 55 | 0 | 13 |
| 1 cup sections w/ juice, 8 oz | 75 | 0 | 18 |
| **Grapes:** Average, 1 cup, 5.5 oz | 105 | 0 | 28 |
| 1 small bunch, 4 oz | 80 | 0 | 20 |
| 1 medium bunch, 7 oz | 140 | 0 | 36 |
| 1 large bunch, 16 oz | 315 | 0 | 82 |
| **Granadilla,** flesh, 3.5 oz | 95 | 0 | 23 |
| **Guava,** 1 medium, 4 oz | 80 | 1 | 16 |
| **Honeydew:** 1 slice, ¾" thick, 3 oz | 30 | 0 | 7 |
| 1 wedge, (⅛ of 7" diam.), 12 oz (with rind) | 80 | 0 | 20 |
| 1 cup cubes/balls, 6 oz | 60 | 0 | 14 |
| ½ small (4½ lb whole) | 180 | 0.5 | 42 |
| ½ medium (6lb whole) | 230 | 1 | 56 |
| **Honey Murcots,** 1 only, 5 oz | 45 | 0 | 11 |
| **Jaboticaba,** flesh, 4 oz | 75 | 2 | 15 |
| **Jackfruit,** flesh, ⅛ average, 4 oz | 105 | 0 | 27 |
| **Java-Plum,** 4 plums, 0.5 oz | 10 | 0 | 2 |
| **Kiwifruit,:** 1 Medium, 2.7 oz | 45 | 0 | 11 |
| 1 Large, 3.2 oz | 55 | 0.5 | 13 |
| **Kumquats,** 5 medium, 3.5 oz | 65 | 1 | 15 |
| **Kiwano,** ½ medium, 5 oz | 35 | 0 | 8 |
| **Langsat,** Duku, 1 medium, 2 oz | 25 | 0 | 5 |
| **Lemon:** 1 medium, 3 oz | 25 | 0 | 8 |
| 1 wedge, 1 oz | 5 | 0 | 1.5 |
| Peel, grated, 1 Tbsp | 5 | 0 | 1 |

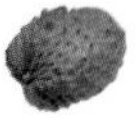

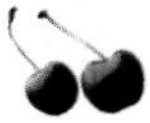

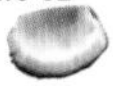

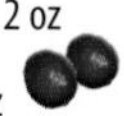

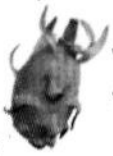

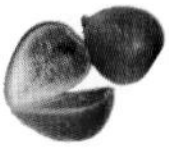

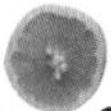

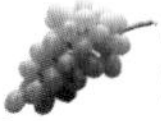

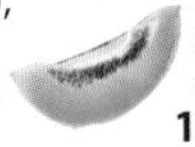

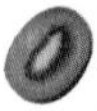

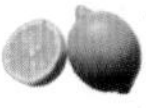

| Weights As Purchased | C | F | Cb |
|---|---|---|---|
| **Limes,** 1 medium (2" diam.), 2.4 oz | 20 | 0 | 7 |
| **Loganberries,** frozen, ½ cup, 2.5 oz | 40 | 0 | 9 |
| **Longans,** 5 fruit, 0.5oz | 10 | 0 | 2.5 |
| **Loquats,** 4 fruit, 2.25 oz | 30 | 0 | 8 |
| **Lychees,** 4 fruit, 2.25oz | 30 | 0 | 7 |
| **Mamey Apple:** ¼ fruit, 7 oz | 100 | 1 | 25 |
| **Mandarin:** 1 small, 3 oz | 35 | 0 | 9 |
| 1 medium, 4 oz | 45 | 0 | 11 |
| 1 large, 6 oz | 50 | 0 | 13 |
| **Mango:** Flesh, ½ cup slices, 3 oz | 55 | 0 | 14 |
| 1 small mango, 7 oz | 90 | 0.5 | 24 |
| 1 medium, 10 oz | 130 | 0.5 | 34 |
| 1 cheek, 4 oz | 60 | 0 | 14 |
| 1 large, 17 oz | 220 | 1 | 58 |
| 1 extra large mango, 24 oz | 310 | 1.5 | 82 |
| **Marionberries,** 1 cup, 5 oz | 75 | 1 | 15 |
| **Melon,** average, 1 c., cubes/balls, 6 oz | 60 | 0 | 14 |
| **Monstera Deliciosa,** (Taxonia), Edible part, 4 oz | 50 | 0 | 11 |
| **Mulberries,** 20 fruit, 1 oz | 15 | 0 | 3 |
| **Nashi Fruit** (Asian Pear), 1 med. 7 oz | 85 | 0 | 21 |
| **Nectarines:** 1 medium, 4 oz | 50 | 0 | 12 |
| 1 large, 5.5 oz | 70 | 0 | 16 |
| **Oheloberries,** ½ cup, 2.5 oz | 20 | 0 | 5 |
| **Olives** (Pickled): Green, 10 lge, 1.5 oz | 60 | 6.5 | 1.5 |
| Ripe, Greek Style, 10 medium, 1 oz | 70 | 6 | 4 |
| Ripe (Black) Californian: | | | |
| 1 small/medium | 5 | 0 | 0.2 |
| 1 large/extra large | 6 | 0.5 | 0.5 |
| 1 jumbo | 7 | 0.5 | 0.5 |
| 1 colossal | 11 | 1 | 0.5 |
| **Oranges:** Average all varieties (weights with skin) | | | |
| 1 small, 5 oz | 45 | 0 | 11 |
| 1 medium (3" diam.), 7 oz | 85 | 0 | 21 |
| 1 large, 10 oz | 130 | 0 | 33 |
| Californian Valencia, 1 medium (2¾" diam.), 6 oz | 60 | 0 | 14 |
| Calif. Navels (3" diameter), 7 oz | 70 | 0 | 17 |
| *Sunkist* Navel, large, 14 oz | 130 | 0 | 30 |
| Florida Orange, 1 med, 7 oz | 70 | 0 | 17 |
| Flesh only, 1 cup, 6 oz | 85 | 0 | 21 |
| Peel, 1 Tbsp | 0 | 0 | 0 |
| **Papaya:** ½ cup, cubed, 2.5 oz | 30 | 0 | 7 |
| 1 medium, (5"x3" diam.), 16 oz | 120 | 0 | 30 |
| Green (unripe), ½ cup, 3.5 oz | 20 | 0 | 5 |
| **Passionfruit,** 1 medium, 1.25 oz | 35 | 0 | 8 |
| **PawPaw** (see Papaya) | | | |
| **Peaches:** 1 small/donut, 3 oz | 30 | 0 | 7.5 |
| 1 medium (4 per lb), 4 oz | 45 | 0 | 11 |
| 1 large, 6 oz | 65 | 0 | 16 |
| 1 extra large, 10 oz | 110 | 0 | 27 |

| Weights As Purchased | C | F | Cb |
|---|---|---|---|
| **Pears,** Average all types: | | | |
| 1 mini, 2.5oz | 35 | 0 | 8 |
| 1 small, 5 oz | 75 | 0 | 18 |
| 1 medium, 7 oz | 105 | 0 | 25 |
| 1 large, 9 oz | 135 | 0 | 33 |
| 1 extra large, 12 oz | 175 | 0 | 42 |
| **Pepino,** ½ medium, 4 oz | 20 | 0 | 4 |
| **Persimmons:** Native, 1 oz | 35 | 0 | 9 |
| Japanese (2½"d. x 2½"h), 7 oz | 120 | 0 | 30 |
| Seedless (Maui), 1 medium, 5 oz | 100 | 0 | 25 |
| **Pineapple** (wts w/out skin): | | | |
| 1 thin slice (½"), 2 oz | 25 | 0 | 6 |
| 1 thick slice (¾"), 3 oz | 40 | 0 | 10 |
| 1 cup, diced, 5.5 oz | 75 | 0 | 19 |
| 1 medium, 1½ lb (peeled) | 325 | 0 | 86 |
| Wedges *(Del Monte)*, 12 oz package | 195 | 0 | 47 |
| **Canned ~ See Page 102** | | | |
| **Pitanga,** (Surinam-Cherry) (5), 1.2 oz | 10 | 0 | 2 |
| **Plantains,** ½ cup slices, 2.5oz | 90 | 0 | 22 |
| **Plums:** Average all types, | | | |
| Mini/Damson, (1" diameter), 0.5 oz | 7 | 0 | 1.5 |
| Small (2" diameter), 2.25oz | 30 | 0 | 7 |
| Med. (2½" diam.), 3.5 oz | 45 | 0 | 10 |
| Large (3" diameter), 5 oz | 60 | 0 | 14 |
| **Pluot** (plum-apricot), 1 med. 5 oz | 80 | 0 | 19 |
| **Pomegranate,** 1 medium, 10 oz | 105 | 0.5 | 25 |
| **Pummelo,** flesh, ½ cup, 3.5 oz | 35 | 0 | 9 |
| **Prickly Pear,** (Nopal): | | | |
| 1 small, 2.5 oz | 20 | 0 | 5 |
| 1 medium, 5 oz | 40 | 0 | 10 |
| **Quince,** 1 medium, 3.5 oz | 55 | 0 | 14 |
| **Rambutan** (Rambotang), Red/Yellow, 1 medium, 2 oz | 15 | 0 | 4 |
| **Raspberries,** ½ cup, 2 oz | 30 | 0 | 7 |
| 10 Raspberries, 0.75 oz | 10 | 0 | 2 |
| 1 Cup, 4.25 oz | 65 | 1 | 15 |
| 1 Pint, 11 oz | 160 | 2 | 37 |
| **Sapodilla** (Chico), 1 med., 7.5 oz | 140 | 2 | 34 |
| **Sapote,** ½ medium, 8 oz | 150 | 0.5 | 38 |
| **Satsuma Tangerine,** 1 medium, 3 oz | 45 | 0 | 11 |
| **Soursop,** 1 cup pulp, 8 oz | 150 | 0.5 | 38 |
| **Starfruit,** 1 medium, 3 oz | 30 | 0 | 6 |
| **Strawberries:** 1 cup, 5.5 oz | 50 | 0.5 | 12 |
| 6 medium/3 large, 2 oz | 20 | 0 | 4 |
| 1 pint, 13 oz | 115 | 1 | 27 |
| Chocolate Dipped, 1 large | 45 | 2.5 | 6 |
| **Sugar Apple,** (Custard Apple) ½ cup pulp, 4 oz | 120 | 0 | 30 |
| **Tamarillo,** 1 med., 3 oz | 20 | 0 | 3 |
| **Tamarind:** 1 fruit (3"x1") | 5 | 0 | 1.5 |
| Pulp, ½ cup, 2 oz | 140 | 0.5 | 37 |

*Weights as Purchased*

| | C | F | Cb |
|---|---|---|---|
| **Tangelo:** 1 small, 4 oz | 55 | 0 | 13 |
| 1 medium, 5 oz | 70 | 0 | 17 |
| 1 large, 7 oz | 95 | 0 | 23 |
| **Tangerine,** 1 med., (2½" diam.), 4 oz | 50 | 0 | 13 |
| **Tangor,** 1 medium, 4 oz | 35 | 0 | 7 |
| **Tomatillos** (3), 3.5 oz | 35 | 1 | 6 |
| **Tomatoes:** | | | |
| 1 small (2¼" diameter), 3 oz | 15 | 0 | 3 |
| 1 medium (2¾" diameter), 5 oz | 25 | 0 | 5 |
| 1 large (3½" diameter), 8 oz | 40 | 0.5 | 9 |
| 1 extra large (3" diameter), 12 oz | 60 | 0.5 | 14 |
| Grape, 5 medium, 2 oz | 10 | 0 | 2 |
| Yellow Tear Drop, 3 medium, 1 oz | 5 | 0 | 2 |
| Cherry: 4 medium, 2 oz | 10 | 0 | 2 |
| 1 cup, 5 oz | 25 | 0 | 6 |
| Slices (Medium Tomato): | | | |
| 2 thin slices, 1 oz | 5 | 0 | 1 |
| 2 thick (⅜"), 2 oz | 10 | 0 | 2 |
| Wedge, ¼ medium tomato, 1.25 oz | 6 | 0 | 1 |
| Chopped, 1 cup, 6.5 oz | 35 | 0.5 | 7 |
| Fried Green Tomato, 2 slices, 2.5 oz | 140 | 11 | 9 |
| **Canned Tomatoes/Products ~ *See Page 144*** | | | |
| **Tree Tomato** (Tamarillo), 3 oz | 20 | 0 | 5 |
| **Ugli Fruit,** Tangelo type, 5 oz | 40 | 0 | 8 |
| **Watermelon:** Flesh only, 1 oz | 8 | 0 | 2 |
| 1 thin slice, (¼ circle, ⅜"), 2 oz | 15 | 0 | 4 |
| 1 cup cubes or balls, 5½ oz | 45 | 0 | 11 |
| 10 balls, 4.3 oz | 35 | 0 | 9 |
| Buffet Slice, thin, 1 oz | 8 | 0 | 2 |
| **Regular,** (Long Shape): | | | |
| 1 thick (1") slice (¼ circle, 4½" radius) | | | |
| 9 oz w. skin (5½ oz no rind) | 50 | 0 | 12 |
| 1 thin (½") slice (¼ circle) | 25 | 0 | 6 |
| 1 thick (1") slice (½ circle) | | | |
| 18 oz with rind | 100 | 1 | 22 |
| 1 whole melon (15" long, 7½"diameter) | | | |
| 20 lb with rind, 10 lb w/o rind | 1360 | 7 | 330 |
| **Seedless,** (Round Shape): | | | |
| Medium size (13 lb, 8¼" diameter) | | | |
| 1 whole, 8½ lb without rind | 1160 | 5 | 280 |
| Wedge (⅛ whole melon), | | | |
| 26 oz with rind | 145 | 1 | 35 |
| Flesh only, without rind, 8 oz | 70 | 0.5 | 17 |
| Mini size (6 lb, 6½" diameter), | | | |
| 1 whole, 3½ lb without rind | 480 | 2.5 | 110 |
| Wedge (⅛ whole), | | | |
| 1.5 lb, with rind | 60 | 0.5 | 14 |

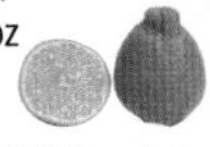

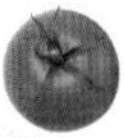

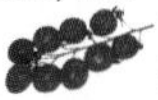

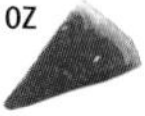

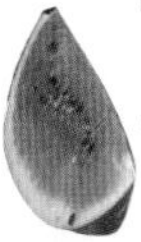

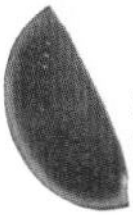

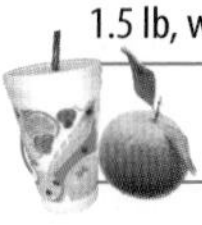

**FRUIT & VEGETABLE JUICES**
~ See Page 41

## Dried Fruit

| | C | F | Cb |
|---|---|---|---|
| **Apples,** 5 rings, 1 oz | 80 | 0 | 19 |
| **Apricots,** 8 halves, 1 oz | 65 | 0 | 16 |
| **Banana Chips,** ½ cup, 1.5 oz | 220 | 14 | 25 |
| **Banana Flakes,** 4 Tbsp, 1 oz | 80 | 0 | 20 |
| **Cranberries** (Craisins): | | | |
| Sweetened, ¼ cup, 1 oz | 100 | 0 | 24 |
| Unsweetened, ¼ cup, 1 oz | 80 | 0 | 19 |
| Choc-coated, 1 oz | 135 | 7.5 | 18 |
| **Currants,** ¼ cup, 1.25 oz | 100 | 0 | 25 |
| **Dates:** 5 medium dates, 1.5 oz | 120 | 0 | 29 |
| Large Calif.: 1 date, 0.7 oz | 55 | 0 | 13 |
| 3 dates, 2 oz | 170 | 0 | 39 |
| ½ cup, chopped, 3 oz | 240 | 0 | 58 |
| Pecan Date Rolls, 1 oz | 100 | 2.5 | 19 |
| **Date Crumbles** (Bob's Redmill), | | | |
| ¼ cup, 1 oz | 90 | 0 | 22 |
| **Figs,** 3 medium figs, 1 oz | 90 | 0 | 23 |
| **Goji Berries,** 3 Tbsp, 1 oz | 100 | 1 | 20 |
| **Longans; Lychees,** 1 oz | 80 | 0 | 20 |
| **Mango Slices,** 5 pieces, 1.4 oz | 25 | 0 | 6 |
| **Papaya Spears,** 2 pieces, 1.4 oz | 120 | 0 | 30 |
| **Peaches,** 2 halves, 1 oz | 60 | 0 | 15 |
| **Pears,** 3 halves, 2 oz | 140 | 0.5 | 34 |
| **Plums** (Sunsweet) (5), 1.4 oz | 100 | 0 | 24 |
| **Prunes,** (dried Plums): With pits, 1 oz | 70 | 0 | 17 |
| 1 medium (60/lb) | 16 | 0 | 4 |
| 1 large (50/lb) | 22 | 0 | 5 |
| 1extra large (40/lb) | 25 | 0 | 6 |
| Without pits, 4 medium, 1 oz | 70 | 0 | 17 |
| Cooked: with sugar, ½ cup, 5 oz | 155 | 0 | 38 |
| without sugar, ½ cup, 4.5 oz | 135 | 0 | 33 |
| **Raisins:** 2 Tbsp, 1 oz pack | 85 | 0 | 20 |
| ½ cup, 2.8 oz | 220 | 0.5 | 56 |

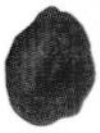

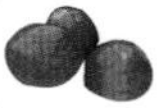

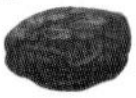

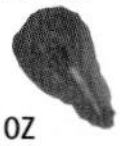

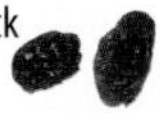

## Candied/Glazed Fruit

| | C | F | Cb |
|---|---|---|---|
| **Apricot,** 1 medium, 1 oz | 70 | 0 | 17 |
| **Cherry,** (Maraschino) (1) | 8 | 0 | 2 |
| **Citron/Fruit Peel,** 1 oz | 85 | 0 | 20 |
| **Ginger,** 1 oz | 90 | 0 | 21 |
| **Pineapple,** 1 slice, 1.25 oz | 120 | 0 | 29 |

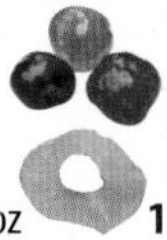

## Fruit Leather/Rolls

| | C | F | Cb |
|---|---|---|---|
| **Average All Brands,** 1 oz | 105 | 1 | 24 |
| Fruit By The Foot, (Betty Crocker) | | | |
| 1 roll, ¾ oz | 80 | 0 | 17 |
| Fruit Gushers, (Betty Crocker), 1 oz | 90 | 1 | 20 |
| Fruit Roll-Ups, (Betty Crocker), 1 roll | 50 | 1 | 12 |
| Leathers (Stretch Island), 2 pcs, 1 oz | 90 | 0 | 24 |

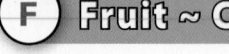
## Canned/Bottled Fruit

| Solids & Liquids: | C | F | Cb |
|---|---|---|---|
| *Per ½ Cup, 4½ oz* | | | |
| **Apricots:** In water/diet | 35 | 0 | 8 |
| In juice/lite | 60 | 0 | 15 |
| In syrup | 105 | 0 | 28 |
| **Black/Blueberries:** Heavy syrup | 120 | 0 | 30 |
| In light syrup | 110 | 0 | 26 |
| **Cherries,** pitted: In water | 55 | 0 | 15 |
| In light syrup | 85 | 0 | 22 |
| In heavy syrup | 105 | 0 | 27 |
| In extra heavy syrup | 135 | 0 | 34 |
| Maraschino, 1 oz | 50 | 0 | 12 |
| Pie Cherries, ⅔ cup, 5 oz | 90 | 0 | 23 |
| **Fruit Salad:** In water/diet | 35 | 0 | 10 |
| In light juice | 60 | 0 | 16 |
| In heavy syrup | 95 | 0 | 25 |
| **Gooseberries,** Light syrup | 90 | 0 | 24 |
| **Grapefruit:** Juice pack | 45 | 0 | 12 |
| In light syrup | 75 | 0 | 20 |
| **Lychees,** ½ cup, 4.5 oz | 105 | 0 | 26 |
| **Mixed Fruit:** In water/diet | 40 | 0 | 10 |
| In fruit juices/light syrup | 70 | 0 | 18 |
| In heavy syrup | 90 | 0 | 24 |
| **Peaches** (halves/slices): In water/diet | 30 | 0 | 7 |
| In juice/light | 55 | 0 | 14 |
| In light syrup | 70 | 0 | 18 |
| Drained, ½ peach | 55 | 0 | 14 |
| In heavy syrup | 100 | 0 | 26 |
| **Pears:** In water/diet | 35 | 0 | 10 |
| In light juice | 60 | 0 | 16 |
| In heavy syrup | 100 | 0 | 26 |
| **Pineapple:** All types | | | |
| In own juice | 75 | 0 | 20 |
| In heavy syrup | 100 | 0 | 26 |
| 1 slice (ring), drained, 1.5 oz | 15 | 0 | 4 |
| **Prunes:** In heavy syrup | 125 | 0 | 33 |
| In Liqueur, ½ cup, 4.4 oz | 280 | 0 | 70 |
| Stewed in Water, ½ cup | 135 | 0 | 35 |
| **Tropical Fruit Salad:** In light syrup | 80 | 0 | 21 |
| In heavy syrup | 110 | 0 | 29 |

## Fruit Snack Cups

| | C | F | Cb |
|---|---|---|---|
| **Deli/Take-Out:** Small, 6 oz | 70 | 0 | 16 |
| Large, 12 oz | 140 | 0 | 32 |
| Yogurt & Fruit Cup, 15 oz | 380 | 4.5 | 75 |
| **Del Monte:** | | | |
| **Bowls:** *Approx. ¼ of 20.5 oz Container, 4.4 oz* | | | |
| Cherry Mixed Fruit | 70 | 0 | 17 |
| Citrus Salad; Grapefrt Duo | 60 | 0 | 16 |
| Red Grapefruit | 60 | 0 | 14 |
| **Fruit Naturals:** *Per ½ Cup* | | | |
| Cherry Mixed Fruit; Peach Chunks, av. | 65 | 0 | 16 |
| Mandarin Orange Segments | 70 | 0 | 17 |
| Pineapple Chunks | 70 | 0 | 18 |
| Red Grapefruit | 60 | 0 | 16 |
| Average others | 70 | 0 | 18 |
| **Pull Top Cans:** In 100% Juice, ½ c. | 65 | 0 | 17 |
| Lite varieties, ½ cup | 60 | 0 | 15 |
| **Snack Cups:** *Per 4 oz Cup* | | | |
| Cherry Mix | 70 | 0 | 18 |
| Average other varieties | 70 | 0 | 17 |
| No Sugar Added, av. all varieties | 40 | 0 | 10 |
| **Super Fruits:** *Per 6 .oz cup* | | | |
| Mixed Fruit Chunks in Juice | 120 | 0 | 29 |
| Peaches/Pears in Juice, av | 100 | 0 | 26 |
| **Dole Fruit Bowls:** | | | |
| **4 oz Bowls:** Diced Peaches | 70 | 0 | 18 |
| Mixed Fruit | 70 | 0 | 17 |
| Pineapple; Tropical Fruit, average | 60 | 0 | 15 |
| **Fruit-n-Gel Bowls,** av. all, 4.3 oz | 85 | 0 | 21 |
| **Safeway (Vons):** | | | |
| **Fruit Cocktail:** *Per ½ Cup, 4.5 oz* | | | |
| In heavy syrup | 100 | 0 | 25 |
| Lite in Pear Juice | 60 | 0 | 14 |

## Apple & Fruit Sauces

| | C | F | Cb |
|---|---|---|---|
| **Apple Sauce:** | | | |
| Regular/sweetened, 2 Tbsp, 1 oz | 20 | 0 | 6 |
| 4 oz package | 85 | 0 | 22 |
| ¼ cup | 50 | 0 | 13 |
| **Fruit Sauces & Purees:** | | | |
| Average all fruit types, 2 Tbsp, 1 oz | 25 | 0 | 6 |
| ½ cup, 4 oz | 100 | 0 | 24 |
| **Mott's:** | | | |
| Apple Sauce: Original, 4 oz | 100 | 0 | 24 |
| Fruit Flavored, average, 4 oz | 90 | 0 | 23 |
| Healthy Harvest, 3.92 oz | 50 | 0 | 13 |
| **Ocean Spray:** *Per ¼ Cup* | | | |
| Jellied Cranberry Sauce | 110 | 0 | 25 |
| Whole Berry Cranberry Sauce | 110 | 0 | 25 |

**Pie Fillings ~ See Page 134**

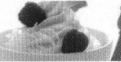 

## Quick Guide  C  F  Cb

### Ice Cream

**Vanilla:** *Average All Brands*
**Other flavors** ~ *See Brand Listings.*
*Counts per USDA food database unless specified*

**Regular (10% fat):**

| | C | F | Cb |
|---|---|---|---|
| 1 scoop, 3 oz | 175 | 9 | 20 |
| ½ cup, 4 oz | 235 | 13 | 27 |
| 1 Pint, 16 oz | 940 | 50 | 107 |
| ½ Gallon (4 pints, 64 oz) | 3755 | 200 | 428 |

**Rich/Premium (16-17% fat):**

| | | | |
|---|---|---|---|
| 1 scoop, 3 oz | 210 | 14 | 19 |
| ½ cup, 4 oz | 285 | 19 | 25 |
| 1 Pint, 16 oz | 1130 | 74 | 101 |
| ½ Gallon (4 pints, 64 oz) | 4525 | 295 | 405 |

**Super Rich (21% fat):**

| | | | |
|---|---|---|---|
| 3 oz scoop | 220 | 15 | 17 |
| ½ cup, 4 oz | 270 | 18 | 21 |
| 1 pint, 16 oz | 1160 | 78 | 91 |

**Reduced-Fat/Light (5% fat):**

| | | | |
|---|---|---|---|
| 1 scoop, 3 oz | 155 | 4 | 25 |
| ½ cup, 4 fl.oz | 205 | 5.5 | 34 |
| 1 Pint, 16 oz | 820 | 22 | 134 |
| ½ gallon (4 pints, 64 oz) | 1090 | 88 | 536 |

**Fat-Free:**

| | | | |
|---|---|---|---|
| 1 scoop, 3 oz | 115 | 0 | 27 |
| ½ cup, 4oz | 155 | 0 | 34 |
| 1 Pint, 16 oz | 625 | 0 | 137 |

**Soft Serve:**

| | | | |
|---|---|---|---|
| Regular: ½ cup, 4 oz | 255 | 15 | 25 |
| 1 cup, 8 oz | 510 | 30 | 50 |
| Light: ½ cup, 4 oz | 145 | 3 | 25 |
| 1 cup, 8 oz | 290 | 6 | 50 |

## Quick Guide  C  F  Cb

### Frozen Yogurt

*Average All Brands*

| | C | F | Cb |
|---|---|---|---|
| **Hard:** Low-Fat, ½ cup | 110 | 3 | 19 |
| Non-Fat, ½ cup | 110 | 0 | 24 |
| **Soft:** Low-Fat, ½ cup | 120 | 4 | 17 |
| Non-Fat, ½ cup | 100 | 0 | 30 |

**Brands** ~ *See Ice Cream & Ices Section*

## Quick Guide  C  F  Cb

### Gelato/Ices/Frozen Custard

**Gelato:** *Per ½ Cup*

| | C | F | Cb |
|---|---|---|---|
| Milk base: Vanilla | 160 | 6 | 25 |
| Chocolate Hazelnut | 230 | 15 | 21 |
| Water base, ½ cup | 100 | 0 | 26 |

**Frozen Custard:** *Per ½ Cup*

| | | | |
|---|---|---|---|
| Chocolate | 140 | 6 | 18 |
| Orange Sherbet | 105 | 2 | 21 |
| Vanilla | 130 | 6 | 16 |

**Ice (Milk base):** *Average all flavors*

| | | | |
|---|---|---|---|
| Hard (4% fat), ½ cup | 100 | 3 | 15 |
| Soft Serve (3% fat), ½ cup | 110 | 2 | 19 |
| **Shaved Ice,** average, 12 fl. oz | 160 | 0 | 40 |
| **Sherbet,** average, ½ cup | 110 | 1.5 | 22 |
| **Sorbet,** Fruit (without fat), ½ cup | 70 | 0 | 19 |
| **Fruit Ice Pops** | 80 | 0 | 20 |

### Sundaes  C  F  Cb

**Baskin Robbins:**

| | C | F | Cb |
|---|---|---|---|
| **Classic:** Banana Royale | 620 | 28 | 87 |
| Banana Split | 1010 | 34 | 173 |
| Brownie | 920 | 47 | 119 |
| **Premium:** | | | |
| Chocolate Chip Cookie Dough | 990 | 43 | 138 |
| Made With Snickers | 1000 | 46 | 138 |
| Reeses Peanut Butter Cup | 1220 | 80 | 109 |

**Denny's:**

| | | | |
|---|---|---|---|
| Oreo Blender Blaster | 890 | 44 | 113 |
| **Topping:** Chocolate, 1.5 oz | 100 | 0 | 9 |
| Other Toppings ~ *See Page 195* | | | |

**McDonald's:**

| | | | |
|---|---|---|---|
| Hot Caramel Sundae | 340 | 8 | 60 |
| Hot Fudge Sundae | 330 | 10 | 54 |
| Strawberry Sundae | 280 | 6 | 49 |
| **Toppings,** Peanuts, ¼ oz | 45 | 3.5 | 2 |

### Ice Cream, Cones & Cups

*Average All Brands*  C  F  Cb

| | C | F | Cb |
|---|---|---|---|
| **Wafer Cone/Cup,** average | 20 | 0 | 4 |
| **Sugar Cone,** average | 50 | 0 | 14 |
| **Waffle Cone:** | | | |
| Small | 50 | 1 | 10 |
| Large | 90 | 0.5 | 19 |
| **Brands:** | | | |
| *Oreo,* Chocolate Cone | 50 | 1 | 10 |
| *Comet,* Sugar Cone | 50 | 0 | 11 |
| *Keebler,* Sugar Cone | 50 | 0 | 10 |

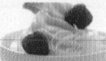

## Brands

| | C | F | Cb |
|---|---|---|---|
| **Baskin-Robbins** ~ *See Fast-Foods Section* | | | |
| **Ben & Jerry's:** | | | |
| **Hand scooped Ice Cream:** *Per ½ Cup* | | | |
| Butter Pecan, 3 oz | 260 | 20 | 17 |
| Cherry Garcia, 3.28 oz | 220 | 11 | 26 |
| Chocolate Fair Trade, 3 oz | 200 | 12 | 21 |
| Choc. Chip Cookie Dough, 3.25 oz | 240 | 12 | 29 |
| Chocolate Therapy, 3 oz | 220 | 12 | 27 |
| Coconut Seven Layer Bar, 3.25 oz | 280 | 18 | 26 |
| Coffee, Coffee BuzzBuzzBuzz, 3.1 oz | 230 | 14 | 23 |
| Imagine Whirled Peace, 3.25 oz | 250 | 15 | 27 |
| Mint Chocolate Chunk, 3.1 oz | 230 | 14 | 23 |
| New York Super Fudge Chunk, 3.25 oz | 270 | 16 | 28 |
| Phish Food, 3.25 oz | 240 | 11 | 32 |
| Strawberry Cheesecake, 3 oz | 220 | 12 | 23 |
| Sweet Cream & Cookies, 3.1 oz | 220 | 13 | 24 |
| Triple Caramel Chunk, 3.25 oz | 230 | 12 | 30 |
| Vanilla Fair Trade, 3.25 oz | 200 | 12 | 20 |
| **1 Pint Tubs:** *Per ½ Cup* | | | |
| Banana Split, 3.85 oz | 250 | 15 | 27 |
| Boston Cream Pie, 3.65 oz | 250 | 13 | 29 |
| Cake Batter, 3.7 oz | 260 | 16 | 27 |
| Cherry Garcia, 3.7 oz | 240 | 13 | 28 |
| Chocolate Chip Cookie Dough, 3.7 oz | 270 | 14 | 33 |
| Dulce Delish', 3.7 oz | 240 | 12 | 29 |
| Everything But The... ,3.85 oz | 290 | 17 | 31 |
| Imagine Whirled Peace | 270 | 16 | 27 |
| Karamel Sutra, 3.75 oz | 260 | 14 | 31 |
| Milk & Cookies, 3.55 oz | 270 | 15 | 30 |
| Mission To Marzipan, 3.6 oz | 260 | 13 | 32 |
| New York Super Fudge Chunk, 3,75 oz | 300 | 20 | 29 |
| Peanut Brittle, 3.65 oz | 260 | 15 | 29 |
| Peanut Butter Cup, 4 oz | 360 | 26 | 27 |
| Phish Food, 3.75 oz | 280 | 13 | 39 |
| Red Velvet Calke, 3.56 oz | 250 | 13 | 30 |
| Triple Caramel Chunk, 3.75 oz | 280 | 16 | 32 |
| Turtle Soup, 3.65 oz | 280 | 16 | 30 |
| **Frozen Yogurt:** *Per ½ Cup* | | | |
| Fro Yo: Cherry Garcia, 3.8 oz | 200 | 3 | 37 |
| Chocolate Fudge Brownie, 3.65 oz | 180 | 2.5 | 35 |
| Half Baked, 3.5 oz | 180 | 3 | 35 |
| Strawberry Banana, 3.35 oz | 150 | 1.5 | 32 |
| **Sorbet,** average all flavors | 120 | 0 | 27 |

| **Blue Bunny:** *Per ½ Cup* | C | F | Cb |
|---|---|---|---|
| **Ice Cream:** | | | |
| **Fat-Free:** *No Added Sugar* | | | |
| (Carbs include 5g sugar alcohol) | | | |
| Brownie Sundae, 2.6 oz | 90 | 0 | 23 |
| Caramel Toffee Crunch, 2.5 oz | 90 | 0 | 24 |
| Vanilla, 2.5 oz | 80 | 0 | 20 |
| **Reduced-Fat:** *No Added Sugar* | | | |
| (Carbs include 3-7g sugar alcohol) | | | |
| Banana Split, 2.5oz | 120 | 5 | 20 |
| Butter Pecan, 2.5 oz | 130 | 6 | 16 |
| Chocolate, 2.5 oz | 110 | 5 | 16 |
| Turtle Sundae, 2.5 oz | 140 | 7 | 20 |
| **Personals:** *Per Container* | | | |
| Cherry Vanilla, 6 oz | `170 | 7 | 25 |
| Double Strawberry, 3.92 oz | 160 | 6 | 26 |
| **Hi Lite:** Chocolate, 2.3 oz | 110 | 3 | 17 |
| Fudge Nut Sundae, 2.3 oz | 120 | 4 | 19 |
| Homemade Van., 2.35 oz | 110 | 3.5 | 18 |
| **Frozen Yogurt,** average all flavors, 2.4 oz | 120 | 3 | 21 |
| **Bars/Pops** ~ *See Page 108* | | | |
| **Breyers:** *Per ½ Cup* | | | |
| **All Natural Ice Cream:** | | | |
| Original: Butter Pecan | 150 | 10 | 14 |
| Cherry Vanilla | 130 | 6 | 18 |
| Cookies & Cream; Rocky Road | 155 | 7 | 20 |
| Vanilla, Chocolate | 130 | 7 | 16 |
| **Smooth & Dreamy:** | | | |
| Half The Fat: Butter Pecan | 130 | 6 | 16 |
| Chocolate Chocolate Chip | 140 | 5 | 21 |
| Cookies & Cream | 130 | 4 | 20 |
| Creamy, Chocolate/Vanilla, av. | 120 | 3.5 | 17 |
| Mint Chocolate Chip | 130 | 4.5 | 18 |
| Strawberry Cheesecake | 130 | 3.5 | 20 |
| Vanilla, Chocolate, Strawberry | 110 | 3.5 | 17 |
| Fat Free: Creamy Van. | 90 | 0 | 20 |
| French Chocolate | 90 | 0 | 22 |
| Strawberry | 90 | 0 | 21 |
| No Added Sugar: | | | |
| (Carbs include 5g sugar alcohol and 4g fiber) | | | |
| Butter Pecan | 110 | 6 | 15 |
| Vanilla/Choc./Strawberry | 90 | 4 | 15 |
| **Blasts!:** Chips Ahoy | 140 | 5 | 22 |
| Mint Fudge Brownie | 140 | 4 | 17 |
| Oreo | 140 | 6 | 21 |
| Snickers | 170 | 8 | 21 |
| Whoppers Malted Van. | 140 | 6 | 23 |
| **CarbSmart:** Choc./Van. | 90 | 6 | 13 |
| (Carbs include 5g sugar alcohol and 4g fiber) | | | |

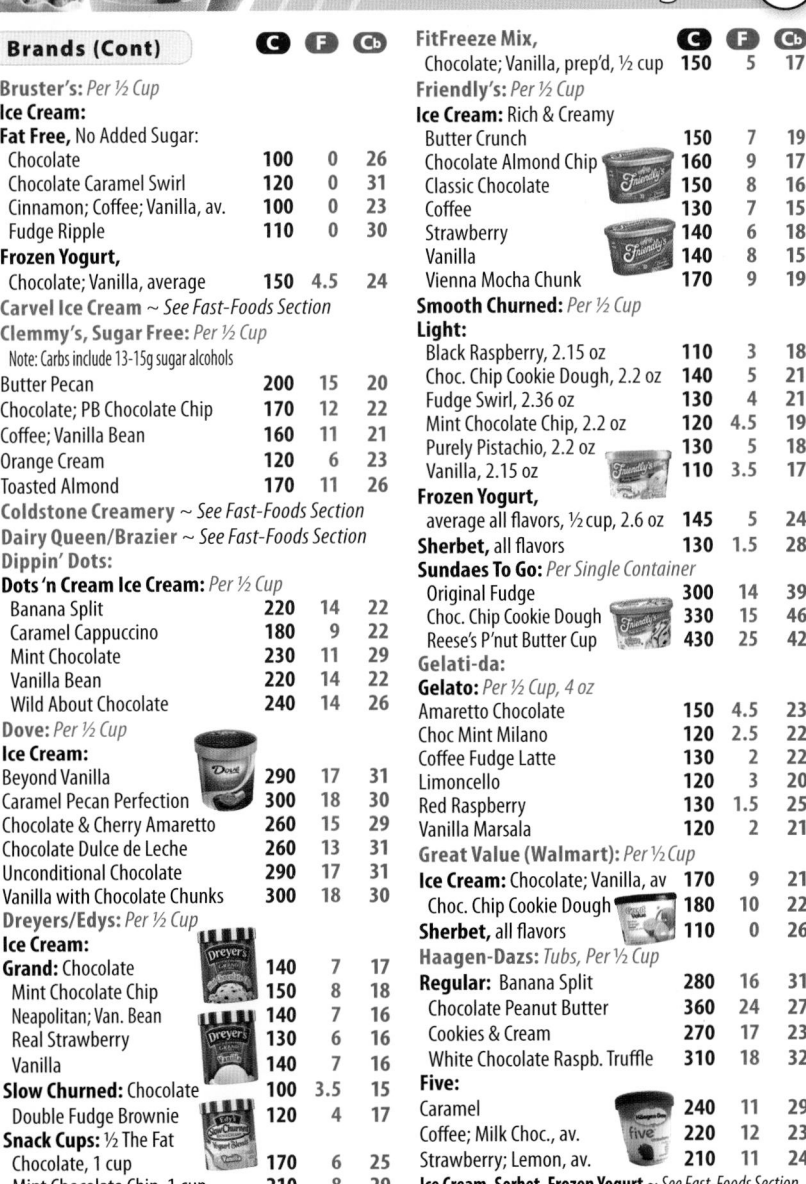

## Brands (Cont)

| | C | F | Cb |
|---|---|---|---|
| **Bruster's:** *Per ½ Cup* | | | |
| **Ice Cream:** | | | |
| **Fat Free,** No Added Sugar: | | | |
| Chocolate | 100 | 0 | 26 |
| Chocolate Caramel Swirl | 120 | 0 | 31 |
| Cinnamon; Coffee; Vanilla, av. | 100 | 0 | 23 |
| Fudge Ripple | 110 | 0 | 30 |
| **Frozen Yogurt,** | | | |
| Chocolate; Vanilla, average | 150 | 4.5 | 24 |
| **Carvel Ice Cream** ~ *See Fast-Foods Section* | | | |
| **Clemmy's, Sugar Free:** *Per ½ Cup* | | | |
| Note: Carbs include 13-15g sugar alcohols | | | |
| Butter Pecan | 200 | 15 | 20 |
| Chocolate; PB Chocolate Chip | 170 | 12 | 22 |
| Coffee; Vanilla Bean | 160 | 11 | 21 |
| Orange Cream | 120 | 6 | 23 |
| Toasted Almond | 170 | 11 | 26 |
| **Coldstone Creamery** ~ *See Fast-Foods Section* | | | |
| **Dairy Queen/Brazier** ~ *See Fast-Foods Section* | | | |
| **Dippin' Dots:** | | | |
| **Dots 'n Cream Ice Cream:** *Per ½ Cup* | | | |
| Banana Split | 220 | 14 | 22 |
| Caramel Cappuccino | 180 | 9 | 22 |
| Mint Chocolate | 230 | 11 | 29 |
| Vanilla Bean | 220 | 14 | 22 |
| Wild About Chocolate | 240 | 14 | 26 |
| **Dove:** *Per ½ Cup* | | | |
| **Ice Cream:** | | | |
| Beyond Vanilla | 290 | 17 | 31 |
| Caramel Pecan Perfection | 300 | 18 | 30 |
| Chocolate & Cherry Amaretto | 260 | 15 | 29 |
| Chocolate Dulce de Leche | 260 | 13 | 31 |
| Unconditional Chocolate | 290 | 17 | 31 |
| Vanilla with Chocolate Chunks | 300 | 18 | 30 |
| **Dreyers/Edys:** *Per ½ Cup* | | | |
| **Ice Cream:** | | | |
| **Grand:** Chocolate | 140 | 7 | 17 |
| Mint Chocolate Chip | 150 | 8 | 18 |
| Neapolitan; Van. Bean | 140 | 7 | 16 |
| Real Strawberry | 130 | 6 | 16 |
| Vanilla | 140 | 7 | 16 |
| **Slow Churned:** Chocolate | 100 | 3.5 | 15 |
| Double Fudge Brownie | 120 | 4 | 17 |
| **Snack Cups:** ½ The Fat | | | |
| Chocolate, 1 cup | 170 | 6 | 25 |
| Mint Chocolate Chip, 1 cup | 210 | 8 | 29 |
| **Yogurt Blends,** av. all flavors | 110 | 4 | 19 |

| | C | F | Cb |
|---|---|---|---|
| **FitFreeze Mix,** | | | |
| Chocolate; Vanilla, prep'd, ½ cup | 150 | 5 | 17 |
| **Friendly's:** *Per ½ Cup* | | | |
| **Ice Cream:** Rich & Creamy | | | |
| Butter Crunch | 150 | 7 | 19 |
| Chocolate Almond Chip | 160 | 9 | 17 |
| Classic Chocolate | 150 | 8 | 16 |
| Coffee | 130 | 7 | 15 |
| Strawberry | 140 | 6 | 18 |
| Vanilla | 140 | 8 | 15 |
| Vienna Mocha Chunk | 170 | 9 | 19 |
| **Smooth Churned:** *Per ½ Cup* | | | |
| **Light:** | | | |
| Black Raspberry, 2.15 oz | 110 | 3 | 18 |
| Choc. Chip Cookie Dough, 2.2 oz | 140 | 5 | 21 |
| Fudge Swirl, 2.36 oz | 130 | 4 | 21 |
| Mint Chocolate Chip, 2.2 oz | 120 | 4.5 | 19 |
| Purely Pistachio, 2.2 oz | 130 | 5 | 18 |
| Vanilla, 2.15 oz | 110 | 3.5 | 17 |
| **Frozen Yogurt,** | | | |
| average all flavors, ½ cup, 2.6 oz | 145 | 5 | 24 |
| **Sherbet,** all flavors | 130 | 1.5 | 28 |
| **Sundaes To Go:** *Per Single Container* | | | |
| Original Fudge | 300 | 14 | 39 |
| Choc. Chip Cookie Dough | 330 | 15 | 46 |
| Reese's P'nut Butter Cup | 430 | 25 | 42 |
| **Gelati-da:** | | | |
| **Gelato:** *Per ½ Cup, 4 oz* | | | |
| Amaretto Chocolate | 150 | 4.5 | 23 |
| Choc Mint Milano | 120 | 2.5 | 22 |
| Coffee Fudge Latte | 130 | 2 | 22 |
| Limoncello | 120 | 3 | 20 |
| Red Raspberry | 130 | 1.5 | 25 |
| Vanilla Marsala | 120 | 2 | 21 |
| **Great Value (Walmart):** *Per ½ Cup* | | | |
| **Ice Cream:** Chocolate; Vanilla, av | 170 | 9 | 21 |
| Choc. Chip Cookie Dough | 180 | 10 | 22 |
| **Sherbet,** all flavors | 110 | 0 | 26 |
| **Haagen-Dazs:** *Tubs, Per ½ Cup* | | | |
| **Regular:** Banana Split | 280 | 16 | 31 |
| Chocolate Peanut Butter | 360 | 24 | 27 |
| Cookies & Cream | 270 | 17 | 23 |
| White Chocolate Raspb. Truffle | 310 | 18 | 32 |
| **Five:** | | | |
| Caramel | 240 | 11 | 29 |
| Coffee; Milk Choc., av. | 220 | 12 | 23 |
| Strawberry; Lemon, av. | 210 | 11 | 24 |
| **Ice Cream, Sorbet, Frozen Yogurt** ~ *See Fast-Foods Section* | | | |
| **Bars** ~ *See Page 109* | | | |

# Ice Cream & Frozen Yogurt

## Brands (Cont)

**C  F  Cb**

**Hood:** *Per ½ Cup*
**Frozen Fat-Free Yogurt:**

| | C | F | Cb |
|---|---|---|---|
| Maine Blueberry & Sweet Cream | 90 | 0 | 19 |
| Mocha Fudge | 100 | 0 | 22 |
| Strawberry | 80 | 0 | 18 |
| Strawberry Banana | 90 | 0 | 20 |
| Tangy, average all flavors | 110 | 1 | 24 |

**Ice Cream:** *Per ½ Cup*

| | C | F | Cb |
|---|---|---|---|
| Birthday Party; Cookies 'N Cream | 150 | 8 | 19 |
| Chocolate | 140 | 6 | 18 |
| Classic Trio | 140 | 7 | 17 |
| Cookie Dough Delight | 160 | 8 | 19 |
| Creamy Coffee | 140 | 7 | 16 |
| Fudge Twister | 140 | 6 | 20 |
| Golden/Natural Vanilla; Patchwork | 140 | 7 | 17 |
| Maple Walnut | 150 | 9 | 17 |

**New England Creamery** ~ *www.CalorieKing.com*
**Bar** ~ *See Page 109*

**Jerseymaid (Vons):** *Per ½ Cup*
**Ice Cream:**

| | C | F | Cb |
|---|---|---|---|
| Cookies & Crm | 160 | 8 | 18 |
| Choc Chip; Mint Choc Chip | 150 | 9 | 16 |
| Heavenly Hash | 165 | 9 | 19 |
| Mocha Almond Fudge; Chocolate | 150 | 9 | 16 |
| Neapolitan; Real Vanilla | 140 | 8 | 15 |
| Strawberry | 130 | 6 | 17 |

**Oberweis:** *Per 6 oz Scoop*
**Super Premium Ice Cream:**

| | C | F | Cb |
|---|---|---|---|
| Chocolate | 480 | 31 | 43 |
| Chocolate Peanut Butter | 550 | 39 | 42 |
| Cookie Dough | 500 | 28 | 56 |
| Vanilla | 460 | 31 | 40 |

**Pinkberry Frozen Yogurt:**
**Original:** *Without Toppings*

| | C | F | Cb |
|---|---|---|---|
| Mini, 3.2 oz | 90 | 0 | 19 |
| Small, 5.3 oz | 150 | 0 | 31 |
| Medium, 8 oz | 230 | 0 | 48 |
| Large, 13.5 oz | 380 | 0 | 80 |
| **Cone,** with 3 oz Frozen Yogurt | 105 | 0 | 23 |

**Other Flavors:** *Per Medium Serving*

| | C | F | Cb |
|---|---|---|---|
| Chocolate | 275 | 3.5 | 53 |
| Coconut | 320 | 1 | 69 |
| Mango; Passionfruit, av. | 230 | 0 | 53 |

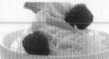 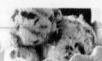

**C  F  Cb**

**Purely Decadent** *(Turtle Mtn):*
**Dairy Free, Soy Based:** *1 Pint Carton, Per 1/1 Cup*

| | C | F | Cb |
|---|---|---|---|
| Belgian Chocolate, 3.5 oz | 180 | 7 | 30 |
| Chocolate Obsession, 3.1 oz | 210 | 7 | 27 |
| **Gluten Free,** Cookie Dough, 3.53 oz | 230 | 8 | 36 |
| **With Coconut Milk:** Chocolate, 3 oz | 150 | 9 | 20 |
| Coconut, 3 oz | 170 | 10 | 19 |
| Mint Chip, 3 oz | 170 | 9 | 20 |
| Vanilla Bean, 3 oz | 150 | 8 | 19 |
| Gluten Free, Cookie Dough, 3 oz | 190 | 9 | 24 |

**Red Mango Frozen Yogurt:** *No Toppings Included*
**Original/Tangomonium:** *3.28 oz*

| | C | F | Cb |
|---|---|---|---|
| *3.28 oz* | 80 | 0 | 19 |
| Small, 4.6 oz | 110 | 0 | 27 |
| Regular, 7.54 oz | 185 | 0 | 21 |
| Large, 11.48 oz | 280 | 0 | 67 |

**Pomegranate:** *3.28 oz*

| | C | F | Cb |
|---|---|---|---|
| *3.28 oz* | 90 | 0 | 21 |
| Small, 4.6 oz | 125 | 0 | 29 |
| Regular, 7.54 oz | 205 | 0 | 53 |
| Large, 11.48 oz | 315 | 0 | 74 |

**Rice Dream (Non-Dairy):**
**Frozen Dessert:** *Per ½ Cup, 2.82 oz*

| | C | F | Cb |
|---|---|---|---|
| Carob Almond | 180 | 10 | 26 |
| Cocoa Marble Fudge | 170 | 6 | 31 |
| Cookies & Dream | 170 | 8 | 27 |
| Neapolitan; Orange Van. Swirl | 160 | 6 | 26 |
| Strawberry | 160 | 8 | 25 |
| Vanilla | 160 | 8 | 26 |

**Bars** ~ *See Page 110*

**Skinny Cow:** *Per Single Serve Cup*

| | C | F | Cb |
|---|---|---|---|
| Choc Fudge; Cookies 'N Cream | 150 | 2 | 29 |
| Caramel Cone | 170 | 3 | 33 |
| Dulce de Leche; Strawb. Cheesecake, av. | 150 | 1 | 32 |

**Bars/Sandwiches/Cones** ~ *See Page 110*

**So Delicious** *(Turtle Mtn):*
**It's Soy Delicious:** *Per ½ Cup, 2.86 oz*

| | C | F | Cb |
|---|---|---|---|
| Almond Pecan | 140 | 4.5 | 24 |
| Choc Almond | 140 | 4.5 | 23 |
| Choc Peanut Butter | 135 | 3.5 | 24 |
| Vanilla | 130 | 1.5 | 24 |

**Coconut Milk Frozen Dessert,**

| | C | F | Cb |
|---|---|---|---|
| Chocolate; Vanilla, av., ½ cup, 3 oz | 150 | 9 | 20 |

**Soy Based:** *Per ½ Cup, 3 oz*

| | C | F | Cb |
|---|---|---|---|
| Butter Pecan | 160 | 7 | 22 |
| Chocolate Velvet | 130 | 3.5 | 23 |
| Creamy Vanilla | 130 | 3 | 24 |
| Dulce de Leche | 140 | 3 | 26 |
| Mint Marble Fudge | 140 | 3 | 27 |
| Mocha Fudge | 130 | 3 | 26 |
| Neapolitan; Strawberry, average | 120 | 3.5 | 23 |

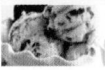 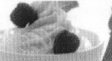 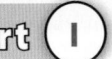

## Brands (Cont)

| | C | F | Cb |
|---|---|---|---|
| **Soy Dream (Non-Dairy):** | | | |
| **Frozen Dessert:** *Per 1/2 Cup, 2.47 oz* | | | |
| Butter Pecan | 190 | 11 | 23 |
| Choc. Fudge Brownie | 170 | 9 | 21 |
| French Vanilla; Vanilla | 140 | 8 | 17 |
| Mocha Fudge | 140 | 9 | 23 |
| Vanilla Fudge | 170 | 9 | 23 |
| **Starbucks:** *Per ½ Cup* | | | |
| **Ice Cream:** Caramel Macchiato | 240 | 13 | 27 |
| Coffee | 210 | 13 | 21 |
| Java Chip Frappuccino | 250 | 15 | 25 |
| Mocha Frappuccino | 220 | 13 | 23 |
| **Stonyfield Farm (Organic):** | | | |
| **Premium Ice Cream:** *Per ½ Cup, 100g* | | | |
| After Dark Chocolate | 240 | 16 | 22 |
| Cookies 'N Cream | 270 | 17 | 27 |
| Creme Caramel | 260 | 14 | 28 |
| Gotta Have Java | 250 | 16 | 22 |
| Vanilla Chai | 240 | 16 | 21 |
| **Stop & Shop:** *Per ½ Cup* | | | |
| **Ice Cream:** | | | |
| Chocolate | 150 | 8 | 18 |
| Neapolitan | 140 | 7 | 17 |
| Vanilla | 140 | 8 | 16 |
| Vanilla Fudge Swirl | 140 | 7 | 18 |

**Tasti D-Lite (Soft Serve):** *Per 4 fl.oz*

Calories will vary with density (air in product) and serving size. Best to weigh product and calculate on 25 cals per 1 oz weight.

| | C | F | Cb |
|---|---|---|---|
| Banana | 70 | 1 | 13 |
| Blueberry Cheesecake | 70 | 1.5 | 14 |
| Brownie Batter | 70 | 1.5 | 13 |
| Buttercrunch Mania | 90 | 3.5 | 13 |
| Chocolate Cookie Dough | 70 | 1.5 | 12 |
| Vanilla Marshmallow | 80 | 1 | 14 |

TCBY ~ See Page 250

| | C | F | Cb |
|---|---|---|---|
| **Tofutti, Non-Dairy Dessert:** *Per ½ Cup* | | | |
| **Premium Pints:** Better Pecan | 210 | 13 | 21 |
| Chocolate Cookie Crunch | 210 | 11 | 26 |
| Chocolate Supreme | 180 | 11 | 18 |
| Vanilla | 210 | 13 | 21 |
| Vanilla Almond Bark | 240 | 15 | 24 |
| Vanilla Fudge; Wild Berry, average | 190 | 9 | 25 |

| | C | F | Cb |
|---|---|---|---|
| **Turkey Hill:** *Per ½ Cup* | | | |
| **Premium Ice Cream:** Black Cherry | 130 | 6 | 18 |
| Butter Pecan | 160 | 10 | 15 |
| Choco Mint Chip | 160 | 9 | 17 |
| Choc. P'Nut Butter Cup | 180 | 11 | 18 |
| Cookies 'n Cream | 150 | 8 | 19 |
| Rocky Road | 170 | 8 | 23 |
| Tin Roof Sundae | 150 | 8 | 19 |
| Vanilla | 140 | 7 | 16 |
| **Light:** Moose Tracks | 130 | 6 | 19 |
| Vanilla Bean | 100 | 2 | 17 |
| Average other flav. | 130 | 4 | 19 |
| **All Natural,** av. all flavors | 150 | 8 | 17 |
| **No Sugar Added:** | | | |
| Cherry Fudge Ripple | 80 | 0 | 22 |
| Dutch Chocolate; Vanilla | 70 | 0 | 20 |
| Moose Tracks | 120 | 5 | 22 |
| **Frozen Yogurt:** | | | |
| Choc. Chip Cookie Dough | 120 | 2 | 23 |
| Fat-Free: Chocolate Marshmallow | 110 | 0 | 24 |
| Average other flavors | 100 | 0 | 19 |
| Sherbet | 120 | 1 | 26 |
| **Walgreens:** | | | |
| **Premium Ice Cream:** *1 Pint Container, Per ½ Cup* | | | |
| Bear Claw | 150 | 6 | 27 |
| Homemade Vanilla | 130 | 7 | 16 |
| Strawberry Cheesecake | 130 | 6 | 18 |
| Toasted Butter Pecan | 170 | 10 | 18 |
| Waffle Cone | 150 | 7 | 19 |
| **Premium:** *1.75 Quarts Container:* | | | |
| Homemade Vanilla, ½ cup | 150 | 8 | 17 |
| Moose Tracks | 170 | 10 | 19 |
| **Old Fashioned:** *1.75 Quarts (Square),* | | | |
| average all flavors, ½ cup | 140 | 7 | 16 |
| **Sherbert:** Orange Citrus | 120 | 1 | 16 |
| Rainbow Swirl | 120 | 1 | 27 |
| **Wawa:** | | | |
| **Premium Ice Cream:** *1 Pint Container, Per ½ cup* | | | |
| Butter Pecan; Mint Choc Chip, av | 180 | 10 | 20 |
| Chocolate | 160 | 8 | 21 |
| Cookies & Cream | 180 | 9 | 21 |
| Strawberry Shortcake | 160 | 7 | 22 |
| Vanilla Bean | 160 | 8 | 19 |

# Ice Cream Bars & Pops

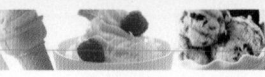

## Bars & Pops
*Per Bar/Serving Unless Indicated*

| | C | F | Cb |
|---|---|---|---|
| **Ben & Jerry's:** | | | |
| **Bars:** Cherry Garcia | 260 | 16 | 23 |
| Fudgy Brownies | 350 | 20 | 38 |
| Half Baked | 360 | 22 | 37 |
| **Big Bear** ~ *See Klondike* | | | |
| **Blue Bunny:** | | | |
| **Pops,** Banana, 1.87 oz | 35 | 0 | 9 |
| **Bars:** Big Fudge, 2.5 oz | 100 | 1 | 20 |
| Big Star, 1.48 oz | 110 | 7 | 11 |
| Caramel Crunch, 1.69 oz | 150 | 10 | 14 |
| Choc. Ice Cream Sundae Crunch | 170 | 9 | 21 |
| Chocolate Raspberry, 2.82 oz | 270 | 18 | 25 |
| English Toffee, 1.38 oz | 130 | 9 | 12 |
| Milk Choc. with Almond, 3.14 oz | 320 | 23 | 25 |
| Orange Dream, 1.86 oz | 70 | 1 | 15 |
| Root Beer Float, 2.22 oz | 90 | 2.5 | 15 |
| Strawberry Crunch, 2.19 oz | 170 | 9 | 20 |
| King Size: Chocolate Eclair, 2.82 oz | 220 | 12 | 27 |
| Cookies 'n Cream, 2.47 oz | 220 | 13 | 24 |
| Crunch with Candy Center, 3 oz | 340 | 28 | 24 |
| Strawberry Shortcake, 2.78 oz | 210 | 11 | 26 |
| **Champ Cones:** Caramel Lovers | 320 | 19 | 34 |
| Caramel Nut | 320 | 19 | 34 |
| Chocolate Lovers | 290 | 15 | 37 |
| Fudge Nut | 330 | 19 | 35 |
| Vanilla | 310 | 19 | 31 |
| King Size, Strawb. Shortcake | 400 | 18 | 54 |
| **FrozFruit:** | | | |
| Banana; Strawb. Cream, average | 160 | 6 | 27 |
| Creamy Pina Colada, 4.3 oz | 190 | 3.5 | 37 |
| Creamy Coconut | 200 | 14 | 19 |
| **Jolly Rancher,** Cool Tubes, 3 oz | 110 | 1 | 25 |
| **Mini Swirls,** Birthday Party, 1.66 oz | 160 | 8 | 22 |
| **Sandwiches:** Big Bopper, 5.01 oz | 460 | 23 | 60 |
| Big Double Strawberry, 3.84 oz | 270 | 10 | 41 |
| Mississippi Mud, 3.75 oz | 280 | 12 | 39 |
| Neapolitan, 3.67 oz | 260 | 1 | 37 |
| Chips Galore, 3.42 oz | 310 | 16 | 40 |

*Per Bar/Serving*

| | C | F | Cb |
|---|---|---|---|
| **Breyers:** | | | |
| **Pure Fruit Bars:** | | | |
| Regular, all flavors | 40 | 0 | 10 |
| No Sugar Added, all flavors | 25 | 0 | 5 |
| *(Carbs include 2g sugar alcohol)* | | | |
| **Carb Smart:** | | | |
| Almond Bar | 180 | 15 | 9 |
| *(Carbs incl. 2g sugar alcohol)* | | | |
| Fudge Bar | 100 | 7 | 9 |
| *(Carbs include 5g sugar alcohol)* | | | |
| Vanilla Ice Cream Bar | 170 | 15 | 9 |
| *(Carbs include 2g sugar alcohol)* | | | |
| **Smooth & Dreamy:** Bars, av. all | 125 | 5 | 18 |
| Sandwiches, all flavors | 160 | 4 | 30 |
| **Butterfinger** *(Nestle):* 1.6 oz bar | 150 | 10 | 15 |
| King Size, 4 oz | 280 | 18 | 27 |
| **Cool Classics:** | | | |
| **Arctic Blasters:** Crispy Bar | 160 | 11 | 15 |
| Fudge Bar | 100 | 1 | 21 |
| Ice Cream Bar | 150 | 10 | 13 |
| Orange Cream | 100 | 2.5 | 18 |
| Strawberry Shortcake | 210 | 11 | 28 |
| Toffee Bar | 160 | 11 | 14 |
| **Icepix:** Grape; Cherry; Orange | 35 | 0 | 8 |
| Honeydew; Watermelon; Cantelope | 35 | 0 | 9 |
| **Swirl Pops,** Mango-Cherry | 80 | 0 | 20 |
| **Creamsicles:** Original, low fat | 100 | 2 | 20 |
| Sugar-Free, all flavors | 40 | 0.5 | 12 |
| **Crunch** *(Nestle),* Vanilla, 1.6 oz | 200 | 13 | 19 |
| **Dove:** *Per 2.6 oz Bar* | | | |
| Caramel Swirl w/ Milk Choc. & Cashews | 250 | 16 | 23 |
| Milk Chocolate with Vanilla | 250 | 16 | 24 |
| Milk Chocolate with Almonds | 250 | 17 | 24 |
| Dark Chocolate with Vanilla | 250 | 17 | 24 |
| 70 Calorie Miniatures (1), 0.61 oz | 60 | 4 | 66 |
| **Dreyer's/Edy's:** | | | |
| **Dibs:** Mint, 4 oz | 340 | 24 | 30 |
| Vanilla, 4 oz | 380 | 27 | 30 |
| **Real Fruit Bars:** | | | |
| Acai Blueb.; Lime, Strawb., Wildb. | 60 | 0 | 15 |
| Creamy Coconut | 120 | 3 | 21 |
| Grape; Lemonade; Lime | 80 | 0 | 20 |
| Peach | 100 | 0 | 24 |
| Pomegranate | 70 | 0 | 17 |
| Average other flavors | 80 | 0 | 20 |

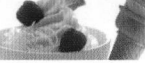 

| **Bars & Pops (Cont)** | **C** | **F** | **Cb** |
|---|---|---|---|
| *Per Bar/Serving* | | | |
| **Drumstick** (Nestlé): Classic Vanilla | 290 | 16 | 33 |
| Vanilla Caramel | 310 | 16 | 37 |
| Vanilla Fudge | 310 | 16 | 37 |
| King Size, Triple Choc. | 390 | 21 | 46 |
| **Simply Dipped:** Vanilla | 270 | 13 | 37 |
| Cookies & Cream | 290 | 14 | 39 |
| Mint | 290 | 14 | 38 |
| **Lil' Drums,** average all flavors | 120 | 6 | 16 |
| **Edy's** ~ *See Dreyer's* | | | |
| **Fat Boy:** | | | |
| **Sundae On A Stick:** | | | |
| Casco Vanilla Nut, 3 oz | 270 | 20 | 22 |
| Peppermint, 3 oz | 280 | 20 | 26 |
| Vanilla, Milk Choc. Dipped | 270 | 20 | 21 |
| **Sandwiches:** Chocolate, 3 oz | 210 | 9 | 31 |
| Cookies n' Cream 3 oz | 220 | 9 | 33 |
| Mint Chocolate Chip, 2.68 oz | 270 | 20 | 21 |
| Rasp. Cheesecake, 3 oz | 220 | 8 | 35 |
| Strawberry, 3 oz | 210 | 9 | 30 |
| Vanilla, 3 oz | 210 | 9 | 30 |
| **Fresh & Easy,** Vanilla Sundae Cone | 260 | 15 | 29 |
| **Fudge Bar** (Nestle): | | | |
| Regular, 2.8 oz | 110 | 2.5 | 21 |
| Super, 5 oz | 230 | 6 | 42 |
| **Fudgesicle:** | | | |
| Fudge Bar | 100 | 2 | 17 |
| Fat-Free | 60 | 0 | 13 |
| No Added Sugar | 40 | 1 | 10 |
| **Good Humor:** Original Vanilla | 160 | 10 | 17 |
| Oreo Bar | 250 | 15 | 28 |
| Candy Center Crunch | 300 | 21 | 27 |
| Chocolate Eclair | 220 | 10 | 30 |
| Reese's Peanut Butter Cups | 310 | 21 | 27 |
| Toasted Almond | 240 | 12 | 30 |
| **Cones:** King | 250 | 13 | 30 |
| Sundae | 260 | 15 | 29 |
| Triple Choc. Brownie | 420 | 19 | 58 |
| Vanilla Chocolate | 390 | 21 | 44 |
| **Sandwiches:** Choc. Chip Cookie | 270 | 10 | 44 |
| Giant Neapolitan | 250 | 9 | 38 |
| Giant Vanilla | 250 | 9 | 38 |
| **Snack Pops,** average all flavors | 210 | 13 | 23 |
| **Great Value** (Walmart): | | | |
| Chocolate Fudge Sticks (2), 3.45 oz | 130 | 1.5 | 28 |
| Ice Cream Cone, Van., Choc Dipped | 270 | 14 | 34 |
| Sandwiches: Vanilla, 2.1 oz | 160 | 5 | 25 |
| Minis, Vanilla, 1.4 oz | 100 | 3.5 | 16 |
| Ice Pops, Assorted, 1.85 oz | 45 | 0 | 11 |

| *Per Bar/Serving* | **C** | **F** | **Cb** |
|---|---|---|---|
| **Haagen-Dazs:** | | | |
| **Milk Chocolate Bars:** | | | |
| Vanilla & Almonds | 310 | 22 | 22 |
| Vanilla | 280 | 20 | 22 |
| **Snack Size:** Coffee & Alm. Crunch | 190 | 13 | 15 |
| Vanilla & Almonds | 190 | 14 | 14 |
| Dark Chocolate: Chocolate | 290 | 20 | 24 |
| Vanilla | 280 | 20 | 21 |
| **Healthy Choice:** Fudge Bar | 80 | 1.5 | 13 |
| Mocha Swirl | 90 | 1 | 17 |
| Sorbet & Cream Bar | 80 | 0.5 | 18 |
| Vanilla Sandwich | 150 | 1.5 | 30 |
| **Hershey's:** | | | |
| **Cones:** Candy Bar Overload | 320 | 12 | 48 |
| Crazy | 120 | 2 | 24 |
| Incredible | 250 | 13 | 28 |
| Moose Tracks | 430 | 27 | 43 |
| P-Nutty | 220 | 13 | 20 |
| **Pops:** Orange/Strawb. Blossom, av | 80 | 2.5 | 12 |
| Average other varieties | 35 | 0 | 10 |
| **Sandwiches:** Chocolate | 230 | 10 | 30 |
| Strawberry | 220 | 8 | 33 |
| Vanilla | 210 | 9 | 30 |
| **Signature Bars:** Choc. Eclair | 230 | 10 | 40 |
| Cotton Candy | 280 | 15 | 33 |
| Strawberry Cheesecake | 230 | 9 | 34 |
| **Hood:** Ice Cream Bar | 150 | 11 | 12 |
| Fudge Stix | 70 | 0 | 14 |
| Orange Cream | 90 | 1.5 | 19 |
| Hoodsie Cups: Vanilla; Chocolate | 100 | 5 | 14 |
| Pops | 60 | 0 | 16 |
| Sundae | 120 | 5 | 19 |
| Sandwiches, Vanilla | 170 | 6 | 28 |
| **Jolly Llama:** *Per 2.7 oz tubes* | | | |
| **Sorbet Squeezups:** Banana Coconut | 100 | 3 | 17 |
| Average other flavors | 75 | 0 | 20 |
| **Klondike:** | | | |
| **Bars:** | | | |
| 100 Calorie: Choc. Fudge | 100 | 3 | 20 |
| English Toffee | 100 | 6 | 12 |
| Dark Chocolate | 250 | 14 | 29 |
| Double Chocolate | 240 | 14 | 27 |
| Heath, English Toffee | 230 | 15 | 25 |
| Krunch | 250 | 14 | 30 |
| Neapolitan | 250 | 14 | 29 |
| Oreo Cookies & Cream | 250 | 15 | 29 |
| Original Vanilla, 3 fl.oz | 250 | 14 | 29 |
| Reese's | 260 | 16 | 26 |
| **Sandwiches:** Oreo | 200 | 7 | 34 |
| Vanilla | 170 | 9 | 21 |
| **Slim-a-Bear S'wich,** | | | |
| Vanilla, no sugar added | 100 | 2 | 20 |

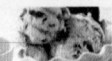

## Bars & Pops (Cont)    C   F   Cb

*Per Bar/Serving*

| | C | F | Cb |
|---|---|---|---|
| **Luigi's Real Italian Ice:** | | | |
| **Cups:** Lemon; Cherry; Mango, 6 fl.oz | 100 | 0 | 26 |
| Watermelon; Blue Rasp., 6 fl.oz | 160 | 0 | 39 |
| **Swirls:** av. all flavors, 6 fl.oz | 150 | 0 | 38 |
| **Mochi** *(Maeda-en):* | | | |
| Ice Cream Bon Bons, 1 piece, 1.5 oz | 150 | 9 | 20 |
| **M&M's:** Cone, Single, 2.8 oz | 250 | 12 | 33 |
| Cookie Ice Cream Sandwich, 3 oz | 260 | 12 | 34 |
| **Magnum:** Almond, 79g | 270 | 18 | 24 |
| Classic, 76g | 240 | 16 | 22 |
| Dark, 77g | 240 | 17 | 20 |
| Double Chocolate, 83g | 340 | 21 | 34 |
| White, 77g | 250 | 16 | 23 |
| **Minute Maid:** | | | |
| Juice Bars | 60 | 0 | 15 |
| Soft Frozen Lemonade | 70 | 0 | 19 |
| **Nestlé:** | | | |
| **Bars:** Crunch Van., 3 oz | 210 | 15 | 20 |
| Toll House, Choc. Chip, 1.7 oz | 150 | 9 | 18 |
| **Drumsticks:** Chocolate | 310 | 17 | 34 |
| Vanilla Fudge | 310 | 16 | 37 |
| **Push Up Pops,** av. | 70 | 1 | 16 |
| **Sandwiches:** Oreo | 250 | 10 | 38 |
| Vanilla: Mini Size | 80 | 1.5 | 15 |
| Regular size | 140 | 3 | 26 |
| **Popsicles:** | | | |
| **Regular:** | | | |
| Firecracker | 35 | 0 | 9 |
| Rainbow | 45 | 0 | 11 |
| Scribblers | 30 | 0 | 8 |
| SpongeBob Pop-Ups | 80 | 1 | 16 |
| Super Heros | 40 | 0 | 11 |
| Sugar Free: Orange Cherry Grape | 15 | 0 | 4 |
| Tropicals | 15 | 0 | 4 |
| **Slow Melts:** Dora The Explorer | 30 | 0 | 7 |
| Mighty Minis, 3 pcs | 40 | 0 | 10 |
| **Creamsicle:** | | | |
| Low Fat, Orange & Raspberry | 70 | 1 | 13 |
| Sugar Free, Orange; Cherry; Berry | 20 | 0 | 6 |
| **Reese's,** Peanut Butter Ice Cream | 310 | 21 | 27 |
| **Rice Dream,** Van. Nutty Bar, 95g | 320 | 24 | 27 |
| **Skinny Cow:** | | | |
| **Bars:** Fudge Bars, low fat | 100 | 1 | 22 |
| Minis Fudge Pops (2) | 100 | 2 | 19 |
| Truffle Bars, av. all flavors | 105 | 2 | 19 |
| **Sandwiches,** average all flavors | 145 | 3 | 30 |
| **Snickers:** | | | |
| **Bars:** Regular, 1.75 oz | 180 | 11 | 18 |
| Mini Bar, 4 pieces | 370 | 23 | 36 |
| **Cone,** 2.9 oz | 280 | 15 | 33 |
| **Ice Cream Brownie,** 4.5 oz | 120 | 14 | 42 |

*Per Bar/Serving*

| | C | F | Cb |
|---|---|---|---|
| **Snow Cone** *(Wonder),* average, 7 fl.oz | 60 | 0 | 15 |
| **So Delicious** *(Turtle Mtn):* | | | |
| **Coconut Based Bars:** Mini Almond | 170 | 15 | 10 |
| Mini Vanilla | 150 | 7 | 14 |
| **Soy Based Bars:** Creamy Fudge | 90 | 2 | 18 |
| Creamy Orange | 80 | 1.5 | 18 |
| **Soy Dream** *(Non-Dairy),* | | | |
| Lil' Dreamers, Vanilla | 100 | 4 | 15 |
| **Sweet Nothings** *(Turtle Mtn),* | | | |
| **Bars,** all flavors | 100 | 0 | 23 |
| **Tampico,** Freezer Pops, 1 pop | 30 | 0 | 8 |
| **Tofutti** *(Non-Dairy):* | | | |
| **Cuties:** Cookies 'N Cream | 130 | 6 | 11 |
| Mint Chocolate Chip | 130 | 6 | 19 |
| Vanilla | 130 | 6 | 17 |
| **Sticks:** | | | |
| Choc. Fudge Treats | 30 | 1.5 | 6 |
| Marry Me Bar | 170 | 8 | 22 |
| Mint By Mintz | 170 | 7 | 7 |
| Totally Fudge Pops | 95 | 1.5 | 19 |
| **Trader Joe's:** | | | |
| **Fruit Floes:** Caribbean | 80 | 0 | 21 |
| Lime | 60 | 0 | 16 |
| Strawberry | 100 | 0 | 24 |
| **Bars:** | | | |
| Coffee Latte & Cream, 1.4 oz | 90 | 6 | 9 |
| Ice Cream Sandwich | 440 | 21 | 60 |
| Mango & Cream, 1.4 oz | 60 | 2 | 10 |
| Mini Mint S'wich, 1.4 oz | 120 | 6 | 18 |
| Peach Pops, 1.75 oz | 45 | 0 | 11 |
| **Turkey Hill:** | | | |
| **Sandwiches:** Double Decker | 190 | 7 | 30 |
| Vanilla Bean: Regular | 190 | 7 | 29 |
| Light | 160 | 3 | 32 |
| **Sundae Cone,** Van. Fdge | 320 | 18 | 33 |
| **Twix Bar,** 2.65 oz | 280 | 16 | 31 |
| **Weight Watchers:** | | | |
| **Bars:** Choc. Dipped Strawberry | 100 | 4 | 18 |
| Dark Chocolate: | | | |
| Dulce de leche | 110 | 4 | 18 |
| Rasp. Cheesecake | 110 | 4 | 18 |
| Giant: | | | |
| Chocolate Cookies & Cream | 130 | 5 | 24 |
| Cookies & Cream | 130 | 5 | 23 |
| Fudge Bar | 110 | 1 | 24 |
| Latte Bar | 90 | 1 | 21 |
| **Cones,** Choc./Vanilla, av. | 140 | 4 | 27 |
| **Cups:** Chocolate Chip Cookie Dough | 150 | 1.5 | 32 |
| Mint Chocolate Chip | 140 | 2.5 | 29 |
| **Sandwiches:** Vanilla | 120 | 2 | 28 |
| Round, Vanilla | 140 | 1.5 | 31 |

## Canned & Packaged Meals

| B & M: Per 16 oz Can, ½ cup, 4.6 oz | C | F | Cb |
|---|---|---|---|
| **Baked Beans:** Original | 170 | 2 | 31 |
| Barbeque | 190 | 0.5 | 39 |
| Vegetarian | 160 | 1 | 28 |
| **Raisin Brown Bread,** ½" slice, 2 oz | 130 | 0.5 | 29 |

**Banquet:**
**Homestyle Bakes:** Per Serving, Prepared

| | C | F | Cb |
|---|---|---|---|
| Asian Style Fried Rice | 240 | 1.5 | 47 |
| Chicken & Dumplings | 220 | 6 | 30 |
| Country Chicken, Mshd Potato & Bisc. | 360 | 17 | 43 |
| Creamy Cheesy Chicken Alfredo | 410 | 21 | 40 |
| Creamy Chicken & Biscuits | 350 | 17 | 39 |
| Lasagna | 330 | 13 | 39 |
| Pasta & Meatballs | 310 | 10 | 42 |

**Betty Crocker:**
**Chicken Helper:** Per Cup, Prepared

| | C | F | Cb |
|---|---|---|---|
| Cheesy Chicken Enchilada | 350 | 7 | 41 |
| Chicken Fried Rice | 280 | 11 | 21 |
| Italian Fettuccini Alfredo | 330 | 11 | 31 |

**Helper Complete Meals:** Per ¼ Pkt· Prepared

| | C | F | Cb |
|---|---|---|---|
| Cheesy Beef Taco | 220 | 5 | 37 |
| Chicken & Buttermilk Biscuits | 260 | 9 | 37 |
| Chicken Cheesy Rice & Broccoli | 230 | 6 | 36 |
| Stroganoff | 230 | 8 | 32 |

**Hamburger Helper:** Per Cup, Prepared

| | C | F | Cb |
|---|---|---|---|
| Beef Pasta | 280 | 11 | 24 |
| Cheeseburger Macaroni | 310 | 12 | 27 |
| Cheesy Baked Potatoes | 310 | 12 | 31 |
| Cheesy Hashbrowns | 340 | 18 | 24 |
| Cheesy Jambalaya | 320 | 13 | 29 |
| Cheesy Nachos | 330 | 12 | 35 |
| Crunchy Taco | 330 | 14 | 32 |
| Salisbury | 280 | 11 | 26 |

**Tuna Helper:** Per Serving

| | C | F | Cb |
|---|---|---|---|
| Creamy Parmesan | 270 | 10 | 30 |
| Average other varieties | 270 | 10 | 30 |

**Side Dishes/Casseroles:** Per Serving, Prepared

| | C | F | Cb |
|---|---|---|---|
| Au Gratin, ½ cup | 150 | 5 | 23 |
| Cheddar & Bacon; Cheesy Scalloped | 145 | 5.5 | 23 |
| Roasted Garlic, ½ cup | 120 | 3.5 | 21 |
| Scalloped Potatoes, ⅔ cup | 130 | 3 | 23 |
| Sour Cream and Chives, ⅔ cup | 140 | 6 | 18 |

**Flavored Potatoes:** Prepared

| | C | F | Cb |
|---|---|---|---|
| Average all flavors, ⅔ cup | 140 | 6 | 18 |

**Betty Crocker (Cont)**  C  F  Cb
**Seasoned Skillets:** Prepared

| | C | F | Cb |
|---|---|---|---|
| Hash Brown, ½ cup | 120 | 4 | 18 |
| Roasted Garlic & Herb, ⅔ cup | 170 | 9 | 21 |
| Traditional, ½ cup | 180 | 9 | 22 |

**Bowl Appetit:** Per Bowl, Prep'd As Directed

| | C | F | Cb |
|---|---|---|---|
| Cheddar Broccoli Rice | 290 | 6 | 52 |
| Homestyle Chicken Pasta | 250 | 5 | 44 |
| Pasta Alfredo | 350 | 9 | 55 |
| Teriyaki Rice | 250 | 1 | 57 |
| Three-Cheese Rotini | 340 | 7 | 59 |

**Biggest Loser:**
**Simply Sensible:** Per ½ Package

| | C | F | Cb |
|---|---|---|---|
| Beef Pot Roast & Gravy | 220 | 5 | 16 |
| Beef Tips & Gravy | 200 | 3.5 | 21 |
| Lasagna | 200 | 5 | 28 |
| Medit.-Style Chicken | 250 | 6 | 36 |
| Zing Chicken | 230 | 1.5 | 38 |

**Bush's Best:** Per ½ Cup

| | C | F | Cb |
|---|---|---|---|
| Black Beans | 105 | 0.5 | 23 |
| Chili Beans, Pinto | 110 | 1 | 20 |
| Dark Red Kidney Beans | 100 | 0 | 22 |
| Garbanzo Beans | 105 | 2 | 20 |
| **Refried Beans:** Traditional | 150 | 3 | 24 |
| Fat Free | 130 | 0 | 24 |
| **Baked Beans:** Original | 140 | 1 | 29 |
| Vegetarian | 130 | 0 | 29 |
| Average other flavors | 150 | 1 | 32 |

**Campbell's:**
**Beans:** Per ½ Cup

| | C | F | Cb |
|---|---|---|---|
| Baked Beans, Sugar & Bacon Flav | 160 | 2.5 | 30 |
| Pork & Beans | 140 | 1.5 | 25 |

**Chunky Microwavable Bowls:** Per Cup

| | C | F | Cb |
|---|---|---|---|
| Firehouse; Roadhouse, Beef & Beans Chili | 230 | 8 | 25 |
| Roasted Beef Tips With Veges | 130 | 1.5 | 20 |

**Spaghetti O's:** Per Cup

| | C | F | Cb |
|---|---|---|---|
| Original | 170 | 1 | 35 |
| With Meatballs | 240 | 7 | 32 |
| With Sliced Franks | 220 | 6 | 32 |

**Chef Boyardee:** Makes Two
**Big:** Per Cup

| | C | F | Cb |
|---|---|---|---|
| Beef Ravioli in Sauce | 250 | 6 | 38 |
| Italian Sausage Ravioli in Sauce | 240 | 5 | 39 |

**Boxed Kits:**

| | C | F | Cb |
|---|---|---|---|
| Cheese Pizza Maker, ⅛ pkg, 4.6 oz | 250 | 4 | 45 |
| Pepperoni Pizza Maker, ⅛ pkg, 4.6 oz | 280 | 7 | 44 |

**Canned:** Per Cup

| | C | F | Cb |
|---|---|---|---|
| Beefaroni in Tomato Sauce | 240 | 9 | 30 |
| Beef Ravioli in Tom. & Meat Sce | 230 | 8 | 31 |
| Cheesy Burger Macaroni | 200 | 6 | 28 |

### Chef Boyardee (Cont):

| | C | F | Cb |
|---|---|---|---|
| **Forkables:** Sports; Sealife: | | | |
| Pasta in Sauce with Meat | 240 | 6 | 37 |
| Mini Size | 210 | 6 | 30 |
| **Microwavable Bowls (40% More):** Per Cup | | | |
| Beef Ravioli | 220 | 7 | 32 |
| Lasagna | 250 | 9 | 33 |
| Macaroni & Cheese | 240 | 10 | 28 |
| **Mini:** Per Cup | | | |
| ABC & 123, with Meatballs | 210 | 9 | 26 |
| Micro Beef Ravioli In Tomato Sauce | 160 | 4 | 26 |
| Beef Ravioli & Meatballs | 240 | 9 | 31 |
| Spaghetti Rings & Meatballs | 220 | 9 | 26 |

### Dennison's Chili: Per Cup

| | C | F | Cb |
|---|---|---|---|
| **Chili Con Carne:** | | | |
| Original: With Beans | 350 | 15 | 31 |
| Without Beans | 310 | 16 | 20 |
| **Chili:** Original, with Beans | 360 | 14 | 38 |
| Chunky; Hot with Beans | 310 | 10 | 32 |
| Vegetarian, 99% fat free | 190 | 1.5 | 34 |

### Dinty Moore: (Hormel Foods)

| | C | F | Cb |
|---|---|---|---|
| **Cans:** Chicken & Noodles, 7.5 oz can | 190 | 9 | 19 |
| Beef Stew, 15 oz can, 1 cup, 8.3 oz | 200 | 10 | 17 |
| **Big Bowl (15 oz):** | | | |
| Chicken & Dumplings, 8.47 oz | 220 | 7 | 29 |
| Scalloped Potatoes & Ham, 8.47 oz | 280 | 16 | 23 |
| **Microwave Ready:** | | | |
| Beef Stew, 10 oz tray | 150 | 6 | 15 |
| Chix & Dumplings, 7.,5 oz cup | 200 | 6 | 26 |
| Meatball Stew, 15 oz can, 8.47 oz | 250 | 15 | 18 |
| Noodles & Chicken, 7.5 oz cup | 190 | 9 | 20 |

### Dr. McDougall's: Per Container

| | C | F | Cb |
|---|---|---|---|
| Curry with Rice & Fruuited Pilaf | 300 | 3 | 60 |
| Vegetarian Chicken flav. Ramen | 200 | 1 | 40 |
| Vegetarian Chicken flav. Pilaf | 260 | 1 | 52 |

### Eden Organics: Per ½ Cup (4.5 oz)

| | C | F | Cb |
|---|---|---|---|
| Baked Navy Beans w/ Sorghum, Mstrd | 150 | 0 | 27 |
| Black Eyed Peas | 90 | 1 | 16 |
| Black Soy Beans | 120 | 6 | 8 |
| Refried: Black Beans | 110 | 1.5 | 18 |
| Pinto; Kidney Beans, av. | 85 | 1 | 19 |

### Farmhouse:

| | C | F | Cb |
|---|---|---|---|
| **Pasta:** Unprepared | | | |
| Herb & Butter, 4.7 oz | 240 | 2 | 45 |
| White Cheddar, 6.2 oz | 260 | 2.5 | 47 |

### Farmhouse (Cont):

| | C | F | Cb |
|---|---|---|---|
| **Rice:** Unprepared | | | |
| Chicken Flavor, 6 oz | 200 | 1 | 43 |
| Long Grain & Wild Herb & Butter | 200 | 1.5 | 42 |
| Mexican, 6 oz | 190 | 0.5 | 42 |
| **French's French Fried Onions:** | | | |
| Original; Cheddar: 2 Tbsp, 0.25 oz | 45 | 3.5 | 3 |
| ¼ cup, 0.5 oz | 90 | 7 | 6 |
| 1 cup, 2 oz | 360 | 28 | 24 |
| **Great Value** (Walmart): | | | |
| Dirty Rice Mix, 1 cup, prep'd | 130 | 0 | 29 |
| Rice & Vermicelli, | | | |
| av. all flavors, 1 cup, prep'd | 320 | 9 | 54 |

### Health Valley:

| | C | F | Cb |
|---|---|---|---|
| **Vegetarian Chili:** Per Cup | | | |
| 3 Bean Chipotle | 200 | 3 | 37 |
| Black Bean & Mango | 210 | 3 | 41 |
| Santa Fe White Bean | 200 | 3 | 39 |
| Tame Tomato | 210 | 2.5 | 41 |

### Heinz,

| | C | F | Cb |
|---|---|---|---|
| Vegetarian Beans, ½ cup | 140 | 0.5 | 27 |

### Hormel: Per Cup

| | C | F | Cb |
|---|---|---|---|
| **Compleats:** Per 10 oz Serving | | | |
| Beef Pot Roast | 270 | 6 | 29 |
| Beef Steak Tips | 270 | 9 | 29 |
| Chicken & Dumplings | 260 | 8 | 34 |
| Chicken & Noodles | 240 | 8 | 27 |
| Chicken & Rice | 280 | 11 | 34 |
| Chicken Alfredo | 330 | 18 | 28 |
| Chicken Breast and Dressing | 270 | 7 | 29 |
| Chicken Breast & Gravy | 210 | 3.5 | 26 |
| Homestyle Beef | 220 | 6 | 30 |
| Lasagne with Meat Sce | 280 | 7 | 42 |
| Meatloaf with Potatoes & Gravy | 310 | 11 | 34 |
| Salisbury Steak | 280 | 11 | 30 |
| Santa Fe Style Chkn | 250 | 4 | 36 |
| Sesame Chicken | 290 | 6 | 41 |
| Spaghetti with Meat Sauce | 290 | 9 | 36 |
| Teriyaki Chicken with Rice | 270 | 1.5 | 50 |
| Turkey & Hearty Vegetables | 180 | 3.5 | 24 |
| Turkey & Dressing | 290 | 9 | 31 |
| **Kid's Kitchen:** Beans & Wieners | 310 | 13 | 37 |
| Cheesy Mac 'N Cheese | 270 | 14 | 24 |
| Mini Beef Ravioli | 240 | 6 | 38 |
| Noodle Rings & Chicken | 140 | 4 | 18 |
| **Chili with Beans:** Per ½ of 15 oz can, 8.5 oz | | | |
| Regular; Hot; Chunky | 260 | 7 | 33 |
| Turkey | 210 | 3 | 28 |
| Vegetarian | 190 | 1 | 35 |
| **Without Beans:** Per 8.3 oz | | | |
| Regular; Hot Chili | 220 | 9 | 18 |
| Turkey | 190 | 3 | 16 |

| Hungry Jack Potatoes, | C | F | Cb |
|---|---|---|---|
| Instant Potato Flakes, ⅓ cup | 80 | 0 | 19 |

**Hunt's,**

| | C | F | Cb |
|---|---|---|---|
| Manwich Sloppy Joe, Orig., ¼ cup | 40 | 0 | 7 |

**Knorr:** *Sides, Prepared As Directed*

| | C | F | Cb |
|---|---|---|---|
| **Asian:** Chicken Fried Rice | 280 | 7 | 48 |
| Teriyaki Noodles | 280 | 9 | 44 |
| Teriyaki Rice | 280 | 7 | 48 |
| **Cajun:** Garlic Butter Rice | 260 | 4 | 49 |
| Red Beans & Rice | 290 | 1 | 62 |
| **Fiesta:** Mexican Rice | 280 | 6 | 51 |
| Spanish Rice | 280 | 6 | 48 |
| Taco Rice | 250 | 1 | 52 |
| **Pasta:** Alfredo | 290 | 10 | 39 |
| Alfredo Broccoli | 300 | 10 | 39 |
| Butter | 260 | 8 | 39 |
| Butter & Herb | 260 | 7 | 40 |
| Cheesy Cheddar | 270 | 7 | 39 |
| Parmesan | 290 | 10 | 39 |
| Stroganoff | 260 | 7 | 39 |
| **Rice:** Cheddar Broccoli | 280 | 6 | 48 |
| Chicken Broccoli | 270 | 5 | 48 |
| Chicken Flavor | 280 | 6 | 48 |

**Sides Plus Veggies:**

| | C | F | Cb |
|---|---|---|---|
| Butter & Herb Rotini with Veges | 300 | 8 | 51 |
| Chedd. Rice w/ Brocc. & Carrots | 300 | 7 | 51 |
| Vegetable Fried Rice | 300 | 8 | 51 |

**Kraft:**

**Macaroni & Cheese Dinner:** *Per 1 Cup Prepared*

| | C | F | Cb |
|---|---|---|---|
| Original, family size, 2.47 oz | 400 | 19 | 47 |
| Cheesy Alfredo, 2.47 oz | 380 | 14 | 50 |
| Easy Mac. av. all varieties, 2 oz | 220 | 4.5 | 39 |
| Premium White Cheddar, 2.47 oz | 400 | 18 | 51 |
| Scooby-Doo, 2.47 oz | 290 | 6 | 50 |
| The Cheesiest, Original flavor, 2.47 oz | 400 | 19 | 47 |
| Thick 'N Creamy, 2.47 oz | 410 | 17 | 50 |

**Bistro Deluxe:** *Dry Mix Only*

| | C | F | Cb |
|---|---|---|---|
| Creamy Portabello Mushroom | 310 | 11 | 40 |
| Sundried Tomato Parmesan | 300 | 11 | 40 |
| **Deluxe:** Four Cheese, 3.45 oz | 320 | 10 | 46 |
| Sharp Cheddar, 3.45 oz | 320 | 9 | 46 |
| **Velveeta,** Shells & Chse, Orig., 3.95 oz | 360 | 12 | 49 |

**Kraft (Cont):**

**Velveeta Potatoes:** *Per ½ Cup, Prepared*

| | C | F | Cb |
|---|---|---|---|
| Cheesy: Au Gratin | 190 | 7 | 26 |
| Bacon Scalloped | 200 | 7 | 26 |
| Cheesy Mashed, Twin Pack | 180 | 9 | 21 |

**Kroger:**

**Kitchen Creation Skillet Dinners:** *1 Cup Prepared*

| | C | F | Cb |
|---|---|---|---|
| Creamy Broccoli | 300 | 12 | 33 |
| Creamy Pasta | 300 | 13 | 33 |
| Double Cheeseburger | 320 | 13 | 30 |
| Lasagna | 280 | 12 | 26 |
| Stroganoff | 320 | 14 | 27 |

**La Choy:**

| | C | F | Cb |
|---|---|---|---|
| Beef Chow Mein, 1 cup | 80 | 1 | 11 |
| Chicken Chow Mein, 1 cup | 100 | 4 | 11 |
| Chop Suey Vegetables, ½ cup | 15 | 0 | 3 |
| Chow Mein Noodles, ½ cup | 130 | 5 | 19 |

**Creations:** *Per Cup, Prepared*

| | C | F | Cb |
|---|---|---|---|
| Sweet & Sour Chicken | 320 | 4.5 | 46 |
| Sweet Sesame Chicken | 340 | 9 | 38 |
| Teriyaki Chicken | 310 | 6 | 40 |

**Lightlife (Vegetarian):**

**Entrees:** *Per Package, with Sauce*

| | C | F | Cb |
|---|---|---|---|
| Asian Teriyaki, 11¾ oz | 310 | 7 | 51 |
| Indian Veggie Masala, 12.5 oz | 390 | 9 | 65 |
| Tuscan Portobello, 11.75 oz | 250 | 5 | 40 |
| Zesty Mexican, 11.5 oz | 330 | 6 | 57 |

**Organic Tempeh:**

| | C | F | Cb |
|---|---|---|---|
| Flax; Soy, average, 4 oz | 225 | 9 | 16 |
| Garden Veggie, 4 oz | 240 | 10 | 17 |
| Three Grain; Wild Rice, av., 4 oz | 235 | 11 | 14 |

**Smart Tenders:**

| | C | F | Cb |
|---|---|---|---|
| Lemon Pepper (3), 3 oz | 110 | 0.5 | 9 |
| Savory Chick'n (3), 3 oz | 110 | 1 | 7 |

**Lunchables** *(Oscar Mayer): Per Pkg., without drink*

| | C | F | Cb |
|---|---|---|---|
| Bologna & American Crackers Stackers | 390 | 22 | 33 |
| Extra Cheesy Pizza | 280 | 9 | 31 |
| Ham & Cheddar/Swiss w/ Crackers, av. | 340 | 19 | 23 |
| Nachos, Cheese Dip & Salsa | 380 | 21 | 40 |
| Pizza with Pepperoni | 310 | 13 | 31 |
| Turkey & American Cracker Stackers | 380 | 19 | 38 |
| Turkey & Cheddar with Crackers | 330 | 17 | 24 |
| Turkey & Cheddar Sub | 230 | 5 | 34 |

**Lunchmakers** *(Armour):*

| | C | F | Cb |
|---|---|---|---|
| Loco Nachos | 400 | 14 | 69 |
| Cheese Pizza | 360 | 9 | 53 |

| Macaroni Grill: Per 1 Cup, Prep'd | C | F | Cb |
|---|---|---|---|
| Chicken Piccata | 280 | 11 | 24 |
| Chicken Marsala | 330 | 13 | 30 |
| Garlic & Herb Chicken | 240 | 7 | 22 |

**Maruchan:**

**Ramen Noodle Soup:**

| | C | F | Cb |
|---|---|---|---|
| Average, 3 oz block/package | 380 | 16 | 52 |
| "35% Less Sodium", av., 1 pkg | 380 | 14 | 54 |
| **Instant Lunch Noodles,** av., 1 pkg | 290 | 11 | 39 |

**Yakisoba:** Per 4 oz Package

| | C | F | Cb |
|---|---|---|---|
| Chicken Flavor | 520 | 22 | 72 |
| Sweet & Sour Chicken | 560 | 22 | 78 |
| Teriyaki Beef Flavor | 520 | 20 | 72 |

**Minute Rice:**

**Ready To Serve:** Per 4.4 oz Container, Prepared

| | C | F | Cb |
|---|---|---|---|
| Brown/Chicken Rice Mix, average | 230 | 3.5 | 40 |
| White Rice | 200 | 3 | 40 |
| Yellow Rice Mix | 190 | 4 | 35 |

**Nissin:**

**Chow Mein:** Per 4 oz Package

| | C | F | Cb |
|---|---|---|---|
| Chicken Flavor | 480 | 18 | 70 |
| Spicy Chicken Flavor | 520 | 22 | 72 |
| Teriyaki Beef; Thai P'nut | 540 | 24 | 72 |
| With Shrimp | 560 | 28 | 64 |

**Cup Noodles:** Per Cup

| | C | F | Cb |
|---|---|---|---|
| Beef/Chicken/Shrimp | 300 | 13 | 38 |
| Beef Flavor Minestrone | 270 | 11 | 37 |
| **Top Ramen,** average, 3 oz pkg | 380 | 14 | 54 |

**Old El Paso:**

**Dinner Kits:** Per Serving, Prepared, without Meat

| | C | F | Cb |
|---|---|---|---|
| Burrito | 260 | 10 | 31 |
| Enchilada | 390 | 16 | 27 |
| **Mexi Beans,** 3.75 oz | 65 | 0.5 | 8 |
| **Refried Beans,** Traditional, 4.23 oz | 90 | 0.5 | 16 |

**Tortilla Stuffers:** Per ⅓ Cup, Includes Meat

| | C | F | Cb |
|---|---|---|---|
| Carne Asada Steak; Mesq. Chkn, 1.94 oz | 90 | 2 | 14 |
| Garlic Chili Chicken, 1.76 oz | 80 | 2 | 11 |

*Most packaged noodle soups are high in calories and fat. Their promotion of '0 Grams Trans Fat' does not make them heart-healthy. They are still high in saturated fat as well as salt/sodium.*

| Pasta Roni: Per Cup, Prepared | C | F | Cb |
|---|---|---|---|
| Angel Hair Pasta varieties, average | 310 | 13 | 41 |
| Butter & Herb Italiano | 300 | 11 | 41 |
| Chicken & Broccoli | 360 | 15 | 49 |
| Chicken Flavor | 300 | 12 | 40 |
| Fettuccine Alfredo | 450 | 24 | 44 |
| Four Cheese Corkscrew | 370 | 15 | 49 |
| Shells & White Cheddar | 290 | 12 | 38 |
| Tomato Parmesan | 270 | 9 | 40 |

**Nature's Way:**

| | C | F | Cb |
|---|---|---|---|
| Creamy Parmesano | 270 | 7 | 43 |
| Mushroom in Cream Sce | 280 | 9 | 41 |
| Olive Oil & Italian Herb | 250 | 8 | 38 |

**Rice-A-Roni:**

**Classic Favorites:** Per Cup, Prepared

| | C | F | Cb |
|---|---|---|---|
| Beef; Herb & Butter; Rice Pilaf, av. | 310 | 9 | 52 |
| Broccoli Au Gratin | 350 | 16 | 46 |
| Chicken | 300 | 9 | 50 |
| Chicken & Broccoli | 220 | 5 | 40 |
| Chicken & Garlic | 250 | 8 | 41 |
| Fried Rice | 310 | 10 | 50 |
| Spanish Rice | 260 | 8 | 44 |

(Reduced Fat Recipe: If only 1 Tbsp fat is used instead of 2 Tbsp, deduct 35 calories and 0.15 oz fat.)

| **Nature's Way:** Ital. Cheese & Herb | 340 | 12 | 52 |
|---|---|---|---|
| Long Grain & Wild Rice | 250 | 7 | 43 |
| Parmesan & Romano Cheese | 280 | 9 | 42 |

**Whole Grain Blends:**

| | C | F | Cb |
|---|---|---|---|
| Chicken & Herb Classico | 260 | 8 | 41 |
| Roasted Garlic Italiano | 270 | 9 | 41 |
| Spanish | 250 | 8 | 42 |

**Rosarita:**

**Refried Beans:** Per ½ Cup

| | C | F | Cb |
|---|---|---|---|
| Traditional; Spicy | 120 | 2 | 18 |
| Vegetarian | 120 | 2 | 19 |
| Non-Fat: Black Bean | 110 | 0 | 19 |
| With Salsa | 100 | 0 | 19 |

**S & W:** Per ½ Cup

| | C | F | Cb |
|---|---|---|---|
| Black Beans, 4.5 oz | 100 | 1 | 17 |
| Chili Beans with Chipotle, 4.55 oz | 110 | 1 | 23 |
| Kidney Beans, 4.66 oz | 120 | 1 | 20 |
| White Beans, 4.48 oz | 110 | 0.5 | 19 |

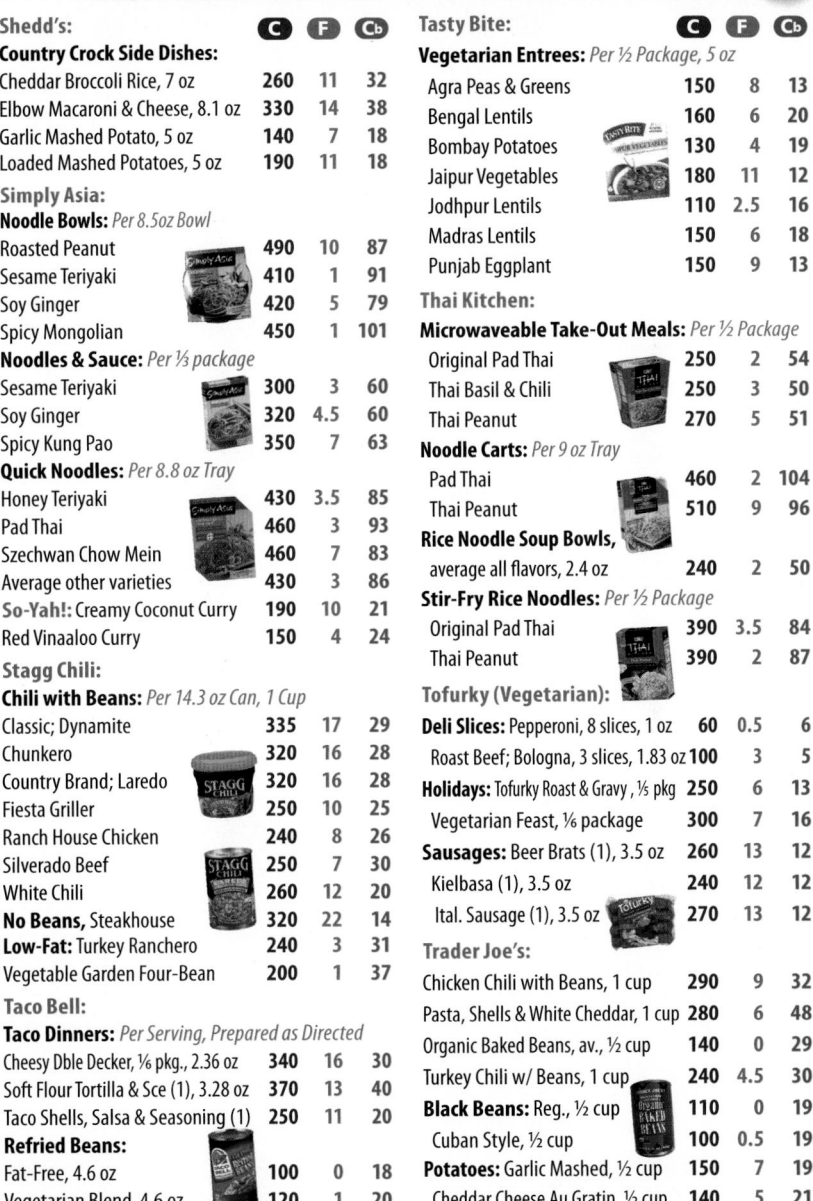

| Shedd's: | **C** | **F** | **Cb** |
|---|---|---|---|
| **Country Crock Side Dishes:** | | | |
| Cheddar Broccoli Rice, 7 oz | 260 | 11 | 32 |
| Elbow Macaroni & Cheese, 8.1 oz | 330 | 14 | 38 |
| Garlic Mashed Potato, 5 oz | 140 | 7 | 18 |
| Loaded Mashed Potatoes, 5 oz | 190 | 11 | 18 |

| Simply Asia: | | | |
|---|---|---|---|
| **Noodle Bowls:** *Per 8.5oz Bowl* | | | |
| Roasted Peanut | 490 | 10 | 87 |
| Sesame Teriyaki | 410 | 1 | 91 |
| Soy Ginger | 420 | 5 | 79 |
| Spicy Mongolian | 450 | 1 | 101 |
| **Noodles & Sauce:** *Per ⅓ package* | | | |
| Sesame Teriyaki | 300 | 3 | 60 |
| Soy Ginger | 320 | 4.5 | 60 |
| Spicy Kung Pao | 350 | 7 | 63 |
| **Quick Noodles:** *Per 8.8 oz Tray* | | | |
| Honey Teriyaki | 430 | 3.5 | 85 |
| Pad Thai | 460 | 3 | 93 |
| Szechwan Chow Mein | 460 | 7 | 83 |
| Average other varieties | 430 | 3 | 86 |
| **So-Yah!:** Creamy Coconut Curry | 190 | 10 | 21 |
| Red Vinaaloo Curry | 150 | 4 | 24 |

| Stagg Chili: | | | |
|---|---|---|---|
| **Chili with Beans:** *Per 14.3 oz Can, 1 Cup* | | | |
| Classic; Dynamite | 335 | 17 | 29 |
| Chunkero | 320 | 16 | 28 |
| Country Brand; Laredo | 320 | 16 | 28 |
| Fiesta Griller | 250 | 10 | 25 |
| Ranch House Chicken | 240 | 8 | 26 |
| Silverado Beef | 250 | 7 | 30 |
| White Chili | 260 | 12 | 20 |
| **No Beans,** Steakhouse | 320 | 22 | 14 |
| **Low-Fat:** Turkey Ranchero | 240 | 3 | 31 |
| Vegetable Garden Four-Bean | 200 | 1 | 37 |

| Taco Bell: | | | |
|---|---|---|---|
| **Taco Dinners:** *Per Serving, Prepared as Directed* | | | |
| Cheesy Dble Decker, ⅙ pkg., 2.36 oz | 340 | 16 | 30 |
| Soft Flour Tortilla & Sce (1), 3.28 oz | 370 | 13 | 40 |
| Taco Shells, Salsa & Seasoning (1) | 250 | 11 | 20 |
| **Refried Beans:** | | | |
| Fat-Free, 4.6 oz | 100 | 0 | 18 |
| Vegetarian Blend, 4.6 oz | 120 | 1 | 20 |

| Tasty Bite: | **C** | **F** | **Cb** |
|---|---|---|---|
| **Vegetarian Entrees:** *Per ½ Package, 5 oz* | | | |
| Agra Peas & Greens | 150 | 8 | 13 |
| Bengal Lentils | 160 | 6 | 20 |
| Bombay Potatoes | 130 | 4 | 19 |
| Jaipur Vegetables | 180 | 11 | 12 |
| Jodhpur Lentils | 110 | 2.5 | 16 |
| Madras Lentils | 150 | 6 | 18 |
| Punjab Eggplant | 150 | 9 | 13 |

| Thai Kitchen: | | | |
|---|---|---|---|
| **Microwaveable Take-Out Meals:** *Per ½ Package* | | | |
| Original Pad Thai | 250 | 2 | 54 |
| Thai Basil & Chili | 250 | 3 | 50 |
| Thai Peanut | 270 | 5 | 51 |
| **Noodle Carts:** *Per 9 oz Tray* | | | |
| Pad Thai | 460 | 2 | 104 |
| Thai Peanut | 510 | 9 | 96 |
| **Rice Noodle Soup Bowls,** | | | |
| average all flavors, 2.4 oz | 240 | 2 | 50 |
| **Stir-Fry Rice Noodles:** *Per ½ Package* | | | |
| Original Pad Thai | 390 | 3.5 | 84 |
| Thai Peanut | 390 | 2 | 87 |

| Tofurky (Vegetarian): | | | |
|---|---|---|---|
| **Deli Slices:** Pepperoni, 8 slices, 1 oz | 60 | 0.5 | 6 |
| Roast Beef; Bologna, 3 slices, 1.83 oz | 100 | 3 | 5 |
| **Holidays:** Tofurky Roast & Gravy , ⅕ pkg | 250 | 6 | 13 |
| Vegetarian Feast, ⅙ package | 300 | 7 | 16 |
| **Sausages:** Beer Brats (1), 3.5 oz | 260 | 13 | 12 |
| Kielbasa (1), 3.5 oz | 240 | 12 | 12 |
| Ital. Sausage (1), 3.5 oz | 270 | 13 | 12 |

| Trader Joe's: | | | |
|---|---|---|---|
| Chicken Chili with Beans, 1 cup | 290 | 9 | 32 |
| Pasta, Shells & White Cheddar, 1 cup | 280 | 6 | 48 |
| Organic Baked Beans, av., ½ cup | 140 | 0 | 29 |
| Turkey Chili w/ Beans, 1 cup | 240 | 4.5 | 30 |
| **Black Beans:** Reg., ½ cup | 110 | 0 | 19 |
| Cuban Style, ½ cup | 100 | 0.5 | 19 |
| **Potatoes:** Garlic Mashed, ½ cup | 150 | 7 | 19 |
| Cheddar Cheese Au Gratin, ½ cup | 140 | 5 | 21 |

**Uncle Ben's:**

| | C | F | Cb |
|---|---|---|---|
| **Country Inn:** *Per Cup, Prepared w/o Margarine* | | | |
| Broccoli Rice Au Gratin | 210 | 2.5 | 41 |
| Chicken & Vegetable Rice | 200 | 1.5 | 41 |
| Mexican Fiesta Rice | 200 | 1 | 42 |
| Oriental Fried Rice | 200 | 1 | 42 |
| **Ready Rice:** *Per 1 Cup, Prepared* | | | |
| Butter & Garlic Flavored Rice | 220 | 4 | 41 |
| Garden Vegetable | 200 | 2.5 | 41 |
| Roasted Chicken | 210 | 3 | 42 |
| Teriyaki Style | 220 | 3 | 42 |
| **Ready Whole Grain Medley:** *Per 1 Cup, Prepared* | | | |
| Brown & Wild | 220 | 3.5 | 42 |
| Chicken Medley | 210 | 3.5 | 41 |
| Roasted Garlic | 200 | 3 | 38 |
| Santa Fe | 220 | 3 | 42 |
| Vegetable Harvest | 220 | 3 | 44 |

**Valley Fresh:**

| | C | F | Cb |
|---|---|---|---|
| **Chicken:** *Per 2 oz* | | | |
| Premium White Breast | 70 | 2 | 0 |
| White & Dark | 80 | 3.5 | 0 |
| **Turkey,** Premium White | 80 | 3 | 0 |

**Van Camp's:**

| | C | F | Cb |
|---|---|---|---|
| Baked Beans, Original, ½ cup, 4.75oz | 160 | 1 | 30 |
| Beanee Weenee, Original, 7.75 oz | 240 | 8 | 29 |
| Pork & Beans, 28 oz can | | | |
| ½ cup, 4.6 oz | 110 | 1 | 23 |

**Worthington/Loma Linda:**

| | C | F | Cb |
|---|---|---|---|
| Big Franks: 1 link, 1.8 oz | 110 | 6 | 3 |
| Low-fat, 1 link, 1.8 oz | 80 | 2.5 | 3 |
| Chili, 1 cup, 8.10 oz | 280 | 10 | 25 |
| Choplets, 2 slices, 3.2 oz | 90 | 1 | 4 |
| Diced Chik, 2 oz | 50 | 0 | 2 |
| FriChik, Original, low fat, 2 pcs, 3 oz | 80 | 2.5 | 4 |
| Linketts, (1), 1¼ oz | 70 | 4 | 1 |
| Little Links (2), 1.6 oz | 90 | 5 | 3 |
| Redi-Burger, ⅝" slice, 3 oz | 120 | 2.5 | 7 |
| Saucettes (1), 1 oz | 90 | 6 | 1 |
| Super Links (1), 1.7 oz | 110 | 8 | 2 |
| Tender Bits (6), 2.8 oz | 120 | 4 | 7 |
| Tender Rounds (6), 2.8 oz | 120 | 4.5 | 6 |

**Worthington/Loma Linda Cont:**

| | C | F | Cb |
|---|---|---|---|
| Vegetable Skallops, ½ cup, 3 oz | 90 | 1 | 4 |
| Vegetarian Burger, ¼ cup, 1.9 oz | 70 | 1.5 | 3 |
| Veja-Links (1), 1 oz | 50 | 3 | 1 |
| Low-Fat Veja-Links (1), 1 oz | 45 | 1.5 | 3 |

**Yves Veggie Cuisine:**

| | C | F | Cb |
|---|---|---|---|
| **Breakfast:** Patties (2), 1.8 oz | 80 | 2 | 4 |
| Canadian Bacon, 3 slices | 80 | 0.5 | 2 |
| **Burgers:** Meatless Beef Burger (1) | 110 | 4 | 8 |
| Meatless Chicken (1) | 100 | 3 | 5 |
| **Deli Slices:** | 80 | 2.5 | 5 |
| Meatless: Bologna, 4 slices | | | |
| Ham, 4 slices | 100 | 2 | 5 |
| Pepperoni, 6 slices | 80 | 1 | 4 |
| Roast without the Beef, 4 slices | 110 | 2.5 | 4 |
| Salami, 4 slices | 80 | 0 | 4 |
| Smoked Chicken, 4 sl. | 100 | 1.5 | 5 |
| Turkey, 4 slices | 100 | 1.5 | 5 |
| **Ground Rounds:** | | | |
| Meatless: Turkey, ⅓ cup, 1.95 oz | 60 | 1 | 4 |
| Taco Stuffers, ⅓ cup, 1.95 oz | 90 | 2.5 | 5 |
| **Hot Dog:** | | | |
| Good Dog (1), 2 oz | 70 | 3.5 | 1 |
| Hot Dog (1), 1.6 oz | 50 | 0.5 | 2 |
| Jumbo Dog (1), 2.7 oz | 110 | 3 | 5 |
| Tofu Dog (1), 1.3 oz | 45 | 1 | 2 |
| **Brats:** | | | |
| Veggie Classic (1), 3.3 oz | 160 | 5 | 9 |
| Zesty Italian (1), 3.3 oz | 150 | 5 | 9 |
| **Skewers,** | | | |
| Lemon Herb Chicken (1), 2.8 oz | 100 | 1 | 7 |
| **Strips:** Meatless Beef, 3 oz | 120 | 1 | 4 |
| Meatless Chicken, 3 oz | 110 | 1 | 3 |

**Zatarain's:**

| | C | F | Cb |
|---|---|---|---|
| **Beans & Rice Mix:** *Per ⅓, Cup Dry Mix Only* | | | |
| Black Beans & Rice | 220 | 0.5 | 47 |
| Black-Eyed Peas & Rice | 220 | 0.5 | 46 |
| Caribbean Rice | 160 | 1.5 | 34 |
| Chicken Creole Rice | 130 | 0.5 | 28 |
| Chicken Flavor Rice | 210 | 1 | 44 |
| Garlic & Herb & Rice | 150 | 0 | 33 |
| Gravy & Rice | 200 | 0.5 | 45 |
| Rice Pilaf | 200 | 0 | 45 |
| Smothered Chicken Rice | 130 | 0 | 28 |
| Yellow Rice | 190 | 0 | 43 |

## Amy's (Vegetarian): *Per Serve* | C | F | Cb
| | C | F | Cb |
|---|---|---|---|
| **Asian Meals:** | | | |
| Stir-Fry: Thai, 9.5 oz | 310 | 11 | 45 |
| Asian Noodle, 10 oz | 300 | 7 | 50 |
| **Bowls:** Pestp Tortellini, 9.5 oz | 430 | 19 | 45 |
| Santa Fe Enchilada, 10 oz | 350 | 11 | 47 |
| **Burritos:** Bean & Cheese, 6 oz | 310 | 9 | 46 |
| Bean & Rice, 6 oz | 300 | 8 | 48 |
| Breakfast Burrito, 6 oz | 270 | 8 | 38 |
| **Entrees:** Cheese Enchilada, 4.5 oz | 240 | 14 | 18 |
| Cheese Lasagna, 10.3 oz | 380 | 14 | 44 |
| Macaroni & Cheese, 9 oz | 410 | 16 | 47 |
| Macaroni & Soy Cheeze, 9 oz | 370 | 15 | 42 |
| Roasted Vegetable Lasagna, 9.8 oz | 350 | 11 | 47 |
| Vegetable Lasagna, 9.5 oz | 310 | 12 | 35 |
| **Whole Meals:** Chse Enchilada, 9 oz | 370 | 15 | 41 |
| Black Bean Enchilada, 10 oz | 330 | 8 | 53 |
| Black Bean Tamale Verde, 10.3 oz | 330 | 10 | 55 |
| Enchilada Verde, 10 oz | 400 | 13 | 54 |
| Veggie Loaf, 10 oz | 290 | 8 | 47 |
| **Light & Lean:** | | | |
| Black Bean & Cheese Enchilada, 8 oz | 240 | 4.5 | 44 |
| Pasta & Veggies, 8 oz | 210 | 5 | 33 |
| Soft Taco Fiesta, 8 oz | 210 | 7 | 20 |
| **Pot Pies:** | | | |
| Broccoli, 7.5 oz | 460 | 24 | 50 |
| Mex. Tamale; Shepherd's Pie, av., 8 oz | 155 | 3 | 27 |
| Vegetable, 7.5 oz | 420 | 19 | 54 |
| **Snacks:** Nacho, Chse & Bean, 5-6 pcs | 220 | 8 | 25 |
| Cheese Pizza, 5-6 pieces | 210 | 7 | 25 |
| **Veggie Burgers,** | | | |
| All American (1), 2.5 oz | 140 | 3.5 | 14 |
| **Wraps:** Indian Samosa, 5 oz | 250 | 9 | 35 |
| Indian Spinach Tofu, 5.5 oz | 270 | 13 | 28 |
| Teriyaki, 5.5 oz | 310 | 7 | 51 |

**Extra Product Listings ~ www.CalorieKing.com**

| Bagel Bites: | C | F | Cb |
|---|---|---|---|
| Three Cheese, 4 pcs, 3 oz | 190 | 5 | 28 |
| Cheese, Ssge & Pepp., 4 pcs | 200 | 7 | 26 |

| Banquet: | C | F | Cb |
|---|---|---|---|
| **Dinners:** Boneless Pork Rib, 10 oz | 320 | 11 | 42 |
| Cheesy Smothered Meat Patty, 7 oz | 280 | 16 | 21 |
| Chicken Fingers, 7 oz | 480 | 21 | 56 |
| Chicken Pasta Marinara, 6.5 oz | 290 | 14 | 29 |
| Fettuccine Alfredo, 8 oz | 280 | 11 | 35 |
| Fish Sticks, 7.5 oz | 310 | 10 | 44 |

| Banquet (Cont): | C | F | Cb |
|---|---|---|---|
| **Dinners:** | | | |
| Fried Beef Steak, 10 oz | 390 | 18 | 43 |
| Honey Mustard Chicken, 9 oz | 340 | 14 | 42 |
| Lasagna w/ Meat Sce, 8 oz | 250 | 7 | 34 |
| Mac & Cheese, 8 oz | 260 | 6 | 39 |
| Macaroni & Beef, 8 oz | 210 | 4.5 | 32 |
| Meat Balls in Tomato Sauce (5), 5 oz | 200 | 13 | 9 |
| Meatloaf, 9.5 oz | 280 | 13 | 28 |
| Mexican Beef Enchil. & Tamale, 8.5 oz | 310 | 10 | 45 |
| Mexican Style Chkn Enchiladas, 8.5 oz | 280 | 8 | 45 |
| Pepperoni Pizza, 5.75 | 340 | 12 | 47 |
| Salisbury Steak, 9.5 oz | 250 | 12 | 25 |
| Savory Pork Patty, 8 oz | 300 | 17 | 26 |
| Spaghetti & Meatballs, 9 oz | 330 | 14 | 35 |
| Swedish Meatballs, 10.25 oz | 440 | 18 | 51 |
| Turkey , 9.25 oz | 250 | 7 | 32 |
| **Pot Pies:** Beef, 7 oz | 390 | 22 | 36 |
| Chicken; Turkey, av., 7 oz | 375 | 21 | 35 |
| Chicken & Brocolli, 7 oz | 360 | 20 | 34 |
| **Select Recipe:** Chicken Parmigian | 350 | 15 | 37 |
| Corn Dog Meal, 7.5 oz | 460 | 16 | 68 |
| Homestyle Pot Roast, 9.6 oz | 170 | 5 | 19 |
| Original Fried Chicken Meal, 9 oz | 440 | 26 | 30 |
| Spag. with Popcorn Chicken, 7 oz | 270 | 8 | 37 |
| Sweet & Sour Chicken, 8 oz | 390 | 14 | 56 |

| Birds Eye: *Per 1 Cup, Unless Indicated* | C | F | Cb |
|---|---|---|---|
| **Voila!:** Heat and Serve | | | |
| Alfredo Chicken, 1½ cups | 280 | 12 | 37 |
| Beef & Broccoli Stir Fry | 160 | 6 | 13 |
| Beef Lo Mein | 230 | 3 | 37 |
| Chicken Florentine | 230 | 6 | 27 |
| Chicken Parmesan | 360 | 11 | 50 |
| Garlic Chicken | 240 | 8 | 29 |
| Garlic Shrimp | 230 | 9 | 30 |
| Shrimp Scampi | 190 | 2.5 | 31 |
| Sweet & Sour Chicken | 200 | 1 | 38 |
| Three Cheese Chicken | 210 | 8 | 21 |

| Boca (Vegetarian): | C | F | Cb |
|---|---|---|---|
| **Burger:** | | | |
| Cheeseburger, 2.5 oz | 120 | 5 | 6 |
| All American Classic, 2.5 oz | 140 | 5 | 9 |
| Grilled Vegetables, 2.5 oz | 80 | 1 | 7 |
| Original Vegan, 3.5 oz | 100 | 1 | 8 |
| **Chik'n:** Orig. Nuggets, 3 oz | 180 | 7 | 17 |
| Patties (1), 2.5 oz | 160 | 6 | 15 |
| **Veggie Patties,** Bruschetta | 90 | 1.5 | 9 |

**Boston Market:**

| | C | F | Cb |
|---|---|---|---|
| **Dinners:** Beef Steak & Noodles, 14 oz | 490 | 13 | 53 |
| Chicken Parmesan | 620 | 24 | 69 |
| Salisbury Steak | 720 | 37 | 62 |
| Swedish Meatballs | 760 | 43 | 57 |
| Turkey Breast Medallions with Potato | 290 | 11 | 27 |
| **Entrees:** Chicken Pot Pie, 8 oz | 530 | 35 | 40 |
| Honey Roasted Chicken, 9.2 oz | 410 | 17 | 46 |

**Buitoni:**

| | | | |
|---|---|---|---|
| Butternut Squash Ravioli, 12 oz | 490 | 16 | 72 |
| Five Chse Cannelloni, 13 oz | 560 | 27 | 52 |
| Main Lobster Ravioli, 8.5 oz | 430 | 20 | 106 |
| Sthrn Italian Meat Lasagna, 12 oz | 500 | 24 | 38 |

**Contessa:**

**On The Stove:** *Per Serving w/ Sauce, Prepared*

| | | | |
|---|---|---|---|
| Beef/Chicken Stir Fry, av., 8 oz | 175 | 3 | 23 |
| Chicken Fried Rice, 8 oz | 250 | 3.5 | 40 |
| Jambalaya, 8 oz | 240 | 7 | 29 |
| Mongolian Beef, 8 oz | 310 | 7 | 48 |
| Shrimp Stir-Fry, 10 oz | 130 | 0 | 22 |

**Microsteam:** *Per 1 Cup Prepared*

| | | | |
|---|---|---|---|
| Chicken Alfredo | 260 | 13 | 24 |
| Italian Sausage Rigatoni | 300 | 11 | 41 |
| Spaghetti Bolognese | 300 | 13 | 34 |

**Fresh & Easy:**

**Family Package:** *Per 1 Cup Serving:*

| | | | |
|---|---|---|---|
| Cheese Tortellini Caprese | 300 | 11 | 34 |
| Lem. Rosemary Chkn | 190 | 6 | 24 |
| Linguini Carbonara | 400 | 19 | 42 |
| Ravioli Bolognese | 310 | 14 | 26 |

**Single Serve:** *Per Package, 9-10 oz*

| | | | |
|---|---|---|---|
| Beef & Broccoli | 270 | 6 | 40 |
| Sweet & Sour Chkn | 270 | 2 | 51 |
| Teriyaki Chicken | 350 | 6 | 52 |
| Turkey with Stuffing | 230 | 4.5 | 37 |

**GardenBurger:**

**Veggie Burgers:** *Per Patty*

| | | | |
|---|---|---|---|
| The Original | 100 | 3 | 18 |
| Portabella | 100 | 2.5 | 17 |
| Sun-Dried Tomato Basil | 100 | 2.5 | 17 |

**garden lites:** *Per 7 oz Serving*

| | | | |
|---|---|---|---|
| Soufles: Butternut Squash | 180 | 2 | 35 |
| Average other varieties | 140 | 1.5 | 28 |
| Zucchini Marinara/Portabella | 110 | 4 | 19 |

**Gorton's:**

**Fish Fillets:**

Battered Pollock:

| | | | |
|---|---|---|---|
| Beer Battered (2), 3.63 oz | 250 | 18 | 16 |
| Crispy Battered (2), 3.81 | 230 | 12 | 22 |
| Lemon Peppered Battered (2), 2.7 oz | 270 | 18 | 20 |

Breaded Pollock:

| | | | |
|---|---|---|---|
| Classic Crunchy Golden (2) | 240 | 12 | 23 |
| Garlic & Herb (2) | 230 | 12 | 22 |
| Lemon Herb Peppered (2) | 240 | 13 | 21 |

**Gorton's (Cont):**

| | C | F | Cb |
|---|---|---|---|
| **Grilled:** Classic Salmon (1), 3.15 oz | 100 | 3 | 2 |
| Garlic Lemon Butter Pollock (1) | 100 | 3 | 1 |
| Signature Tilapia (1), 3.15 oz | 80 | 2.5 | 2 |

**Shrimp:**

| | | | |
|---|---|---|---|
| Butterfly (5), 3.5 oz | 250 | 11 | 27 |
| Shrimp Scampi, 4 oz | 120 | 6 | 8 |
| Grilled: Classic, 4 oz | 110 | 1.5 | 5 |
| Shrimp Scampi, 4oz | 130 | 4.5 | 3 |

**Great Value:**

**Breakfast Bowls:** *Per 8 oz*

| | | | |
|---|---|---|---|
| Bacon/Sausage, Eggs & Pot., av. | 490 | 34 | 21 |
| Maple P'cakes & Ssg Griddle S'wch | 380 | 22 | 36 |

**Complete Skillet Meals:** *Per ½ Package*

| | | | |
|---|---|---|---|
| Chkn Florentine & Farfalle | 570 | 32 | 40 |
| Italian Ssg & Rigatoni | 500 | 26 | 46 |

**Lean Cafe:** *Per Container*

| | | | |
|---|---|---|---|
| Cheese Ravioli, 8.5 oz | 220 | 5 | 32 |
| Chicken Fettuccni Entree, 9.25 oz | 265 | 6 | 33 |
| Salisbury Steak, 9.5 oz | 260 | 9 | 21 |

**Meals:** *Per ¼ 32 oz Package, 8 oz*

| | | | |
|---|---|---|---|
| Cheese Manicoti | 320 | 16 | 24 |
| Lasagna | 280 | 9 | 36 |

**Healthy Choice:**

**All Natural Entrees:**

| | | | |
|---|---|---|---|
| Asian Potstickers, 10 oz | 340 | 4.5 | 66 |
| Portabella Spin. Parm., 9.4 oz | 270 | 7 | 39 |
| Ravioli: Lobster Cheese, 9 oz | 270 | 6 | 41 |
| Pumpkin Squash, 9.2 oz | 300 | 6 | 52 |
| Tortellini Primavera Parm., 9 oz | 240 | 5 | 37 |

**Asian/Cafe/Mediterranean Steamers:**

| | | | |
|---|---|---|---|
| Chicken Margherita, 10 oz | 330 | 8 | 42 |
| Grilled Whiskey Steak, 9.5 oz | 290 | 4 | 47 |
| Lem. Garlic Chkn & Shrimp, 10 oz | 260 | 6 | 35 |

**Complete Meals:**

| | | | |
|---|---|---|---|
| Beef Pot Roast, 11 oz | 280 | 4.5 | 41 |
| Chkn Parmigiana,11.5 oz | 350 | 10 | 49 |
| Homestyle Salisbury Steak, 12.5 oz | 310 | 6 | 46 |
| Lemon Pepper Fish, 10.7 oz | 300 | 5 | 49 |

**Select Entrees:**

| | | | |
|---|---|---|---|
| Bacon & Smokey Cheddar Chicken | 240 | 6 | 28 |
| Ravioli Florentine Marinara, 8.5 oz | 230 | 4 | 37 |
| Spicy Caribbean Chicken, 8.5 oz | 310 | 2 | 56 |

**Hot Pockets:**

**Calzones:** *Per ½ Calzone, 4.2 oz*

| | | | |
|---|---|---|---|
| 4 Meat & 4 Cheese | 300 | 13 | 34 |
| Pepperoni & 3 Chse | 320 | 16 | 34 |
| Supreme | 280 | 12 | 33 |

**Mexican Style:** *Per Sandwich*

| | | | |
|---|---|---|---|
| Beef Taco | 290 | 12 | 35 |
| Jalap. Steak & Cheese | 280 | 11 | 35 |
| Steak Fajita | 290 | 12 | 34 |
| Three Cheese & Chicken Quesadilla | 270 | 9 | 36 |

| Hot Pockets (Cont): | C | F | Cb |
|---|---|---|---|
| **Paninis:** *Per ½ Panini* | | | |
| Bruschetta Chicken | 190 | 6 | 25 |
| Steak & Cheddar | 260 | 11 | 26 |
| **Pizzeria:** Four Cheese | 320 | 12 | 40 |
| Pepperoni | 340 | 17 | 37 |
| Sausage | 340 | 16 | 39 |
| **Sandwiches:** *Per 4 oz Sandwich* | | | |
| Barbeque Recipe Beef | 340 | 13 | 44 |
| Cheeseburger | 310 | 12 | 39 |
| Meatballs & Mozzarella | 340 | 15 | 39 |
| Philly Steak & Cheese | 310 | 13 | 37 |
| **Snackers:** *Per 4 Pieces* | | | |
| Fiesta Nacho Bites | 220 | 8 | 28 |
| Grilled Italian Style Bites | 210 | 6 | 28 |
| Loaded Potato Skins Bites | 230 | 10 | 25 |
| Toasted Five Cheese Ravoli | 220 | 6 | 33 |
| **Hungry Man:** | | | |
| **Dinners:** | | | |
| Boneless Fried Chkn | 860 | 39 | 85 |
| Boneless Pork | 810 | 36 | 98 |
| Classic Fried Chkn | 1030 | 62 | 62 |
| Country Fried Chkn | 570 | 27 | 53 |
| Homestyle Meatloaf | 660 | 35 | 61 |
| Mexican Style Fiesta | 600 | 22 | 89 |
| **Pub Favorites:** | | | |
| Beer Battered Chicken | 790 | 33 | 79 |
| Bourbon Steak Strips | 480 | 11 | 70 |
| Chopped Beef Steak | 590 | 37 | 40 |
| Honey Bourbon Chicken Strips | 620 | 24 | 56 |
| **XXL Sandwiches:** *Per 1 Box Serving* | | | |
| Angus Beef Charbroil | 740 | 47 | 52 |
| BBQ Chicken | 490 | 14 | 64 |
| Buffalo Fried Chicken | 660 | 27 | 70 |
| Chicken Parmesan | 610 | 29 | 63 |
| Crispy Fried Chicken | 670 | 32 | 64 |
| **José Olé:** | | | |
| **Breakfast Burritos:** | | | |
| Egg & Bacon, 4 oz | 260 | 9 | 33 |
| Egg & Ham, 4 oz | 250 | 8 | 34 |
| Egg & Sausage, 4 oz | 270 | 10 | 34 |
| **Premium Burritos:** | | | |
| Steak & Cheese (1) | 300 | 10 | 40 |
| Chicken Monterey (1) | 270 | 6 | 41 |
| **Premium Chimichangas:** | | | |
| Chicken & Cheese (1), 5 oz | 330 | 11 | 45 |
| Steak & Cheese (1), 5 oz | 350 | 14 | 41 |
| **Snacks:** | | | |
| Chimichangas, Steak & Ched., Mini (3) | 370 | 20 | 37 |
| Quesadillas: Grilled Chkn & 3 Chse (1) | 270 | 9 | 31 |
| Grilled Steak & 3 Cheese (1) | 260 | 9 | 32 |
| Tacos, Beef & Cheese Mini, (4) | 230 | 12 | 23 |
| **Taquitos:** Chicken, Corn Tortillas, (3) | 200 | 8 | 26 |
| Steak & Cheese, Flour Tortillas, (2) | 250 | 12 | 26 |

| Kids Cuisine: *Per Meal* | C | F | Cb |
|---|---|---|---|
| All American Fried Chicken | 540 | 24 | 53 |
| All Star Chicken Breast Nuggets | 410 | 15 | 52 |
| Home Run Blast Mac & Cheese | 420 | 11 | 69 |
| Magical Cheese Stuffed Crust Pizza | 390 | 7 | 66 |
| Pop Star Popcorn Chicken | 410 | 11 | 64 |
| Twist & Twirl Spaghetti w/ Meatballs | 410 | 10 | 61 |
| **Kroger:** | | | |
| **Meals Made Simple:** | | | |
| Beef Stir Fry, 1¾ cups | 180 | 4 | 26 |
| Chicken Florentine, 2¼ cups, 6.9 oz | 330 | 19 | 25 |
| Chicken Stir Fry, 1½ cups | 200 | 2 | 30 |
| Shrimp Fried Rice, 1¼ cups, 8 oz | 190 | 0.5 | 36 |
| **Oven Ready:** | | | |
| Breaded Calamari Rings (10), 3 oz | 200 | 10 | 21 |
| Coconut Shrimp w/ Dipping Sauce | 350 | 21 | 27 |
| **Pot Pies:** Beef, (1), 7 oz | 450 | 27 | 36 |
| Chicken (1), 7 oz | 370 | 20 | 38 |
| Turkey (1), 7 oz | 380 | 22 | 36 |
| **Lean Cuisine:** | | | |
| **Cafe Cuisine:** *Per Complete Meal* | | | |
| Beef & Broccoli | 270 | 5 | 43 |
| Beef Chow Fun | 320 | 5 | 54 |
| Beef Portabello | 200 | 6 | 24 |
| Chicken with Almonds | 250 | 4 | 38 |
| Sun Dried Tomato Pesto Chicken | 270 | 9 | 28 |
| Thai Style Chicken | 220 | 4 | 35 |
| **Casual Cuisine:** *Each Unless Indicated* | | | |
| Flatbread Melts: Chicken Ranch Club | 370 | 9 | 52 |
| Steakhouse Ranch | 360 | 9 | 50 |
| Sun-Dried Tom. Basil Chkn | 360 | 8 | 49 |
| Snacks, | | | |
| Dips with Pita Bread, av. all var., 8 oz | 195 | 5 | 29 |
| Paninis: Chicken Club Panini | 360 | 9 | 45 |
| Chicken, Spinach & Mushroom | 310 | 7 | 42 |
| Philly-Style Steak & Cheese | 320 | 9 | 39 |
| Steak, Cheddar & Mushroom | 340 | 9 | 43 |
| Spring Rolls: Fajita Style Chicken (2) | 200 | 7 | 20 |
| Garlic/Thai Chicken, (2), average | 200 | 8 | 24 |
| **Comfort Cuisine:** *Per Complete Meal* | | | |
| Baked Chicken | 240 | 7 | 30 |
| Beef Pot Roast | 210 | 6 | 26 |
| Roasted Turkey & Veges | 200 | 7 | 18 |
| **Dinnertime Selects:** | | | |
| Chicken Fettuccini | 330 | 6 | 42 |
| Lemon Garlic Shrimp | 280 | 6 | 39 |
| Salisbury Steak | 270 | 9 | 27 |

## Lean Cuisine (Cont):

| | C | F | Cb |
|---|---|---|---|
| **Market Creations:** | | | |
| Asiago Cheese Tortellini | 270 | 7 | 39 |
| Chicken Margherita | 300 | 8 | 38 |
| Shanghai Style Shrimp | 250 | 3 | 41 |
| Sweet & Spicy Ginger Chicken | 280 | 2.5 | 43 |
| **Simple Favorites:** | | | |
| Asian Style Pot Stickers | 260 | 3.5 | 49 |
| Cheese Ravioli | 220 | 5 | 33 |
| Macaroni and Cheese | 290 | 7 | 41 |
| **Spa Cuisine:** | | | |
| Butternut Squash Ravioli | 260 | 7 | 40 |
| Lemongrass Chicken | 250 | 4.5 | 35 |
| Salmon with Basil | 210 | 5 | 25 |
| **Pizzas ~** See Page 136 | | | |

## Lean Pockets: Per Single Pocket

| | C | F | Cb |
|---|---|---|---|
| **Sandwiches:** | | | |
| Breakfast, Bacon, Egg & Cheese | 260 | 9 | 37 |
| Culinary Creations: | | | |
| Chicken Bacon Dijon | 270 | 8 | 38 |
| Chipotle Chicken | 260 | 7 | 39 |
| Garlic Chkn White Pizza | 270 | 8 | 38 |
| Originals: Cheeseburger | 290 | 9 | 42 |
| Italian Style Meatballs & Mozz. | 300 | 9 | 40 |
| Average other varieties, | 270 | 6 | 41 |
| Pretzel Bread, average | 280 | 9 | 35 |
| **Stuffed Quesadillas:** | | | |
| B'fast, Turkey, Ssg, Egg & Cheese | 250 | 7 | 32 |
| Grilled Chicken & Three Cheese | 180 | 4 | 24 |
| Grilled Chicken Jajita | 170 | 4 | 24 |

## Macaroni Grill:

**Frozen Entrees:** Per 1½ Cups Prepared Unless Indicated

| | C | F | Cb |
|---|---|---|---|
| Basil Parmesan Chicken | 480 | 22 | 44 |
| Grilled Chicken Florentine | 560 | 19 | 57 |
| Roasted Garlic Shrimp Scampi | 410 | 16 | 51 |
| **Restaurant Favorites,** | | | |
| Classic Lasagna, 1 cup | 390 | 19 | 30 |

## Marie Callender's:

**Bakes:** Per 1 Cup

| | C | F | Cb |
|---|---|---|---|
| 3 Meat 4 Cheese Lasagna | 290 | 12 | 31 |
| Chicken & Spinach Lasagna | 290 | 11 | 32 |
| Scallop Potatoes & Ham | 320 | 18 | 23 |
| Southwest Chipotle Chicken | 280 | 11 | 33 |
| **Complete Dinners:** Per Meal | | | |
| Country Fried Chicken & Gravy | 570 | 27 | 60 |
| Golden Battered Fish Fillet | 400 | 13 | 50 |
| Grilled Chicken Bake | 500 | 26 | 34 |
| Honey Roasted Chicken | 320 | 10 | 38 |
| Honey Roasted Turkey | 320 | 11 | 31 |
| Old Fashioned Beef Pot Roast | 260 | 6 | 31 |

## Marie Callender's (Cont):

| | C | F | Cb |
|---|---|---|---|
| **Pasta Al Dente:** | | | |
| Cavatappi Genovese, 11 oz | 410 | 15 | 44 |
| Fettuccine Chkn Balsamic, 10.5 oz | 440 | 18 | 46 |
| Penne Chicken Modesto, 10 oz | 410 | 17 | 43 |
| Rigatoni: Con Pesce, 10.5 oz | 340 | 12 | 44 |
| Marinara Classico, 10.5 oz | 460 | 24 | 41 |
| Tortellini Romano, 10 oz | 430 | 14 | 59 |
| **Pot Pies:** Per Pie | | | |
| Chicken, 16.5 oz pie | 1040 | 62 | 90 |
| Turkey, 1 pie, 10 oz | 630 | 36 | 58 |

## Michael Angelo's: Per Single Serve Package

| | C | F | Cb |
|---|---|---|---|
| Chicken Alfredo, 11 oz | 480 | 17 | 57 |
| Chicken Piccata, 10 oz | 510 | 24 | 52 |
| Eggplant Parmesan, 11oz | 430 | 28 | 26 |
| Four Cheese Lasagna, 11 oz | 480 | 18 | 51 |
| Lasagna with Meat Sauce, 11 oz | 420 | 13 | 51 |
| Manicotti with Sauce, 11 oz | 410 | 18 | 39 |
| Shrimp Scampi, 11 oz | 540 | 28 | 46 |
| Vege. Lasagna, 11 oz | 390 | 15 | 44 |

## Morningstar Farms (Vegetarian):

| | C | F | Cb |
|---|---|---|---|
| **Biscuits:** Bacon, Egg & Cheese | 270 | 8 | 40 |
| Sausage, Egg & Biscuit | 270 | 8 | 39 |
| **Burgers:** Per Patty | | | |
| Grillers Original (1) | 130 | 6 | 5 |
| Mushroom Lovers (1) | 110 | 6 | 8 |
| Spicy Black Bean (1) | 120 | 4 | 13 |
| **Entrees:** Per Serving | | | |
| Chik'n Enchilada (1) | 280 | 7 | 47 |
| Sesame Chik'n, 9½ oz | 310 | 9 | 46 |
| Three Bean Chili w/ Gr. Crumbles, 1 c. | 270 | 4 | 52 |
| **Chik'n:** Buffalo Wings (5) | 200 | 8 | 20 |
| Chik'n Nuggets (4) | 190 | 9 | 19 |
| **Patties:** Breakfast (1) | 80 | 3 | 4 |
| Chik'n Veggie Pattie (1) | 80 | 3 | 7 |

## P.F. Chang's: Per ½ Package

| | C | F | Cb |
|---|---|---|---|
| Beef with Broccoli | 360 | 18 | 26 |
| General Chang's Chicken | 410 | 13 | 54 |
| Ginger Chicken & Broccoli | 320 | 12 | 23 |
| Orange Chicken | 450 | 16 | 61 |
| Shanghai Style Beef | 320 | 12 | 38 |
| Shrimp in Garlic Sauce | 290 | 9 | 33 |
| Shrimp Lo Mein | 360 | 12 | 40 |
| Sweet & Sour Chicken | 410 | 10 | 66 |

## Pillsbury:

**Egg Scrambles:** Per Package

| | C | F | Cb |
|---|---|---|---|
| Bacon & Veggies | 290 | 15 | 22 |
| Sausage & Cheese | 300 | 16 | 25 |
| Sausage & Veggies | 280 | 16 | 21 |

| Safeway Select: | C | F | Cb |
|---|---|---|---|
| Beef Salisbury Steak, 9.35 oz | 410 | 28 | 23 |
| Chicken Cacciatore, 8.75 oz | 290 | 10 | 34 |
| Fettucini Alfredo, 11.5 oz | 380 | 12 | 55 |
| Five Vegetable Lasagna, 10.6 oz | 330 | 8 | 48 |
| Homestyle Baked Chicken, 9 oz | 260 | 11 | 31 |
| Orange Chicken, 9 oz | 360 | 7 | 61 |
| Penne Pasta, 8 oz | 300 | 11 | 42 |
| Pot Roast, 9 oz | 270 | 11 | 23 |
| Spaghetti with Meat Sauce, 12 oz | 450 | 16 | 61 |
| Swedish Meat Balls, 11.5 oz | 470 | 24 | 43 |
| Three Cheese Tortellini, 7.5 oz | 350 | 16 | 38 |
| Triple Cheese Enchilada, 9 oz | 410 | 14 | 57 |

**Seapak** ~ *See www.calorieking.com*

**Stouffer's:**

**Corner Bistro:** *Per Single Serve Package*

| Flatbread Melts: | C | F | Cb |
|---|---|---|---|
| Chicken Quesadilla | 370 | 15 | 41 |
| Steak, Mushr. Cheddar | 390 | 17 | 40 |
| Stromboli: | | | |
| Italian-Style Suprme | 430 | 19 | 45 |
| Pepperoni & Prov. | 430 | 17 | 45 |
| Toasted Subs: | | | |
| Meatball Italiano | 400 | 18 | 42 |
| Philly-Style Stk & Chse | 370 | 16 | 39 |
| Zesty Italian | 470 | 25 | 40 |

**Easy Express Skillets:** *Per Serving*

| | C | F | Cb |
|---|---|---|---|
| Broccoli & Beef, 12.5 oz | 350 | 6 | 57 |
| Teriyak Chicken, 12.5 oz | 270 | 4 | 41 |
| Yankee Pot Roat, 12 oz | 300 | 8 | 38 |

**Farmers' Harvest:** *Per Single Serve Package*

| | C | F | Cb |
|---|---|---|---|
| Chicken Fettuccini Alfredo, 12 oz | 510 | 29 | 44 |
| Chicken-Parm. Pasta Bake, 12 oz | 310 | 8 | 39 |
| Rstd Chicken & Bow Tie Pasta w/ Veg | 430 | 18 | 46 |
| Made With Whole Grain Pasta: | | | |
| Lasagna w/ Meat & Sce, 10 oz | 360 | 12 | 40 |
| Spag. & M'balls w/ Veges, 12 oz | 320 | 9 | 41 |
| Vegetable Lasagna, 10.5 oz | 400 | 19 | 43 |

**Satisfying Servings:** *Per Single Serve Package*

| | C | F | Cb |
|---|---|---|---|
| Bourbon Steak Tips, 14 oz | 490 | 17 | 61 |
| Macaroni & Cheese, 20 oz | 680 | 32 | 72 |
| Monterey Chkn, 14.5 oz | 530 | 21 | 54 |
| Sesame Chicken, 15 oz | 590 | 16 | 87 |
| Shrimp Scampi, 14 oz | 400 | 12 | 56 |

| Stouffer's (Cont): | C | F | Cb |
|---|---|---|---|
| **Signature Classics:** *Per Package* | | | |
| Beef Pot Roast, 16 oz | 320 | 8 | 41 |
| Chicken Pot Pie, 10 oz | 670 | 38 | 64 |
| Creamed Chipped Beef, 11 oz | 280 | 14 | 18 |
| Five Cheese Lasagna, 10.75oz | 370 | 14 | 39 |
| Green Pepper Steak, 10.5 oz | 240 | 4 | 32 |
| Meatloaf, 16 oz | 530 | 26 | 40 |
| Roast Turkey Breast, 9.5 oz | 270 | 9 | 30 |
| Turkey Pot Pie, 10 oz | 710 | 41 | 61 |
| Veal Parmigiana, 11.6 oz | 430 | 18 | 46 |

**Starkist:**

**SeaSations Fillets:** *Per 1 Fillet, 4.6 oz*

| | C | F | Cb |
|---|---|---|---|
| Mediterranean Tomato Basil | 90 | 3 | 3 |
| Savory Lemon Herb | 100 | 4 | 4 |
| Teriyaki & Orange Ginger | 100 | 2.5 | 7 |
| **SeaSations Entrees:** | | | |
| Creamy Tuna Casserole, 9 oz | 300 | 9 | 35 |
| Garlic Butter Shrimp, 9 oz | 260 | 7 | 35 |
| Lemon Dill Salmon, 9 oz | 290 | 5 | 45 |
| Orange Miso Tilapia, 9 oz | 280 | 4 | 45 |

**Swansons:**

| Pot Pies: Beef (1), 7 oz | 390 | 24 | 33 |
|---|---|---|---|
| Chicken/Turkey (1), 7 oz | 380 | 22 | 34 |

**TGI Friday's:**

| | C | F | Cb |
|---|---|---|---|
| Beer Battered Onion Rings (3) | 180 | 8 | 26 |
| Buffalo Popcorn Chkn & Sce, | 230 | 7 | 15 |
| Buffalo Wings (3) | 180 | 11 | 4 |
| Honey BBQ Wings (3) | 200 | 11 | 10 |
| Mozzarella Sticks & Sauce, 1 stick | 110 | 5 | 9 |
| Potato Skins, Chedd. & Bacon, 3 pieces | 210 | 12 | 17 |
| **Complete Skillet Meals:** | | | |
| Sizzling Chicken Fajitas,1¼ cups | 360 | 14 | 34 |
| Sizzling Shrimp Stir Fry, 1⅓ cups | 300 | 6 | 54 |

**Trader Joe's:**

**Meals:** *Per Serving*

| | C | F | Cb |
|---|---|---|---|
| Butter Chkn w/ Basmati Rice, 1 cup | 270 | 8 | 33 |
| Chicken Chow Mein, ⅓ pkg, 6.35 oz | 210 | 2 | 35 |
| Chicken Quesadilla (1), 6 oz | 320 | 16 | 26 |
| Citrus Glazed Chicken w/ Rice, 8 oz | 270 | 5 | 40 |
| Mac & Cheese, 1 cup, 7 oz | 360 | 15 | 42 |
| Mac & Chees, Reduced Guilt, 7 oz | 270 | 6 | 40 |
| Shrimp Stir Fry, 6.4 oz | 70 | 0.5 | 6 |
| Spaghetti & Beef Meatballs, 1 cup | 380 | 13 | 48 |
| Spicy Beef & Broccoli, 1.75 cups | 430 | 13 | 64 |
| Thai Vegetale Kao Soi, 12.6 oz | 430 | 20 | 55 |
| Vegan Pad Thai, 11 oz | 600 | 7 | 114 |
| **Pies:** Chicken Pot Pie, ½ pie, 8 oz | 360 | 22 | 28 |
| Shepherd's Pie, 1 cup | 170 | 3 | 22 |

## Tyson:

### Refrigerated Entrees:

**Beef:** *Per 5 oz Serving Unless Indicated*

| | C | F | Cb |
|---|---|---|---|
| Brisket in Fire Roasted Onion Sauce | 140 | 4 | 6 |
| Pot Roast in Gravy | 170 | 8 | 2 |
| Steak Tips: In Bourbon Sauce | 180 | 5 | 12 |
| In Burgundy Sauce | 180 | 9 | 6 |
| Grilled & Ready, Beef Strips, 3 oz | 140 | 6 | 1 |

### Chicken:

Any'tizers:

| | C | F | Cb |
|---|---|---|---|
| Chkn Brst Chunks: With 2 T. TSO Sauce | 240 | 6.5 | 35 |
| With 2 Tbsp Sweet & Sour Sauce | 260 | 6 | 42 |
| Fajita QuesaDippers, with 2 Tbsp Cilantro Lime Salsa | 200 | 0 | 19 |
| Grilled & Ready: |  |  |  |
| Fajita Chkn Strips, 3 oz | 110 | 4 | 1 |
| Sthwstrn Chkn Breast Strips, 3 oz | 120 | 3 | 3 |
| Nuggets: Fun Shaped, 5 pieces | 280 | 18 | 16 |
| Southern Style, 6 pieces | 270 | 21 | 11 |
| Stuffed Chkn Cordon Bleu Minis, 3 pcs | 200 | 11 | 9 |
| Stuffed Chkn Pepperoni Minis, 3 pcs | 200 | 11 | 10 |
| Wings: Buffalo Style, Hot, 3 oz | 190 | 13 | 3 |
| Honey BBQ, 3 oz | 190 | 12 | 9 |
| Hot & Spicy, 3 pieces | 220 | 15 | 1 |

**Pork:** *Per 5 oz Serving*

| | C | F | Cb |
|---|---|---|---|
| Maple & Br. Sugar Glazed Ham, 5 oz | 180 | 4.5 | 14 |
| Pork Loin in Sweet & Tangy Sce, 5 oz | 180 | 7 | 13 |
| Pork Roast in Gravy, 5 oz | 190 | 10 | 5 |

## Van De Kamp's:

| | C | F | Cb |
|---|---|---|---|
| Crispy Halibut Fillets (3) | 280 | 13 | 24 |
| Crunchy Fish Sticks, 18 Count Box (6) | 240 | 11 | 22 |
| Fish Shaped Nuggets (4), 4.25 oz | 280 | 13 | 25 |
| **Fried,** Beer Battered Fillets (2) | 240 | 13 | 18 |
| **Breaded:** Butterfly Shrimp, 7 pcs | 330 | 16 | 31 |
| Popcorn Fish, 8 pieces, 4.13 oz | 270 | 13 | 25 |

## Weight Watchers:

**Smart Ones:** *Entrees: Per Meal*

| | C | F | Cb |
|---|---|---|---|
| Angel Hair Marinara | 230 | 4 | 40 |
| Chkn & Broccoli Alfredo | 300 | 4 | 39 |
| Chicken Carbonara | 260 | 5 | 32 |
| Chicken Enchiladas Suiza | 290 | 5 | 49 |
| Chicken Oriental | 230 | 1.5 | 41 |
| Chicken Fettuccini | 290 | 6 | 40 |
| Chicken Parmesan | 290 | 5 | 35 |
| Chicken Teriyaki Stir Fry | 340 | 6 | 49 |
| Cranberry Turkey Medallions | 250 | 2 | 43 |
| Lasagna Bake with Meat Sauce | 270 | 4 | 46 |
| Lasagna Florentine | 310 | 11 | 40 |
| Lemon Herb Chicken Piccata | 230 | 1.5 | 41 |

## Weight Watchers Smart Ones (Cont):

**Entrees cont:** *Per Meal*

| | C | F | Cb |
|---|---|---|---|
| Macaroni & Cheese | 270 | 2 | 52 |
| Meatloaf w/ Pot. & Gravy | 240 | 8 | 22 |
| Orange Sesame Chicken | 320 | 8 | 48 |
| Pasta Primavera | 250 | 4 | 41 |
| Pasta with Ricotta & Spinach | 280 | 6 | 43 |
| Ravioli Florentine | 270 | 5 | 43 |
| Salisbury Steak, 9.5 oz | 280 | 9 | 33 |
| Sesame Chicken | 360 | 7 | 49 |
| Shrimp Marinara | 180 | 2.5 | 32 |
| Spaghetti with Meat Sauce | 290 | 5 | 44 |
| Spicy Szechuan Style Vege. & Chkn | 240 | 5 | 38 |
| Stuffed Turkey Breast | 260 | 5 | 39 |
| Swedish Meatballs | 270 | 6 | 35 |
| Teriyaki Chicken & Veges | 230 | 2.5 | 39 |
| Three Cheese Macaroni | 300 | 6 | 48 |
| Three Cheese Ziti Marinara | 300 | 8 | 44 |
| Traditional Lasagna w/ Meat Sce | 300 | 7 | 41 |
| Tuna Noodle Gratin | 240 | 4.5 | 43 |
| Ziti with Meatballs & Cheese | 390 | 9 | 52 |

**Morning Express:** *Per Meal*

| | C | F | Cb |
|---|---|---|---|
| Breakfast Quesadilla | 230 | 7 | 29 |
| Canad. Bacon Eng. Muffin | 210 | 6 | 27 |
| English Muffin S'wich | 210 | 5 | 28 |
| Stuffed Breakfast Sandwich | 240 | 7 | 30 |

**Satisfying Selections** (30% Larger): *Per Meal*

| | C | F | Cb |
|---|---|---|---|
| Chicken & Broccoli, 11.67 oz | 300 | 4 | 39 |
| With Cheese, 11.67 oz | 340 | 8 | 37 |
| Chicken Teriyaki, 11.67 oz | 340 | 6 | 49 |
| Sesame Chicken, 11.67 oz | 360 | 7 | 49 |
| Ziti with M'balls & Cheese, 11.67 oz | 390 | 9 | 52 |

## Worthington/Loma Linda (Vegetarian):

| | C | F | Cb |
|---|---|---|---|
| Chic-ketts, 2 slices | 110 | 5 | 3 |
| Dinner Roast, ¾" slice | 180 | 11 | 6 |
| Fried Chik'n w/ Gravy, 2 pcs | 150 | 10 | 5 |
| FriPats, 1 pattie, 2.25 oz | 130 | 6 | 5 |
| Leanies, 1 link, 1.4 oz | 100 | 7 | 2 |
| Meatless: |  |  |  |
| Chicken Style Roll, ⅜" slice | 90 | 4.5 | 2 |
| Smoked Turkey Roll, ⅜" slice | 130 | 8 | 4 |
| Prosage Links (2), 1.6 oz | 80 | 3 | 3 |
| Stakelets, 2.5 oz piece | 150 | 7 | 7 |
| Stripples, 2 strips, 0.56 oz | 60 | 4.5 | 2 |
| Swiss Stake, with Gravy, 1 piece | 130 | 6 | 9 |

## Zatarains:

*Per 12oz Package Unless Indicated*

| | C | F | Cb |
|---|---|---|---|
| Blackened Chicken Alfredo, 10.5 oz | 510 | 24 | 50 |
| Jambalaya Pasta w/ Chkn & Ssge | 380 | 10 | 56 |
| Jambalaya flavored with Sausage | 500 | 14 | 79 |
| Red Beans & Rice with Sausage | 510 | 20 | 68 |

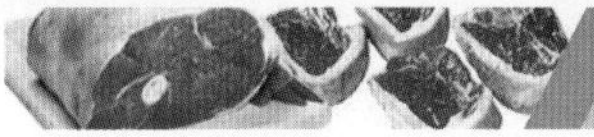

Note: Cooking reduces weight of meat by 20-45% due to water and fat losses. Average weight loss is 30%. Actual loss depends on cooking method and cooking time.

Examples:

4 oz raw weight = approx. 3 oz cooked weight

4 oz cooked weight = approx. 5½ oz raw weight

**What 3 oz Cooked Meat Looks Like**

• Rectangular piece (4" x 2½" x ½" thick)

• Deck of cards (3½" x 2½" x ⅝" thick)

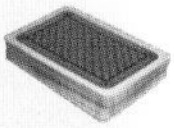

### STEAK QUICK GUIDE

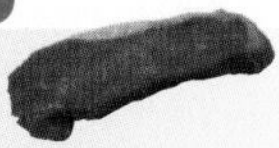

**Sirloin (Choice Grade):**
**External fat trimmed to ⅛"**
*Broiled, Edible Portion (no bone)*

**C  F  Cb**

**Small/Regular Serving, 3 oz (cooked):**

(from 4-4½ oz raw)

| | C | F | Cb |
|---|---|---|---|
| Lean + external fat (⅛"), 3 oz | 220 | 13 | 0 |
| Lean + marbling, 3 oz | 185 | 9 | 0 |
| Lean only, 3 oz | 160 | 6 | 0 |
| (No external fat or marbling) | | | |

**Medium Serving, 5 oz (cooked wt):**

(from approximately 7 oz raw)

| | | | |
|---|---|---|---|
| Lean + external fat (⅛"), 5 oz | 365 | 22 | 0 |
| Lean + marbling, 5 oz | 310 | 15 | 0 |
| Lean only, 5 oz | 265 | 10 | 0 |

**Large Serving, 8 oz (cooked wt):**

(from 11-12 oz raw)

| | | | |
|---|---|---|---|
| Lean + external fat (⅛"), 8 oz | 585 | 36 | 0 |
| Lean + marbling, 8 oz | 500 | 24 | 0 |
| Lean only, 8 oz | 425 | 15 | 0 |

**Extra Large Serving, 12 oz (cooked wt):**

(from approximately 16-17 oz raw)

| | | | |
|---|---|---|---|
| Lean + external fat (⅛"), 12 oz | 875 | 54 | 0 |
| Lean + marbling, 12 oz | 745 | 36 | 0 |
| Lean only, 12 oz | 640 | 22 | 0 |

**Pan Fried:**

Sirloin (Choice), medium serving,

| | | | |
|---|---|---|---|
| Lean + external fat (⅛"), 5 oz | 445 | 30 | 0 |

### Other Steaks

**C  F  Cb**

**Filet Mignon (Tenderloin):**
1 Medium steak (6 oz raw weight)
Broiled, with ¼" fat trim

| | C | F | Cb |
|---|---|---|---|
| Lean + fat (¼"), 4 oz | 360 | 27 | 0 |
| Lean only, 3½ oz | 230 | 12 | 0 |

**New York/Club Steak:**
Top Loin/Short Loin
1 steak, regular (9¼ oz raw, ¼" fat)
Broiled:

| | | | |
|---|---|---|---|
| Lean + fat (¼"), 6.25 oz | 580 | 43 | 0 |
| Lean + marbling, 5.5 oz | 400 | 25 | 0 |
| Lean only, 5.25 oz | 360 | 20 | 0 |

**Porterhouse Steak:**
1 Medium, 6 oz raw weight (no bone), broiled

| | | | |
|---|---|---|---|
| Lean + fat (¼"), 4.25 oz | 410 | 33 | 0 |
| Lean only, 3.5 oz | 210 | 11 | 0 |

1 Large, 12 oz raw weight (no bone), broiled

| | | | |
|---|---|---|---|
| Lean + fat (¼") 8.5 oz cooked | 820 | 66 | 0 |
| Lean only, 7 oz cooked | 420 | 22 | 0 |

**T-Bone Steak:** *Broiled or Grilled*
**Medium Size:** *8 oz raw weight*
Approximately 6 oz cooked

| | | | |
|---|---|---|---|
| Lean + Fat (¼"), 5 oz (no bone) | 400 | 28 | 0 |
| Lean only, 4 oz (no bone) | 265 | 12 | 0 |

**Large Size:** *12 oz raw weight*
(Approximately 9 oz cooked)

| | | | |
|---|---|---|---|
| Lean + fat (¼"), 7 oz (no bone) | 560 | 39 | 0 |
| Lean only, 6 oz (no bone) | 400 | 18 | 0 |

**Extra Large Size:** *20 oz raw weight*
(Approximately 16 oz cooked)

| | | | |
|---|---|---|---|
| Lean + Fat (¼"), 12 oz (no bone) | 960 | 66 | 0 |
| Lean Only, 10 oz (no bone) | 660 | 30 | 0 |

**Also See Fast-Foods & Restaurants Section ~**
*Lone Star Steakhouse ; Outback Steakhouse*

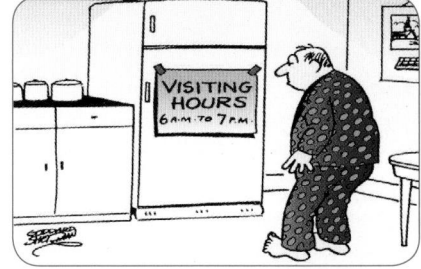

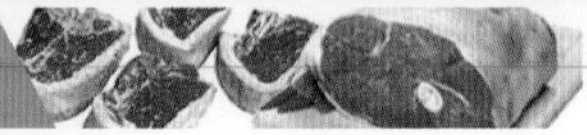

### Beef – Individual Cuts

*Average All Grades*
Edible Weight (no bone)

| | C | F | Cb |
|---|---|---|---|
| **Brisket, whole, braised:** | | | |
| Lean + fat (¼" trim), 3 oz | 330 | 27 | 0 |
| Lean + marbling, 3 oz | 250 | 17 | 0 |
| Lean only, 3 oz | 185 | 9 | 0 |
| **Chuck blade, braised:** | | | |
| Lean + fat (¼"), 3 oz | 310 | 24 | 0 |
| Lean + marbling, 3 oz | 295 | 22 | 0 |
| Lean only, 3 oz | 245 | 13 | 0 |
| **Flank:** Raw, 4 oz | 175 | 8 | 0 |
| Braised, 3 oz | 225 | 14 | 0 |
| Broiled, 3 oz | 155 | 6 | 0 |
| **Round, bottom, braised:** | | | |
| Lean + marbling, 3 oz | 190 | 7.5 | 0 |
| Lean only, 3 oz | 185 | 6.5 | 0 |
| **Round, eye/tip, rstd:** | | | |
| Lean + fat (¼"), 3 oz | 205 | 11 | 0 |
| Lean (w/ marbling), 3 oz | 150 | 5 | 0 |
| **Round, top:** *Per 3 oz (cooked wt)* | | | |
| Braised, Lean + fat | 210 | 10 | 0 |
| Lean only | 170 | 4 | 0 |
| Broiled, Lean + fat | 180 | 8 | 0 |
| Lean only | 160 | 5 | 0 |
| Pan-fried, Lean + fat | 235 | 13 | 0 |
| Lean only | 195 | 7 | 0 |

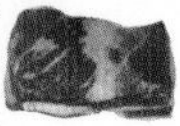

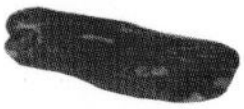

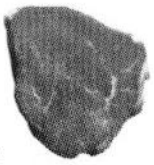

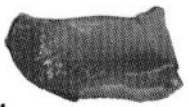

### Beef Ribs

| | C | F | Cb |
|---|---|---|---|
| **Back Ribs:** *7" long, visible fat trimmed to ¼"* | | | |
| 10.3 oz raw w/ bone or 3.5 oz cooked, braised, w/o bone | | | |
| 1 average rib | 410 | 34 | 0 |
| 3 ribs | 1230 | 102 | 0 |
| **Short Ribs:** *2½" long, visible fat trimmed to ¼"* | | | |
| 6 oz raw with bone or 2.5² oz cooked, braised, w/o bone | | | |
| 1 average rib | 320 | 28 | 0 |
| 3 ribs | 960 | 85 | 0 |

### Ground Beef

| | C | F | Cb |
|---|---|---|---|
| **Ground Beef, Raw:** *Per 4 oz* | | | |
| 70% lean (30% fat) | 380 | 34 | 0 |
| 75% lean (25% fat) | 335 | 29 | 0 |
| 80% lean (20% fat) | 290 | 23 | 0 |
| 85% lean (15% fat) | 245 | 17 | 0 |
| 90% lean (10% fat) | 200 | 12 | 0 |
| 95% lean (5% fat) | 155 | 6 | 0 |
| **Baked/Broiled:** Reg. (70%), 3 oz | 230 | 16 | 0 |
| Lean (80%), 3 oz | 215 | 14 | 0 |
| Extra lean (90%), 3 oz | 185 | 10 | 0 |
| **Pan-Broiled:** | | | |
| Reg. (70%), 3 oz | 230 | 15 | 0 |
| Lean (80%), 3 oz | 210 | 14 | 0 |
| Extra lean (90%), 3 oz | 195 | 10 | 0 |
| **Ground Beef Patties:** *Average, 23% Fat* | | | |
| Raw, 4 oz | 330 | 25 | 0 |
| Broiled, 3 oz (from 4 oz raw) | 250 | 19 | 0 |

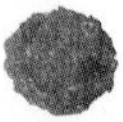

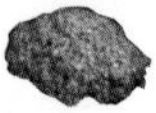

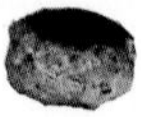

### Quick Guide

**Roast Beef**

**Round (Eye/Tip, average):** *Average All Cuts*

| | C | F | Cb |
|---|---|---|---|
| **Small/Regular Serving:** *3 oz* | | | |
| (2 thin slices/1 thick slice) | | | |
| Lean + fat (⅛" fat trim) | 180 | 9 | 0 |
| Lean only | 145 | 4 | 0 |
| **Medium Serving:** *5 oz* | | | |
| (3-4 thin slices) | | | |
| Lean + fat (⅛" fat trim) | 300 | 15 | 0 |
| Lean only | 245 | 6.5 | 0 |
| **Large Serving, 8 oz:** *3 thick slices* | | | |
| Lean + fat (⅛" fat trim) | 480 | 24 | 0 |
| Lean only | 385 | 11 | 0 |

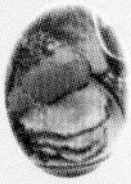

### Roast Dinner Extras

| | C | F | Cb |
|---|---|---|---|
| **Gravy:** Thin, 2 Tbsp | 20 | 0.5 | 3.5 |
| Thick, 2 Tbsp | 50 | 2 | 0.5 |
| 1 Ladle/4 Tbsp | 100 | 4 | 1 |
| **Veggies:** Beans, green, ½ cup | 20 | 0 | 5 |
| Cauliflower w/ chse sauce, 4 oz | 135 | 9 | 15 |
| Corn, kernels, ¼ cup | 35 | 0 | 9 |
| Carrots, ¼ cup | 20 | 0 | 3 |
| Peas, ¼ cup | 35 | 0 | 6 |
| **Potato:** Rstd w/ fat, 1 small | 155 | 8 | 30 |
| Baked in Jacket, 1 large | 280 | 0 | 63 |
| with 1 Tbsp whipped butter | 350 | 8 | 63 |
| with Sour Cream, 2 Tbsp | 270 | 5 | 64 |
| **Sweet Potato/Yam,** 1 medium | 105 | 1 | 24 |

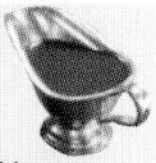

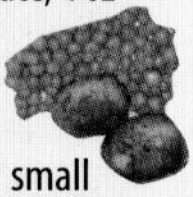

| | C | F | Cb |
|---|---|---|---|
| **Beef Kebab:** *Cooked* | | | |
| Beef & Veggies, 2 oz | 160 | 10 | 4 |
| If very lean meat | 100 | 4 | 4 |

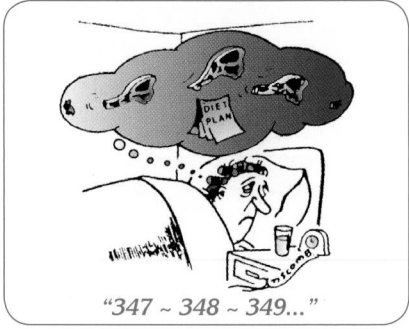

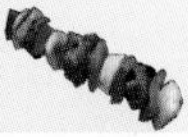

*"347 ~ 348 ~ 349..."*

## Lamb

|  | C | F | Cb |
|---|---|---|---|

**Choice Grade:**

**Leg (Whole), roasted:**

| | | | |
|---|---|---|---|
| Lean + fat, 3 oz | 220 | 14 | 0 |
| Lean only, 3 oz | 160 | 7 | 0 |

**Leg (Sirloin Half), roasted:**

| | | | |
|---|---|---|---|
| Lean + fat, 3 oz | 250 | 18 | 0 |
| Lean only, 3 oz | 175 | 8 | 0 |

**Leg (Shank Half), roasted:**

| | | | |
|---|---|---|---|
| Lean + fat, 3 oz | 190 | 11 | 0 |
| Lean only, 3 oz | 155 | 6 | 0 |

**Loin Chop, broiled:**

| | | | |
|---|---|---|---|
| 1 chop (raw weight, 4.25 oz): | 250 | 17 | 0 |
| Lean + fat (2.25 oz edible) | 180 | 12 | 0 |
| Lean only (1.6 oz edible) | 85 | 3.5 | 0 |

**Rib Chop, broiled:**

| | | | |
|---|---|---|---|
| 1 chop (raw wt., 3.5 oz) | | | |
| Lean + fat (2.5 oz edible) | 255 | 21 | 0 |
| Lean only (1.75 oz edible) | 105 | 6 | 0 |

**Shoulder (Arm/Blade):**

| | | | |
|---|---|---|---|
| Braised: Lean + fat, 3 oz | 295 | 21 | 0 |
| Lean only, 3 oz | 240 | 12 | 0 |
| Broiled: Lean + fat, 3 oz | 240 | 17 | 0 |
| Lean only, 3 oz | 170 | 8 | 0 |
| Roasted: Similar to Broiled | | | |

**Cubed Lamb (Leg/Shoulder):**

For stew or kebab

| | | | |
|---|---|---|---|
| Braised, lean only, 3 oz | 190 | 8 | 0 |
| Broiled, lean only, 3 oz | 160 | 6 | 0 |

## Veal

**Edible Weights:**

|  | C | F | Cb |
|---|---|---|---|

**Leg (Top Round):**

| | | | |
|---|---|---|---|
| Braised: Lean + fat, 3 oz | 180 | 6 | 0 |
| Lean only, 3 oz | 175 | 5 | 0 |
| Pan-fried, breaded: | | | |
| Lean + fat, 3 oz | 195 | 8 | 9 |
| Lean only, 3 oz | 185 | 6 | 9 |
| Pan-fried, not breaded: | | | |
| Lean + fat, 3 oz | 180 | 7 | 0 |
| Lean only, 3 oz | 155 | 4 | 0 |
| Roasted: Lean + fat, 3 oz | 135 | 4 | 0 |
| Lean only, 3 oz | 130 | 3 | 0 |

## Veal (Cont)

|  | C | F | Cb |
|---|---|---|---|

**Loin Chop:** *1 chop, 7 oz raw weight*

| | | | |
|---|---|---|---|
| Braised: Lean + fat, 3 oz | 240 | 15 | 0 |
| Lean only, 3 oz | 190 | 8 | 0 |
| Roasted: Lean + fat, 3 oz | 185 | 11 | 0 |
| Lean only, 3 oz | 150 | 6 | 0 |

**Rib, roasted:** *Lean + fat, 3 oz*

| | | | |
|---|---|---|---|
| | 195 | 12 | 0 |
| Lean only, 3 oz | 150 | 7 | 0 |

**Shoulder, Arm/Blade, roasted:**

| | | | |
|---|---|---|---|
| Lean + fat, 3 oz | 155 | 7 | 0 |
| Lean only, 3 oz | 140 | 5 | 0 |

**Sirloin, roasted:**

| | | | |
|---|---|---|---|
| Lean + fat, 3 oz | 170 | 9 | 0 |
| Lean only, 3 oz | 145 | 6 | 0 |

**Cubed for Stew, braised:**

| | | | |
|---|---|---|---|
| Leg/Shoulder, lean only, 3 oz | 160 | 4 | 0 |
| (1 lb raw yields approx. 9.25 oz cooked) | | | |

## Pork

**Fresh Pork:** *Cooked Weight, no bone):*
*4 oz raw weight = approx. 3 oz cooked weight*

**Blade Steak, broiled:**

| | | | |
|---|---|---|---|
| Lean + fat, 3 oz | 220 | 15 | 0 |
| Lean only, 3 oz | 190 | 11 | 0 |

**Country Style Ribs, broiled/roasted:**

| | | | |
|---|---|---|---|
| Lean + fat, 3 oz | 280 | 22 | 0 |
| Lean only, 3 oz | 210 | 13 | 0 |

**Spareribs,** braised: *lean & fat, 6 oz*

| | | | |
|---|---|---|---|
| (from 1 lb raw weight) | 675 | 52 | 0 |

**Leg (Ham), whole, roasted:**

| | | | |
|---|---|---|---|
| Lean + fat, 3 oz | 230 | 15 | 0 |
| Lean only, 3 oz | 180 | 8 | 0 |

**Loin Chops, broiled:** *Average*

| | | | |
|---|---|---|---|
| (From 1 chop: 5 oz raw weight with bone or 4 oz raw weight, without bone) | | | |
| Lean + fat, 3 oz | 200 | 11 | 0 |
| Lean only, 3 oz | 165 | 7 | 0 |

**Loin Roast, roasted:**

| | | | |
|---|---|---|---|
| Lean + fat, 3 oz | 210 | 13 | 0 |
| Lean only, 3 oz | 180 | 8 | 0 |

**Rib Chops, (Boneless), broiled:**

| | | | |
|---|---|---|---|
| Lean + fat, 3 oz | 220 | 14 | 0 |
| Lean only, 3 oz | 185 | 9 | 0 |

**Rib Roast:**

| | | | |
|---|---|---|---|
| Lean + fat, 3 oz | 215 | 13 | 0 |
| Lean only, 3 oz | 180 | 9 | 0 |

## Pork (Cont)

| | C | F | Cb |
|---|---|---|---|
| **Sirloin Chop, broiled:** | | | |
| Lean + fat, 3 oz | 180 | 8 | 0 |
| Lean only, 3 oz | 165 | 6 | 0 |
| **Sirloin Roast, roasted:** | | | |
| Lean + fat, 3 oz | 175 | 8 | 0 |
| Lean only, 3 oz | 170 | 7 | 0 |
| **Tenderloin (Boneless), roasted:** | | | |
| Lean + fat, 3 oz | 125 | 4 | 0 |
| Lean only, 3 oz | 120 | 3 | 0 |
| **Ground Pork:** | | | |
| Raw: Average, ¼ lb, 4 oz | 300 | 24 | 0 |
| Broiled, 3 oz | 250 | 18 | 0 |
| Pan-fried, drained, 3 oz | 260 | 19 | 0 |

## Bacon

| | C | F | Cb |
|---|---|---|---|
| **Raw:** 1 med. slice, 0.75 oz | 95 | 9 | 0 |
| 1 thick slice, 1⅓ oz | 175 | 17 | 0 |
| (1 lb raw yields approximately 5 oz cooked) | | | |
| **Broiled/Pan-Fried:** | | | |
| 1 medium slice, 0.3 oz | 40 | 3 | 0 |
| 3 medium slices, 0.8 | 125 | 10 | 0 |
| 2 thin slices, 0.5 oz | 75 | 6 | 0 |
| 1 thick slice, 0.85 oz | 65 | 5 | 0 |
| **Canadian Bacon:** | | | |
| Cooked, 1 slice, 1 oz | 45 | 2 | 0.5 |
| Pkg, 3 slices, 2 oz | 90 | 4 | 1 |
| **Bacon Bits,** 1 T., 0.25 oz | 35 | 2 | 0 |
| **Breakfast Strips,** Broiled, 1 sl.,, 0.42 oz | 50 | 4 | 0 |

## Ham

| | C | F | Cb |
|---|---|---|---|
| **Boneless Ham,** cooked: | | | |
| Regular, (approximately 13% fat): | | | |
| Roasted, 3 oz | 150 | 8 | 0 |
| Extra Lean (5% fat), | | | |
| Roasted, 3 oz | 125 | 5 | 0 |
| **Whole Ham,** cooked: | | | |
| Lean + fat (as purchased) | | | |
| Roasted, 3 oz | 210 | 15 | 0 |
| Lean only, Roasted, 3 oz | 135 | 5 | 0 |
| **Canned Ham:** *Similar to boneless ham* | | | |
| Chopped, canned, 3 oz | 200 | 16 | 0 |
| Ham Patties, cooked, 1 pattie, 2.25 oz | 220 | 20 | 1 |
| Ham Steak, extra lean, 2 oz | 70 | 2.5 | 0 |
| **Lunch Slices ~** *See Deli Meats, Page 128* | | | |

## Game & Other Meats

| | C | F | Cb |
|---|---|---|---|
| **Bison Steak,** | | | |
| lean, 6 oz (raw) | 205 | 4 | 0 |
| **Boar (wild),** roasted, 3 oz | 140 | 4 | 0 |
| **Buffalo Steak:** *New West Foods,* 4 oz | 70 | 3 | 0 |
| *Trader Joe's,* 1 pattie | 430 | 30 | 1 |
| **Caribou,** roasted, 3 oz | 140 | 4 | 0 |
| **Deer/Venison,** roasted 3 oz | 135 | 3 | 0 |
| **Goat (Capretto):** | | | |
| Raw, 3 oz | 95 | 2 | 0 |
| Roasted, 3 oz | 120 | 2.5 | 0 |
| **Ostrich:** *Blackwing Ostrich Meats,* | | | |
| Sport Jerky, 0.5 oz piece | 25 | 0 | 0 |
| Sausage Patties (2) 2 oz | 60 | 0.5 | 0 |
| *New West Foods:* | | | |
| Ground Ostrich, 4 oz | 165 | 7 | 0 |
| Ostrich Steak, 4 oz steak | 130 | 2.5 | 0 |
| **Rabbit:** Roasted, 3 oz | 165 | 7 | 0 |
| Stewed, 1 cup, diced, 5 oz | 290 | 12 | 0 |

## Variety & Organ Meats

| | C | F | Cb |
|---|---|---|---|
| **Brain (Lamb):** Braised, 3 oz | 125 | 9 | 0 |
| Pan-fried, 3 oz | 230 | 19 | 0 |
| **Chitterlings,** pork, simmered, 3 oz | 260 | 25 | 0 |
| **Ears,** pork, simmered, 1 ear, 4 oz | 185 | 12 | 0 |
| **Feet,** pork: Simmered, 3 oz | 200 | 14 | 0 |
| Cured, pickled, 3 oz | 170 | 14 | 0 |
| *Hormel,* 2 oz | 80 | 6 | 0 |
| **Head Cheese (Pork Snouts/Ears/Vinegar/Spices):** | | | |
| 1 oz slice | 50 | 4 | 0 |
| **Heart,** Beef, braised, 3 oz | 140 | 4 | 0 |
| **Jowl,** pork, raw, 4 oz | 750 | 80 | 0 |
| **Kidneys,** braised, 3 oz | 140 | 5 | 0 |
| **Liver (beef):** Raw, 4 oz | 150 | 4 | 4 |
| Braised, 3 oz | 140 | 4 | 3 |
| Pan-fried, 3 oz | 185 | 7 | 7 |
| **Pancreas,** pork, braised, 3 oz | 185 | 8 | 0 |
| **Pork Cracklins,** 0.5 oz | 80 | 6 | 0 |
| **Pork Hocks,** 1 piece, 6 oz | 340 | 23 | 0 |
| **Scrapple,** pork, 2 oz | 120 | 8 | 8 |
| **Spleen,** pork, braised, 3 oz | 130 | 3 | 0 |
| **Stomach,** pork, raw, 4 oz | 185 | 12 | 0 |
| **Sweetbreads:** | | | |
| Beef, cooked, 3 oz | 125 | 9 | 0 |
| Lamb, cooked, 3 oz | 125 | 9 | 0 |
| **Tail,** pork, simmered, 3 oz | 340 | 31 | 0 |
| **Tongue,** raised, Veal, 3 oz | 170 | 9 | 0 |
| Beef/Lamb/Pork, av., 3 oz | 235 | 17 | 0 |
| **Tripe,** beef, raw, 3 oz | 85 | 3.5 | 0 |

### Quick Guide

**Franks & Weiners**
*Average All Brands*

| | C | F | Cb |
|---|---|---|---|
| **Regular (Pork Mix):** *Per Frank* | | | |
| Regular (10/16 oz package), 1.5 oz | 140 | 13 | 1 |
| Bun Length/Jumbo, 2 oz | 185 | 17 | 2 |
| Extra Long, 2.75 oz | 255 | 24 | 2 |
| Small/Cocktail (50/lb), each | 30 | 3 | 0.5 |
| **Beef Franks:** *Per Frank* | | | |
| Regular (10/16 oz package), 1.5 oz | 140 | 13 | 2 |
| Bun Length/Jumbo, 2 oz | 175 | 16 | 2.5 |
| ¼ lb Dog, 4 oz | 375 | 33 | 5 |

### Franks & Weiners

| | C | F | Cb |
|---|---|---|---|
| **Ball Park:** *Per 2 oz Frank Unless Indicated* | | | |
| **Angus Beef:** | | | |
| Original; Bun Size | 170 | 15 | 3 |
| Lower Fat, 1.87 oz | 130 | 10 | 2 |
| **Beef:** Original | 190 | 16 | 4 |
| Fat Free, 1.75 oz | 50 | 0 | 7 |
| Lite, 1.75 oz | 110 | 7 | 5 |
| Deli Style | 140 | 12 | 2 |
| **Cheese,** with Turkey, Beef & Pork | 190 | 16 | 5 |
| **GrillMaster:** Hearty Beef (1), 2.9 oz | 250 | 21 | 3 |
| Beef: Fat Free, 1.75 oz | 50 | 0 | 7 |
| Lite, 1.75 oz | 110 | 7 | 6 |
| **Meat:** Original; Bun Size | 180 | 15 | 5 |
| Lite, 1.75 oz | 100 | 7 | 4 |
| Singles, 1.6 oz | 140 | 12 | 3 |
| **Turkey:** Original | 110 | 7 | 6 |
| Smoked White, 1.75 oz | 45 | 0 | 5 |
| **Foster Farms:** *Per Frank* | | | |
| Chicken;Turkey, 2 oz | 140 | 12 | 1 |
| **Hebrew National:** *Per Frank* | | | |
| **Beef:** Regular, 1.72 oz | 150 | 14 | 1 |
| ¼ Pounder (4 oz) | 360 | 33 | 3 |
| Jumbo, 2 oz | 270 | 25 | 2 |
| 97% Fat-Free, 1.6 oz | 40 | 1 | 3 |
| Beef Frank in a Blanket, 5 pcs, 3 oz | 300 | 24 | 12 |
| **Jennie-O:** *Per Frank* | | | |
| **Turkey Franks:** 1.2 oz | 70 | 5 | 1 |
| Jumbo, 2 oz | 120 | 9 | 2 |
| **Oscar Mayer:** *Per Frank* | | | |
| **Beef,** 1.6 oz | 130 | 12 | 1 |
| **Cheese Dogs,** 1.6 oz | 140 | 13 | 1 |
| **Turkey:** Classic, 1.6 oz | 100 | 8 | 2 |
| Classic Bun Length, 2 oz | 120 | 10 | 3 |
| **Shelton's:** *Per Frank* | | | |
| Chicken, 1.2 oz | 80 | 6 | 0.5 |
| Smoked Chicken, 3 oz | 190 | 17 | 2 |
| Turkey, 1.2 oz | 60 | 4.5 | 1 |
| **Zacky Farms,** Chicken; Turkey, av | 115 | 10 | 4 |

### Quick Guide

**Fresh Sausages**
**Pork/Beef:** *Average All Types*

| | C | F | Cb |
|---|---|---|---|
| **Small:** Raw, 4" link, 1 oz | 85 | 7.5 | 0 |
| Broiled/Pan-fried | 80 | 7 | 0 |
| **Medium:** Raw, 2 oz | 170 | 15 | 0 |
| Broiled/Pan-fried | 165 | 14 | 0 |
| **Large:** Raw, 3 oz | 255 | 22 | 0 |
| Broiled/Pan-fried | 245 | 21 | 0 |
| **Italian:** Raw, 3.2 oz | 315 | 28 | 0.5 |
| Cooked, 2.4 oz | 230 | 18 | 3 |
| **Chorizo:** Beef Chorizo, 2.5 oz piece | 250 | 23 | 5 |
| Pork Chorizo, 2 oz piece | 250 | 23 | 5 |

**Note:** Fat is lost in broiling/pan frying.
(Cooked weight = approx. 60-70% raw weight)

### Smoked Sausage

| | C | F | Cb |
|---|---|---|---|
| **Average All Brands:** | | | |
| 2 oz link | 170 | 15 | 0 |
| 3 oz link | 255 | 22 | 0 |
| **Ball Park,** | | | |
| Smoked White Turkey, Bun Size, 1.75 oz | 45 | 0 | 5 |
| **Butterball,** | | | |
| Turkey, 2.8 oz | 150 | 8 | 7 |
| **Eckrich,** Grillers, av.,2 oz | 180 | 15 | 4 |
| **Hillshire Farm:** Beef, 2 oz | 170 | 15 | 3 |
| Hardwood Smoked Chicken, 2 oz | 90 | 5 | 3 |
| Italian Style, 2 oz | 190 | 16 | 3 |
| Turkey, 2 oz | 90 | 5 | 3 |

### Breakfast Sausages/Patties

| | C | F | Cb |
|---|---|---|---|
| **Butterball:** | | | |
| Turkey: B'fast Ssg Links, cooked (3) | 110 | 6 | 2 |
| Sausae Patties (2), cooked | 110 | 6 | 2 |
| **Jennie-O:** | | | |
| Breakfast Sausages, uncooked | | | |
| Turkey (2), lean, | 90 | 5 | 0 |
| Turkey Pattie, uncooked, | | | |
| white, extra lean, 3.95 oz | 140 | 5 | 0 |
| **Jimmy Dean:** | | | |
| **Heat 'N Serve:** Sausage Links (3) | 210 | 19 | 1 |
| Sausage Patties (2) | 200 | 17 | 1 |
| Maple Sausage Links (3) | 220 | 18 | 4 |
| **Breakfast Sandwiches** ~ *See Page 92* | | | |
| **Jones Golden Brown:** | | | |
| **All Natural:** Beef Sausage Links (3) | 200 | 18 | 2 |
| Maple Sausage (3) | 240 | 22 | 2 |
| Sausage Patties, All Natural (1) | 120 | 12 | 0 |

**Vegetarian Patties:**
Boca ~ *See Page 117*
Garden Burger ~ *See Page 118*

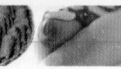

## Bagel, Corn & Hot Dogs

### Hot Dogs, Ready-To-Go:

| (Includes Ketchup/Relish; w/o Mayo) | **C** | **F** | **Cb** |
|---|---|---|---|
| **Regular,** 1.5 oz frank, 1.5 oz bun | 260 | 15 | 22 |
| **Bun Length,** 2 oz frank, 1.5 oz bun | 290 | 18 | 21 |
| **Jumbo Dog,** 2 oz frank, 2 oz bun | 360 | 20 | 36 |
| **¼ lb Beef Dog,** 2 oz bun | 480 | 15 | 36 |
| **Mile Long Dog,** 2.6 oz dog, 1.5 oz bun | 360 | 24 | 23 |

### Corn Dogs:

| | | | |
|---|---|---|---|
| Beef/Pork Frank, average, 2.6 oz | 170 | 10 | 16 |
| **Foster Farms,** Corn Dogs: 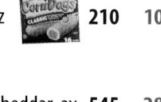 | | | |
| Chili Cheese (1), 2.7 oz | 190 | 9 | 21 |
| Honey Crunchy (1), 2.7 oz | 180 | 9 | 19 |
| Mini (4), 2.7 oz | 210 | 12 | 18 |
| **State Fair with Ball Park Franks:** | | | |
| Beef Corn Dog (1), 2.7 oz | 220 | 10 | 25 |
| Classic Corn Dog (1), 2.7 oz | 210 | 10 | 23 |

### Bagel Dogs:

| **Einstein Bros,** | | | |
|---|---|---|---|
| Asiago/Original with Cheddar, av | 545 | 28 | 56 |
| **Vienna Beef:** Bageldog (1), 5 oz | 420 | 17 | 33 |
| Mini (1), 2.8 oz | 150 | 4 | 20 |

### Hot Dog Toppings/Extras:

| **American Cheese,** 1 slice, 1 oz | 110 | 9 | 1 |
|---|---|---|---|
| **Chili,** with Beans, ¼ cup | 70 | 3.5 | 9 |
| **Ketchup,** 1 Tbsp | 15 | 0 | 4 |
| **Mustard,** 1 Tbsp | 20 | 0 | 1 |
| **Onions,** chopped, 1 Tbsp | 5 | 0 | 1 |
| **Pickle Relish,** 1 Tbsp | 20 | 0 | 5 |
| **Sauerkraut,** ½ cup | 20 | 0 | 5 |

## Deli & Lunch Meats

| **Beef Jerky/Meat Snacks,** | **C** | **F** | **Cb** |
|---|---|---|---|
| Berliner (pork/beef), 1 oz | 65 | 5 | 1 |
| **Beerwurst (Beef):** | | | |
| Small (2¾"diam), ¹⁄₁₆" sl. | 20 | 2 | 0 |
| Large (4" diam), ⅛" slice | 75 | 7 | 0.5 |
| **Beerwurst (Pork):** | | | |
| Small (2.75"diameter), ¹⁄₁₆" slice | 15 | 1 | 0 |
| Large (4"diameter), ⅛" Slice | 55 | 4 | 0.5 |
| **Blood Sausage,** 1 oz | 100 | 9 | 0.5 |

## Deli & Lunch Meats (Cont)

| **Bologna:** | **C** | **F** | **Cb** |
|---|---|---|---|
| 1 Slice, 1 oz | 65 | 6 | 1 |
| Fat-Free, 1 slice, 1 oz | 20 | 0 | 2 |
| Beef Bologna: 1 slice, 1 oz | 90 | 8 | 1 |
| Light, 1 slice, 1 oz | 60 | 4 | 2 |
| Light *(Oscar Mayer)*, 1 slice, 1 oz | 60 | 4 | 2 |
| 98% Fat Free *(Oscar Mayer)*, 1 oz | 25 | 0.5 | 3 |
| Ring *(Boar's Head)*, 2 oz | 150 | 13 | 0 |
| Turkey, average, 1 oz | 60 | 5 | 0.5 |
| **Bratwurst:** Average, 1 oz | 80 | 7 | 1 |
| *Bob Evan's,* Beer, 2.6 oz link | 270 | 21 | 1 |
| **Braunschweiger,** (Pork/Liver/Sausage), | | | |
| *Oscar Mayer,* 2 oz slice | 190 | 17 | 1 |
| **Chicken:** *Average All Brands* | | | |
| 1 thick or 2 thin slices, 1 oz | 30 | 1 | 1 |
| *Hillshire Farm,* Oven Rstd, Ultra Thin, 2 oz | 60 | 1 | 2 |
| **Corned Beef,** average, full fat, 1 oz | 60 | 5 | 0.5 |
| **Ham, Sliced:** | | | |
| Baked/Boiled, sliced, 1 oz | 30 | 1 | 0.5 |
| *Oscar Mayer,* 1 oz slice | 60 | 2 | 0.5 |
| Honey/Brown Sugar, av., 1 oz | 35 | 1 | 1 |
| Prosciutto, average, 1 oz | 70 | 5 | 0 |
| **Ham & Cheese Loaf,** average, 1 oz | 70 | 5 | 1 |
| **Italian Sausage,** 2.6 oz | 250 | 20 | 3 |
| **Kielbasa,** Polish Sausage, 2 oz | 65 | 5 | 1 |
| Beef, 2 oz link | 190 | 17 | 1 |
| *Boar's Head,* 1 oz | 60 | 5 | 0 |
| *Hillshire Farm,* 2.68 oz | 250 | 22 | 4 |
| **Knockwurst,** av., 1 oz | 90 | 8 | 0.5 |
| **Linguica** *(Gaspar's)*, 2 oz | 180 | 8 | 1 |
| **Liverwurst,** 1 oz | 65 | 5 | 2 |
| **Liver Pate,** fresh, average, 1 oz | 90 | 8 | 1 |
| **Luncheon Loaf** *(Armour)*, 1 oz | 70 | 5.5 | 2 |
| **Mortadella,** 1 oz | 105 | 9 | 0 |
| **Olive Loaf:** Average, 1 oz | 70 | 5 | 3 |
| *Oscar Mayer,* 1 oz | 80 | 6 | 3 |
| **Pancetta,** (Boars Head), 1 slice | 50 | 4.5 | 0 |

## Deli & Lunch Meats (Cont)

| | C | F | Cb |
|---|---|---|---|
| **Pastrami (Beef):** | | | |
| *Healthy Deli*, 2 oz | 70 | 2 | 1 |
| *Hillshire*, DeliSelect, 6 slice, 2 oz | 60 | 1 | 0 |
| *Boar's Head*, Round, 2 oz | 80 | 3.5 | 1 |
| **Peppered Beef**, 1 oz slice | 40 | 2 | 1 |
| **Pepperoni**, 5 slices, 1 oz | 140 | 13 | 0 |
| **Pickle Loaf**, av., 1 oz | 70 | 5 | 5 |
| **Pickle & Pepper Loaf,** | | | |
| *Boars Head*, 2 oz | 150 | 13 | 2 |
| **Proscuitto/Proscuitti**, av., 1 oz | 70 | 5 | 1 |
| **Roast Beef**, Lean, 1 oz | 40 | 2 | 0 |
| **Salami:** Beef, average, 1 oz | 80 | 7 | 1 |
| *Kraft*, 1 slice, 1.76 oz | 150 | 13 | 0 |
| Beer Salami, average, 1 oz | 50 | 4 | 0.5 |
| *Kraft*, Cotto, 1 slice, 1 oz | 60 | 5 | 1 |
| Dry: Hard, av., 4 slices, 1 oz | 100 | 8 | 1 |
| Genoa: Average, 1 oz | 100 | 8 | 1 |
| Stick, 1.75 oz | 175 | 14 | 2 |
| *Bridgford*, Italian, 1 oz | 120 | 11 | 0 |
| *Louis Rich*, Turkey,1 oz | 40 | 2.5 | 0.5 |

**SPAM (Hormel):** *Per 2 oz Serving*

| | C | F | Cb |
|---|---|---|---|
| Classic: 2 oz serving | 180 | 16 | 1 |
| 7 oz can | 630 | 56 | 3.5 |
| 12 oz can | 1080 | 96 | 6 |
| Spam Lite: 2 oz | 110 | 8 | 1 |
| 12 oz can | 660 | 48 | 6 |

**Other Spam Products:**

| | C | F | Cb |
|---|---|---|---|
| Hickory Smoked, 2 oz | 170 | 15 | 2 |
| Hot & Spicy, 2 oz | 180 | 16 | 2 |
| Oven Roastd Turkey, 2 oz | 80 | 4 | 2 |
| Spam with Bacon, 2 oz | 180 | 16 | 1 |
| Spam with Cheese, 2 oz | 170 | 15 | 1 |
| Spam Spread, 2 oz | 140 | 12 | 1 |
| 25% Less Sodium | 180 | 16 | 1 |

**Spam Singles:**

| | C | F | Cb |
|---|---|---|---|
| Classic, 3 oz package | 250 | 22 | 2 |
| Lite, 3 oz package | 160 | 11 | 2 |

## Deli & Lunch Meats (Cont)

| | C | F | Cb |
|---|---|---|---|
| **Summer Sausage:** | | | |
| *Armour*, 1 oz | 95 | 9 | 1 |
| *Hillshire Farm*, 2 oz | 190 | 16 | 0.5 |
| **Treet** *(Armour)*, canned, 2 oz | 140 | 11 | 4 |
| **Turkey:** Average, 1 oz slice | 30 | 1 | 0.5 |
| ¾ oz slice | 22 | 0.5 | 0.5 |
| **Turkey Breast:** | | | |
| *Butterball*, oven roasted, 1 sl, 1.1 oz | 30 | 0.5 | 1 |
| *Hillshire Deli Select*, 6 slice, 2 oz | 50 | 0.5 | 3 |
| **Turkey Ham,** 1 slice, 1 oz | 35 | 1.5 | 0.5 |
| **Turkey Pastrami,** 1 oz | 35 | 1.5 | 1 |
| **Turkey Roll,** 1 oz | 40 | 2 | 0.5 |
| **Turkey Loaf,** 1 oz | 30 | 1 | 0.5 |
| **Vegetarian Deli** ~ *See Page 118* | | | |

## Meat Spreads

**Average All Brands:** *Per ¼ Cup, 2 oz*

| | C | F | Cb |
|---|---|---|---|
| Chicken, white meat | 130 | 10 | 2 |
| Ham, Deviled | 140 | 11 | 0 |
| Liverwurst | 190 | 16 | 2 |
| Roast Beef | 130 | 10 | 2 |
| Sandwich Spread | 140 | 10 | 9 |
| Turkey | 110 | 7 | 2 |

**Underwood:** *Per 2 oz*

| | C | F | Cb |
|---|---|---|---|
| Chicken, White Meat | 130 | 10 | 2 |
| Deviled Ham | 180 | 15 | 1 |
| Liverwurst | 160 | 13 | 4 |
| Roast Beef | 130 | 10 | 2 |

## Paté

| | C | F | Cb |
|---|---|---|---|
| **Boar's Head,** | | | |
| Strassburger Liverwurst, 2 oz | 170 | 15 | 1 |
| Braunschweiger, Light, 2 oz | 120 | 8 | 1 |
| **Les Trois Petit Cochons:** *Per 2 oz* | | | |
| Black Peppercorn | 200 | 19 | 1 |
| Chicken & Pork Livers with Truffle | 140 | 11 | 2 |
| Country Pate | 200 | 22 | 1 |
| Smoked Salmon | 110 | 9 | 2 |
| **Marcel Henri:** | | | |
| Pate de Champagne | 210 | 19 | 1 |
| Chicken Liver with Port Wine, 2 oz | 200 | 19 | 1 |
| Duck Truffle with Port Wine, 2 oz | 240 | 24 | 1 |
| **Old Wisconsin Paté,** | | | |
| Braunschweiger, 2 oz | 210 | 18 | 3 |

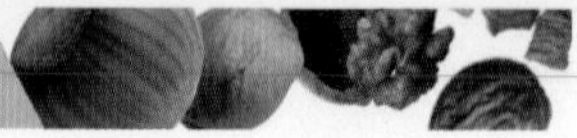

| Nuts | C | F | Cb |
|---|---|---|---|
| *Per 1 oz Unless Indicated* | | | |
| **Acorns,** raw 1 oz | 110 | 7 | 12 |
| **Almonds:** dried/dry roasted: | | | |
| Whole, 24-28 medium, 1 oz | 170 | 15 | 5.5 |
| ½ cup, 2½ oz | 420 | 37 | 13 |
| Chopped,½ cup, 2.25 oz | 380 | 34 | 12 |
| Sliced, ½ cup, 1.65 oz | 280 | 25 | 9 |
| Choc. coated (5-6), 1 oz | 150 | 10 | 15 |
| **Oil Rsted** *(Blue Diamond)*, 1 oz | 170 | 16 | 5 |
| Honey Roasted, 1 oz | 170 | 14 | 8 |
| Almond Meal (partially defattened) | | | |
| 1 cup (not packed), 2.25 oz | 260 | 11 | 11 |
| **Brazil Nuts,** 8 medium, 1 oz | 185 | 19 | 3.5 |
| **Cashews:** dry or oil roasted: | | | |
| 14 large/18 med./26 small, 1 oz | 165 | 14 | 9 |
| ½ cup, 2.4 oz | 375 | 31 | 20 |
| Honey Roasted, 1 oz | 165 | 13 | 10 |
| **Chestnuts,** av. all: Dried, 1 oz | 105 | 1 | 22 |
| Raw/Fresh, 5-6 nuts, 1 oz | 60 | 0 | 13 |
| Canned, water chestnuts, | | | |
| sliced/whole/drained, 1 oz | 30 | 0 | 7 |
| **Coconut:** fresh | | | |
| 1 piece, 2"x2"x ½", 1 oz | 100 | 10 | 4.5 |
| Shredded, fresh, ½ cup, 1.4 oz | 140 | 13 | 6 |
| Dried (Desiccated): | | | |
| Unsweetened, 1 oz | 185 | 18 | 7 |
| Sweetened: Shredded, 1 oz | 140 | 10 | 13 |
| Grated, ½ cup, 1.3 oz | 185 | 12 | 18 |
| Cream (canned), ½ cup, 5.2 oz | 285 | 26 | 12 |
| Milk (canned), ½ cup, 4 oz | 225 | 24 | 3 |
| Water (center liquid), ½ cup,4.25 oz | 25 | 0 | 4.5 |
| **Filberts or Hazelnuts:** | | | |
| Shelled, 18-20 nuts | 180 | 17 | 4.5 |
| Chopped, ¼ cup, 1 oz | 180 | 18 | 5 |
| Ground, ¼ cup, 0.6 oz | 120 | 12 | 3 |
| **Ginkgo Nuts,** canned, 14 med., 1 oz | 32 | 0.5 | 6.5 |
| **Hickory,** 30 small nuts, 1 oz | 200 | 18 | 5 |
| **Macadamia Nuts:** shelled: | | | |
| Raw, 7 medium/14 small, 1 oz | 200 | 21 | 4 |
| ½ cup, 2.3 oz | 480 | 51 | 10 |
| Dry Roasted, 1 oz | 205 | 22 | 4 |
| ½ cup, 2.4 oz | 480 | 51 | 9 |
| Choc. coated, 2-3 pieces, 1 oz | 170 | 12 | 14 |
| **Mixed Nuts:** 18-22 nuts, 1 oz | 170 | 15 | 7 |
| *Planters:* Dry Roasted/Honey | 160 | 12 | 9 |
| Oil Roasted, all types | 170 | 16 | 6 |
| Sweet Roasts, 26 pieces, 1 oz | 160 | 12 | 10 |
| **Nut Toppings,** chopped, 1 Tbsp, 0.25 oz | 40 | 4 | 1.5 |

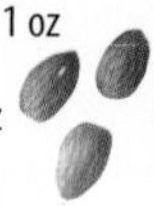

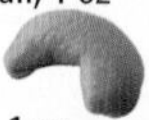

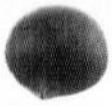

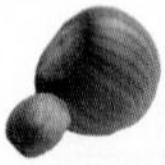

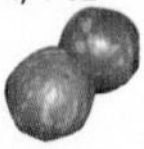

| *Per 1 oz Unless Indicated* | C | F | Cb |
|---|---|---|---|
| **Peanuts:** | | | |
| **Raw/Dried:** | | | |
| In shell, 1 oz | 117 | 10 | 3 |
| Shelled, 1 oz | 160 | 14 | 4.5 |
| **Boiled,** shelled, ½ cup, 3.1 oz | 285 | 20 | 19 |
| **Roasted:** 30 large/60 small | 165 | 14 | 6 |
| 1 cup, 5.1 oz | 860 | 76 | 22 |
| Chopped, 3 Tbsp | 165 | 14 | 6 |
| *Planters:* Cocktail | 170 | 14 | 5 |
| Rich Roasted in Milk Choc., 2.5 oz | 210 | 15 | 18 |
| Dry Roasted, Lightly Salted | 160 | 14 | 5 |
| Dry Roasted | 160 | 13 | 6 |
| Honey Roasted | 160 | 13 | 7 |
| Spanish Redskins, 1 oz | 170 | 15 | 4 |
| Sweet N' Crunchy | 140 | 8 | 15 |
| **Pecans:** Kernel halves | 195 | 20 | 4 |
| (20 jumbo or 31 large halves) | | | |
| 1 cup halves, 3.8 oz | 755 | 78 | 15 |
| Chopped, ½ cup, 2 oz | 380 | 39 | 7.5 |
| Oil Roasted, 15 halves | 205 | 20 | 4 |
| Honey Roasted, 1 oz | 200 | 21 | 4 |
| **Pilinuts,** dried, ¼ cup, 1 oz | 215 | 24 | 1 |
| **Pine Nuts,** dried, 1 Tbsp, 0.3 oz | 70 | 7 | 1.5 |
| **Pistachios:** Unshelled, ½ c., 2 oz | 165 | 14 | 7 |
| Shelled, ¼ cup, 45 nuts, 1 oz | 170 | 14 | 8.5 |
| *Lance,* 1.1 oz package | 95 | 7 | 4 |
| **Sesame Nut Mix,** 1 oz | 160 | 13 | 9 |
| **Soy Nuts:** Dry Roasted | 130 | 6 | 9 |
| ½ cup, 3 oz | 390 | 18 | 28 |
| *Dr Soy:* Chocolate coated, 1 oz pkg | 140 | 7 | 13 |
| Average other flavors | 150 | 8 | 8 |
| **Trail Mix** *(Planters)* | | | |
| Berry Almond | 130 | 5 | 19 |
| Energy Mix, 1.5 oz | 250 | 20 | 14 |
| Fruit & Nut | 140 | 9 | 14 |
| Mixed Nuts & Raisins | 160 | 12 | 11 |
| Nut & Chocolate, 1 oz | 150 | 9 | 14 |
| Nuts, Seeds & Raisins | 160 | 11 | 11 |
| Spicy Nuts & Cajun Sticks | 150 | 11 | 10 |
| Sweet & Nutty, 1 oz | 160 | 9 | 15 |
| **Walnuts:** | | | |
| Black: 15-20 halves, 1 oz | 175 | 17 | 3 |
| Chopped, ¼ cup, 1.1 oz | 195 | 18 | 3 |
| English/Persian: | | | |
| 14 halves, 1 oz | 185 | 18 | 4 |
| Chopped, ¼ cup, 1 oz | 190 | 19 | 4 |
| Ground, ¼ cup, 0.7 oz | 130 | 13 | 3 |

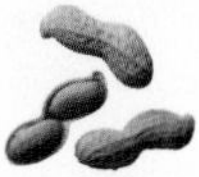

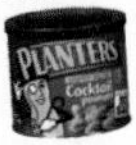

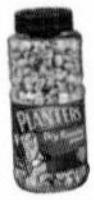

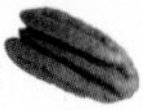

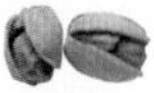

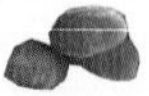

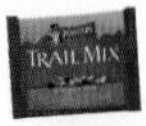

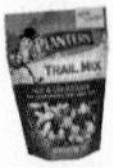

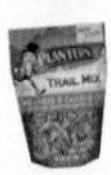

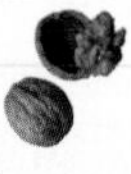

## Quick Guide

| | C | F | Cb |
|---|---|---|---|
| **Peanut Butter:** *Average All Brands* | | | |
| 1 level tsp, 0.2 oz | 35 | 3 | 1 |
| 1 level Tbsp, 0.6 oz | 100 | 8.5 | 3.5 |
| 2 level Tbsp, 1.2 oz | 200 | 17 | 7 |
| 1 oz Quantity | 165 | 14 | 6 |
| ½ cup, 5 oz | 835 | 72 | 29 |
| **Jif:** Reduced Fat, 2 Tbsp | 190 | 12 | 13 |
| Natural, | | | |
| Crmy; Crnchy; Simply, 2 T. | 190 | 16 | 8 |
| Peanut Butter & Honey, 2 T | 180 | 14 | 10 |
| **Laura Scudder's:** | | | |
| Smooth; Nutty, 2 Tbsp | 200 | 16 | 6 |
| **Peanut Wonder,** Original, 2 T. | 100 | 2 | 13 |
| **Peter Pan:** | | | |
| Natural: Creamy; Crunch, av., 2 Tbsp | 210 | 17 | 6 |
| Whipped, Creamy, 2 Tbsp | 150 | 12 | 5 |
| **Smucker's Goober:** | | | |
| Chocolate, 3 Tbsp | 230 | 11 | 27 |
| Grape/Strawberry 3 Tbsp | 240 | 13 | 24 |
| **Skippy:** Natural with Honey, 2 T. | 200 | 16 | 9 |
| Reduced Fat, all var., 2 T. | 180 | 12 | 15 |
| Roasted Honey Nut, all var., 2 Tbsp | 190 | 16 | 7 |

## Peanut Butter & Jelly Sandwich

| | C | F | Cb |
|---|---|---|---|
| **1 sandwich,** with 2 oz Bread: | | | |
| **Light Spread:** | 310 | 10 | 48 |
| (1 Tbsp Peanut Butter + 1 Tbsp Jelly) | | | |
| **Thick Spread:** | 480 | 19 | 67 |
| (2 T. Peanut Butter + 2 Tbsp Jelly) | | | |
| **With Goober Grape,** 3 Tbsp, 2 oz | 380 | 15 | 52 |

## Nutella

| | C | F | Cb |
|---|---|---|---|
| **Nut & Chocolate Spread:** | | | |
| 1 Tbsp, 0.7 oz | 100 | 5.5 | 11 |
| 2 Tbsp, 1.3 oz | 200 | 11 | 22 |

**Note:** *Nutella* contains approximately 50% sugar and only 13% hazelnuts

## Other Nut & Seed Butters

| | C | F | Cb |
|---|---|---|---|
| **Almond Butter,** 1 Tbsp, 0.5 oz | 100 | 10 | 3.5 |
| **Almond Butter,** Honey Rstd, 1 T. | 90 | 7 | 5.5 |
| **Beanut Butter,** 1 Tbsp, 0.5 oz | 90 | 5.5 | 7 |
| **Cashew Butter,** 1 Tbsp, 0.5 oz | 95 | 8 | 4.5 |
| **Hazelnut Butter,** 1 Tbsp, 0.5 oz | 105 | 10 | 2.5 |
| **Pecan Butter,** 1 Tbsp, 0.5 oz | 110 | 10 | 2 |
| **Pistachio Butter,** 1 Tbsp, 0.5 oz | 90 | 6.5 | 4.5 |
| **Sesame Butter (Tahini),** 1 T., 0.5 oz | 90 | 8 | 3 |
| **Soy Nut Butter,** 1 Tbsp, 0.5 oz | 75 | 5 | 4 |
| **Tahini** ~ *See Sesame Butter* | | | |

## Seeds

| | C | F | Cb |
|---|---|---|---|
| **Alfalfa Seeds,** | | | |
| sprouted, ½ cup, 0.5 oz | 5 | 0 | 1 |
| **Caraway/Fennel,** 1 tsp | 7 | 0.5 | 1 |
| **Chia Seeds:** 1 Tbsp, 0.35 oz | 45 | 3 | 4 |
| 3 Tbsp, 1 oz | 140 | 8.5 | 12 |
| **Cottonseed Kernels,** | | | |
| roasted, 1 Tbsp | 50 | 3.5 | 2 |
| **Flax Seeds,** | | | |
| 3 Tbsp, 1 oz | 140 | 9 | 9 |
| **Lotus Seeds,** | | | |
| dried, ½ cup, 0.5 oz | 55 | 0.5 | 10 |
| **Poppy Seeds,** 1 tsp | 15 | 1 | 1 |
| **Pumpkin & Squash Seeds,** whole: | | | |
| Roasted/Tamari, 1 oz | 150 | 12 | 4 |
| ½ cup, 4 oz | 590 | 48 | 15 |
| Dried, (hulled), ¼ cup, 1 oz | 155 | 13 | 5 |
| **Safflower Kernels,** | | | |
| dried, 1 oz | 150 | 11 | 10 |
| **Sesame Seeds:** | | | |
| Dried, 1 Tbsp, 0.3 oz | 50 | 4.5 | 2 |
| Roasted/Toasted, 1 oz | 160 | 14 | 7.5 |
| **Sunflower Kernels/Seeds:** | | | |
| Dried, ¼ cup w/out hulls, 0.25 oz | 200 | 18 | 7 |
| Dry Roasted, 1 Tbsp, 0.3 oz | 45 | 4 | 2 |
| ¼ cup, 1 oz | 165 | 14 | 7 |
| Oil Roasted, ⅓ cup, 1 oz | 170 | 14 | 6.5 |
| **Watermelon Seeds,** dried, | | | |
| ¼ cup, 1 oz | 150 | 13 | 4 |

*N*ut eaters are healthier and live longer, say scientists.

Nuts are a nutritious source of protein, vitamins, minerals, fiber, healthy fats, and antioxidants.

The fat and fiber of nuts can help reduce blood cholesterol. Their protein and fiber also promotes meal satiety (fullness) and reduces hunger levels – of benefit in weight control.

Eat nuts instead of high-sugar snacks, candy and soft drinks. Add chopped nuts to breakfast cereals.

### Quick Guide — C · F · Cb

**Pancakes:**

| | C | F | Cb |
|---|---|---|---|
| **Plain:** *Average All Types* | | | |
| Small (3" diameter), 0.75 oz | 50 | 2 | 6 |
| Medium (4" diameter), 1.25 oz | 85 | 3.5 | 11 |
| Large (6" diameter), 2.5 oz | 175 | 7.5 | 22 |
| *Add Extra for Syrups/Butter* | | | |
| **Pancake Syrup:** Regular, 1 Tbsp | 50 | 0 | 12 |
| ¼ cup, 4 Tbsp | 185 | 0 | 49 |
| Lite, 1 Tbsp | 25 | 0 | 6.5 |
| ¼ cup, 4 Tbsp | 100 | 0 | 27 |
| **Butter/Margarine:** | | | |
| Regular, 1 Tbsp | 100 | 11 | 0 |
| Whipped, 1 Tbsp | 65 | 7.5 | 0 |
| **Waffles:** | | | |
| **Homemade,** 7" waffle, 2.5 oz | 220 | 11 | 25 |
| **Frozen + Toasted,** (4" diam.), 1 oz | 105 | 3 | 16 |

### Frozen Breakfasts

| | C | F | Cb |
|---|---|---|---|
| **Aunt Jemima:** | | | |
| **Pancakes:** Blueberry (3) | 260 | 6 | 44 |
| Buttermilk (3) | 250 | 6 | 41 |
| Low-Fat (3) | 200 | 2 | 41 |
| Homestyle (3) | 250 | 6 | 41 |
| Whole Grain (3) | 240 | 6 | 42 |
| Mini Pancakes (10) | 280 | 8 | 45 |
| **Frozen Breakfasts:** | | | |
| French Toast: Cinnamon, 2 slices | 220 | 4.5 | 37 |
| Homestyle, 2 slices | 220 | 4.5 | 37 |
| Sticks, Cinn., (4) | 270 | 10 | 41 |
| **Eggo** *(Kellogg's):* | | | |
| **French Toaster Sticks,** (2), av | 220 | 6 | 35 |
| **Pancakes:** Blueberry (3) | 260 | 8 | 42 |
| Buttermilk Minis (11) | 260 | 8 | 42 |
| **Jimmy D's** *(Jimmy Dean):* | | | |
| French Toast Griddlers, 1 sandwich | 210 | 8 | 27 |
| Griddle Sticks, 1 stick | 160 | 6 | 21 |
| Pancake Griddlers, 1 sandwich | 230 | 8 | 33 |
| **Krusteaz:** | | | |
| **Pancakes:** | | | |
| Premium Mini (4) | 80 | 1 | 15 |
| Buttermilk (3) | 270 | 4 | 52 |
| **French Toast,** Cinn. Swirl, thick, (2) | 170 | 3 | 30 |
| **Pillsbury:** | | | |
| **Pancakes:** H'Style Orig.; B'milk (3) | 240 | 4 | 47 |
| Mini (11) | 240 | 4 | 45 |
| **Toaster Strudels,** w/ Icing, av. all, (1) | 180 | 9 | 24 |

### Pancake Brands — C · F · Cb

| | C | F | Cb |
|---|---|---|---|
| **Aunt Jemima Mixes:** *Prepared as Directed* | | | |
| Original, 4 x 4" | 250 | 8 | 36 |
| Original Complete, 2 x 4" | 160 | 1.5 | 32 |
| Buttermilk, 4 x 4" | 180 | 6.5 | 23 |
| Whole Wheat Blend, 3 x 4" | 200 | 6.5 | 30 |
| **Betty Crocker Pancake Mixes:** *Just Add Water* | | | |
| Complete Orig./Buttermilk (3) | 200 | 2.5 | 40 |
| Bisquick (Shake 'N Pour), (3) | 220 | 3 | 43 |
| **Hungry Jack Pancakes:** | | | |
| **Mixes:** *Per ⅓ Cup, Prepared as Directed* | | | |
| Complete: Buttermilk, 3 x 4" | 150 | 1.5 | 31 |
| Extra Light & Fluffy, 3 x 4" | 150 | 2 | 31 |
| Original, with 2% Milk, Oil, Egg | 250 | 8 | 37 |
| With Skim Milk, Oil, Egg Whites | 180 | 1 | 37 |
| **Easy Packs:** *Per ⅓ Cup Dry Mix, Prepared* | | | |
| Blueberry Wheat | 160 | 2.5 | 32 |
| Buttermilk | 150 | 1.5 | 31 |
| **Northern Pines,** | | | |
| (3), 3 x 4", 3.5 oz | 200 | 3.5 | 38 |

### Frozen Waffles

| | C | F | Cb |
|---|---|---|---|
| **Aunt Jemima:** Buttermilk (2) | 165 | 4.5 | 27 |
| Homestyle; Blueberry (2) | 175 | 5 | 28 |
| Low-Fat (2) | 160 | 3 | 27 |
| **Eggo** *(Kellogg's):* Blueberry (2) | 190 | 6 | 29 |
| Chocolate Chip (2) | 210 | 7 | 32 |
| French Toast (1) | 140 | 6 | 20 |
| Homestyle (2) | 190 | 7 | 27 |
| Nutri-Grain: | | | |
| Wholewheat; Blueberry (2), av. | 175 | 6 | 29 |
| Low-Fat (2) | 140 | 2.5 | 27 |
| **Kashi,** Go-Lean, average (1) | 150 | 5 | 25 |
| **Nature's Path:** Flax Plus (2), av. | 190 | 8 | 27 |
| Homestyle (2) | 270 | 10 | 44 |
| Mesa Sunrise (2) | 200 | 7 | 34 |
| **Smucker's,** | | | |
| Snack'nWaffles, av. all var., (1) | 215 | 8 | 32 |
| **Van's:** Belgian Homestyle (2) | 210 | 9 | 29 |
| **Mini:** Chocolate Chip (8) | 150 | 4 | 27 |
| Totally Natural (8) | 140 | 3.5 | 25 |
| Wheat Free Minis (8) | 150 | 5 | 25 |
| **Sticks:** Chocolate (1) | 80 | 2 | 14 |
| Vanilla (1) | 70 | 1 | 14 |

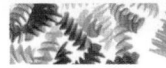 

- Pasta includes all shapes and sizes; (e.g. spaghetti, fettuccini, elbows, shells, twists, sheets, cannelloni, tubes, ziti).
- All regular pasta products have the same cals/fat/carbs on a weight basis.
- 1 oz Dry = approximately 2.5 -3 oz cooked.

### Dry Spaghetti/Pasta

| | C | F | Cb |
|---|---|---|---|
| **1 oz quantity** | 105 | 0.5 | 21 |
| **1lb box/package,** 16 oz | 1685 | 7 | 339 |
| **Elbows,** 1 cup, 3.75 oz | 380 | 2 | 80 |
| **Shells,** small, 1 cup, 3¼ oz | 330 | 1.5 | 69 |
| **Spirals,** 1 cup, 3 oz | 305 | 1.5 | 64 |

### Cooked Spaghetti/Pasta

| | C | F | Cb |
|---|---|---|---|
| **Plain, All Types (no added fat):** | | | |
| Firm/Al Dente (8-10 minutes), 1 oz | 42 | 0.5 | 8.5 |
| Medium (11-13 minutes), 1 oz | 37 | 0.5 | 7.5 |
| Tender (14-20 minutes), 1 oz | 32 | 0.5 | 7 |
| (Longer cooking increases water absorbed) | | | |
| **Spaghetti:** ½ cup, 2.5 oz | 90 | 0.5 | 18 |
| Medium serving, 1 cup, 5 oz | 225 | 1.5 | 44 |
| Large Serving, 2 cups, 10 oz | 450 | 3 | 88 |
| Extra Large, 3 cups, 15 oz | 675 | 5 | 132 |
| **Elbows/Spirals,** 1 cup, 5 oz | 220 | 1.5 | 43 |
| **Small Shells,** 1 cup, 4 oz | 180 | 1 | 36 |
| **Protein-fortified:** Dry, 1 c., 3.35 oz | 350 | 2 | 63 |
| Cooked, 1 cup, 5 oz | 230 | 0.5 | 45 |
| **Spinach/Vegetable:** Dry, 1 cup, 3 oz | 310 | 1 | 61 |
| Cooked, 1 cup, 5 oz | 180 | 0.5 | 38 |
| **Whole-wheat:** Dry, 1 cup, 3.75 oz | 365 | 1.5 | 79 |
| Cooked, 1 cup, 5 oz | 175 | 1 | 37 |

### Fresh Pasta (Refrigerated)

| | C | F | Cb |
|---|---|---|---|
| **Plain/Spinach/Tomato:** *Average:* | | | |
| As purchased, 4.5 oz | 370 | 3 | 70 |
| Cooked, 1 cup, 5 oz | 185 | 1.5 | 35 |
| **Home-made,** without egg, | | | |
| Cooked, 1 cup, 5 oz | 175 | 1 | 35 |
| **Buitoni:** | | | |
| **Cut Pasta:** *Per ⅓ of 9 oz Pkg* | | | |
| Angel Hair | 230 | 1.5 | 44 |
| Fettuccine | 240 | 2.5 | 44 |
| Linguine | 250 | 1.5 | 45 |
| **Ravioli:** Four Cheese, 3.7 oz | 340 | 12 | 42 |
| Light Four Cheese, 3.3 oz | 250 | 6 | 38 |
| Whole Wheat Four Cheese, 3.7 oz | 330 | 12 | 40 |

### Fresh Pasta (Refrigerated Cont.)

**Buitoni (Cont):**

| | C | F | Cb |
|---|---|---|---|
| **Tortellini:** Herb Chicken, 4 oz | 350 | 10 | 52 |
| Spinach Cheese, 1 cup, 3.7 oz | 320 | 7 | 49 |
| Three Cheese, 3.7 oz | 330 | 9 | 46 |
| **Tortelloni** | | | |
| Chse & Rsted Garlic, 3.15 oz | 270 | 8 | 37 |
| Av. other varieties, 3.75 oz | 340 | 10 | 49 |

**Pasta Sauces ~** *See Page 148*

### Macaroni & Cheese

**Packaged (Hormel/Kraft) ~** *See Page 112*

| **Restaurant:** *Average* | C | F | Cb |
|---|---|---|---|
| Side, 6 oz | 265 | 13 | 26 |
| Medium serving, 1 cup, 9 oz | 350 | 17 | 34 |
| Large serving, 2 cups, 18 oz | 700 | 34 | 68 |

### Noodles

| | C | F | Cb |
|---|---|---|---|
| **Plain/Egg:** Dry, 1 oz | 110 | 1.5 | 20 |
| 1 cup, 1.35 oz | 145 | 1.5 | 27 |
| **Cooked:** 1 oz | 40 | 0.5 | 7 |
| ½ cup, 2.75 oz | 110 | 1.5 | 20 |
| 1 cup, 5.5 oz | 220 | 3.5 | 40 |
| **Stir-Fried:** 1 cup, 5.5 oz | 270 | 9 | 40 |
| 2 cup serving, 11 oz | 540 | 18 | 80 |
| **Yolk Free (Cooked):** *Per Cup* | | | |
| 'No Yolks' *(Foulds)*, 2 oz | 210 | 0.5 | 41 |
| Passover Gold *(Manischewitz)* | 200 | 0 | 41 |
| **Chinese:** Cellophane/Rice, dry, 1 oz | 100 | 0 | 25 |
| Chow Mein/hard, dry, 1 oz | 150 | 9 | 16 |
| **Japanese:** Soba: Dry, 1 oz | 95 | 0.5 | 21 |
| Cooked, 1 cup, 4 oz | 115 | 0.5 | 24 |
| Somen: Dry, 1 oz | 100 | 0.5 | 21 |
| Cooked, 1 cup, 6 oz | 230 | 0.5 | 49 |
| **Japanese Style Pan Fried,** | | | |
| *Maruchan's,* Yaki-Sobu, 5.6 oz cup | 260 | 3 | 50 |
| **Ramen Noodles ~** *See Page 114* | | | |
| **Rice Noodles:** Dry, 3.5 oz | 365 | 0.5 | 83 |
| Cooked, 1 cup, 6.2 oz | 190 | 0.5 | 44 |
| Stir Fry (Yakisoba), 3.5 oz | 430 | 6 | 52 |
| *House Foods,* Tofu Shirataki, 4 oz | 20 | 0.5 | 3 |
| *Chikara,* Udon, average, 7.5 oz pkt | 250 | 1 | 52 |
| *Simply Asia/Thai Kitchen ~ Page 115* | | | |

### Egg Roll/Won Ton Wrappers

| | C | F | Cb |
|---|---|---|---|
| Egg/Spring Roll (1), 0.8 oz | 65 | 0 | 15 |
| Won Ton Wrapper (1), 0.25 oz | 20 | 0 | 4 |

## Quick Guide

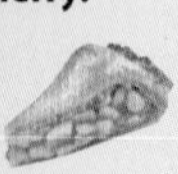

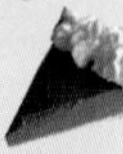

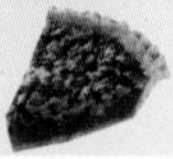

| Fruit Pies: *Average All Brands, 9"* | C | F | Cb |
|---|---|---|---|
| **Apple; Blueberry; Cherry:** | | | |
| Small, ⅛ pie, 4.75 oz | 350 | 16 | 49 |
| Med., ⅙ pie, 6.35 oz | 465 | 22 | 65 |
| Large, ¼ pie, 9.5 oz | 700 | 33 | 98 |
| Whole Pie (9"), 38oz | 2800 | 131 | 392 |
| **Other Pies:** *Per Serving, ⅙ of 8" Pie* | | | |
| Chocolate Cream Pie | 345 | 22 | 38 |
| Custard: Egg | 220 | 12 | 22 |
| Coconut | 270 | 14 | 31 |
| Lemon Meringue | 305 | 10 | 53 |
| Peach | 260 | 12 | 39 |
| Pecan | 440 | 23 | 57 |
| Pumpkin Pie | 315 | 14 | 41 |

## Brands

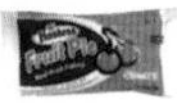

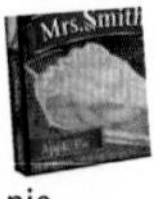

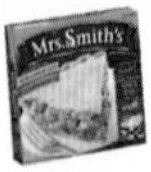

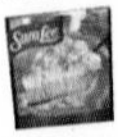

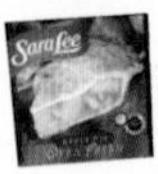

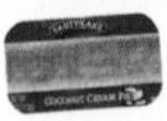

| | C | F | Cb |
|---|---|---|---|
| **Denny's:** Apple Pie, 7 oz | 480 | 22 | 67 |
| Chocolate French Silk Pie, 7 oz | 770 | 57 | 59 |
| **Hostess:** Cherry Pie, 4.5 oz | 480 | 20 | 69 |
| Lemon Pie, 4.5 oz | 490 | 22 | 69 |
| **Long John Silver's:** | | | |
| Chocolate Cream Pie | 280 | 17 | 28 |
| Pineapple Cream Pie | 300 | 17 | 35 |
| **Marie Callender's,** | | | |
| Banana Cream, ⅑ slice , 4.2 oz | 310 | 17 | 37 |
| **Mrs Smith's:** | | | |
| **Classic Pies:** | | | |
| Apple, ⅙ pie | 320 | 14 | 47 |
| Cherry, ⅙ pie | 300 | 14 | 40 |
| Dutch Apple Crumb, ⅙ pie | 340 | 14 | 52 |
| **Deep Dish,** Apple, ⅒ pie | 290 | 13 | 41 |
| **Pre Baked:** *Per ⅛ Pie* | | | |
| Apple Raisin Spiced | 370 | 16 | 55 |
| Dutch Apple Crumb | 390 | 16 | 53 |
| **Sara Lee:** | | | |
| **Pies:** *Per ⅛ Unless Indicated* | | | |
| French Silk , ⅕ pie | 460 | 28 | 51 |
| Key West Lime | 380 | 18 | 50 |
| Southern Pecan | 470 | 23 | 62 |
| Tropical Coconut Cream, ⅕ pie | 450 | 27 | 49 |
| **Oven Fresh Pies (9", 37 oz Box):** *Per Slice, 4.6 oz* | | | |
| Apple, ⅛ pie | 340 | 16 | 47 |
| Cherry, ⅛ pie | 340 | 16 | 45 |
| Mince, ⅛ pie | 380 | 17 | 53 |
| Peach, ⅛ pie | 320 | 15 | 42 |
| Pumpkin, ⅛ pie | 260 | 10 | 39 |
| **Tastykake:** Apple | 270 | 11 | 40 |
| Coconut Cream | 370 | 20 | 42 |
| Lemon | 300 | 14 | 44 |
| Strawberry | 340 | 12 | 55 |

## Croissants

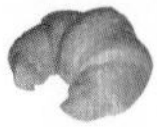

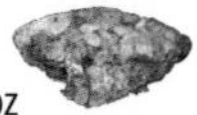

| Average all Brands | C | F | Cb |
|---|---|---|---|
| **Plain/Butter/Cheese:** Mini, 1 oz | 115 | 6 | 13 |
| Small, 1½ oz | 170 | 9 | 19 |
| Medium, 2 oz | 230 | 12 | 26 |
| Large, 2½ oz | 290 | 15 | 32 |
| Extra Large, 3 oz | 330 | 19 | 37 |
| **Sweet Croissants:** | | | |
| Almond Filled, 3 oz | 330 | 18 | 39 |
| Chocolate Filled, 3 oz | 360 | 19 | 43 |
| **Dunkin' Donuts,** Plain Croissant | 310 | 16 | 35 |
| **Sara Lee:** French Style: Orig, 1¾ oz | 185 | 9 | 21 |
| Mini, 1 oz | 230 | 11 | 26 |

**Croissant Sandwiches ~** See Page 165

## Pastry & Pie Crust

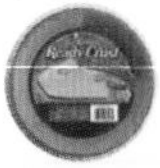

| | C | F | Cb |
|---|---|---|---|
| **Pie Crust:** Baked, 9" diameter shell | | | |
| 1 Pie Shell, 6½ oz | 970 | 64 | 87 |
| 2-crust Pie, 9", 11¼ oz | 1660 | 109 | 150 |
| **Filo Pastry:** 4 sheets, 2½ oz | 210 | 2.5 | 40 |
| *Athens,* 14"x18", 2½ sheets, 2 oz | 180 | 1.5 | 37 |
| **Puff** *(Pepp.Farm),* ½ sheet, 4.5 oz | 510 | 33 | 42 |
| Bake & Fill Shell, 1.7 oz | 190 | 13 | 16 |
| **Arrowhead Mills,** | | | |
| Graham Cracker Pie Crust, ⅛ of 9" | 110 | 5 | 14 |
| **Bisquick:** Baking Mix, | | | |
| Original, ⅓ cup, 1½ oz | 160 | 4.5 | 26 |
| Heart Smart, ⅓ cup, 1½ oz | 140 | 2.5 | 27 |
| **Keebler:** | | | |
| **Ready Crust:** *Per ⅛ of 9" Crust* | | | |
| Chocolate | 100 | 4.5 | 14 |
| Graham: Regular | 110 | 5 | 14 |
| Reduced Fat | 100 | 3.5 | 15 |
| Shortbread Crust | 110 | 5 | 14 |
| **Marie Callenders,** Deep Dish Pie Shell, | | | |
| ⅛ pie, 1 oz | 140 | 10 | 11 |
| **Mrs Smith's,** Homestyle, | | | |
| Deep Dish, 9", ⅛ | 130 | 7 | 15 |
| **Nabisco:** | | | |
| Honey Maid Graham, ⅙ of 9", 1 oz | 150 | 8 | 18 |
| Nilla Pie Crust, ⅙ of 9", 1 oz | 140 | 8 | 18 |
| **Pillsbury,** Rolled, ⅛,1 oz | 100 | 6 | 12 |
| **Trader Joe's,** Pie Crust, ⅛ pie, 1.2 oz | 190 | 13 | 17 |

## Pie Fillings (Canned)

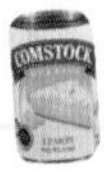

| **Fruit:** *Average all Fruits* | C | F | Cb |
|---|---|---|---|
| (Apple/Blueberry/Cherry/Strawberry) | | | |
| Sweetened: ⅓ cup, 3.2oz | 90 | 0 | 22 |
| 1 cup, 9½ oz | 270 | 0 | 66 |
| 1 can, 21 oz | 600 | 0 | 150 |
| Light/Lite, ⅓ cup, 3.2 oz | 60 | 0 | 15 |
| Unsweetened, ⅓ cup, 3.2 oz | 35 | 0 | 8 |
| **Lemon Cream/Creme,** ⅓ cup, 3.2 oz | 130 | 1.5 | 28 |

## Pizzas ~ Ready-To-Eat

*Average All Retail Outlets/Restaurants*

### Cheese Pizza:
*Medium Size (12"):*

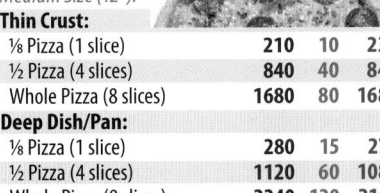

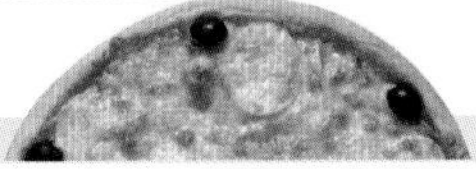

**Thin Crust:**

| | C | F | Cb |
|---|---|---|---|
| ⅛ Pizza (1 slice) | 200 | 8 | 22 |
| ½ Pizza (4 slices) | 800 | 32 | 88 |
| Whole Pizza (8 slices) | 1600 | 64 | 172 |

**Deep Dish/Pan:**

| | | | |
|---|---|---|---|
| ⅛ Pizza (1 slice) | 270 | 13 | 27 |
| ½ Pizza (4 slices) | 1080 | 52 | 108 |
| Whole Pizza (8 slices) | 2160 | 104 | 216 |

### Pepperoni:
*Medium Size (12"):*

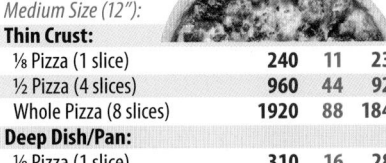

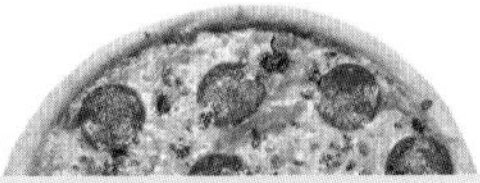

**Thin Crust:**

| | | | |
|---|---|---|---|
| ⅛ Pizza (1 slice) | 210 | 10 | 23 |
| ½ Pizza (4 slices) | 840 | 40 | 84 |
| Whole Pizza (8 slices) | 1680 | 80 | 168 |

**Deep Dish/Pan:**

| | | | |
|---|---|---|---|
| ⅛ Pizza (1 slice) | 280 | 15 | 27 |
| ½ Pizza (4 slices) | 1120 | 60 | 108 |
| Whole Pizza (8 slices) | 2240 | 120 | 216 |

### Supreme:
*Medium Size (12"):*

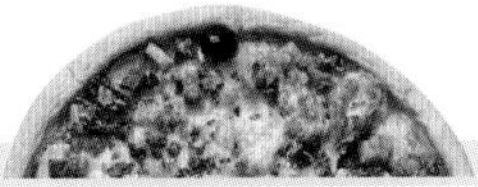

**Thin Crust:**

| | | | |
|---|---|---|---|
| ⅛ Pizza (1 slice) | 240 | 11 | 23 |
| ½ Pizza (4 slices) | 960 | 44 | 92 |
| Whole Pizza (8 slices) | 1920 | 88 | 184 |

**Deep Dish/Pan:**

| | | | |
|---|---|---|---|
| ⅛ Pizza (1 slice) | 310 | 16 | 28 |
| ½ Pizza (4 slices) | 1240 | 64 | 112 |
| Whole Pizza (8 slices) | 2480 | 128 | 224 |

### Meat Deluxe:
*Medium Size (12"):*

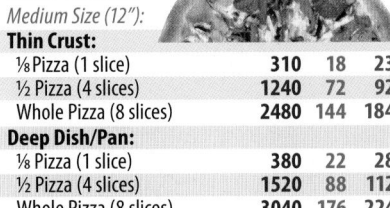

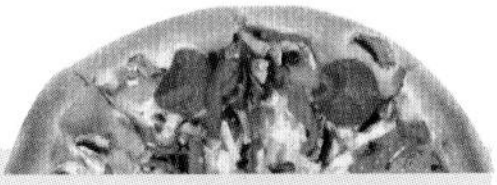

**Thin Crust:**

| | | | |
|---|---|---|---|
| ⅛ Pizza (1 slice) | 310 | 18 | 23 |
| ½ Pizza (4 slices) | 1240 | 72 | 92 |
| Whole Pizza (8 slices) | 2480 | 144 | 184 |

**Deep Dish/Pan:**

| | | | |
|---|---|---|---|
| ⅛ Pizza (1 slice) | 380 | 22 | 28 |
| ½ Pizza (4 slices) | 1520 | 88 | 112 |
| Whole Pizza (8 slices) | 3040 | 176 | 224 |

### Hawaiian: *Ham & Pineapple*
*Medium Size (12"):*

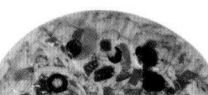

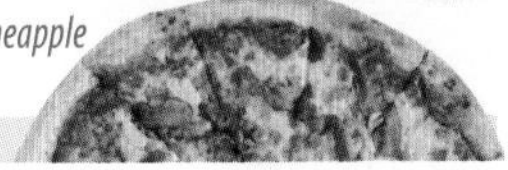

**Thin Crust:**

| | | | |
|---|---|---|---|
| ⅛ Pizza (1 slice) | 190 | 7 | 23 |
| ½ Pizza (4 slices) | 760 | 28 | 92 |
| Whole Pizza (8 slices) | 1520 | 56 | 184 |

**Deep Dish/Pan:**

| | | | |
|---|---|---|---|
| ⅛ Pizza (1 slice) | 250 | 11 | 28 |
| ½ Pizza (4 slices) | 1000 | 44 | 112 |
| Whole Pizza (8 slices) | 2000 | 88 | 224 |

### Veggie:
Similar to Hawaiian

### Single Slices:
*(Extra Large):*
*(Example: Sbarro's)*

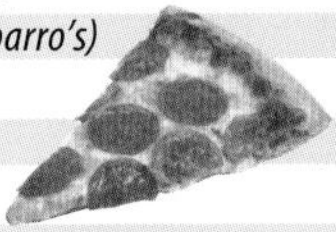

| | C | F | Cb |
|---|---|---|---|
| Cheese | 460 | 13 | 60 |
| Pepperoni | 730 | 37 | 61 |
| Sausage | 670 | 31 | 60 |
| Supreme | 630 | 27 | 63 |

### Individual Pizza: *(6")*
**Deep Dish/Pan:**
*(Approx. 9 oz weight):*

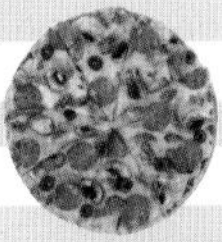

| | | | |
|---|---|---|---|
| Cheese | 600 | 24 | 69 |
| Hawaiian | 570 | 21 | 70 |
| Meat Deluxe | 900 | 50 | 70 |
| Pepperoni | 650 | 30 | 67 |
| Veggie | 560 | 22 | 70 |

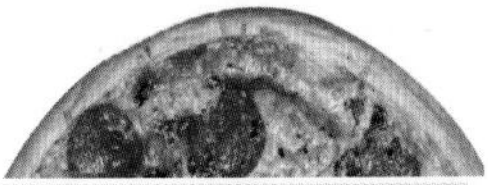

### Large: *(14") Thin Crust*

| | | | |
|---|---|---|---|
| **Cheese:** ⅛ Pizza | 290 | 12 | 30 |
| ½ Pizza | 1160 | 48 | 120 |
| **Hawaiian:** ⅛ pizza | 260 | 9 | 33 |
| ½ Pizza | 1040 | 36 | 132 |
| **Pepperoni:** ⅛ Pizza | 310 | 15 | 30 |
| ½ Pizza | 1240 | 60 | 120 |
| **Supreme:** ⅛ Pizza | 340 | 17 | 32 |
| ½ Pizza | 1360 | 68 | 128 |
| **Meat Deluxe:** ⅛ Pizza | 440 | 26 | 31 |
| ½ Pizza | 1760 | 104 | 124 |
| **Veggie:** ⅛ Pizza | 260 | 10 | 32 |
| ½ Pizza | 1040 | 40 | 128 |

## Frozen Pizzas

| | C | F | Cb |
|---|---|---|---|
| **Amy's:** *Per ⅓ Pizza* | | | |
| Cheese Pizza | 290 | 12 | 33 |
| Mushroom & Olive | 260 | 10 | 33 |
| Pesto | 310 | 12 | 39 |
| Roasted Vegetable | 280 | 9 | 42 |
| Whole Wheat Crust, Cheese & Pesto | 360 | 18 | 37 |
| **California Pizza Kitchen:** | | | |
| **Crispy Thin Crust:** *Per ⅓ Pizza* | | | |
| Margherita | 290 | 13 | 31 |
| Sicilian Recipe | 310 | 14 | 30 |
| Spinach & Artichoke | 350 | 19 | 34 |
| White | 290 | 12 | 31 |
| **Self Rising Crust:** *Per ⅓ Pizza* | | | |
| BBQ Chicken, 4.3 oz | 270 | 9 | 33 |
| Five Cheese & Tomato, 4.3 oz | 390 | 17 | 41 |
| Garlic Chicken, 4.3 oz | 280 | 11 | 30 |
| **Traditional Crust:** *Per Small Pizza* | | | |
| Four Cheese, 6.9 oz | 510 | 17 | 69 |
| Margherita, 6 oz | 420 | 18 | 45 |
| Sicilian, 5.5 oz | 440 | 21 | 43 |
| Celeste: | | | |
| **Pizza For One:** Original, 1 pizza | 340 | 16 | 39 |
| Deluxe; Pepperoni | 365 | 18 | 39 |
| Meatball | 420 | 22 | 40 |
| Sausage & Pepperoni; Suprema | 420 | 23 | 40 |
| Zesty 4 Cheese; Four Cheese | 350 | 16 | 38 |
| **DiGiorno:** *Per Slice Unless Indicated* | | | |
| **Cheese Stuffed Crust:** | | | |
| Four Cheese, 4.23 oz | 330 | 15 | 33 |
| Pepperoni, 4.23 oz | 340 | 16 | 33 |
| Three Meat, 5 oz | 360 | 18 | 34 |
| **Classic Thin Crust,** average all | 340 | 16 | 35 |
| **Crispy Flatbread Pizza:** | | | |
| Italian Sausage & Onion, 5½ oz | 400 | 26 | 27 |
| Pepperoni & Rstd Peppers, 4½ oz | 340 | 20 | 26 |
| Tuscan Style Chicken, 4.7 oz | 280 | 14 | 25 |
| **Deep Dish:** Four Cheese, 3¾ oz | 300 | 17 | 26 |
| Italian, 3¾ oz | 310 | 18 | 26 |
| Pepperoni, 3¾ oz | 300 | 17 | 26 |
| **Flatbread Melts:** | | | |
| Chicken & Bacon Ranch, 6 oz | 420 | 18 | 44 |
| Chicken Parmesan, 6 oz | 380 | 14 | 45 |
| Italian Meatballs & Four Chse, 5.9 oz | 400 | 17 | 46 |
| **Garlic Bread:** | | | |
| Four Cheese, 5 oz | 350 | 14 | 41 |
| Pepperoni, 5.1 oz | 380 | 17 | 40 |
| Supreme, 4.27 oz | 300 | 14 | 31 |

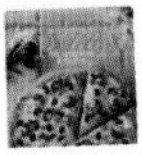

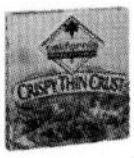

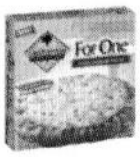

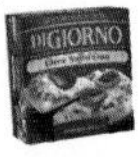

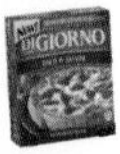

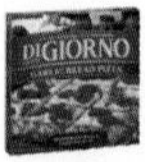

| | C | F | Cb |
|---|---|---|---|
| **DiGiorno (Cont):** | | | |
| **Traditional Crust:** *Per Whole Pizza* | | | |
| Four Cheese, 9.17 oz | 720 | 30 | 84 |
| Pepperoni, 9.28 oz | 770 | 35 | 83 |
| Supreme, 9.98 oz | 790 | 36 | 85 |
| **Ultimate Toppings:** *Per Slice* | | | |
| Cheese, 4.6 oz | 320 | 13 | 34 |
| Four Meat, 5 oz | 380 | 19 | 34 |
| Pepperoni, 4.8 oz | 370 | 19 | 34 |
| Supreme 5.3 oz | 360 | 18 | 35 |
| **Freschetta:** | | | |
| **Naturally Rising:** *Per ⅕ of Large Pizza Unless Indicated* | | | |
| 4 Cheese Medley | 360 | 13 | 43 |
| Can. Bacon P'apple | 310 | 9 | 44 |
| Meat Medley | 380 | 15 | 44 |
| Pepperoni | 360 | 14 | 44 |
| Supreme, ⅙ | 320 | 13 | 37 |
| **Simply Inspired:** *Per ⅓ pizza* | | | |
| Chicken Bianco | 360 | 19 | 30 |
| Classic Bruschetta | 380 | 23 | 32 |
| Harvest Supreme | 350 | 18 | 32 |
| Rustic Pepp. Pomodoro | 390 | 22 | 30 |
| Tuscan Farmhouse | 300 | 15 | 31 |
| **Jeno's:** *Per Pizza, 7 oz* | | | |
| **Crispy 'N Tasty:** Cheese | 460 | 22 | 50 |
| Sausage | 480 | 24 | 50 |
| **Home Run Inn (Chicago):** *Per ⅙ Pizza* | | | |
| **Classic Large 12":** Cheese, 4.5 oz | 340 | 18 | 30 |
| Sausage, 5 oz | 360 | 19 | 29 |
| Sausage & Pepperoni, 5.15 oz | 380 | 20 | 30 |
| **Signature,** Sausage Supreme, 5½ oz | 360 | 18 | 31 |
| **Kashi:** | | | |
| **Thin Crust:** *Per ⅓ Pizza* | | | |
| Mediterranean | 290 | 9 | 37 |
| Mshrm Trio & Spin.; Rstd Vege | 250 | 9 | 28 |
| **Kroger:** | | | |
| **3 Minute Microwave:** *Per 8 oz Pizza* | | | |
| 3-Meat | 500 | 17 | 64 |
| Cheese | 490 | 16 | 66 |
| Combination | 520 | 20 | 64 |
| Pepperoni | 530 | 20 | 65 |
| Supreme | 490 | 18 | 63 |
| **French Bread,** Pepperoni, 5 oz | 380 | 17 | 42 |
| **Lean Cuisine:** | | | |
| **Casual Cuisine:** *Per Pizza* | | | |
| Deep Dish: Roasted Vegetable | 320 | 5 | 52 |
| Spinach & Mushroom | 340 | 7 | 52 |
| Three Meat | 390 | 9 | 55 |
| Traditional: Four Chse | 350 | 6 | 55 |
| Mushroom | 300 | 5 | 50 |
| Pepperoni | 380 | 9 | 55 |
| Wood Fired: BBQ Recipe Chicken | 340 | 7 | 48 |
| Margherita | 310 | 7 | 46 |
| Roasted Garlic Chicken | 350 | 8 | 47 |

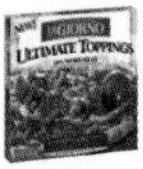

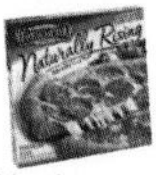

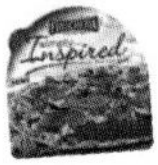

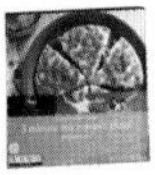

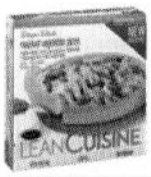

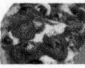

## Frozen Pizzas (Cont)

| | C | F | Cb |
|---|---|---|---|
| **Red Baron:** | | | |
| **Classic Crust:** | | | |
| 4 Cheese, ¼ pizza | **380** | 16 | 40 |
| Pepperoni, ¼ pizza | **370** | 16 | 40 |
| Sausage & Pepperoni, ¼ pizza | **400** | 19 | 41 |
| Supreme, ⅕ pizza | **310** | 14 | 34 |
| **Fire Baked:** | | | |
| Original Crust: | | | |
| 4-Cheese, ¼ pizza | **360** | 15 | 40 |
| Pepperoni, ¼ pizza | **370** | 17 | 40 |
| Thin Crust: | | | |
| 5 Cheese, ⅓ pizza | **360** | 16 | 40 |
| Pepperoni, ⅓ pizza | **400** | 19 | 40 |
| **Pan:** | | | |
| 4 Cheese, ⅕ pizza | **390** | 18 | 40 |
| Meat Trio; Supreme, ⅙ pizza, av | **355** | 18 | 35 |
| Pepperoni, ⅕ pizza | **400** | 19 | 41 |
| **Pizza By The Slice:** *Per Slice* | | | |
| 4 Cheese | **340** | 13 | 41 |
| Meat Trio | **380** | 17 | 41 |
| Pepperoni; Supreme, av. | **355** | 15 | 41 |
| **Singles:** *Per Pizza* | | | |
| Deep Dish: 4 Chse; Meat Trio, av | **405** | 18 | 46 |
| Pepperoni; Supreme, average | **420** | 19 | 46 |
| French Bread: Extra Cheese | **360** | 12 | 43 |
| 5 Cheese & Garlic | **430** | 23 | 41 |
| Pepperoni | **380** | 15 | 43 |
| Supreme | **380** | 15 | 44 |
| **Safeway Select:** | | | |
| **Pizzeria Crust:** | | | |
| Cheese Trio, ¼ pizza | **340** | 15 | 34 |
| Fajita Chicken Ole, ⅕ pizza | **250** | 10 | 29 |
| Pepperoni & Sausage, ⅕ pizza | **320** | 17 | 30 |
| **Self Rising:** *Per ⅙ Pizza* | | | |
| Four Cheese | **300** | 9 | 41 |
| Pepperoni | **350** | 14 | 41 |
| Sausage & Pepperoni | **340** | 13 | 41 |
| **Ultra Thin Crust:** *Per ⅓ Pizza Unless Indicated* | | | |
| BBQ Chicken, ¼ pizza | **250** | 10 | 23 |
| Garlic Chicken | **320** | 12 | 31 |
| Margherita | **330** | 17 | 28 |
| Primo Italiano Meat | **330** | 16 | 27 |

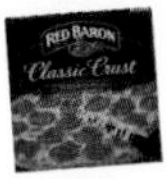

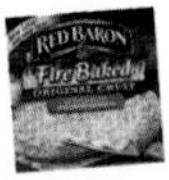

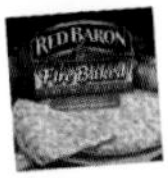

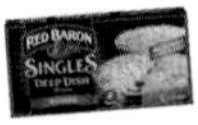

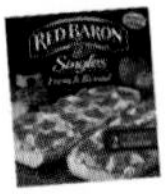

| | C | F | Cb |
|---|---|---|---|
| **Stouffer's:** *Each* | | | |
| **French Bread Pizzas:** | | | |
| **Two Per Box:** Deluxe (1), 6 .19 oz | **430** | 21 | 44 |
| Sausage & Pepperoni (1), 6.25 oz | **460** | 24 | 43 |
| **Nine Per Box:** Extra Chse(1), 5.88 oz | **400** | 18 | 44 |
| Pepperoni, 5.68 oz | **430** | 21 | 44 |
| **Tombstone:** | | | |
| **Original:** *Per ⅕ of Large 12" Pizza Unless Indicated* | | | |
| 4 Meat | **310** | 14 | 30 |
| Canadian Style Bacon, ¼ pizza | **320** | 12 | 37 |
| Deluxe | **290** | 12 | 31 |
| Extra Cheese, ¼ pizza | **350** | 15 | 36 |
| Pepperoni, ⅓ pizza | **280** | 14 | 28 |
| Pepperoni & Sausage, ¼ pizza | **370** | 17 | 37 |
| Sausage & Mushroom | **290** | 13 | 30 |
| Supreme | **300** | 14 | 31 |
| **Thin Crust:** Three Cheese, ¼ pizza | **310** | 15 | 28 |
| Pepperoni; Sausage, av., ¼ pizza | **315** | 16 | 28 |
| **Brick Oven Style:** Cheese, ⅓ pizza | **350** | 15 | 37 |
| Pepperoni; Supreme, av., ¼ pizza | **315** | 16 | 29 |
| **Tony's:** | | | |
| **Original Crust:** Cheese, ⅓ pizza | **290** | 12 | 37 |
| Pepperoni, ⅓ pizza | **310** | 14 | 36 |
| Ssg & Pepperoni; Supreme, av., ⅓ | **340** | 17 | 37 |
| **Pizza For One:** *Microwavable* | | | |
| Cheese (1) | **380** | 14 | 50 |
| Pepperoni (1) | **410** | 18 | 48 |
| **Totino's:** | | | |
| **Crisp Crust Party Pizza:** *Per ½ Pizza* | | | |
| Cheese | **330** | 16 | 35 |
| Classic Pepperoni | **370** | 20 | 35 |
| **Pizza Rolls:** Cheese (6), 3 oz | **200** | 8 | 26 |
| Pepperoni (6), 3 oz | **210** | 10 | 24 |
| **Stuffers,** average all, 1 piece | **260** | 12 | 32 |
| **Trader Joe's:** | | | |
| 3 Cheese, ⅓ pizza | **310** | 9 | 42 |
| Parlanno, ¼ pizza | **340** | 16 | 34 |
| Pizza 4 Formaggi, ⅓ pizza | **310** | 9 | 42 |
| Spinach, ⅓ pizza | **300** | 12 | 38 |
| **Weight Watchers (Smart Ones):** *Per Pizza* | | | |
| Fajita Chicken | **380** | 7 | 58 |
| Four Cheese | **370** | 7 | 57 |
| Pepperoni | **390** | 8 | 58 |
| **Wolfgang Puck:** | | | |
| **Rustica Pizzas:** *Per ¼ Pizza* | | | |
| 4 Cheese Tomato & Pesto | **350** | 18 | 35 |
| BBQ Chicken | **340** | 11 | 42 |
| Chicken Poblamo | **310** | 10 | 39 |
| Meditteranean Vege. | **300** | 11 | 40 |

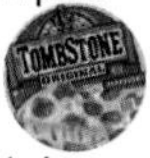

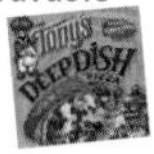

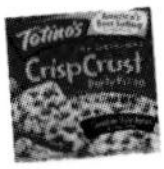

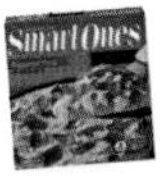

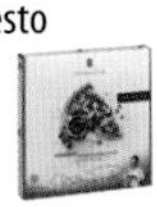

## Quick Guide

### Chicken
From 1lb ready-to-cook chicken

| | **C** | **F** | **Cb** |
|---|---|---|---|
| **Breast:** | | | |
| **Roasted:** With skin, 2 oz | 115 | 4.5 | 0 |
| Without skin, 1.8 oz | 85 | 2 | 0 |
| **Fried,** batter dipped, 3 oz | 220 | 11 | 8 |
| **Leg Quarter:** | | | |
| **Thigh & Drumstick:** | | | |
| **Roasted:** With skin, 2.4 oz | 160 | 10 | 0 |
| Without skin, 2 oz | 110 | 5 | 0 |
| **Fried,** batter dipped, 3.3 oz | 260 | 15 | 9 |
| **KFC** ~ See Fast-Foods Section | | | |

## Per 4 oz Edible Portion

**Average of Light Meat:** *Per 4 oz (no bone)*

| | C | F | Cb |
|---|---|---|---|
| Roasted: With skin | 250 | 12 | 0 |
| Without skin | 175 | 4.5 | 0 |
| Stewed: With skin | 230 | 12 | 0 |
| Without skin | 180 | 4.5 | 0 |
| Fried: Batter-dipped, 4 oz | 315 | 17 | 11 |
| Flour-coated, 4 oz | 280 | 14 | 2 |

**Average of Dark Meat:** *Per 4 oz (no bone)*

| | | | |
|---|---|---|---|
| Roasted: With skin | 290 | 18 | 0 |
| Without skin | 235 | 11 | 0 |
| Stewed: With skin | 265 | 17 | 0 |
| Without skin | 220 | 10 | 0 |
| Fried: Batter-dipped, 4 oz | 340 | 21 | 11 |
| Flour-coated, 4 oz | 325 | 19 | 5 |

## Chicken Parts

**Broilers or Fryers:** *Edible Weights (no bone)*

**Breast:** *Per ½ Breast*

| | | | |
|---|---|---|---|
| Raw: With skin, 5 oz | 250 | 14 | 0 |
| Without skin, 4.25 oz | 130 | 1.5 | 0 |
| Roasted: With skin, 3.5 oz | 195 | 8 | 0 |
| Without skin, 3 oz | 140 | 3 | 0 |
| Stewed: With skin, 4 oz | 200 | 8 | 0 |
| Without skin, 3.25 oz | 145 | 3 | 0 |
| Fried: Batter-dipped, 5 oz | 365 | 19 | 13 |
| Flour-coated, with skin, 3.5 oz | 220 | 9 | 2 |

**Drumstick:** *Per Drumstick*

| | | | |
|---|---|---|---|
| Roasted: With skin, 2 oz | 115 | 6 | 0 |
| Without skin, 1.5 oz | 75 | 2.5 | 0 |
| Fried: Batter-dipped, 2.5 oz | 195 | 11 | 6 |
| Flour-coated, 1.75 oz | 120 | 7 | 1 |
| Stewed: With skin, 2 oz | 115 | 6 | 0 |
| Without skin, 1.5 oz | 80 | 3 | 0 |

## Chicken Parts (Cont)

| | **C** | **F** | **Cb** |
|---|---|---|---|
| **Thigh Portion:** *Edible Weight (no bone)* | | | |
| Raw: With skin, 3.3 oz (4¼ oz with bone) | 200 | 14 | 0 |
| Without skin, 2.4 oz | 80 | 3 | 0 |
| Roasted: With skin, 2¼ oz | 155 | 10 | 0 |
| Without skin, 2 oz | 110 | 6 | 0 |
| Stewed: With skin, 2.5 oz | 160 | 10 | 0 |
| Without skin, 2 oz | 105 | 5 | 0 |
| Fried: Batter-dipped, 3 oz | 240 | 14 | 8 |
| Flour-coated, 2.25 oz | 165 | 9 | 2 |
| **Wing:** *Per Wing* | | | |
| Raw Weight, 3.2 oz, (with bone) | | | |
| Raw: With skin | 110 | 8 | 0 |
| Without skin | 35 | 1 | 0 |
| Roasted: With skin | 100 | 7 | 0 |
| Without skin | 45 | 2 | 0 |
| Fried: Batter-dipped | 160 | 11 | 5 |
| Flour-coated | 105 | 7 | 1 |
| Stewed, with skin, 4 oz | 100 | 7 | 0 |
| **Buffalo Wings** ~ See Fast-Foods Section | | | |
| **Neck:** Simmered, with skin | 95 | 7 | 0 |
| Without skin | 30 | 2 | 0 |
| **Skin Only:** *Skin from ½ Chicken* | | | |
| Raw skin, 2.75 oz | 275 | 26 | 0 |
| Roasted skin, 2 oz | 255 | 23 | 0 |
| Stewed skin, 2.52 oz | 260 | 24 | 0 |
| Fried, Flour-coated, 2 oz | 280 | 24 | 5 |
| Fried, Batter-dipped, 6.75 oz | 750 | 55 | 44 |
| **Roasters:** *Average of Light & Dark Meat:* | | | |
| Roasted: With skin, 4 oz | 250 | 15 | 0 |
| Without skin, 4 oz | 190 | 8 | 0 |
| Light Meat, without skin, roasted | 175 | 5 | 0 |
| Dark Meat, without skin, roasted | 200 | 10 | 0 |
| **Stewing Chicken:** | | | |
| *Average of Light & Dark Meat: Per 4 oz* | | | |
| Stewed: With skin | 325 | 22 | 0 |
| Without skin | 270 | 14 | 0 |
| Light Meat, without skin | 240 | 9 | 0 |
| Dark Meat, without skin | 290 | 17 | 0 |
| **Capon Chicken:** | | | |
| Roasted: With skin, 4 oz | 260 | 13 | 0 |
| ½ Chicken, with skin | 1460 | 74 | 0 |

**Chicken Offal & Stuffing:**

| | | | |
|---|---|---|---|
| **Giblets:** Simmered, 1 cup | 230 | 7 | 0.5 |
| Fried, flour-coated, 1 cup | 400 | 20 | 6 |
| **Gizzard,** simmered, 1 cup | 210 | 4 | 0 |
| **Heart,** simmered, 1 cup | 270 | 12 | 0.2 |
| **Liver:** Raw, 4 oz | 130 | 5.5 | 0 |
| Simmered, 1 cup | 215 | 8.5 | 1 |
| **Liver Pate,** Fresh, 1 Tbsp, 0.5 oz | 30 | 2 | 1 |
| **Stuffing,** average, ½ cup | 180 | 9 | 22 |

## Chicken Products
**C  F  Cb**

**Bumble Bee:**
**Chicken In Water:** *Per 5 oz Can*

| | C | F | Cb |
|---|---|---|---|
| Premium White, drained 2 oz | 70 | 3 | 1 |
| Premium Breast, drained 2 oz | 70 | 1 | 1 |
| **Foster Farms:** | | | |
| Grilled Chicken Breast Strips, 3 oz | 100 | 1.5 | 2 |
| Wings: Chipotle, 4 wings, 3 oz | 190 | 14 | 1 |
| Honey BBQ Glazed, 4 wings, 2.9 oz | 170 | 10 | 5 |
| Hot 'n' Spicy, 4 wings, 2.9 oz | 170 | 13 | 1 |
| **Tyson:** | | | |
| **Any'tizers:** | | | |
| Bites: Buffalo Style Popcorn, 8 pcs | 80 | 9 | 12 |
| Honey BBQ Boneless, 3 pieces | 200 | 8 | 20 |
| Popcorn, 7 pieces | 180 | 9 | 11 |
| Wings: Buffalo style Hot (3) | 190 | 10 | 3 |
| Honey BBQ Boneless (3) | 200 | 8 | 20 |
| **Canned,** Premium Chunk, 2 oz | 60 | 1 | 0 |
| **Pouch,** Chunk Breast, 5 oz | 175 | 4 | 0 |

## Duck, Goose, Quail

| | C | F | Cb |
|---|---|---|---|
| **Duck:** Roasted, | | | |
| With skin, 3 oz | 290 | 24 | 0 |
| Without skin, 3 oz | 170 | 10 | 0 |
| ½ duck, with skin, 13.5 oz | 1290 | 108 | 0 |
| **Goose:** Roast, with skin, 3 oz | 260 | 19 | 0 |
| Without skin, 3 oz | 200 | 11 | 0 |
| **Pheasant,** cooked, 3 oz | 210 | 10 | 0 |
| **Quail,** cooked, 1 whole, 6 oz | 400 | 24 | 0 |

## Turkey

**Fryer-Roasters:** *Per 3 oz Serving*
**Roasted:**

| | C | F | Cb |
|---|---|---|---|
| Light Meat: With skin | 140 | 4 | 0 |
| Without skin | 120 | 1 | 0 |
| Dark Meat: With skin | 155 | 6 | 0 |
| Without skin | 140 | 4 | 0 |

**½ of Whole Turkey:** (Approx. 3.25 lbs raw weight)
Without neck and giblets; 1.8 lbs cooked weight)

| | C | F | Cb |
|---|---|---|---|
| **Roasted:** With skin | 1650 | 74 | 0 |
| Without skin | 1125 | 31 | 0 |
| **Ground Turkey,** Raw: (4 oz raw wt. = 3 oz ckd wt.) | | | |
| Regular (85% lean), 4 oz | 170 | 10 | 0 |
| Lean (93% lean), average, 4 oz | 160 | 8 | 0 |
| *Foster Farms,* (94% lean), 4 oz | 150 | 7 | 0 |
| *Jennie-O,* (93% lean), 4 oz | 170 | 8 | 0 |
| *Trader Joe's,* (93% lean), 4 oz | 150 | 8 | 0 |
| Breast, no skin, 4 oz | 115 | 1 | 0 |
| Patties: Small, 3 oz | 130 | 7 | 0 |
| Medium, 4 oz | 170 | 10 | 0 |
| Large, 5.3 oz | 225 | 13 | 0 |

## Turkey Parts
**C  F  Cb**

**Roasted, Edible Weights, without bone:**
**Breast (½):** (from 17¼ oz raw weight with bone)

| | C | F | Cb |
|---|---|---|---|
| With skin, 12 oz (no bone) | 525 | 11 | 0 |
| Without skin, 10.75 oz | 415 | 2 | 0 |
| **Back (½):** With skin, 4.5 oz | 265 | 13 | 0 |
| Without skin, 3.5 oz | 165 | 6 | 0 |

**Leg (Thigh & Drumstick):**
(from 1 lb raw weight with bone)

| | C | F | Cb |
|---|---|---|---|
| With skin, 8.5oz (without bone) | 410 | 13 | 0 |
| Without skin, 7.75 oz | 355 | 8.5 | 0 |

**Wing:** (From 7.25 oz raw weight)

| | C | F | Cb |
|---|---|---|---|
| With skin, 3 oz (without bone) | 185 | 9 | 0 |
| Without skin, 2 oz (with bone) | 100 | 2 | 0 |
| **Neck:** Simmered, 1 neck, | | | |
| (9 oz with bone) | 275 | 11 | 0 |
| **Giblets,** simmered, 1 cup, 5 oz | 240 | 7 | 3 |

## Young Hens (Roasted)

**Light Meat:**

| | C | F | Cb |
|---|---|---|---|
| With skin, 3 oz | 175 | 8 | 0 |
| Without skin, 3 oz | 135 | 3 | 0 |
| **Dark Meat:** With skin, 3 oz | 200 | 11 | 0 |
| Without skin, 3 oz | 165 | 7 | 0 |

**Young Toms ~** *Similar to Young Hens*

## Turkey Products

**Banquet ~** *See Frozen Meals, Page 117*
**Foster Farms:** *Cooked, Frozen*

| | C | F | Cb |
|---|---|---|---|
| Meatballs: Homestyle (3) | 150 | 7 | 8 |
| Italian Style (3) | 160 | 8 | 5 |
| Homesyle Cutlets (1), 3 oz | 180 | 8 | 14 |

**Hormel:** *Turkey Chunks (canned), cooked:*

| | C | F | Cb |
|---|---|---|---|
| Chunk Turkey, 2 oz | 70 | 2.5 | 0 |
| White Turkey, 2 oz | 60 | 1.5 | 0 |

**Jennie-O:**

| | C | F | Cb |
|---|---|---|---|
| All Natural, White Burgers, 5.25 oz | 160 | 5 | 0 |
| Fully Cooked: Italian Meatballs, 3 oz | 190 | 12 | 3 |
| Home Style Meatballs, 3 oz | 190 | 11 | 5 |
| Turkey Bacon, 1 slice | 35 | 3 | 1 |
| Turkey Bratwurst, | | | |
| Lean, 3.85 oz | 170 | 10 | 2 |
| **Spam,** Oven Roasted Turkey, 2 oz | 80 | 4 | 2 |

**Swanson ~** *Frozen Meals, Page 121*

| | C | F | Cb |
|---|---|---|---|
| **Trader Joe's,** Turkey Meatloaf, 3 oz | 140 | 8 | 5 |

## White Rice

| | C | F | Cb |
|---|---|---|---|
| **Raw:** Short Grain, 1 cup, 7 oz | 715 | 1 | 158 |
| Long Grain, 1 cup, 6.5 oz | 675 | 1 | 148 |
| Glutinous, 1 cup, 6.5 oz | 685 | 1 | 151 |
| **Cooked Rice:** *(Boiled/Steamed):* | | | |
| **Short/Medium Grain:** | | | |
| ½ cup, 3.25 oz | 140 | 0 | 30 |
| 1 cup (½ Pint), 7.2 oz | 265 | 0.5 | 59 |
| 2 cups (1 Pint), 13 oz | 480 | 1 | 106 |
| **Long Grain:** ½ cup, 2.75 oz | 100 | 0 | 22 |
| 1 cup, 5.5 oz | 205 | 0.5 | 44 |
| **Glutinous/Sticky,** cooked, 1 c., 6 oz | 170 | 0.5 | 37 |
| **Parboiled,** cooked, ½ cup, 3 oz | 105 | 0.5 | 22 |
| **Precook./Instant:** Dry, ½ cup, 3.5 oz | 380 | 1 | 82 |
| Cooked, ½ cup, 3 oz | 95 | 0.5 | 21 |
| **Wild Rice:** Raw, 1 cup, 5.5 oz | 570 | 2 | 120 |
| Cooked, 1 cup, 5.75 oz | 165 | 0.5 | 35 |

## Brown Rice

| | C | F | Cb |
|---|---|---|---|
| *Average of Short or Long Grain* | | | |
| **Raw/Dry:** ½ cup, 3.25 oz | 340 | 2.5 | 71 |
| 1 cup, 6.5 oz | 685 | 5.5 | 143 |
| **Cooked:** ½ cup, 3.5 oz | 110 | 1 | 22 |
| 1 cup, 7 oz | 220 | 2 | 46 |

## Rice Dishes

| | C | F | Cb |
|---|---|---|---|
| **Chinese Fried Rice:** | | | |
| ½ cup, 2.5 oz | 140 | 4.5 | 21 |
| 1 cup, (½ Pint), 5 oz | 280 | 9 | 42 |
| 2 cups, (1 Pint), 10 oz | 565 | 18 | 84 |
| **Mexican Rice:** 1 cup | 500 | 12 | 90 |
| *Taco John's,* 1 serving (6 oz) | 250 | 5 | 45 |
| *Taco Time,* 1 serving (4 oz) | 160 | 2 | 30 |
| **Rice-A-Roni** ~ *See Page 114* | | | |
| **Rice with Raisins/Pinenuts,** 1 cup | 400 | 11 | 60 |
| **Rice Pilaf:** Restaurant, 1 cup | 275 | 7.5 | 46 |
| *O'Charley's,* 1 order | 190 | 5 | 30 |
| **Rice Pudding** *(Kozy Shack),* | | | |
| Original, ½ cup | 130 | 3 | 22 |
| **Risotto,** 1 cup | 420 | 12 | 70 |
| **Saffron Rice,** 4 oz | 175 | 7 | 25 |
| **Spanish Rice:** 1 cup, 5 oz | 390 | 9 | 72 |
| *El Pollo Loco,* small, 4.5 oz | 170 | 2.5 | 32 |
| *Taco Cabana,* 4 oz | 180 | 5 | 30 |
| **Sticky Rice,** 1 cup, 5 oz | 155 | 0.5 | 34 |
| **Sushi Rice:** 1 Tbsp | 25 | 0 | 5 |
| 1 cup, 5.2 oz | 390 | 0 | 77 |
| **Other Packaged Rice Products:** | | | |
| **Uncle Ben's / Zatarain's** ~ *See Page 116* | | | |

# CalorieKing.com Recipes

See the CalorieKing website for a salubrious selection of healthy recipes – all analyzed for calories, fat, protein, carbohydrate, fiber and sodium.

*Choose from:*
- *Starters/Appetizers*
- *Salads*
- *Entrees: Meat, Fish and Chicken*
- *Vegetarian*
- *Desserts*
- *Cakes, Cookies*
- *Drinks*

**www.CalorieKing.com/recipes**

## HEALTHY RECIPE TIPS

- **Use non-fat milk** in place of whole or 2% milk
- **Use low-fat yogurt** in place of sour cream
- **Skim fat** from surface of soups and casseroles after cooling
- **Add extra vegetables** to soups and hot entrees
- **Cakes/cookies/muffins:** Replace most or all the fat/oil with applesauce and/or prune puree (Example: *Sunsweet Lighter Bake*)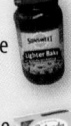
- **Drinks:** Replace sugar with no-calorie sweeteners such as *Equal, Stevia, Splenda* and *Sweet 'N Low*

## Deli Salads

**C F Cb**

*General Average, All Outlets*

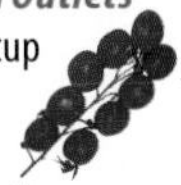

| | C | F | Cb |
|---|---|---|---|
| **Antipasto Salad,** ½ cup | 135 | 8 | 13 |
| **3-Bean Salad,** ½ cup | 90 | 4.5 | 12 |
| **Bulgur Salad,** ½ cup | 70 | 2 | 12 |
| **Caesar Salad,** Classic, 1 cup | 200 | 14 | 15 |
| **Side Salad,** without Dressing | 25 | 0 | 6 |
| **Carrot Raisin:** With Dressing, ½ cup | 135 | 12 | 6 |
| Without Dressing, ½ cup | 20 | 0 | 5 |
| **Chef's Salad:** Regular, w/o Dressing | 620 | 37 | 8 |
| With 2 oz 1000 Island | 860 | 61 | 8 |
| **Chicken Salad,** ½ cup/scoop, 4 oz | 280 | 21 | 2 |
| **Coleslaw:** Traditional, ½ cup | 150 | 8 | 18 |
| W/ Low Cal Dressing, ½ c. | 50 | 2 | 8 |
| **Corn,** Mexican, ½ cup | 240 | 12 | 33 |
| **Cucumber:** Non-Oil Dressing, ½ c. | 60 | 0 | 14 |
| With Oil Dressing, ½ cup | 140 | 12 | 8 |
| **Eggplant Salad,** ½ cup | 75 | 5 | 7 |
| **Fettucini,** with veges, ½ cup | 135 | 6 | 16 |
| **Garden Salad,** without Dressing, 1 c. | 10 | 0 | 2 |
| **Greek Salad,** 1 cup | 105 | 8 | 7 |
| **Greek Vegetables,** 1 cup | 110 | 8 | 6 |
| **Lobster Salad,** ½ cup, 4 oz | 250 | 21 | 11 |
| **Macaroni Salad,** ½ cup, 5 oz | 360 | 26 | 26 |
| **Nicoise,** 1 cup | 450 | 32 | 18 |
| **Pasta Salad,** ½ cup | 200 | 11 | 19 |
| **Potato Salad:** Dijon, 3 oz | 120 | 7 | 13 |
| With Mayonnaise, ½ cup, 4 oz | 215 | 15 | 17 |
| Lowfat, ½ cup | 110 | 1.5 | 21 |
| **Rice Salad,** ½ cup | 150 | 10 | 13 |
| **Saffron Rice,** 4 oz | 175 | 7 | 25 |
| **Spinach Salad,** 1 cup | 180 | 13 | 13 |
| **Tabouli,** ½ cup | 125 | 7 | 13 |
| **Three Bean Salad,** ½ cup | 90 | 4.5 | 12 |
| **Tomato & Mozzarella,** ½ cup | 180 | 14 | 10 |
| **Tortellini,** with Basil Pesto, ½ cup | 150 | 9 | 15 |
| **Waldorf,** with Mayo, ½ cup | 110 | 7 | 12 |

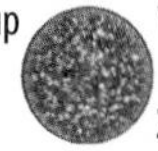

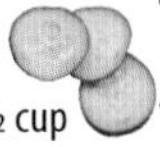

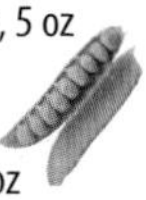

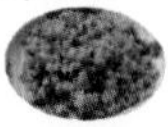

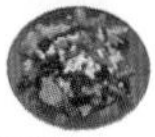

**Signature Salads:** *Per 6 oz Serving*
(Supplied to Deli's and Institutions)

| | C | F | Cb |
|---|---|---|---|
| Antipasto Salad | 510 | 50 | 4 |
| Artichoke Salad, marinated | 400 | 41 | 8 |
| California Medley | 120 | 7 | 15 |
| Cheese Agnolotti | 250 | 8 | 23 |
| Chicken Salad | 420 | 33 | 11 |
| Crabmeat Flavored | 450 | 38 | 20 |

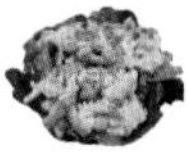

**C F Cb**

**Signature Salads (Cont):** *Per 6 oz Serving*

| | C | F | Cb |
|---|---|---|---|
| Egg Salad | 300 | 23 | 14 |
| Fresh Button Mushroom | 190 | 16 | 6 |
| Garden Olive | 630 | 67 | 3 |
| Ham Salad | 400 | 32 | 14 |
| Prima Pasta Salad | 360 | 30 | 18 |
| Seafood Pasta Del Mar | 170 | 10 | 21 |
| Seafood with Crab & Shrimp | 420 | 34 | 20 |
| Shrimp Salad | 360 | 32 | 8 |
| Tuna Salad | 450 | 36 | 14 |

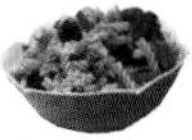

*~ Also See Fast-Foods & Restaurants Section*

## Fresh Salad Packs

**C F Cb**

*Pre-Packaged (Supermarkets)*
**Dole:**
**Kits:** *Per 3½ oz, Includes Dressing*

| | C | F | Cb |
|---|---|---|---|
| Asian Island Crunch | 130 | 7 | 15 |
| Caesar | 150 | 12 | 8 |
| Perfect Harvest | 160 | 12 | 11 |
| Southwest | 140 | 10 | 10 |

**Salad Blends:** *Without Dressing*

| | C | F | Cb |
|---|---|---|---|
| American; Mediterranean, 3 oz | 15 | 0 | 3 |
| Arugula; Baby Spinach, 3 oz | 20 | 0 | 3 |

**Fresh Express:**
**Complete Salad Kits:** *Per 3½ oz, Prepared*

| | C | F | Cb |
|---|---|---|---|
| Asian | 120 | 5 | 17 |
| Caesar: Regular | 120 | 11 | 7 |
| Chicken | 90 | 5 | 5 |
| Lite | 90 | 7 | 7 |
| Pear Gorganzola | 130 | 6 | 17 |
| Strawberry Fields | 200 | 13 | 17 |
| Supreme | 140 | 12 | 6 |
| **Gourmet Cafe:** Tuscan Pesto Chkn | 140 | 9 | 8 |
| Waldorf Chicken | 170 | 91 | 19 |

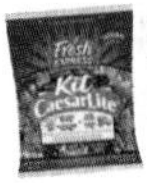

## Salad Toppings

**C F Cb**

| | C | F | Cb |
|---|---|---|---|
| **Bac'n Pieces:** McCormick, 1T, ¼ oz | 30 | 1 | 2 |
| **Bacon Bits:** | | | |
| *Bacos,* 1 Tbsp | 30 | 1.5 | 2 |
| *Hormel,* 1 Tbsp | 25 | 1.5 | 0 |
| **Chow Mein Noodles,** dry, ½ cup | 120 | 7 | 13 |
| **Croutons,** 2 Tbsp, 0.3 oz | 40 | 1 | 7 |
| **Olives,** 5 medium | 25 | 2 | 0 |
| **Salad Toppins:** | | | |
| *McCormick,* 4 tsp, ¼ oz | 35 | 1.5 | 3 |
| **Sunflower Seeds,** 1 T., 0.3 oz | 45 | 4 | 1.5 |
| **Toasted Sliced Almonds,** 2 T., 0.5 oz | 85 | 7 | 3 |
| **Tortilla Chips,** 12 chips, 1 oz | 140 | 7 | 19 |

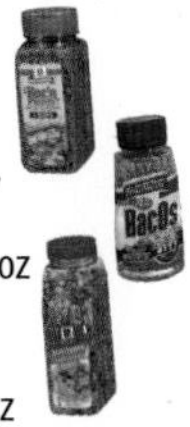

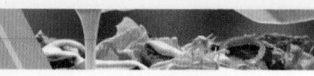

| Quick Guide | C | F | Cb |
|---|---|---|---|
| **Salad Dressings** | | | |
| *Average All Brands: Per 2 Tbsp, Approx 1 fl.oz* | | | |
| **Balsamic Vinaigrette:** | | | |
| Regular | 90 | 9 | 3 |
| Light, 2 Tbsp | 45 | 4 | 2 |
| Fat Free, 2 Tbsp | 25 | 0 | 6 |
| **Blue Cheese:** Reg., 2 Tbsp | 145 | 15 | 1.5 |
| Regular, ¼ cup, 2 oz | 280 | 30 | 3 |
| Light, 2 Tbsp | 30 | 1 | 4 |
| **Caesar:** Regular, 2 Tbsp | 165 | 17 | 1 |
| Regular, ¼ cup, 2 oz | 310 | 34 | 2 |
| Light, 2 Tbsp | 35 | 1.5 | 5.5 |
| **Coleslaw:** Regular, 2 Tbsp | 125 | 11 | 8 |
| Regular, ¼ cup, 2 oz | 245 | 21 | 15 |
| Light, 2 Tbsp | 110 | 7 | 14 |
| **French:** Regular | 145 | 14 | 5 |
| Regular, ¼ cup, 2 oz | 260 | 25 | 9 |
| Light, 2 Tbsp | 65 | 4 | 9 |
| Fat/Oil-Free, 2 Tbsp | 40 | 0 | 10 |
| **Italian:** Regular, 2 Tbsp | 85 | 8.5 | 3 |
| Regular, ¼ cup, 2 oz | 165 | 16 | 6 |
| Light, 2 Tbsp | 55 | 5.5 | 2 |
| Fat/Oil-Free, 2 Tbas | 15 | 0 | 2.5 |
| **Ranch:** Regular, 2 Tbsp | 145 | 16 | 2 |
| Regular, ¼ cup, 2 oz | 290 | 30 | 4 |
| Light, 2 Tbsp | 60 | 4 | 6.5 |
| Fat-Free, 2 Tbsp | 35 | 0.5 | 8 |
| **Thousand Island:** Reg. | 115 | 11 | 4.5 |
| Regular, ¼ cup, 2 oz | 210 | 20 | 9 |
| Light, 2 Tbsp | 60 | 3.5 | 7 |
| Fat-Free, 2 Tbsp | 40 | 0.5 | 10 |

*Enjoy a healthy salad but don't drown it in high-fat salad dressings. Use 'light' dressings to halve the fat and calories.*

## Brands ~ Salad Dressings

| | C | F | Cb |
|---|---|---|---|
| **Annie's Naturals:** *Per 2 Tbsp* | | | |
| Organic: Buttermilk | 70 | 6 | 1 |
| French | 110 | 11 | 3 |
| Oil & Vinegar | 120 | 13 | 1 |
| Papaya & Poppy Seed | 90 | 8 | 5 |
| Red Wine & Olive Oil | 130 | 14 | 0 |
| Thousand Island | 90 | 8 | 5 |
| Vinaigrettes: Pomegranate | 70 | 7 | 2 |
| Sesame Ginger | 90 | 8 | 4 |
| Shitake Sesame | 120 | 13 | 1 |
| **Bernstein's:** *Per 2 Tbsp* | | | |
| Creamy Caesar | 120 | 13 | 1 |
| Herb Garden French | 130 | 12 | 6 |
| Italian | 110 | 12 | 1 |
| Restaurant Recipe Italian | 120 | 12 | 1 |
| Sweet Herb Italian | 130 | 11 | 8 |
| **Fat-Free,** Cheese & Garlic Italian | 10 | 0 | 2 |
| **Light Fantastic:** Cheese Fantastico | 25 | 1.5 | 3 |
| Roasted Garlic Balsamic | 45 | 3.5 | 3 |
| **Best Foods:** | | | |
| **Dijonnaise,** 1 tsp | 5 | 0 | 0.5 |
| **Mayonnaise:** *Per 1 Tbsp* | | | |
| Canola | 40 | 4.5 | 0 |
| Low-Fat | 15 | 1 | 2 |
| Light | 35 | 3.5 | 1 |
| Mayonesa, Lemom-Lime | 90 | 10 | 0 |
| Olive Oil, 2 Tbsp | 50 | 5 | 0.5 |
| Real Mayonnaise | 90 | 10 | 0 |
| **Tartar Sauce,** 2 Tbsp | 80 | 7 | 4 |
| **Cardini's:** *Per 2 Tbsp* | | | |
| Aged Parmesan Ranch | 150 | 16 | 1 |
| Caesar Original | 160 | 17 | 1 |
| Fat-Free Caesar | 40 | 0 | 9 |
| Light Caesar | 80 | 7 | 5 |
| Honey Mustard | 140 | 13 | 5 |
| Italian | 100 | 8 | 7 |
| Roasted Asian Sesame | 120 | 10 | 7 |
| Vinaigrette Dressing: | | | |
| Balsamic | 100 | 8 | 5 |
| Lite Balsamic | 50 | 3 | 5 |
| **Great Value:** *Per 2 Tbsp* | | | |
| Buttermilk Ranch; Caesar, av | 115 | 12 | 2 |
| Thousand Island | 90 | 7 | 6 |
| Light: Buttermilk Ranch | 80 | 7 | 3 |
| Balsamic/Raspberry Vinaig., av. | 50 | 3.5 | 4 |
| **Hidden Valley:** *Per 2 Tbsp* | | | |
| Cole Slaw | 150 | 15 | 5 |
| **Ranch:** Original | 140 | 14 | 2 |
| Light Original | 80 | 7 | 3 |

## Brands ~ Salad Dressings (Cont)

### Hidden Valley (Cont)

| | C | F | Cb |
|---|---|---|---|
| **Other Ranch Flavors:** | | | |
| Bacon | 140 | 14 | 1 |
| Cracked Peppercorn | 120 | 12 | 2 |
| Old-Fashioned Buttermilk | 130 | 14 | 2 |

### Kraft: *Per 2 Tbsp*

| | C | F | Cb |
|---|---|---|---|
| **Regular Dressings:** | | | |
| Caesar Vinaigrette with Parmesan | 70 | 5 | 3 |
| Catalina Dressing & Dip | 90 | 6 | 9 |
| Creamy Italian | 100 | 11 | 2 |
| Greek Vinaigrette | 110 | 12 | 2 |
| Honey Dijon Vinaigrette | 90 | 7 | 6 |
| Ranch Dressing & Dip | 130 | 13 | 3 |
| Roka Blue Cheese | 120 | 13 | 1 |
| Sweet Honey Catalina | 130 | 10 | 8 |
| Tangy Tomato Bacon | 100 | 6 | 10 |
| Thousand Island | 130 | 12 | 4 |
| Tuscan House Italian | 130 | 13 | 3 |
| **Kraft Free (Fat-Free):** Italian | 20 | 0 | 4 |
| Classic Caesar; Honey Dijon | 50 | 0 | 11 |
| **Light:** Asian Tst'd Sesame | 50 | 2.5 | 7 |
| Balsamic Vinaigrette | 30 | 1 | 4 |
| Creamy Caesar | 35 | 2 | 4 |
| Zesty Italian | 25 | 1.5 | 3 |
| **Seven Seas:** | | | |
| Green Goddess | 130 | 13 | 2 |
| Red Wine Vinaig.; Viva Robust Ital. | 90 | 9 | 2 |
| Reduced Fat: Viva Italian | 45 | 4 | 2 |
| Red Wine Vinaigrette | 45 | 4 | 3 |
| **Signature,** Raspb. Vinaig. | 60 | 4 | 5 |
| **Special Collection,** | | | |
| Parmesan Romano | 140 | 14 | 2 |

### Marie's: *Per 2 Tbsp*

| | C | F | Cb |
|---|---|---|---|
| Caesar; Creamy Ranch | 170 | 19 | 1 |
| Chunky Blue Cheese | 160 | 17 | 0 |
| Honey Dijon | 130 | 12 | 5 |
| Poppy Seed | 150 | 13 | 8 |
| Potato Salad Dressing: | | | |
| Classic | 170 | 19 | 0 |
| Dijon Herb | 140 | 15 | 1 |
| German Style | 110 | 11 | 3 |
| Sesame Ginger | 100 | 8 | 7 |
| Spinach Salad | 60 | 1.5 | 11 |
| Thousand Island | 150 | 15 | 4 |

### Marzetti's:

| | C | F | Cb |
|---|---|---|---|
| Organic: Caesar | 150 | 16 | 1 |
| Blue Cheese | 130 | 14 | 1 |
| Raspberry Cranberry | 100 | 8 | 6 |
| Chunky Blue Cheese | 150 | 15 | 1 |
| Classic Ranch | 160 | 17 | 1 |

### Marzetti's (Cont)

| | C | F | Cb |
|---|---|---|---|
| Thousand Island | 150 | 15 | 5 |
| Simply Dressed: Champagne | 80 | 8 | 2 |
| Greek Feta | 110 | 12 | 2 |

### Newman's Own: *Per 2 Tbsp*

| | C | F | Cb |
|---|---|---|---|
| **Regular:** Balsamic Vinaigrette | 90 | 9 | 3 |
| Creamy Caesar | 170 | 18 | 1 |
| Family Recipe Italian | 130 | 13 | 1 |
| Olive Oil & Vinegar | 150 | 16 | 1 |
| Parmesan Roasted Garlic | 110 | 11 | 2 |
| Ranch | 150 | 16 | 2 |
| **Lighten Up:** Light Italian | 60 | 6 | 1 |
| Light Raspberry & Walnut | 70 | 5 | 7 |
| **Organic:** Light Balsamic Vinaig. | 45 | 4 | 3 |
| Low Fat Asian | 35 | 2 | 5 |
| Tuscan Italian | 100 | 11 | 2 |

### Spectrum: *Per 2 Tbsp*

| | C | F | Cb |
|---|---|---|---|
| Organic Omega-3: | | | |
| Asian Ginger | 130 | 13 | 2 |
| Creamy Garlic Ranch | 120 | 13 | 1 |
| Golden Balsamic Vin. | 120 | 13 | 1 |
| Pomegranate Chipotle | 120 | 13 | 1 |
| Vegan Caesar | 100 | 9 | 2 |

### Wish-Bone:

| | C | F | Cb |
|---|---|---|---|
| **Creamy:** Chunky Blue Cheese | 150 | 15 | 1 |
| Creamy Caesar | 180 | 18 | 1 |
| Creamy Italian | 110 | 10 | 4 |
| Deluxe French | 120 | 11 | 5 |
| Ranch | 130 | 13 | 2 |
| Russian | 110 | 6 | 14 |
| Sweet 'n Spicy | 140 | 12 | 7 |
| Thousand Island | 130 | 12 | 5 |
| **Light:** Blue Cheese | 70 | 6 | 2 |
| Creamy Caesar | 70 | 6 | 2 |
| Honey Dijon | 70 | 5 | 6 |
| Italian | 35 | 2.5 | 3 |
| Parm. Peppercorn Ranch | 60 | 5 | 2 |
| Ranch | 70 | 5 | 4 |
| Thousand Island | 60 | 5 | 4 |
| **Fat-Free:** | | | |
| Chunky Blue Cheese | 30 | 0 | 7 |
| Italian | 15 | 0 | 3 |
| Ranch | 30 | 0 | 6 |
| **Oil & Vinegar:** Bals. Vinaig. | 60 | 5 | 3 |
| House Italian | 110 | 10 | 3 |
| Red Wine Vinaigrette | 70 | 5 | 6 |
| Robusto Italian | 80 | 7 | 4 |
| **Light Vinaigrette:** Balsamic & Basil | 60 | 5 | 3 |
| Asian with Sesame & Ginger | 70 | 5 | 5 |
| Raspberry Walnut | 80 | 5 | 7 |
| **Salad Spritzers,** average all flavors | | | |
| 10 sprays (¼ fl.oz) for 1 cup salad | 10 | 1 | 1 |

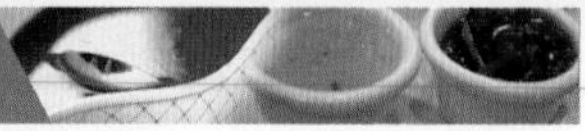

| Gravy | C | F | Cb |
|---|---|---|---|
| **Homemade Gravy,** average: | | | |
| Thin, little fat, 2 Tbsp, 1 oz | 20 | 1 | 3 |
| Thick: 2 Tbsp, 1.25 oz | 50 | 2 | 9 |
| ¼ cup, 2.5 oz | 100 | 4 | 18 |
| **McCormick Gravy Mix:** *Per Tbsp, mix with water* | | | |
| Brown | 20 | 0 | 3 |
| Turkey | 20 | 0.5 | 4 |

### Gravy-In-Jars-Homestyle

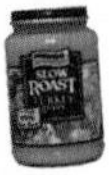

| | C | F | Cb |
|---|---|---|---|
| **Boston Market,** ¼ cup, 2 oz | 40 | 2 | 3 |
| **Franco-American,** Slow Roast, 99% Fat Free, ¼ cup, 2 oz | 25 | 0.5 | 4 |
| **Heinz:** | | | |
| Regular, all flav., ¼ cup, 2 oz | 25 | 2 | 4 |
| Fat Free, all flavors, ¼ cup, 2 oz | 20 | 0 | 4 |
| **Safeway,** all flavors, ¼ cup, 2 oz | 20 | 0.5 | 4 |

### Tomato Products

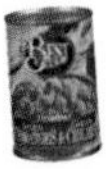

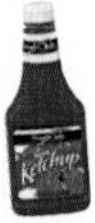

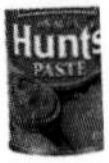

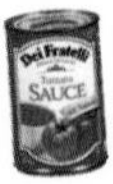

| Whole/Chopped/Crushed/Diced: | C | F | Cb |
|---|---|---|---|
| 1 cup, 8.5 oz | 50 | 0 | 10 |
| In Aspic, ½ cup | 50 | 0 | 12 |
| With Green Chili, 1 cup, 8.5 oz | 60 | 0 | 16 |
| Stewed, ½ cup, 1.7 oz | 40 | 1.5 | 6.5 |
| Wedges in Tomato Juice, 1 cup | 70 | 0.5 | 18 |
| Salsa, average, 1 Tbsp | 15 | 0 | 3.5 |
| **Tomato Ketchup:** | | | |
| Regular: 1 Tbsp, 0.5 oz | 15 | 0 | 4 |
| Single Serve, 1 packet | 10 | 0 | 3 |
| *One-Carb (Heinz),* 1 Tbsp, 0.5 oz | 5 | 0 | 1 |
| **Tomato Paste:** | | | |
| Regular: 2 Tbsp, 1 oz | 25 | 0 | 6 |
| ¾ cup, 6 oz | 140 | 1 | 32 |
| **Tomato Puree,** ½ cup, 4.5 oz | 50 | 0 | 10 |
| **Tomato Sauce:** | | | |
| Regular, ½ cup, 4.4 oz | 50 | 0 | 11 |
| Spanish Style, ½ cup, 4.3 oz | 40 | 0 | 9 |
| With Mushr., ½ cup, 4.3 oz | 45 | 0 | 10 |
| With Onions, ½ cup, 4.3 oz | 50 | 0 | 12 |
| **Tomato Seasoning,** 3 tsp | 20 | 0 | 4 |
| **Sundried Tomatoes:** | | | |
| Natural, 5-6 pieces, 0.4 oz | 22 | 0 | 5 |
| In Oil, drained, 6 pieces,0.5 oz | 40 | 2.5 | 4 |

### Sauces ~ Brands

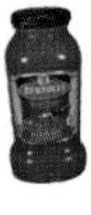

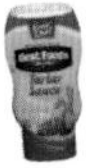

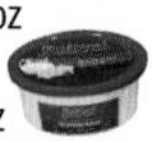

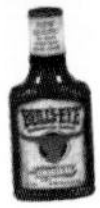

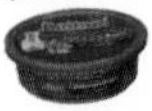

| | C | F | Cb |
|---|---|---|---|
| **A-1:** | | | |
| **Steak Sauces & Marinades:** *Per Tablespoon, ½ oz* | | | |
| Original | 15 | 0 | 3 |
| Bold & Spicy | 20 | 0 | 5 |
| Cracked Peppercorn | 15 | 0 | 0 |
| Kobe Sesame Teriyaki | 25 | 0 | 4 |
| Smokey Mesquite | 30 | 0 | 8 |
| Supreme Garlic | 25 | 0 | 5 |
| Sweet Hickory | 20 | 0 | 5 |
| Thick & Hearty | 25 | 0 | 6 |
| **Barilla:** *Per ½ Cup* | | | |
| Arrabbiata, Spicy Marinara | 60 | 1.5 | 11 |
| Basilico, Tomato & Basil | 80 | 3 | 11 |
| Calabrese, Sweet Peppers | 70 | 1.5 | 11 |
| Formaggi, Three Cheese | 70 | 1.5 | 11 |
| Marinara, Traditional | 90 | 3.5 | 12 |
| **Bertolli:** *Per ½ Cup* | | | |
| Traditional: Italian Sausage | 90 | 3 | 14 |
| Olive Oil & Garlic | 80 | 3 | 14 |
| Tomato & Basil | 70 | 2 | 13 |
| Vineyard Collection: Marinara | 80 | 2 | 14 |
| Portobello Mushroom, with Merlot | 80 | 2.5 | 12 |
| **Best Foods/Hellmann's,** Tartar Sauce, 2 Tbsp | 80 | 7 | 4 |
| **Buitoni:** | | | |
| **Pasta Sauces:** *Per ½ Cup Unless Indicated* | | | |
| Alfredo, ¼ cup, 2.15 oz | 140 | 12 | 4 |
| Light Alfredo, ¼ c., 2.15 oz | 90 | 6 | 5 |
| Marinara, 4.4 oz | 70 | 3 | 10 |
| With Rsted Garlic, 4.4 oz | 60 | 1 | 11 |
| Pesto: With Basil, ¼ c., 2.2 oz | 270 | 23 | 6 |
| Reduced Fat, ¼ cup, 2.2 oz | 230 | 17 | 8 |
| Tomato Herb Parmesan, 4,4 oz | 130 | 8 | 10 |
| Vodka, 4.23 oz | 90 | 6 | 5 |
| **Bull's Eye:** *Per 2 Tbsp* | | | |
| Original BBQ Sauce | 60 | 0 | 14 |
| Sweet & Tangy | 60 | 0 | 13 |
| Texas Style | 45 | 0 | 10 |
| **Catelli:** *Per ½ Cup* | | | |
| Pizza Sauce, average, 4 fl.oz | 60 | 1.5 | 11 |
| Meat Sauce, 4 fl.oz | 80 | 2.5 | 11 |
| **Garden Select 6 Vege Sauce:** *Per ½ Cup* | | | |
| Parmesan & Romano | 70 | 2.5 | 14 |
| Thick & Smooth, Diced Tom. & Basil | 70 | 1 | 12 |

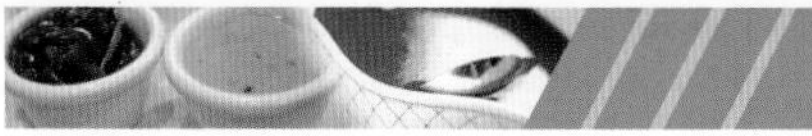

### Brands (Cont)

| | C | F | Cb |
|---|---|---|---|
| **Cento:** *Per ½ Cup* | | | |
| **Sauces:** | | | |
| All Natural: Pasta | 70 | 4 | 8 |
| Pizza | 30 | 0 | 5 |
| Arrabbiata | 70 | 3.5 | 6.5 |
| Marinara | 100 | 9 | 6 |
| Porcini | 70 | 3.5 | 4 |
| Puttanesca | 100 | 9 | 6 |
| White Clam | 160 | 2 | 3 |
| **Classico:** | | | |
| **Alfredo:** Creamy, ¼ cup | 100 | 9 | 3 |
| Roasted Red Pepper, ¼ cup | 60 | 5 | 3 |
| **Traditional Favorites Sauce:** *Per ½ Cup* | | | |
| Four Cheese | 80 | 3 | 12 |
| Italian Sausage w/ Peppers & Onions | 80 | 3 | 10 |
| Roasted Garlic | 60 | 2 | 9 |
| Sweet Basil | 70 | 1 | 13 |
| **Signature Recipes Sauce:** | | | |
| Basil Pesto, ¼ cup, 2.1 oz | 230 | 21 | 6 |
| Caramelized Onion & Rstd Garlic | 80 | 3 | 11 |
| Fire Roasted Tomato & Garlic | 50 | 1 | 8 |
| Florentine Spin. & Cheese | 80 | 4 | 9 |
| Mushrooms & Ripe Olives | 60 | 2 | 10 |
| Spicy Tomato & Pesto | 90 | 5 | 10 |
| Sun-Dried Tomato | 80 | 4 | 11 |
| **Colgin,** Liquid Smoke | 0 | 0 | 0 |
| **Contadina:** *Per ¼ Cup* | | | |
| **Pizza Sauce:** Flavored w/ Pepperoni | 35 | 1 | 5 |
| Original; Four Cheese | 30 | 0.5 | 6 |
| **Tomato Sauce,** average | 20 | 0 | 4 |
| **Crosse & Blackwell:** | | | |
| **Meat:** Ham Glaze, 1 Tbsp | 30 | 0 | 7 |
| Mint Sauce, 1 tsp | 5 | 0 | 1 |
| **Seafood:** Cocktail, ¼ cup, | 90 | 0 | 21 |
| Creole, 2 Tbsp | 45 | 0 | 9 |
| Remoulade, 2 Tbsp | 70 | 3 | 10 |
| **Dave's Gourmet:** *Per ½ Cup* | | | |
| Butternut Squash | 100 | 4 | 17 |
| Organic: Red Heirloom | 45 | 1.5 | 7 |
| Roasted Garli & Sweet Basil | 45 | 1.5 | 7 |
| **Del Monte:** | | | |
| **Spaghetti Sauces:** *Per ½ Cup* | | | |
| With Four Cheeses | 80 | 1 | 14 |
| Meat; Mushrooms | 70 | 1 | 14 |
| Average other varieties | 75 | 1 | 16 |
| **Sloppy Joe Sauce,** Orig. ¼ cup | 50 | 0 | 11 |

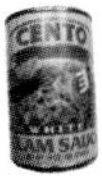

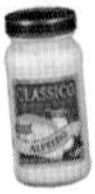

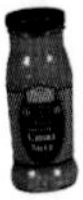

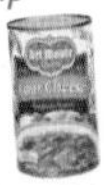

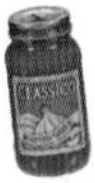

| | C | F | Cb |
|---|---|---|---|
| **Emeril's:** | | | |
| **Pasta Sauces:** *Per ½ Cup* | | | |
| Homestyle Marinara | 90 | 3 | 14 |
| Kicked Up Tomato | 80 | 3.5 | 11 |
| Roasted Gaaahlic | 80 | 3.5 | 12 |
| Roasted Red Pepper | 70 | 3.5 | 9 |
| Vodka Sauce | 110 | 7 | 12 |
| **Francesco Rinaldi:** *Per ½ Cup* | | | |
| **Traditional:** Original | 80 | 3 | 14 |
| Meat Flavored; Mushroom, average | 85 | 3 | 14 |
| **Hearty:** Super Mushroom | 100 | 4.5 | 15 |
| Three Cheese | 90 | 2 | 16 |
| **French's,** | | | |
| Worcestershire Sauce, 1 tsp | 60 | 0 | 1 |
| **Heinz:** *Per 1 Tbsp* | | | |
| 57 | 20 | 0 | 5 |
| Barbecue Sauces, all flavors | 35 | 0 | 9 |
| Chili Sauce | 20 | 0 | 5 |
| Horseradish Sauce | 75 | 6 | 3 |
| Tomato Ketchup: Regular | 20 | 0 | 5 |
| Reduced Sugar | 5 | 0 | 1 |
| Worcestershire Sauce, 1 Tbsp | 10 | 0 | 1 |
| **Original Cocktail Sauce,** | | | |
| ¼ cup, 2.2 oz | 60 | 0 | 15 |
| **House of Tsang:** *Per 1 Tbsp (Approx. ½ oz)* | | | |
| Bangkok Padang Peanut | 45 | 2.5 | 4 |
| Ginger Soy | 10 | 0 | 2 |
| General Tsao | 45 | 0.5 | 10 |
| Hibachi Grill: Kobe Steak | 50 | 4 | 3 |
| Hunan Smokehut | 40 | 1 | 8 |
| Sweet Ginger Sesame | 40 | 1 | 8 |
| Thai Peanut | 50 | 3 | 5 |
| Hoisin, 1 tsp | 15 | 0 | 3 |
| Imperial Citrus Stir-Fry | 25 | 0 | 5 |
| Korean Teriyaki Stir-Fry | 35 | 1.5 | 5 |
| Mandarin Marinade | 25 | 0 | 6 |
| Oyster Flavored | 30 | 0 | 7 |
| Sweet & Sour Stir-Fry | 35 | 0 | 9 |
| Szechuan Spicy Stir-Fry | 25 | 1 | 4 |
| **Hunt's:** | | | |
| **BBQ Sauce:** Original, 2 Tbsp | 60 | 0 | 15 |
| Hickory & Brown Sugar, 2 Tbsp | 70 | 0 | 18 |
| Manwich Sloppy Joe Sauce, ¼ cup | 40 | 0 | 9 |
| **Spaghetti Sauce:** *Per ½ Cup* | | | |
| Classic Italian: Four Cheese | 60 | 1 | 10 |
| Garlic & Herb | 40 | 1 | 8 |
| Meat Flavor | 60 | 1 | 10 |
| Traditional | 50 | 1 | 11 |
| Zesty & Spicy | 60 | 1.5 | 11 |

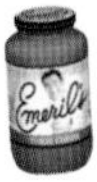

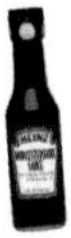

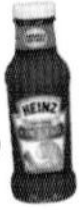

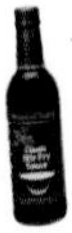

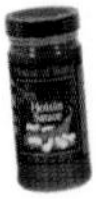

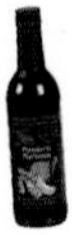

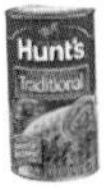

## Brands (Cont)

| Kikkoman: | C | F | Cb |
|---|---|---|---|
| Black Bean Sauce, w/ Garlic 2 T. | 50 | 1 | 6 |
| Hoisin Sauce, 2 Tbsp | 80 | 1.5 | 17 |
| Honey Mustard, 1Tbsp | 30 | 0 | 6 |
| Roasted Garlic & Herbs, 1 Tbsp | 20 | 0 | 4 |
| Teriyaki, 1 Tbsp | 15 | 0 | 2 |
| Teriyaki Roasted Garlic, 1 Tbsp | 25 | 0 | 4 |
| **Knorr:** | | | |
| **Classic Sauce:** *Per Whole Package* | | | |
| Bearnaise, dry mix only | 100 | 0 | 20 |
| Hollandaise, dry mix only | 100 | 0 | 20 |
| **Classic Brown Gravy,** av., ¼ cup | 20 | 0.5 | 3 |
| **Kraft:** | | | |
| **Specialty Sauce:** Cocktail, 2 Tbsp | 60 | 0.5 | 13 |
| Coleslaw Dressing, 1 oz | 110 | 8 | 9 |
| Horseradish, 1 tsp | 15 | 1.5 | 1 |
| Sandwich Spread, 1 Tbsp | 35 | 2.5 | 3 |
| Sweet 'n Sour, 2 Tbsp | 60 | 0 | 14 |
| **Tartar,** Original, 1 Tbsp | 60 | 4.5 | 4 |
| **Barbecue Sauces,** average, 2 Tbsp | 65 | 0 | 15 |
| **Las Palmas:** | | | |
| Red Chile Sauce, ¼ cup, 2 oz | 15 | 0.5 | 2 |
| **Enchilada Sauce:** | | | |
| Green Chili, 2oz | 25 | 1.5 | 3 |
| Red Chili, hot, 2 oz | 15 | 0.5 | 2 |
| **La Victoria,** Enchilada Sce, ¼ c, 2 oz | 20 | 0 | 4 |
| **Lawry's:** | | | |
| **30 Minute Marinade:** *Per Tbsp* | | | |
| Caribbean Jerk; Teriyaki, av. | 25 | 0 | 5 |
| Herb & Garlic; Lemon Pepper | 10 | 0 | 2 |
| Mesquite; Steak & Chop | 5 | 0 | 1 |
| Sesame Ginger | 30 | 0 | 7 |
| **Packet Seasonings:** *Dry* | | | |
| Fajitas; Taco, average, 2 tsp | 15 | 0 | 3 |
| Average other flavors, 2 tsp | 20 | 0 | 4 |
| **Lea & Perrins:** | | | |
| Worcestershire Sauce: 1 tsp | 5 | 0 | 1 |
| Thick, Classic, 2 Tbsp | 30 | 0 | 8 |
| **McCormicks:** | | | |
| **Seafood Sauces:** *Per ¼ Cup* | | | |
| Cajun Seafood Sauce, 2 T., 1.1 oz | 15 | 0 | 3 |
| Cocktail Sauce, Original/Extra Hot | 90 | 0.5 | 19 |
| Tartar Sauce: Original, 2 Tbsp | 140 | 14 | 3 |
| Fat Free, 2 T., 1 oz | 30 | 0 | 7 |
| Scampi Seafood Sauce, 2 T., 1 oz | 160 | 17 | 2 |

| Mrs. Dash: | C | F | Cb |
|---|---|---|---|
| **Marinades (Salt-Free):** *Per 1 Tbsp* | | | |
| Garlic Lime | 30 | 1.5 | 4 |
| Lemon Herb Peppercorn | 25 | 2 | 2 |
| Southwestern Chipotle | 25 | 1.5 | 2 |
| Spicy Teriyaki | 25 | 0.5 | 4 |
| **Newman's Own:** *Per ½ Cup* | | | |
| Regular: Bombolina | 90 | 4.5 | 13 |
| Five Cheese | 80 | 3 | 10 |
| Fra Diavolo | 70 | 3 | 10 |
| Marinara; Sockarooni | 70 | 2 | 12 |
| Roasted Garlic & Peppers | 70 | 2.5 | 11 |
| Vodka | 110 | 5 | 11 |
| **O Organics:** *Per ½ Cup* | | | |
| Marinara; Roasted Garlic, average | 60 | 1.5 | 9 |
| Mushroom; Tomato Basil | 50 | 1.5 | 8 |
| Roasted Garlic | 60 | 1.5 | 8 |
| **Old El Paso:** | | | |
| Enchilada Sauce: | | | |
| Green Chile, ¼ cup | 25 | 1.5 | 4 |
| Other varieties, ¼ cup | 20 | 0 | 4 |
| Salsas, Thick & Chunky, all var., 2 T. | 10 | 0 | 2 |
| Taco Sauce, 1 Tbsp | 5 | 0 | 1 |
| **Pace:** *Per 2 Tbsp* | | | |
| Chunky Salsa | 10 | 0 | 3 |
| Picante Sauce | 10 | 0 | 3 |
| Mexican Four Cheese, | | | |
| Salsa Con Queso | 90 | 7 | 5 |
| **Prego:** *Per ½ Cup* | | | |
| **100% Natural:** Marinara | 80 | 3 | 10 |
| Flavored with Meat | 80 | 2.5 | 13 |
| Fresh Mushroom; Traditional | 70 | 1.5 | 13 |
| Italian Sausage & Garlic | 90 | 3 | 13 |
| Mini Meatball | 100 | 3 | 13 |
| Mushroom & Garlic | 80 | 2.5 | 13 |
| Pizza Sauce | 70 | 1.5 | 13 |
| Roasted Garlic Parmesan | 70 | 1 | 13 |
| Three Cheese; Tom. Basil & Garlic, av. | 80 | 2 | 13 |
| **Chunky Garden:** | | | |
| Combo | 70 | 1.5 | 13 |
| Mushroom Supreme | 90 | 3 | 13 |
| Average other varieties | 90 | 3 | 13 |
| **Heart Smart:** Traditional; Mushroom | 70 | 1.5 | 13 |
| **Veggie Smart,** average | 90 | 1.5 | 17 |
| **Premier Japan:** | | | |
| Hoisin; Teriyaki, 1 Tbsp | 15 | 0 | 3 |
| Tamari, Ginger, 1 Tbsp | 5 | 0 | 1 |

## Brands (Cont)    C F Cb

**Ragu:** *Per ½ cup Unless Indicated*

| Item | C | F | Cb |
|---|---|---|---|
| **Pizza Quick Sauce,** | | | |
| Traditional, ¼ cup | 45 | 2 | 6 |
| **Pizza Sauce,** Homemade Style, ¼ cup | 30 | 1 | 5 |
| **White:** *Per ¼ Cup* | | | |
| Classic Alfredo | 110 | 10 | 2 |
| Light Parmesan | 60 | 5 | 2 |
| Roasted Garlic Parmesan | 110 | 10 | 3 |
| **Chunky:** | | | |
| Mushroom & Green Pepper | 80 | 2.5 | 13 |
| Average other varieties | 80 | 2.5 | 12 |
| Light varieties, average | 55 | 1 | 10 |
| **Old World Style:** Marinara | 80 | 3 | 10 |
| Flavored with Meat | 70 | 3 | 9 |
| Mushroom | 70 | 2.5 | 10 |
| Traditional | 80 | 2.5 | 11 |
| **Organic:** Garden Veggie | 80 | 2.5 | 12 |
| Traditional | 80 | 3 | 11 |
| **Robusto!:** 7-Herb Tomato | 80 | 3 | 12 |
| Chopped Tomato, Olive Oil & Garlic | 90 | 4 | 12 |
| Roasted Garlic | 80 | 2.5 | 13 |
| Sauteed Onion & Garlic | 90 | 3.5 | 12 |
| Six Cheese | 90 | 3 | 12 |
| **Safeway Select:** | | | |
| **Salsa,** average all flavors, 2 Tbsp | 15 | 0 | 3 |
| **Select Sauces:** *Per ½ Cup* | | | |
| Arrabbiata | 110 | 8 | 10 |
| Artichoke Pesto | 60 | 2 | 9 |
| Four Cheese | 80 | 3.5 | 11 |
| Garlic Basil | 70 | 4.5 | 7 |
| Marinara | 60 | 2 | 10 |
| Spicy Red Bell Pepper | 50 | 1 | 9 |
| Sundried Tomato & Olive | 60 | 1.5 | 11 |
| Tomato Alfredo; Vodka | 130 | 10 | 9 |
| **Taco Bell,** Jalapeno Sce, 2 Tbsp | 110 | 11 | 3 |
| **Tony Roma's:** | | | |
| Bold & Spicy, 2 Tbsp | 50 | 0 | 12 |
| Wing Sauce, 1 Tbsp | 15 | 1 | 0 |
| **Trader Joe's:** | | | |
| BBQ Sauce, Kansas City Style, 2 Tbsp | 60 | 0 | 15 |
| Tomato & Basil, ½ cup, 4.4 oz | 80 | 4.5 | 10 |
| **Walnut Acres:** *Per ½ Cup, 125g* | | | |
| Marinara & Zinfandel | 50 | 1 | 9 |
| Tomato & Basil: Regular | 50 | 1 | 9 |
| Low Sodium | 40 | 0 | 9 |
| Tomato & Mushroom | 50 | 1 | 9 |

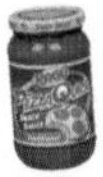

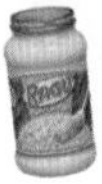

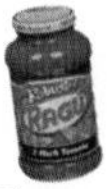

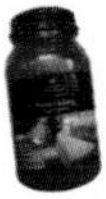

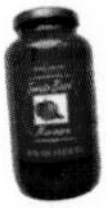

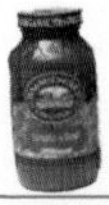

## Seasonings & Flavorings   C F Cb

| Item | C | F | Cb |
|---|---|---|---|
| *Accent,* Flavor Enhancer, 1 tsp | 0 | 0 | 0 |
| *Angostura Bitters,* 1 tsp | 15 | 0 | 4 |
| Bacon Bits, average, 1 Tbsp | 35 | 2 | 2 |
| Bacon Chips *(Durkee),* 1 Tbsp | 30 | 1 | 2 |
| Bac-Os *(Betty Crocker),* 1½ Tbsp | 20 | 1 | 1.5 |
| Butter Buds, 1 tsp | 5 | 0 | 2 |
| Garlic Bread Sprinkle, 1 tsp | 8 | 0.5 | 1 |
| Garlic Salt, 1 tsp | 2 | 0 | 0 |
| Italian Seasoning, 1 tsp | 4 | 0 | 1 |
| Lemon Pepper Seasoning, 1 tsp | 7 | 0 | 1 |
| Liquid Aminos *(Bragg),* 1 tsp | 0 | 0 | 0 |
| Meat Tenderizer, average, 1 tsp | 7 | 0 | 1 |
| *Molly McButter,* 1 tsp | 5 | 1 | 1 |
| *Mrs Dash,* Blends, 1 tsp | 0 | 0 | 0 |
| Salad Crunchies *(McCormick),* 1 tsp | 10 | 0.5 | 2 |
| Salt, Reg., Sea Salt, Lite Salt | 0 | 0 | 0 |
| Seasoning *(Old Bay),* ¼ tsp | 0 | 0 | 0 |
| Seasoning Mix *(Vegit),* ¼ tsp | 0 | 0 | 0 |
| Seasoning Mixes, av., ¼ pkg | 70 | 1 | 9 |
| Taco Seasoning, av., ¼ pkg | 30 | 0.5 | 4 |
| *Old El Paso:* Chili Season. Mix, 1 T. | 8 | 0.5 | 1.5 |
| Cheesy Taco Seasoning Mix, 1 Tbsp | 10 | 0.5 | 2 |
| Taco/Burrito Seasoning Mix, 2 tsp | 15 | 0 | 4 |
| Fajita Seasoning Mix, 1 tsp | 5 | 0 | 1.5 |

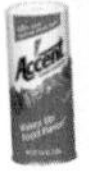

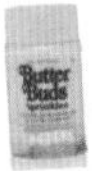

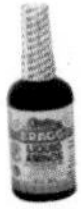

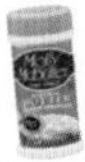

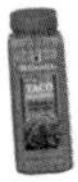

## Spices & Herbs

| Per Teaspoon: Average all types | C | F | Cb |
|---|---|---|---|
| Average all types | 5 | 0 | 1 |
| All Purpose, 1 tsp | 0 | 0 | 0 |
| Allspice, ground | 5 | 0 | 1 |
| Chili Powder | 8 | 0 | 1 |
| Cinnamon, ground | 6 | 0 | 2 |
| Curry Powder | 6 | 0 | 1 |
| Garlic Powder | 9 | 0 | 2 |
| Nutmeg, ground | 12 | 0 | 1 |
| Onion Powder | 7 | 0 | 2 |
| Parsley, dried | 4 | 0 | 1 |
| Pepper, average | 6 | 0 | 1 |
| Saffron | 2 | 0 | 0 |
| Salt-Free Blends, 1 tsp | 0 | 0 | 0 |
| Tumeric, ground | 8 | 0 | 1 |
| **Seeds:** Fenugreek | 12 | 1 | 2 |
| Mustard, Poppyseed | 15 | 1 | 1 |
| Other types, average | 7 | 0 | 1 |

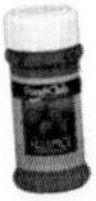

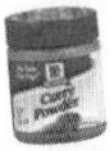

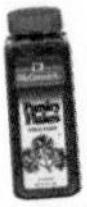

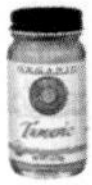

## Home-Popped Popcorn

| | C | F | Cb |
|---|---|---|---|
| **Popping Corn Kernels:** | | | |
| 2 Tbsp, 1 oz | 110 | 1 | 26 |
| (makes approximately 5 cups) | | | |
| **Air-popped,** w/o oil: Plain, 1 oz | 110 | 1 | 22 |
| 1 cup, 0.2 oz | 20 | 0 | 5 |
| **Oil-popped:** Plain, 1 oz | 145 | 8 | 16 |
| 1 cup, 0.4 oz | 55 | 3 | 6 |
| **Popcorn Oil,** 1 Tbsp | 120 | 14 | 0 |

## Microwave Popcorn

*Average all Brands: Per 1 Cup Popped, Unless Indicated*

| | C | F | Cb |
|---|---|---|---|
| Butter: Regular | 35 | 2 | 4 |
| Light | 25 | 1 | 4 |
| **Act II Popcorn:** | | | |
| Butter: 1 cup | 35 | 2 | 4 |
| 4½ cups, 1 oz | 160 | 9 | 18 |
| 94% Fat-Free Butter: 1 cup | 20 | 0.5 | 4 |
| 7 cups, 1 oz | 130 | 2.5 | 28 |
| Butter Lovers: 1 cup | 40 | 2 | 4 |
| 4 cups, 1 oz | 160 | 9 | 19 |
| Xtreme Butter: 1 cup | 45 | 3 | 4.5 |
| 4 cups | 180 | 12 | 18 |
| **American Fare (K-Mart):** | | | |
| **Smart Sense:** Butter: 0.3 oz | 40 | 2 | 5 |
| 3½ cups, 1 oz | 130 | 4.5 | 19 |
| Kettle Corn;Theatre Butter: 1 cup | 40 | 2 | 5 |
| 3½ cups | 130 | 6 | 18 |
| **Jolly Time:** | | | |
| American's Best | 20 | 0 | 4 |
| Blast O Butter: Regular | 45 | 3 | 5 |
| Light | 30 | 1.5 | 4 |
| Healthy Pop: Butter Flavor | 20 | 0 | 6 |
| Caramel Apple | 20 | 0 | 6 |
| Newman's Own: Butter Flavor, 3½ c. | 130 | 5 | 18 |
| Light Butter Flavor, 3½ cups | 140 | 4.5 | 22 |
| **Orville Redenbacher's:** | | | |
| Movie Theater Butter: 1 cup | 35 | 2 | 3 |
| 4½ cups, popped | 170 | 12 | 16 |
| Pop Up Bowls: Butter, 4 cups | 170 | 12 | 17 |
| Ultimate Butter, 4 cups | 170 | 12 | 16 |
| Pour Over Caramel, 2 cups | 170 | 8 | 24 |
| Smart Pop!, | | | |
| Tender White, 3½ cups | 170 | 12 | 15 |
| **Pop Secret:** | | | |
| 1-Step, Cheddar | 40 | 2.5 | 3 |
| 100 Calorie Pop, Butter | 15 | 0.5 | 3 |
| Butter; Extra Butter, av | 30 | 2 | 3 |
| Homestyle; Movie Theatre Butter, av | 35 | 2.5 | 3 |
| 94% Fat-Free: Butter | 15 | 0 | 3 |

## Bagged Popcorn

*Average All Brands (Ready-to-Eat)*

| | C | F | Cb |
|---|---|---|---|
| **Regular/Plain:** ½ oz package | 80 | 5 | 8 |
| 1 oz package | 160 | 10 | 16 |
| 4 oz package | 640 | 40 | 64 |
| 2 oz Box (store/airport) | 320 | 16 | 32 |
| 3 oz Bag (9" high x 5" wide) | 480 | 24 | 48 |
| **Caramel Popcorn,** | | | |
| with nuts, 1 cup, 1.5 oz | 230 | 12 | 39 |

## Brands ~ Bagged Popcorn

| | C | F | Cb |
|---|---|---|---|
| **Boston's:** Lite, 3½ cups, 1 oz | 130 | 4.5 | 20 |
| Homestyle, 2½ cups, 1 oz | 160 | 9 | 18 |
| **Cracker Jack:** Original, | | | |
| 1 cup, 1.5 oz | 180 | 3 | 35 |
| 4.25 oz pkg (Hunger Grab) | 510 | 8 | 98 |
| **Crunch 'N Munch:** | | | |
| Buttery Toffee: ⅔ cup, 1.1 oz | 150 | 6 | 22 |
| 1 cup, 1.6 oz | 220 | 9 | 32 |
| Caramel: ⅔ cup, 1.1 oz | 160 | 8 | 20 |
| 1 cup, 1.6 oz | 230 | 12 | 29 |
| 12 oz box | 1745 | 87 | 218 |
| **Fiddle Faddle:** | | | |
| Av. all varieties: 1 oz | 120 | 2 | 24 |
| 1 cup, 2 oz | 240 | 4 | 48 |
| 6 oz box | 720 | 12 | 144 |
| **Korn Krunch** *(Kornfections & Treasures)*, | | | |
| Almond Pecan (Sugar Free), 1 oz | 125 | 6 | 28 |
| **PopCorners,** Butter/Kettle, 1 oz | 120 | 3.5 | 21 |
| **Poppycock:** | | | |
| Original/Pecan Delight: ½cup, 1 oz | 150 | 8 | 20 |
| 1 cup, 2 oz | 300 | 16 | 40 |
| Original Clusters, 1 oz | 160 | 8 | 20 |
| Chocolate Lovers, 1.15 oz | 160 | 7 | 22 |

## Movie Theater Popcorn

| | C | F | Cb |
|---|---|---|---|
| **Small,** (7 cups): Plain | 385 | 21 | 44 |
| With Butter (3 pumps, 0.75 oz) | 570 | 42 | 44 |
| **Medium,** (15 cups): Plain | 825 | 45 | 94 |
| With Butter (4 pumps, 1 oz) | 1075 | 73 | 94 |
| **Large,** (20 cups): Plain | 1100 | 60 | 124 |
| With Butter (6 pumps, 1.5 oz) | 1485 | 102 | 124 |
| **Butter:** 1 Pump, 0.25 oz | 65 | 7 | 0 |
| 4 Pumps (2 Tbsp), 1 oz | 250 | 28 | 0 |

## Corn & Tortilla Chips

| Average All Brands | C | F | Cb |
|---|---|---|---|
| **Corn Chips:** | | | |
| Average all types: 1 oz | 150 | 8 | 18 |
| 8 oz bag | 1200 | 64 | 144 |
| *Fritos,* Original, 32 chips, 1 oz | 160 | 10 | 15 |
| **Tortilla Chips:** Average, 1 oz | 140 | 7 | 18 |
| *(1 oz = approx. 12 chips or 13 strips)* | | | |
| *Doritos:* Regular, 13 chips, 1 oz | 140 | 7 | 18 |
| Reduced Fat (13), 1 oz | 130 | 5 | 19 |
| White Nacho Cheese, 1 oz | 150 | 8 | 17 |
| Baked! Nacho Cheese (15), 1 oz | 120 | 3.5 | 21 |
| *Kettle:* Tias, av. all flavors, 1 oz | 145 | 8 | 17 |
| Salsa Picante, 1 oz | 140 | 8 | 17 |
| *Snyder's:* White/Yellow Corn | 140 | 4.5 | 23 |
| Restaurant Style, 1 oz | 130 | 5 | 20 |
| *Utz:* White/Yellow Corn | 140 | 7 | 18 |
| Restaurant Style | 130 | 6 | 18 |
| **Tostitos:** | | | |
| Average all, 1 oz | 145 | 7 | 19 |
| Baked! Scoops, 1 oz | 120 | 3 | 22 |
| Blue Corn, 1 oz | 140 | 7 | 19 |

## Potato Chips/Crisps

| Average All Brands | C | F | Cb |
|---|---|---|---|
| **Regular:** | | | |
| Plain or flavored, (2 chips) | 15 | 1 | 1.5 |
| 1 oz package (20 chips) | 150 | 10 | 15 |
| 4 oz quantity | 600 | 40 | 60 |
| 14 oz package | 2100 | 140 | 210 |
| **Brands:** | | | |
| *Lay's,* Regular, av. all 1 oz | 160 | 10 | 15 |
| *Lay's Stax,* av. all, 1 oz | 150 | 9 | 15 |
| *Pringles:* Original; Xtreme | 150 | 9 | 15 |
| Large, 6.41 oz can | 960 | 58 | 96 |
| Minis, 1 bag, 0.8 oz | 140 | 9 | 16 |
| Snack Stacks, av., 1 tub | 140 | 9 | 12 |
| Multi Grain, all flav., 1 oz | 140 | 8 | 16 |
| *Ruffles,* Reg., av., 1 oz | 160 | 11 | 15 |
| **Reduced Fat:** | | | |
| *Lay's,* Kettle, 1 oz | 140 | 6 | 19 |
| *Pringles,* all flavors, 16 Chips, 1 oz | 130 | 7 | 17 |
| *Sun Chips:* Original | | | |
| 16 chips, 1 oz | 140 | 6 | 19 |
| **Low-Fat/Baked:** | | | |
| *Lay's Baked!,* Original (15), 1 oz | 120 | 2 | 23 |
| *Ruffles Baked!,* Average all, | 120 | 3.5 | 21 |
| Baked! Tostitos Scoops, (15) 1 oz | 120 | 3 | 22 |
| **Fat Free:** *Lay's Light,* Original, 1 oz | 75 | 0 | 17 |
| *Pringles,* (Fat-Free) (15). 1 oz | 70 | 0 | 15 |

## Pretzels

| Average All Brands | C | F | Cb |
|---|---|---|---|
| **Hard-Baked Pretzels:** *Each* | | | |
| 1 oz quantity | 110 | 1 | 23 |
| Sticks, thin, 2¼" (9/oz) | 12 | 0 | 3 |
| Twists, thin, ¼" thick, (5/oz) | 25 | 0 | 5 |
| Dutch (2¾"x 2⅝"), 0.5 oz | 55 | 1 | 11 |
| Sourdough *(Snyder's)*, 0.75 oz | 100 | 0 | 22 |
| **Soft Pretzels** *(Twists)* average: Each | | | |
| Plain: Small, 2 oz | 210 | 2 | 43 |
| Medium, 4 oz | 390 | 3.5 | 80 |
| Large, 5 oz | 485 | 4.5 | 100 |
| New York Street Vendors, 7 oz | 660 | 6 | 135 |
| Big Cheese, 1.76 oz | 130 | 3 | 22 |
| **Peanut Butter filled** *(Tr. Joe's)*, 1 oz | 150 | 8 | 14 |
| **Milk Choc-Coated** *(Snyders)*, 1 oz | 140 | 6 | 19 |
| **White Choc covered,** 7 pieces, 1 oz | 130 | 6 | 19 |

## Brands ~ Pretzels

| | C | F | Cb |
|---|---|---|---|
| *Flipz:* Milk Choc, 8 pcs, 1 oz | 140 | 5.5 | 22 |
| White Fudge, 7 pcs, 1 oz | 130 | 5 | 20 |
| *Rold Gold (Frito-Lay):* | | | |
| Braided Twists, | | | |
| Honey Wheat (8), 1 oz | 110 | 1 | 24 |
| Classic: Pretzel Sticks, 1 oz | 100 | 0 | 23 |
| Rods/Tiny Twists, av., 1 oz | 110 | 1 | 23 |
| Fat-Free, Tiny Twists, 1 oz | 110 | 0 | 23 |
| Sourdough, 1 pretzel | 90 | 1 | 19 |
| **Snyder's of Hanover Pretzels:** | | | |
| 100 Calorie Pack, Snaps, 0.9 oz | 100 | 0.5 | 22 |
| Gluten Free Pretzel Sticks (30) | 120 | 1.5 | 25 |
| Homestyle (15), 1 oz | 120 | 1 | 25 |
| Organic Sticks: | | | |
| Honey Whole Wheat | 110 | 2 | 20 |
| Whole Wheat & Oat | 110 | 1.5 | 21 |
| Pretzel Chips, Original, (14) | 110 | 0.5 | 24 |
| Rods (3), 1 oz | 120 | 1.5 | 24 |
| Thins, 1 oz | 110 | 0 | 23 |
| **SuperPretzel:** | | | |
| Soft Pretzels (1) | 160 | 1 | 34 |
| Softstix (2) | 130 | 3 | 22 |
| Soft Pretzel Bites (5) | 150 | 0.5 | 32 |
| **Pretzelfils:** Pizza (2) | 120 | 2 | 20 |
| Pepperjack; Mozzarella, (2),av. | 130 | 4.5 | 19 |
| *Utz:* Chocolate covered, 2 pcs | 110 | 4 | 17 |
| Average other varieties , 1 oz | 110 | 1 | 21 |

## Snacks    C   F   Cb

Note: Actual weight of packaged snacks is usually 5-10% more than label Net Wt. For accuracy, weigh snack and allow extra calories, fat and carbs for any extra weight.

| Item | C | F | Cb |
|---|---|---|---|
| **Apple Chips** (Seneca), av., 1 oz | 140 | 7 | 20 |
| **Bagel Crisps** (N.Y. Style) 6 crisps, 1 oz | 130 | 6 | 17 |
| **Banana Chips,** (T.Joe's), 13 chips, 1 oz | 160 | 11 | 13 |
| **Beef Jerky** (Jack Link's), av., 1 oz | 80 | 1 | 5 |
| **Beef Sticks:** (Slim Jim), Orig., 0.28 oz | 40 | 3.5 | 0 |
| (Jack Links), Original, 1 oz | 110 | 9 | 1 |
| **Bugles,** Orig.; Nacho, 1⅓ cup, 1 oz | 160 | 9 | 18 |
| **Cheese Balls,** 1 oz package | 130 | 7 | 16 |
| **Cheese Nips,** 1.25 oz package | 170 | 7 | 22 |
| **Cheese Puffs:** Average, 1 oz | 160 | 10 | 15 |
| Snyder's, Multigrain, 1 oz | 130 | 6 | 20 |
| **Cheese Twists,** 1 oz | 140 | 8 | 15 |
| **Cheerios,** Snack Mix, average, ⅔ cup, 1.1 oz | 130 | 3.5 | 22 |
| **Cheetos:** Av. all flav., 1 oz | 160 | 10 | 15 |
| 4 oz package | 640 | 40 | 60 |
| Baked!; Fantastix, av. 1 oz | 130 | 5 | 19 |
| Natural White Cheddar Puffs, 1 oz | 150 | 9 | 16 |
| **Cheez Balls,** 27 balls, 1 oz | 150 | 9 | 11 |
| **Cheez-It Crackers:** | | | |
| Original, 1.23 oz package | 180 | 9 | 20 |
| Baked, reduced fat, av., 1 oz | 130 | 4.5 | 21 |
| Big (13) | 150 | 8 | 17 |
| Party Mix, 1 pouch, 0.74 oz | 100 | 3 | 15 |
| **Chester's,** Fries, 1 oz | 150 | 8 | 17 |
| **Chex Mix** (General Mills): | | | |
| 100 Calorie, av., 1 bag, 0.81 oz | 100 | 3 | 18 |
| **Snack Mix:** BBQ; Tradt'nl, av., 1 oz | 120 | 4 | 21 |
| Chipotle Cheddar, 1.2 oz | 140 | 4.5 | 24 |
| **Chips Ahoy!:** Choc Chip Cookies: | | | |
| 1.4 oz Single Serve Pack | 190 | 9 | 27 |
| Mini: 3 oz package | 410 | 20 | 57 |
| Go-Pak!, 4 oz cup | 570 | 27 | 77 |
| **Churros** (Rubio's) 9", 1.6 oz | 170 | 8 | 22 |
| **Combos,** | | | |
| Crackers: ⅓ cup, 1 oz | 140 | 6 | 18 |
| Snack size, 1.7 oz pkg | 240 | 11 | 31 |
| Pretzels: ⅓ cup, 1 oz | 130 | 4.5 | 19 |
| Single snack bag, average, 1.7oz | 235 | 8 | 34 |
| **Cookies** ~ See Pages 81 | | | |
| **Cool Cuts,** Carrot & Ranch, 2.3 oz | 70 | 5 | 5 |
| **Corn Chips** ~ See Page 149 | | | |
| **Corn Nuts:** ⅓ cup, 1 oz | 120 | 4.5 | 20 |
| 1.7 oz bag | 210 | 8 | 34 |
| **Corn Puffs/Twists,** (32 approx), 1 oz | 160 | 11 | 15 |
| **Dunkin Stixs** (Hostess), (3) 4oz | 490 | 25 | 63 |

## Snacks (Cont)    C   F   Cb

| Item | C | F | Cb |
|---|---|---|---|
| **Edamame** (Seapointe), dry rstd, 1 oz pkg | 130 | 4 | 10 |
| Choc. Covered (Trader Joe's), 1.5 oz | 200 | 11 | 21 |
| **Fig Newtons:** | | | |
| Regular, 2 oz pkg | 200 | 4 | 40 |
| Fat-Free, 2.1 oz pkg | 200 | 0 | 44 |
| Minis, Fig/Strawb., av., 1.34 oz pkg | 130 | 3 | 27 |
| **Flipz** ~ See page 149 | | | |
| **Fritos,** av. all, (30), 1oz | 160 | 10 | 15 |
| Flavor Twists (23), 1 oz | 150 | 9 | 16 |
| **Funyuns,** 1⅛ oz package | 220 | 11 | 27 |
| **Goldfish** (Pepp. Farm), 1 oz | 140 | 5 | 20 |
| **Gold-N-Chees** (Lance), 1.25 oz | 190 | 10 | 19 |
| **Hot Peanuts** (Lays), 1.65 oz | 310 | 25 | 10 |
| **Lance S'wich Crackers:** Per Pack, 6 pcs | | | |
| Nip Chee/Toasty, average | 185 | 9 | 21 |
| Toast Chee | 220 | 12 | 23 |
| Whole Grain: Cheese | 190 | 9 | 25 |
| Peanut Butter | 180 | 9 | 23 |
| **Munchies Snack Mix** (Frito-Lay): | | | |
| Cheese Fix, ¾ cup | 140 | 7 | 18 |
| Flaming; Totally Ranch, ¾ c. | 140 | 6 | 19 |
| **Munchos,** 16 pieces, 1 oz | 160 | 10 | 16 |
| **Nabisco,** Toasted Chips: | | | |
| Ritz, average all flavors, 1 oz | 130 | 5.5 | 20 |
| Wheat Thins, 1 oz | 125 | 4.5 | 20 |
| **Nutter Butter,** Sandwich Cookies: | | | |
| Singles, 1.9 oz pkg | 250 | 10 | 37 |
| Bites: 1.25 oz pkg | 170 | 7 | 24 |
| Milk Choc-Covered, 2.54 oz pkg | 350 | 17 | 48 |
| **Onion Rings** (T.G.I. Friday), 1 oz | 130 | 6 | 19 |
| **Oreo Cookies:** | | | |
| Double Stuf: 1.5 oz pkg | 210 | 10 | 30 |
| Mini Bite Size: (9 cookies), 1.25 oz | 170 | 7 | 25 |
| Go-Pak, 4 oz cup | 530 | 22 | 81 |
| Snak-Saks, 8 oz pkg | 1040 | 48 | 168 |
| **Oreo Cakesters,** soft, 2 oz | 250 | 12 | 36 |
| **Oriental Mix** (Rice Snacks), 1 oz | 125 | 3.5 | 21 |
| **Peanut Butter Nuggets,** (10), 1 oz | 140 | 6 | 15 |
| **Pirate's Booty:** | | | |
| 1 oz bag | 130 | 5 | 19 |
| 4 oz bag | 520 | 20 | 76 |
| With Caramel, 2.75 oz bag | 330 | 5.5 | 63 |
| **Pita Chips,** average, (9) 1 oz | 130 | 4 | 18 |
| **PopCorners,** Butter/Kettle, 1 oz | 120 | 5.5 | 21 |
| **Popcorn** ~ See Page 148 | | | |
| **Pork Cracklins,** 1 oz | 160 | 12 | 0 |
| **Pork Skins/Rinds:** 1 oz | 160 | 10 | 0 |
| Baken-ets, 99c pkg, 1.25 oz | 200 | 13 | 0 |
| Mission, Chicharrones, 3 oz pkt | 480 | 27 | 0 |

## Snacks (Cont)

| | C | F | Cb |
|---|---|---|---|
| Potato Chips ~ *See Page 149* | | | |
| Potato Skins *(TGI Friday)*, (16), 1 oz | 130 | 9 | 24 |
| Pretzels ~ *See Page 149* | | | |
| Quakes Rice Snacks, average, 1 oz | 130 | 4 | 26 |
| Rice Cakes: *Lundberg*, (1), av, 0.7 oz | 75 | 0.5 | 16 |
| Quaker (1), average, 0.4 oz | 50 | 1 | 9 |
| Rice Chips *(Lundberg)*, av., 1 oz | 140 | 7 | 18 |
| **Ritz Bits S'wiches:** | | | |
| Cheese: 1.5 oz package | 220 | 13 | 24 |
| Go-Pak: 13 crackers, 1 oz | 150 | 9 | 17 |
| 3½ oz Pak | 520 | 29 | 58 |
| P'nut Butter: 1.25 oz pkg | 170 | 10 | 20 |
| Big Bag (99cents), 3 oz | 420 | 23 | 48 |
| Sabritones, 2⅛ oz pkg | 300 | 16 | 34 |
| **Sandwich Crackers** *(Austin):* | | | |
| Cheese Cracker w/ Cheddar, 1.38 oz | 190 | 10 | 23 |
| Cheese Cracker w/ Pnut Butter, 1.3 oz | 190 | 10 | 23 |
| PB & J Flavored, 1.38 oz | 190 | 8 | 26 |
| Sesame Sticks *(SunRidge Farm)*, 1.1 oz | 170 | 11 | 14 |
| Smart Puffs *(Pirates Booty)*, 1.1 oz | 150 | 8 | 18 |
| Snack Mix *(Quaker)*, Kids Mix, 1 pkg | 110 | 4 | 18 |
| Snackwell's, Cookies,Crm S'wich (1) | 110 | 3 | 20 |
| Soy Crisps, average,1 oz | 120 | 3 | 17 |
| Soy Nuts: Dry Roasted, ¼ cup, 1 oz | 130 | 6 | 9 |
| Choc-coated, 1 oz | 140 | 7 | 13 |
| **Sun Chips** *(Fritolay)*, | | | |
| average (15 chips), 1 oz | 140 | 6 | 19 |
| Takis: Fajitas (12), 1 oz | 140 | 7 | 17 |
| 4 oz package | 560 | 28 | 68 |
| **TastyKake:** | | | |
| Koffee Kake Jr., 2.5 oz | 280 | 10 | 45 |
| Chocolate Jr., 3 oz | 320 | 13 | 48 |
| Creme Filled Koffee Kakes (2) | 230 | 10 | 25 |
| Tings *(Robert's)*, 2 oz bag | 300 | 16 | 36 |
| Toasted Cheese Crackers, 1 package | 220 | 11 | 23 |
| Tortilla Chips ~ *Page 149* | | | |
| **Tostitos:** | | | |
| Blue; Yellow; Scoops; | | | |
| average, 1 oz | 140 | 7 | 19 |
| Multigrain, 1 oz | 150 | 8 | 18 |
| **Trail Mix (Nuts/Seeds/Dried Fruit):** | | | |
| Regular, 3 Tbsp, 1 oz | 140 | 9 | 13 |
| Tropical, 3 Tbsp, 1 oz | 130 | 7 | 16 |
| Turkey Jerky: Teriyaki, 1 oz | 80 | 1 | 8 |
| Original *(Trader Joe's)*, 1 oz | 60 | 0.5 | 6 |
| Veggie Crisps *(Snyder's)*, 1 oz | 140 | 7 | 20 |
| Wasabi Peas, ¼ cup, 1 oz | 120 | 3 | 19 |
| Yogurt Pretzels, (7), 1.5 oz | 190 | 7 | 30 |
| Yogurt Raisins *(Sun-Maid)*, 1 oz | 120 | 4.5 | 20 |

## Fruit Snacks

| | C | F | Cb |
|---|---|---|---|
| **Betty Crocker:** Fruit Gushers, 0.9 oz | 90 | 1 | 20 |
| Fruit by the Foot, 1 roll, 0.75 oz | 80 | 1 | 17 |
| Fruit Roll Ups, 1 roll, 0.5 oz | 50 | 1 | 12 |
| Fruit Flavored Shapes: | | | |
| Dora The Explorer, 0.9 oz | 80 | 0 | 19 |
| Scooby Doo, 0.9 oz | 80 | 0 | 19 |
| All other varities, 0.9 oz | 80 | 0 | 19 |
| **Sunkist:** Fruit Snacks, 1 pouch | 80 | 0 | 19 |
| Fruit Smoothie Blitz, 1.3 oz | 140 | 1 | 32 |

## Vending Machines

| | C | F | Cb |
|---|---|---|---|
| Bugles, Nacho Cheese, 1.5 oz | 220 | 12 | 25 |
| Cheese Balls *(Utz)*, 1 oz | 150 | 9 | 16 |
| Cheetos, Crunchy, 2 oz | 325 | 20 | 30 |
| Cheeze-It, Snack Mix, 1.5 oz | 195 | 6.5 | 30 |
| Chex Mix, average, 1.75 oz | 220 | 5 | 42 |
| Chester's Fries, 1.75 oz | 260 | 14 | 29 |
| Choc Chip Cookies: *Chips Ahoy*, 1.4 oz | 190 | 9 | 27 |
| Famous Amos, 2 oz | 280 | 13 | 38 |
| Grandma's (2), 2⅞ oz | 350 | 14 | 53 |
| **Chocolate Bars:** *Hershey's*, 1.55 oz | 210 | 13 | 26 |
| Kit Kat, 1.5 oz | 210 | 11 | 28 |
| Milky Way, 2 oz | 260 | 10 | 41 |
| Snickers, 2.07 oz bar | 280 | 14 | 35 |
| Donut, plain, 1.4 oz | 160 | 9 | 18 |
| Doritos, 1.75 oz | 245 | 12 | 32 |
| Fritos Corn Chips, Orig., 1.75 oz | 280 | 17 | 26 |
| Fruit Pie *(Hostess)*, 4.5 oz | 480 | 20 | 68 |
| Granola/Cereal Bars, av., 1 oz | 140 | 3 | 26 |
| **M & M's,** Milk Chocolate, 1.69 oz | 240 | 10 | 34 |
| Peanuts, 1.74 oz | 250 | 13 | 30 |
| Oreo Cookies, 1.8 oz | 250 | 10 | 37 |
| **Peanut Butter Cups,** | | | |
| Reese's, 1.5 oz | 230 | 13 | 23 |
| Popcorn, plain, 1 oz | 160 | 10 | 16 |
| Pop Chips, 0.8 oz | 100 | 3 | 16 |
| Pork Skins, 1.5 oz | 240 | 15 | 0 |
| Potato Chips: 1 oz | 150 | 10 | 15 |
| Baked! *(Ruffles)*, 1.12 oz | 140 | 4 | 24 |
| Potato Skins *(TGI Friday's)*, 1.5 oz | 225 | 12 | 29 |
| Pretzels *(Snyder's)*, Old Time, 2.25 oz | 110 | 1 | 23 |
| Raisins, ½ oz package | 45 | 0 | 11 |
| Rice Krispies Treat | 90 | 2.5 | 17 |
| Skittles, 2.17 oz | 250 | 2.5 | 56 |
| Starburst, Fruit Chews, Orig., 2.07 oz | 240 | 4.5 | 48 |
| Tortilla Chips, 1 oz | 140 | 7 | 18 |
| Soft Drinks, av.: 12 fl.oz | 145 | 0 | 40 |
| 20 fl.oz bottle | 245 | 0 | 62 |

## Homemade & Restaurant

| Restaurant & Take-Out: Average All Preparations, Per 8 fl.oz | C | F | Cb |
|---|---|---|---|
| Bean Medley | 200 | 3 | 34 |
| Beef Consomme | 30 | 0 | 2 |
| Borscht (with Sour Cream) | 130 | 8 | 14 |
| Bouillabaisse | 400 | 15 | 10 |
| Chicken & Corn | 290 | 14 | 20 |
| Chicken & Wild Rice | 80 | 4 | 9 |
| Chicken Consomme | 50 | 0 | 2 |
| Chicken Curry | 180 | 8 | 18 |
| Chicken Jambalaya | 160 | 7 | 8 |
| Chicken Noodle | 80 | 2 | 12 |
| with Chicken | 160 | 4 | 12 |
| Chicken Soup | 80 | 2 | 6 |
| Chili with Beans | 250 | 12 | 25 |
| Clam Chowder | 240 | 15 | 17 |
| Corn & Crab | 120 | 3 | 18 |
| Corn Chowder | 150 | 8 | 16 |
| Cream of Broccoli | 200 | 12 | 20 |
| Cream of Potato | 150 | 6.5 | 17 |
| Cream of Mushroom | 200 | 13 | 15 |
| Fish Chowder | 220 | 15 | 6 |
| French Onion | 420 | 15 | 25 |
| Gazpacho | 50 | 0 | 5 |
| Lentil Soup | 250 | 9 | 28 |
| Lobster Bisque | 320 | 15 | 10 |
| Matzo Ball (with 1 large ball) | 180 | 7 | 24 |
| Minestrone | 125 | 2.5 | 20 |
| Mulligatawny | 300 | 15 | 8 |
| Pea & Ham | 240 | 10 | 25 |
| Potato & Bacon | 170 | 7 | 19 |
| Pumpkin, Creamy | 210 | 10 | 26 |
| Shark Fin Soup | 100 | 4 | 8 |
| Spicy Shrimp Soup, 1 bowl | 160 | 7 | 10 |
| Split Pea Soup | 180 | 2.5 | 30 |
| Vegetable (Fat Free) | 75 | 0 | 18 |
| Vegetable Beef | 80 | 2 | 10 |
| Vichyssoise | 200 | 9 | 15 |
| Watercress | 90 | 4 | 13 |

**Other Soups** ~ See International & Fast-Foods Sections (Arby's, Au Bon Pain, Boston Market, Dunkin' Donuts, Denny's, Schlotzsky's, Sizzler, Souplantation,Sweet Tomatoes, Zoup!)
**Homemade Soups:** Calculate calories, fat and carbohydrates from recipe ingredients.

## Bouillon Cubes & Powders

| Bouillon Cubes: Average all Types | C | F | Cb |
|---|---|---|---|
| Regular, 1 cube | 5 | 0 | 1 |
| Granulate, sodium fre | 10 | 0 | 2 |
| **Powders,** average, 1 tsp | 10 | 0 | 1 |
| **Herb-Ox:** | | | |
| Instant Broth & Seasoning, Beef, 1 envelope | 5 | 0 | 1 |
| Chicken; Vegetarian | 5 | 0 | 1 |

## Soup

| Amy's: | C | F | Cb |
|---|---|---|---|
| **Heat & Serve:** Per ½ Can, 1 Cup, Unless Indicated | | | |
| Organic: Alphabet | 80 | 0 | 16 |
| Chunky Vegetable | 60 | 0 | 13 |
| Cream of Mushroom, ¾ cup, 6 fl.oz | 150 | 9 | 13 |
| Cream of Tomato | 110 | 2.5 | 19 |
| Curried Lentil | 230 | 8 | 30 |
| Fire Roasted Southwestern Vege | 140 | 4 | 21 |
| Indian Golden Lentil | 220 | 9 | 25 |
| Lentil Vegetable | 160 | 4 | 24 |
| Rustic Italian Vegetable | 140 | 6 | 18 |
| Split Pea | 100 | 0 | 19 |
| Thai Coconut | 140 | 10 | 10 |
| Tuscan Bean & Rice | 160 | 4.5 | 25 |
| Vegetable Barley | 70 | 1 | 13 |
| **Andersen's:** Per ½ Can, 1 Cup | | | |
| Lentil | 110 | 2 | 19 |
| Split Pea | 130 | 0 | 24 |
| Split Pea with Bacon | 140 | 1 | 23 |
| Tomato | 130 | 3.5 | 22 |
| **Campbell's:** | | | |
| **Chunky:** Per 8 fl.oz Cup | | | |
| Baked Potato w/ Ched. & Bacon Bits | 200 | 9 | 24 |
| Chicken Corn Chowder | 290 | 10 | 20 |
| Classic Chicken Noodle | 120 | 3 | 14 |
| Hearty Beef Noodle | 110 | 1 | 17 |
| Hearty Style Ital. Wedding | 140 | 2.5 | 21 |
| Hearty Tomato with Pasta | 140 | 1 | 30 |
| **Condensed Soup:** Per ½ Cup Soup | | | |
| Bean with Bacon | 160 | 3 | 25 |
| Beef w/ Vegs & Barley | 90 | 1.5 | 16 |
| Cheddar Cheese | 100 | 5 | 11 |
| Chicken Won Ton | 50 | 1 | 8 |
| Cream of Broccoli | 90 | 5 | 12 |

### Campbell's (Cont):

**Condensed Soup (Cont):** *Per ½ Cup Soup*

| | C | F | Cb |
|---|---|---|---|
| Cream of Mushroom | 100 | 6 | 9 |
| Cream of Potato | 90 | 2 | 15 |
| Cream of Shrimp | 100 | 6 | 8 |
| French Onion | 70 | 1.5 | 12 |
| Harvest Orange Tomato | 100 | 1 | 22 |
| Manhattan Clam Chowder | 60 | 0.5 | 12 |
| New England Clam Chowder | 90 | 2 | 15 |
| Split Pea with Ham & Bacon | 180 | 2 | 30 |
| Tomato | 90 | 0 | 20 |

**Healthy Kids Condensed Soup:** *Per ½ Cup Soup*

| | C | F | Cb |
|---|---|---|---|
| Dora The Explorer | 70 | 2 | 12 |
| Chicken Alphabet | 70 | 2 | 12 |
| Chicken & Stars | 70 | 2 | 11 |
| Chicken NoodleO's | 90 | 2.5 | 15 |
| Goldfish Pasta | 80 | 2 | 12 |

**Select Harvest:** *Per Cup*

| | C | F | Cb |
|---|---|---|---|
| Beef with Roasted Barley | 130 | 1 | 22 |
| Carmelized French Onion | 70 | 2 | 10 |
| Chicken Vegetable Medley | 120 | 1.5 | 20 |
| Chicken w/ Egg Noodles | 90 | 3 | 10 |
| Creamy Chicken Alfredo | 220 | 13 | 15 |
| Creamy Potato with Roasted Garlic | 180 | 10 | 20 |
| Italian-Style Wedding | 100 | 2.5 | 13 |
| New Eng. Clam Chowder | 190 | 10 | 19 |
| Potato Broccoli Cheese | 180 | 10 | 18 |
| Split Pea w/ Roasted Ham | 120 | 1 | 20: |

**Classic Bowls:** *Per 8 fl.oz Cup*

| | C | F | Cb |
|---|---|---|---|
| Chicken Noodle | 70 | 2 | 10 |
| Tomato | 100 | 0 | 23 |
| Vegetable | 100 | 0.5 | 22 |
| Vegetable Beef | 80 | 0.5 | 15 |

**Soup at Hand:** *Per 10¾ oz Container*

| | C | F | Cb |
|---|---|---|---|
| Chicken & Stars | 70 | 2 | 10 |
| Chicken with Mini Noodles | 80 | 2 | 11 |
| Creamy Chicken | 150 | 9 | 13 |
| Cream of Broccoli | 160 | 10 | 15 |
| Creamy Tomato Parmesan Bisque | 220 | 7 | 35 |
| New England Clam Chowder | 150 | 10 | 13 |
| Vegetable Beef | 70 | 1 | 11 |

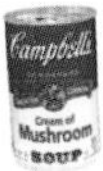

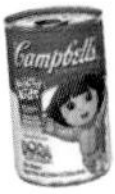

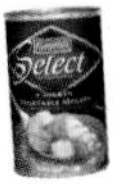

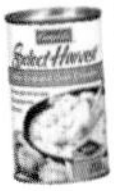

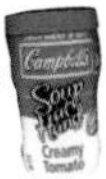

### Dr McDougall's:

**Big Cup Soups/Meals:** *Per Container*

| | C | F | Cb |
|---|---|---|---|
| Black Bean & Lime | 340 | 2 | 60 |
| Hot & Sour Noodle | 320 | 1 | 34 |
| Minestrone & Pasta | 200 | 1 | 40 |
| Pad Thai Noodle | 200 | 1 | 42 |
| Split Pea with Barley | 240 | 1 | 42 |
| Tamale/Tortilla with Baked Chips | 200 | 2 | 35 |

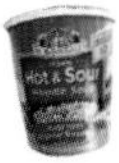

### Dr McDougall's (Cont):

**Ready To Serve:** *Per Cup*

| | C | F | Cb |
|---|---|---|---|
| Black Bean | 120 | 1 | 23 |
| Lentil | 115 | 0.5 | 21 |
| Roasted Pepper Tomato | 80 | 0 | 19 |
| Split Pea | 100 | 0 | 19 |
| Vegetable | 75 | 0.5 | 14 |

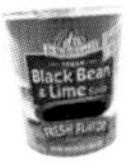

### Fresh & Easy:

**Refrigerated Tubs:** *Per ½ Tub*

| | C | F | Cb |
|---|---|---|---|
| Black Bean | 190 | 1 | 30 |
| Chicken Noodle | 150 | 4.5 | 20 |
| Clam Chowder | 275 | 30 | 25 |
| Lentil | 150 | 1 | 20 |
| Minestrone | 175 | 2 | 35 |
| Tomato | 115 | 4.5 | 14 |
| Tomato Basil | 225 | 15 | 19 |

**Jars:** *Per ½ Jar, 8 oz*

| | C | F | Cb |
|---|---|---|---|
| Chicken Tortilla | 120 | 3 | 11 |
| Potato & Corn Chowder | 180 | 5 | 27 |
| Tomato, Carrot & Zucchini | 110 | 2.5 | 15 |

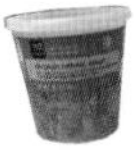

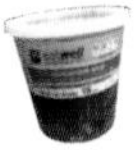

### Health Valley:

**Fat Free Broths:** *Per Cup*

| | C | F | Cb |
|---|---|---|---|
| 40% less sodium, all varieties | 25 | 0 | 0 |
| No Added Salt: Beef | 10 | 0 | 0 |
| Chicken | 35 | 1.5 | 0 |

**Org. Microwavable Soup Cups:**

| | C | F | Cb |
|---|---|---|---|
| Chicken Flavored Noodle, ½ cup | 110 | 0 | 24 |
| Zesty Black Bea, ⅓ cup | 100 | 0 | 22 |

### Healthy Choice:

**Canned:** *Per Cup*

| | C | F | Cb |
|---|---|---|---|
| Chicken & Dumplings | 150 | 3 | 22 |
| Chicken Tortilla | 140 | 1.5 | 23 |
| Country Vegetable | 100 | 0.5 | 20 |
| New England Clam Chowder | 110 | 1.5 | 20 |
| Old Fashioned Chicken Noodle | 90 | 1 | 12 |

**Microwavable Bowls:** *Approx ½ Bowl, 1 Cup*

| | C | F | Cb |
|---|---|---|---|
| Hearty Vegetable Barley | 140 | 1 | 30 |
| Tomato Basil | 110 | 0.5 | 25 |

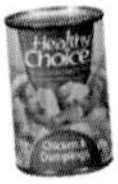

### Imagine:

**Bistro Bisque, Organic:** *Per 8 fl.oz Cup*

| | C | F | Cb |
|---|---|---|---|
| Corn Chipotle | 100 | 1 | 22 |
| Cuban Black Bean | 170 | 3.5 | 30 |
| Fire Rsted Tom. Bisque | 120 | 2.5 | 24 |

**Canned Organic:** *Per Cup*

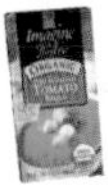

| | C | F | Cb |
|---|---|---|---|
| Chicken Pot Pie | 160 | 4.5 | 22 |
| Country Split Pea | 180 | 2.5 | 30 |
| Minestrone | 160 | 3.5 | 20 |

## Imagine (Cont):

| | C | F | Cb |
|---|---|---|---|
| **Creamy:** *Per 8 fl.oz Cup* | | | |
| Acorn Squash & Mango; Chicken | 70 | 1.5 | 14 |
| Harvest Corn | 110 | 3 | 20 |
| Portobello Mushroom | 80 | 3 | 10 |
| Potato Leek | 70 | 1.5 | 12 |
| Sweet Pea | 80 | 1.5 | 14 |
| Tomato | 90 | 2 | 18 |
| **Kettle Cuisine** *(Gluten Free): Per 10 oz* | | | |
| Angus Beef Steak Chili with Beans | 250 | 9 | 21 |
| Chicken: Chili with White Beans | 320 | 15 | 23 |
| With Rice Noodles | 140 | 3 | 15 |
| Southwest and Corn Chowder | 230 | 10 | 21 |
| Thai Curry | 330 | 11 | 44 |
| New England Clam Chowder | 310 | 17 | 26 |
| Organic Mushroom & Potato | 170 | 6 | 25 |
| Roasted Vegetable | 190 | 9 | 23 |
| Three Bean Chili | 220 | 3.5 | 36 |
| Tomato with Garden Vegetables | 110 | 3.5 | 16 |

## Knorr:

| | C | F | Cb |
|---|---|---|---|
| **Cubes:** *Per ½ Cube, 1 Cup, Prepared* | | | |
| Beef; Chicken, av. | 15 | 1.5 | 1 |
| Vegetable | 20 | 1 | 1 |
| **Homestyle Stock:** *Per 1 Tsp* | | | |
| Beef | 10 | 1 | 0 |
| Chicken | 10 | 2 | 0 |

## Lipton:

| | C | F | Cb |
|---|---|---|---|
| **Cup-a-Soup:** *Per Envelope* | | | |
| Cream of Chicken | 60 | 1.5 | 12 |
| Chicken Noodle, Original | 50 | 1 | 8 |
| **Recipe Secrets:** *Per 1 Tbsp Dry Mix* | | | |
| Beefy Onion | 25 | 0.5 | 5 |
| Onion | 20 | 0 | 4 |
| Onion Mushroom | 25 | 0 | 7 |

## Manischewitz:

| | C | F | Cb |
|---|---|---|---|
| **Condensed:** *Per ½ Cup Soup* | | | |
| Chicken Consume, Clear | 15 | 0 | 2 |
| Chicken Kreplach | 40 | 1 | 6 |
| Chicken Noodle | 60 | 1.5 | 7 |
| **Quart Jars:** *Per 6 fl.oz* | | | |
| Borscht with Beets | 50 | 0 | 13 |
| Borscht, Low Calorie | 15 | 0 | 4 |
| **Ready To Serve,** | | | |
| Matzo Balls Chicken Soup, 1 cup | 120 | 4.5 | 12 |

## Maruchan:

| | C | F | Cb |
|---|---|---|---|
| **Instant Lunch,** | | | |
| average all flavors, 1 pkg | 290 | 12 | 38 |
| **Ramen,** all flavors:, 1 pkg, 3 oz | 380 | 14 | 52 |

## Nile Spice: *Per Cup*

| | C | F | Cb |
|---|---|---|---|
| Black Bean; Lentil | 195 | 1.5 | 35 |
| Couscous Minestrone | 180 | 1.5 | 34 |
| Potato Leek | 120 | 3 | 17 |
| Low-Fat, Split Pea | 200 | 1 | 35 |

## Nissin:

| | C | F | Cb |
|---|---|---|---|
| **Souper Meal:** *Per ½ of 4.3 oz Container* | | | |
| Chicken | 290 | 13 | 38 |
| Picante Shrimp | 270 | 11 | 36 |
| **Top Ramen:** *Per ½ 3 oz Container* | | | |
| Beef/ Chicken Flavor, average | 190 | 7 | 27 |

## Pacific Foods:

| | C | F | Cb |
|---|---|---|---|
| **Condensed Soups:** *Per ½ cup, 4.65 oz* | | | |
| Cream of Celery | 70 | 2.5 | 11 |
| Cream of Mushroom | 100 | 2.5 | 18 |
| **Creamy Organic:** *Per ¼ of 32 fl.oz Container, 8 fl.oz* | | | |
| French Onion | 30 | 1 | 5 |
| Cashew Carrot Ginger | 120 | 5 | 19 |
| Curried Red Lentil | 140 | 4.5 | 19 |
| Tomato | 100 | 2 | 16 |

## Progresso:

| | C | F | Cb |
|---|---|---|---|
| **Rich & Hearty:** *Per Cup* | | | |
| Chicken & Homestyle Noodles | 110 | 2.5 | 14 |
| Chicken Corn Chowder | 200 | 9 | 23 |
| Chicken Pot Pie Style | 140 | 4 | 19 |
| Loaded Potato w/ Bacon | 180 | 10 | 19 |
| New Engl. Clam Chowder | 180 | 8 | 22 |
| Savory Beef Barley Vege. | 130 | 2.5 | 17 |
| Steak & HomeStyle Ndles | 110 | 2.5 | 14 |
| **Traditional (99% Fat Free):** *Per Cup* | | | |
| Chicken Noodle | 100 | 2.5 | 12 |
| Homstyle Chicken | | | |
| w/ Vege & Pasta | 100 | 2 | 14 |
| Italian-Style Wedding | 120 | 4 | 11 |
| Split Pea with Ham | 140 | 1 | 24 |
| **Vegetable Classic:** *Per Cup* | | | |
| French Onion | 50 | 1 | 9 |
| Green Split Pea w/ Bacon | 160 | 2 | 28 |
| Garden Vegetable | 90 | 0 | 20 |
| Minestrone | 100 | 2 | 20 |
| Tomato Rotini | 130 | 0.5 | 28 |
| **Light, Low-Fat/Low-Carb:** *Per Cup* | | | |
| Beef Pot Roast | 80 | 2 | 10 |
| Italian Style Wedding | 70 | 0 | 16 |
| Vegetable & Noodle, 8.75 oz | 60 | 0.5 | 13 |
| **World Recipes:** *Per Cup* | | | |
| Black Bean Jalapeno | 130 | 1 | 30 |
| Chicken & Vegetable | 90 | 1.5 | 14 |
| Chicken Tortitlla | 110 | 2.5 | 17 |

| Safeway (Vons): | C | F | Cb |
|---|---|---|---|
| **Signature Soups:** *Per Cup* | | | |
| Broccoli & Cheesy Cheddar | 270 | 18 | 18 |
| Chunky Chicken Noodle | 160 | 5 | 14 |
| Fiesta Chicken Tortilla | 110 | 2 | 15 |
| Italian-Style Wedding | 120 | 4 | 14 |
| Pacific Coast Clam Chowder | 330 | 24 | 27 |
| Savory Chicken & Orzo | 90 | 0.5 | 13 |
| Tuscan Tomato & Basil Bisque | 330 | 22 | 27 |
| **Swanson:** | | | |
| **Broth:** *Per Cup* | | | |
| Chicken, 99% Fat-Free | 10 | 0.5 | 1 |
| Vegetable | 15 | 0 | 3 |
| **Organic,** Beef/Chkn, | | | |
| 100% Fat-Free | 15 | 0 | 1 |
| **Tabatchnick:** | | | |
| **Dairy:** *Per 15 oz Pouch* | | | |
| Corn Chowder | 130 | 4.5 | 21 |
| Cream of Broccoli | 90 | 4 | 12 |
| New England Potato | 140 | 4 | 24 |
| **Gluten Free:** *Per 15 oz Pouch* | | | |
| Split Pea | 140 | 0 | 34 |
| Southwest Bean | 220 | 5 | 35 |
| Vegetarian Chili | 180 | 3.5 | 28 |
| **Low Sodium:** *Per 15 oz Pouch* | | | |
| Barley Mushroom | 80 | 1 | 17 |
| Split Pea | 140 | 0 | 34 |
| Vegetable | 90 | 1.5 | 17 |
| **Meat:** *Per 15 oz Pouch* | | | |
| Frenchman's Onion | 60 | 1.5 | 11 |
| Wilderness Wild Rice | 80 | 0.5 | 16 |
| **Parve:** *Per 15 oz Pouch* | | | |
| Balsamic Tomato & Rice | 110 | 3.5 | 18 |
| Black Bean | 230 | 2.5 | 39 |
| Minestrone | 100 | 1.5 | 18 |
| **Thai Kitchen:** | | | |
| **Rice Noodle Soup Bowls:** *Per Bowl* | | | |
| Hot & Sour | 250 | 4 | 51 |
| Lemongrass & Chili | 250 | 3.5 | 52 |
| Spring Onion | 260 | 4.5 | 50 |
| Roasted Garlic | 250 | 3 | 52 |
| Thai Ginger | 260 | 3 | 52 |

| Trader Joe's: | C | F | Cb |
|---|---|---|---|
| **28 fl. oz Cans:** *Per Cup* | | | |
| Chunky, Low Fat: | | | |
| Lentil with Vegetables | 140 | 3 | 21 |
| Minestrone | 110 | 2.5 | 19 |
| **14½ oz Cans:** *Per Cup* | | | |
| Organic:: Black Bean | 130 | 1.5 | 25 |
| Lentil Vegetable, ½ can | 130 | 3.5 | 19 |
| Split Pea | 100 | 0 | 19 |
| **10¾ oz Can:** *Per Can* | | | |
| Low Sodium, Minestrone | 200 | 4 | 37 |
| **15 oz Can,** | | | |
| Low Fat, Chicken Noodle, 1 cup | 90 | 1 | 14 |
| **32 fl oz. Cartons:** *Per Cup* | | | |
| Butternut Squash | 90 | 2 | 16 |
| Carrot & Ginger | 80 | 1 | 17 |
| Crmy Corn & Rstd Pepper | 110 | 2 | 23 |
| Latin Style Black Bean | 70 | 1 | 12 |
| Sweet Potato Bisque | 130 | 1 | 28 |
| Organic: Butternut Squash | 70 | 0 | 17 |
| Tom. & Rstd Red Pepper | 100 | 2 | 16 |
| Low Sodium, Crmy Tomato | 90 | 3.5 | 15 |
| Light Sodium, Tomato Bisque | 130 | 4 | 21 |
| **17.6 fl. oz Cartons:** *Per Cup* | | | |
| Beef, Barley with Veggies | 100 | 0.5 | 16 |
| Chicken Noodle with Veggies | 100 | 1 | 16 |
| **Whole Foods:** *Per Cup* | | | |
| **365 Organic:** Black Bean | 150 | 1 | 25 |
| Chicken Noodle | 90 | 2 | 11 |
| Cream of Mushroom | 100 | 6 | 11 |
| Minestrone | 120 | 2 | 21 |
| Tomato | 90 | 3.5 | 14 |
| Vegetable | 70 | 1 | 11 |
| **Wolfgang Puck:** *Per Cup* | | | |
| **Organic:** | | | |
| Butternut Squash | 200 | 11 | 22 |
| Chicken & Dumplings | 140 | 7 | 14 |
| Corn Chowder | 210 | 13 | 20 |
| Classic Tomato with Basil | 150 | 6 | 21 |
| Creamy Tomato | 250 | 16 | 23 |
| Free Range Chicken with | | | |
| White & Wild Rice | 110 | 4 | 15 |
| Hearty Garden Vegetable | 130 | 4 | 22 |
| Hearty Lentil & Vegetable | 150 | 1 | 58 |
| Tortilla | 160 | 3.5 | 27 |

## Soybean Products | C | F | Cb

| | C | F | Cb |
|---|---|---|---|
| Cheeses (Soy) ~ See Page 78 | | | |
| **Miso Soy Bean Paste:** | | | |
| Cold Mountain: Light Yellow, 1 tsp | 10 | 0 | 1 |
| Mellow Red, 1 tsp | 15 | 0 | 3 |
| Red, 1 tsp | 10 | 0 | 1 |
| **Miso Soup (dry mix):** | | | |
| 1 Tbsp., dry mix | 35 | 1 | 5 |
| 1 cup, prepared | 35 | 1 | 5 |
| **Natto,** ½ cup, 3 oz | 160 | 7 | 14 |
| **Okara (Tofu fiber residue),** ½ c., 2 oz | 47 | 1 | 8 |
| **Tempeh:** 1 piece, 3 oz | 180 | 8 | 12 |
| Fried, 3 oz | 250 | 14 | 14 |
| **Seitan** (Westsoy), Strips, 3 oz | 120 | 2 | 4 |
| **Soybean Protein** (TVP), 1 oz | 95 | 0 | 8 |
| **Soy Bean Paste,** 1 tsp | 10 | 0 | 2 |
| Soy Beans ~ See Page 160 | | | |
| Soy Drinks ~ See Page 49 | | | |

## Tofu ~ Packaged | C | F | Cb

| | C | F | Cb |
|---|---|---|---|
| **Azumaya Tofu:** | | | |
| Extra Firm; Firm, 3 oz | 70 | 4 | 2 |
| Soft (Silken), 3.2 oz | 40 | 2 | 1 |
| **House Foods:** Per 3 oz | | | |
| Premium Tofu: Extra Firm | 80 | 4 | 1 |
| Firm | 70 | 3.5 | 2 |
| Medium Firm (Regular) | 60 | 3 | 1 |
| Soft (Silken) | 50 | 2.5 | 2 |
| Organic Tofu: Firm, 3 oz | 60 | 3.5 | 0 |
| Extra Firm, 3 oz | 70 | 4 | 0 |
| House Tofu: Tokusen Kinugoshi, 3 oz | 90 | 4 | 3 |
| Sukui; Soon (Extra Soft), 3 oz | 45 | 2 | 2 |
| Yaki Tofu (Broiled), 3 oz | 90 | 5 | 2 |
| Seasoned Tofu Steak: Grilled, 3 oz | 90 | 5 | 1 |
| Garlic & Pepper, 3 oz | 90 | 4 | 1 |
| **Mori-Nu Tofu:** | | | |
| Silken: Soft, 3 oz, 1" slice | 45 | 2.5 | 2 |
| Firm, 3 oz, 1" slice | 50 | 2.5 | 2 |
| Extra Firm, 3 oz, 1" slice | 45 | 1.5 | 2 |
| Organic, Firm 3 oz, 1" slice | 60 | 2.5 | 2 |
| Lite, Firm, 3 oz, 1" slice | 30 | 1 | 1 |
| **Nasoya:** Soft, 2.8 oz | 60 | 3 | 1 |
| Silken, 3.2 oz | 45 | 2 | 1 |
| Firm, ⅕ pkg., 2.8 oz | 70 | 3 | 2 |
| Extra Firm, ⅕ pkg., 2.8 oz | 80 | 4 | 2 |
| **Tofuplus:** Extra Firm, 3 oz | 80 | 4 | 2 |
| Firm, 3 oz | 70 | 3 | 2 |
| Sprouted, 3 oz | 100 | 5 | 3 |
| **WestSoy:** Firm, 2.8 oz | 95 | 5 | 3 |
| Firm, Fat Reduced, 3.2 oz | 90 | 4 | 4 |

## Supplements | C | F | Cb

| | C | F | Cb |
|---|---|---|---|
| **Aloe Vera Juice,** undiluted, 2 fl.oz | 5 | 0 | 1 |
| **Brewer's Yeast:** Tablets, 2 tabs | 4 | 0 | 0.5 |
| Flakes, 1 heaping Tbsp, 0.3 oz | 30 | 0.5 | 4 |
| Powder, 1 heaping Tbsp, 0.5 oz | 50 | 0.5 | 6 |
| **Calcium Chews:** CVS, 1 chew | 20 | 0 | 3 |
| Trader Joe's, Choc., 1 chew | 20 | 1 | 3 |
| **Cod Liver Oil,** 1 Tbsp | 125 | 13 | 0 |
| Fiber Choice, 2 tabs | 15 | 0 | 4 |
| Fibersure, 1 heaping tsp | 25 | 0 | 6 |
| **Fish Oil Capsules,** av., 1 | 10 | 1 | 0 |
| **Flax Oil:** Capsules, 2 | 10 | 1 | 0 |
| Barlean's, 3 softgels | 110 | 11 | 0 |
| **Garlic Tablets/Capsules,** each | 3 | 0 | 1 |
| **Glowelle:** | | | |
| Beauty Drink, 8 fl.oz | 100 | 0 | 24 |
| Powder Stick (1) | 50 | 0 | 12 |
| **Lecithin Granules,** 1 Tbsp | 55 | 4 | 0.5 |
| Metamucil, Powder: | | | |
| Orange (Smooth Texture), | | | |
| 1 rounded Tbsp | 45 | 0 | 12 |
| Sugar-Free, 1 rounded tsp | 20 | 0 | 5 |
| Pink Lemonade, Sugar-Free, | | | |
| 1 rounded tsp | 20 | 0 | 5 |
| **Fiber Wafers,** (2) | 120 | 5 | 17 |
| **Capsules:** | | | |
| Heart & Digestive (6) | 10 | 0 | 3 |
| Strong Bones (5) | 10 | 0 | 3 |
| **Protein,** Powders, average, 1 oz | 100 | 0.5 | 0 |
| **Seaweed:** Dried, 1 oz | 85 | 0.5 | 22 |
| Soaked, drained, 1 oz | 15 | 0.5 | 3 |
| **Spirulina,** 1 tablet | 2 | 0 | 0.5 |
| **Vitamins/Minerals:** Tabs/Caps, 1 | 2 | 0 | 0 |
| Vitamin E Capsules, each | 5 | 0.5 | 0 |
| **Viactiv Chews,** (1) | 20 | 0.5 | 4 |

## Cough & Pharmaceutical

| | C | F | Cb |
|---|---|---|---|
| **Antacids:** Av., 1 tablet | 4 | 0 | 1 |
| Liquid, 1 Tbsp | 6 | 0 | 1 |
| *Antacid Sodium Counts* ~ See Page 280 | | | |
| **Cough/Cold Syrups:** | | | |
| Regular: With sugar, 1 Tbsp | 35 | 0 | 9 |
| With alcohol, 1 Tbsp | 46 | 0 | 9 |
| Sugar-Free (Diabetic Tussin), 1 T. | 0 | 0 | 0 |
| Cough Drops/Lozenges ~ See Page 75 | | | |
| *Sudafed Syrup,* 1 tsp | 14 | 0 | 3 |
| *Tylenol Liquid:* Child, 1 tsp | 17 | 0 | 4 |
| Extra Strength, 1 tsp | 11 | 0 | 3 |

## Sugar

| | C | F | Cb |
|---|---|---|---|
| **White Sugar, granulated:** | | | |
| 1 level teaspoon | 15 | 0 | 4 |
| 1 heaping teaspoon | 25 | 0 | 6 |
| 1 Tablespoon | 50 | 0 | 12 |
| 1 ounce, 1 oz | 110 | 0 | 28 |
| 1 cup, 7 oz | 775 | 0 | 200 |
| 1 pound | 1760 | 0 | 454 |
| Single Portion Packages: | | | |
| 1 stick | 15 | 0 | 4 |
| 1 packet, 0.1 oz | 10 | 0 | 3 |
| 1 cube, 0.08 oz | 10 | 0 | 2.5 |
| **Brown Sugar:** 1 Tbsp | 50 | 0 | 13 |
| 1 ounce, 1 oz | 110 | 0 | 28 |
| 1 cup, not packed, 5 oz | 550 | 0 | 140 |
| 1 cup, packed, 7.75 oz | 835 | 0 | 216 |
| **Powdered/Confectioners:** | | | |
| Sifted, 1 cup, 3.5 oz | 390 | 0 | 100 |
| Unsifted, 1 cup, 4.25 oz | 465 | 0 | 120 |
| **Cinnamon Sugar,** 1 tsp | 15 | 0 | 4 |
| **Dextrose,** 1¼ tsp | 15 | 0 | 4 |
| **Fructose:** Dry, 1 tsp | 15 | 0 | 4 |
| Liquid, 1 oz | 80 | 0 | 21 |
| **Glucose,** 1 oz | 110 | 0 | 27 |
| **Glucose Tablets,** (1) | 20 | 0 | 5 |
| **Palm Sugar,** 3 Tbsp | 45 | 0 | 11 |
| **Piloncillo (Brown Sugar),** 3oz | 325 | 0 | 81 |
| **Turbinado Sugar,** 2 Tbsp, 1 oz | 110 | 0 | 27 |
| **Unrefined Cane Sugar,** 1 oz | 110 | 0 | 27 |

## Sugar Substitutes

| | C | F | Cb |
|---|---|---|---|
| **DiabetiSweet,** 1 teaspoon | 9 | 0 | 4 |
| (Carbohydrate as Sugar Alcohol) | | | |
| **Equal:** Tablet (2) | 4 | 0 | 0.5 |
| Granular, 1 tsp | 4 | 0 | 0.5 |
| Packet (1) | 4 | 0 | 0.5 |
| Flavored, 1 stick | 4 | 0 | 0.5 |
| **Natra Taste; Sweet One,** 1 packet | 4 | 0 | 1 |
| **NutraSweet,** 1 tsp | 4 | 0 | 0 |
| **Splenda:** | | | |
| Granular: 1 tsp | 5 | 0 | 0.5 |
| 1 cup | 95 | 0 | 24 |
| Packet, all flavors | 5 | 0 | 0.5 |
| Sugar Blend, Orig/Brown, ½ cup | 385 | 0 | 96 |
| **Stevia,** single serving | 0 | 0 | 0 |
| **Sugar Twin,** 1 packet | 3 | 0 | 0.5 |
| **Sweet 'N Low,** 1 packet | 2 | 0 | 0.5 |
| **Truvia,** 1 packet | 0 | 0 | 3 |
| **Walgreens,** Wal-Sweet, 1 packet | 0 | 0 | 0 |
| **Weight Watchers,** 1 packet | 4 | 0 | 1 |
| **Whey Low,** 1 tsp | 3 | 0 | 3 |

## Syrups, Molasses, Agave

**Syrups:** *Average All Brands*
*(Corn/Rice/Maple/Pancake/Sundae/Waffle)*
*Includes Aunt Jemima, Cary's, Karo, Hershey's,*
*Hungry Jack, Log Cabin, Mrs Butterworth's*

| **Regular/Dark/Light Color:** | C | F | Cb |
|---|---|---|---|
| 1 Tbsp, ½ fl.oz | 55 | 0 | 14 |
| ¼ cup (4 Tbsp) | 220 | 0 | 55 |
| **Single Portion:** 1½ oz pkg | 170 | 0 | 42 |
| **Lite:** 1Tbsp | 25 | 0 | 6 |
| ¼ cup (4 Tbsp) | 100 | 0 | 25 |
| **Sugar-Free:** 2 Tbsp, 1 oz | 18 | 0 | 5 |
| *Cozy Cottage,* 2 Tbsp, 1 oz | 10 | 0 | 3 |
| *Da Vinci,* 2 Tbsp, 1 oz | 5 | 0 | 1 |
| **Honey Cream Syrup,** ¼ c., 2 oz | 220 | 0 | 55 |
| **Molasses:** Dark/Light: 1 T., 0.75 oz | 55 | 0 | 14 |
| 1 cup, 11.5 oz | 880 | 0 | 224 |
| **Blackstrap,** 1 Tbsp, 0.75 oz | 47 | 0 | 13 |
| **Agave Nectar,** av. all flavors | | | |
| 1 Tablespoon, 0.75 oz | 60 | 0 | 15 |

## Ice Cream Toppings

| | C | F | Cb |
|---|---|---|---|

**Average All Types & Brands:** *Per 2 Tbsp*
*(Hershey's, Smuckers):*

| | C | F | Cb |
|---|---|---|---|
| Butterscotch; Caramel | 115 | 0 | 29 |
| Chocolate: Hot Fudge, av. | 110 | 4 | 22 |
| Fat Free Chocolate | 100 | 0 | 23 |
| Pineapple, Strawberry | 100 | 0 | 26 |
| Honey, 1 Tbsp, ¾ oz | 65 | 0 | 17 |
| *Smuckers:* Hot Fudge, sugar free | 90 | 0.5 | 23 |
| Magic Shell, average | 210 | 15 | 18 |

## Honey, Jam, Preserves

| **Average All Brands** | C | F | Cb |
|---|---|---|---|
| **Honey:** 1 tsp, 0.25 oz | 22 | 0 | 5.5 |
| 1 Tbsp, 0.75 oz | 65 | 0 | 17 |
| 1 ounce, 1 oz | 85 | 0 | 23 |
| 1 cup, 12 oz | 1030 | 0 | 269 |
| Single Portion, 0.5 oz package | 45 | 0 | 11 |
| **Jams/Jellies/Marmalade/Preserves:** | | | |
| Regular: 1 tsp, 0.25 oz | 20 | 0 | 5 |
| 1 Tbsp, 0.75 oz | 55 | 0 | 14 |
| 1 ounce, 1 oz | 80 | 0 | 20 |
| Single Portion, 0.5 oz pkg | 40 | 0 | 11 |
| **Apple/Fruit Butters,** 1 T., 0.6 oz | 20 | 0 | 6 |
| **Fruit Spreads:** Regular, 1 tsp | 15 | 0 | 4 |
| Low Sugar, 1 tsp | 8 | 0 | 2 |
| Low Calorie *(Featherweight),* 1 tsp | 8 | 0 | 2 |
| **Jelly:** Regular, average, 1 tsp | 18 | 0 | 4.5 |
| Imitation, Low Calorie, 1 tsp | 4 | 0 | 1 |

# V Vegetables & Legumes

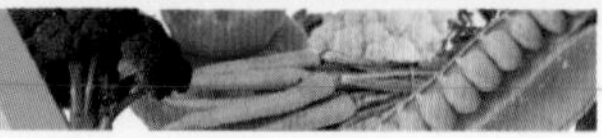

## Vegetables

| Vegetables | C | F | Cb |
|---|---|---|---|
| **Alfalfa Sprouts,** ½ cup ,0.5 oz | 5 | 0 | 0.5 |
| **Artichokes,** Globe/French: | | | |
| 1 medium, 4.5 oz | 60 | 0 | 13 |
| 1 large, 5.7 oz | 75 | 0 | 17 |
| **Artichoke Heart,** plain, 2 pces | 15 | 0 | 3 |
| **Asparagus,** raw/frozen: | | | |
| 3 medium spears | 10 | 0 | 2 |
| Cuts & Tips *(Del Monte),* ½ cup, 4.3 oz | 20 | 0 | 3 |
| **Bamboo Shoots,** cooked, ½ c., 2 oz | 7 | 0 | 1 |
| **Beans:** Green/Snap/String, ½ ., 2 oz | 20 | 0 | 4 |
| 10 beans (4" long), 2 oz | 20 | 0 | 4 |
| **Dried,** average all types: | | | |
| (Kidney, Brown, Lima, Navy, Pinto, White) | | | |
| Raw: 2 Tbsp, 1 oz | 95 | 0.5 | 18 |
| 1 cup, 7 oz | 665 | 3 | 126 |
| Cooked: 1 oz | 35 | 0 | 7 |
| ½ cup, 3 oz | 105 | 0 | 21 |
| **Bean Sprouts,** average, ½ c., 2 oz | 15 | 0 | 3.5 |
| **Beets (Beetroot):** | | | |
| Raw, 1 beet (2" diam), 4 oz | 35 | 0 | 8 |
| Cooked, 1 cup, slices, 3 oz | 35 | 0 | 8 |
| **Canned** ~ *See Page 168* | | | |
| **Beet Greens,** cooked, ½ cup, 2.5 oz | 20 | 0 | 4 |
| **Bell Pepper** ~ *See Peppers* | | | |
| **Bitter Melon/Gourd,** 1 cup, 1.5 oz | 15 | 0 | 1.5 |
| **Blackeye Peas,** cooked, ½ cup, 3 oz | 100 | 0.5 | 18 |
| **Bok Choy (Chinese Chard),** ckd, 3 oz | 10 | 0 | 1.5 |
| **Breadfruit,** ¼ small fruit, 3 oz | 100 | 0 | 26 |
| **Broadbeans (Fava Beans):** | | | |
| Green (in pod), raw: 4 pods | | | |
| (3½ oz w/ shells; 1.2 oz beans) | 30 | 0 | 6 |
| 1 cup beans (w/o shell), 4.5 oz | 110 | 1 | 22 |
| Mature Seeds: Raw, 1 cup, 5.3 oz | 510 | 2.5 | 87 |
| Cooked, ½ cup, 3 oz | 95 | 0 | 17 |
| **Broccoflower,** ⅕ head, 3.5 oz | 35 | 0 | 7 |
| **Broccoli:** Raw, chopped, 1 cup, 3 oz | 30 | 0 | 6 |
| 3 Florets, 2.5 oz | 25 | 0 | 5 |
| 1 Spear (5" long), 1.1 oz | 10 | 0 | 2 |
| 1 Whole: Medium, 14 oz | 135 | 1.5 | 26 |
| Large, 21 oz | 205 | 2 | 40 |
| 1 Head (no stalk), 11 oz | 105 | 1 | 21 |
| 1 Stalk, small (5" long), 5.3 oz | 50 | 0.5 | 10 |
| **Brocco Sprouts,** ½ cup, 1 oz | 15 | 0 | 2 |
| **Brussels Sprouts:** Cooked, ½ c., 2.8 oz | 30 | 0.5 | 6 |
| 2 Sprouts, 1.5 oz | 15 | 0 | 3 |
| **Butterbeans,** cooked, ½ cup, 3 oz | 90 | 0 | 16 |
| **Cabbage,** all types, average: | | | |
| Raw: 1 Leaf, large, 1 oz | 5 | 0 | 2 |
| Shredded, 1 cup, 2.5 oz | 15 | 0 | 4 |
| ½ Large Head (7" diam), 22 oz | 150 | 1 | 35 |
| Cooked, shredded, ½ cup, 2.5 oz | 15 | 0.5 | 3.5 |

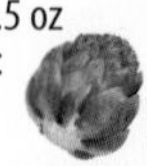
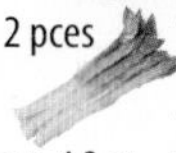
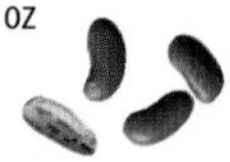
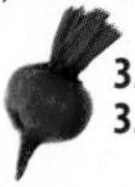
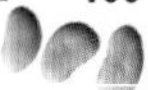
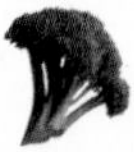
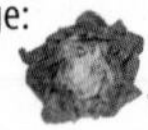

## Vegetables (Cont)

| Vegetables (Cont) | C | F | Cb |
|---|---|---|---|
| **Cactus Leaf (Nopales):** | | | |
| 1 leaf, 4½ oz | 20 | 0 | 4 |
| 1 cup (slices), 3 oz | 15 | 0 | 3 |
| **Carrots, Regular thick variety:** | | | |
| 1 small, 4 oz | 45 | 0 | 11 |
| 1 medium, 6 oz | 70 | 0 | 16 |
| 1 large, 8 oz | 95 | 0 | 22 |
| Chopped, 1 cup, 4.5 oz | 50 | 0 | 12 |
| Grated, 1 cup, 4 oz | 45 | 0 | 11 |
| Slices, 1 cup, 4.5 oz | 50 | 0 | 12 |
| Sticks (4"), 4-5, 1.5 oz | 20 | 0 | 4 |
| Long thin variety, 1 medium, 2.2 oz | 25 | 0 | 6 |
| Baby: Snack size, 3 medium, 1 oz | 10 | 0 | 2.5 |
| Snack Pack, 3 oz | 30 | 0 | 7 |
| **Cauliflower:** Raw: 1 cup (pieces), 3.5 oz | 25 | 0 | 5 |
| ½ medium head, 10 oz | 70 | 0 | 15 |
| Cooked, 3 florets, 2 oz | 10 | 0 | 2 |
| **Celeriac,** ½ cup, raw, 2.75 oz | 35 | 0 | 7 |
| **Celery:** 1 large stalk, 11", 2.2 oz | 10 | 0 | 2 |
| 1 small stalk, 5", 0.5 oz | 2 | 0 | 0.5 |
| 4 Strips, thin sticks, 0.5 oz | 5 | 0 | 1 |
| Chopped, 1 cup, 3.5 oz | 15 | 0 | 3 |
| **Chard (Swiss),** ½ cup, cooked, 3 oz | 20 | 0 | 3.5 |
| **Chayote Squash:** 1 medium, 7 oz | 40 | 0 | 9 |
| 1 cup (pieces), 4.5 oz | 25 | 0 | 6 |
| **Chick Peas:** | | | |
| Dry, 1 cup, 7 oz | 730 | 12 | 121 |
| Cooked, 1 cup, 6 oz | 270 | 4 | 45 |
| **Chicory Greens,** 1 cup, 1 oz | 7 | 0 | 1.5 |
| **Chili Peppers** ~ *See Peppers* | | | |
| **Chinese Long Bean,** sl., 1 cup, 3.2 oz | 45 | 0 | 8 |
| **Chives,** chopped, 1 Tbsp | 1 | 0 | 0 |
| **Choy Sum,** 3 oz | 15 | 0 | 3 |
| **Cilantro (Coriander),** 1 cup | 5 | 0 | 0.5 |
| **Collards,** cooked, ½ cup, 3 oz | 25 | 0 | 5 |
| **Corn:** Yellow/White | | | |
| Raw: Kernels, ½ cup, 3 oz | 80 | 0.5 | 19 |
| Ear (5"x 1¾"), 5.5 oz | 155 | 1 | 37 |
| Cooked, Kernels, ½ cup, 3 oz | 77 | 0.5 | 18 |
| Cob, cooked: Small, 2.25 oz | 60 | 0.5 | 14 |
| Large ear, 5.5 oz | 120 | 1 | 28 |
| **Courgette** ~ *See Zucchini* | | | |
| **Cowpeas** ~ *See Blackeye Peas* | | | |
| **Cress,** garden, raw, 1 cup, 1.75 oz | 15 | 0 | 3 |
| **Cucumber:** 1 whole, 11 oz | 45 | 0.5 | 11 |
| ½ cup slices, 2 oz | 10 | 0 | 2 |
| Mini/Lebanese (1), 3 oz | 15 | 0 | 3 |
| **Daikon Radish,** ½ cup, slices, 2 oz | 9 | 0 | 2 |
| **Dandelion Greens,** raw, ½ cup, 1 oz | 10 | 0 | 2.5 |
| **Edamame** *(Immature green soybeans):* | | | |
| Shelled, ½ cup, 2.6 oz | 110 | 5 | 8 |
| With shells, 10 pods, 1.25 oz | 30 | 1 | 3 |

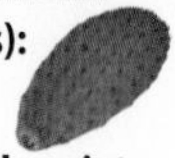
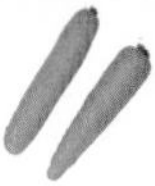
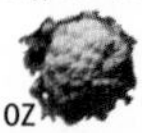
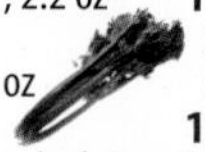
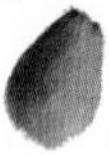
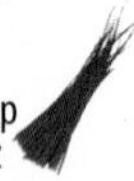
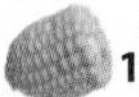
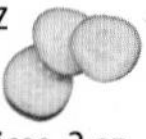

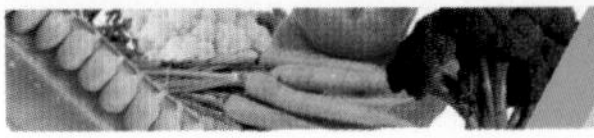

| Vegetables (Cont) | C | F | Cb |
|---|---|---|---|
| **Eggplant:** Raw, ¼ medium, 4 oz | 30 | 0 | 7 |
| Raw, ½ cup, 1" pieces, 1.5 oz | 10 | 0 | 2 |
| 1 slice, fried, 1 oz | 75 | 4 | 10 |
| **Endive, Belgian/French:** Raw, | | | |
| 1 medium head (6"), 2.5 oz | 12 | 0 | 3 |
| **Fennel,** 1 cup, sliced, 3 oz | 25 | 0 | 7 |
| **Gai Choy Cabbage,** ckd, 1 c. 6 oz | 20 | 0 | 3 |
| **Gai Lan (Chinese Kale),** cooked, 1 c. | 35 | 0.5 | 7 |
| **Garlic,** 1 clove | 4 | 0 | 1 |
| **Ginger:** ¼ cup slices, 1 oz | 20 | 0 | 5 |
| Crystallized (sugared), 7 pieces, 1.5 oz | 130 | 0 | 35 |
| **Horseradish,** raw, 1 pod, 0.5 oz | 5 | 0 | 1 |
| **Jerusalem Artichoke,** raw, ½ cup | 55 | 0 | 13 |
| **Jicama,** raw, sliced, ½ cup, 2.25 oz | 25 | 0 | 6 |
| **Kale,** 1 cup, chopped, 2.5 oz | 35 | 0.5 | 7 |
| **Kohlrabi,** ½ cup, cooked, 1.75 oz | 17 | 0 | 5 |
| **Leek,** cooked, 1 whole, 4.5 oz | 40 | 0 | 9 |
| **Lentils, green/brown:** Dry, 1 oz | 100 | 0.5 | 17 |
| 1 cup, 6.75 oz | 675 | 3 | 115 |
| Cooked, ½ cup, 3.5 oz | 115 | 0.5 | 20 |
| **Lettuce:** 1 cup, chopped/shred., 2 oz | 7 | 0 | 1 |
| Butterhead, 2 leaves, 0.5 oz | 2 | 0 | 0.5 |
| Cos/Romaine, shredded, 1 c. | 10 | 0 | 2 |
| Iceberg: 1 outer leaf, 0.5 oz | 2 | 0 | 0.5 |
| 1 meium head, 16 oz | 75 | 1 | 16 |
| **Lima Beans,** baby, cooked, ½ c., 3 oz | 105 | 0 | 20 |
| **Lotus Root,** 10 slices, cooked, 3 oz | 60 | 0 | 14 |
| **Mung Bean Sprouts,** ½ cup, 2 oz | 15 | 0 | 3 |
| **Mushrooms:** Raw, 1 med., 0.6 oz | 4 | 0 | 0.5 |
| 1 large, sliced, 0.75 oz | 5 | 0 | 1 |
| ½ cup pieces, 1.25 oz | 8 | 0 | 1 |
| Cooked, ½ cup pieces, 2.5 oz | 20 | 0.5 | 4 |
| Fried/Sauteed, 6 oz | 220 | 16 | 11 |
| **Mustard Greens,** raw, ½ cup, 1 oz | 7 | 0 | 2 |
| **Nopales:** See Cactus Leaf | | | |
| **Okra:** Raw, 8 pods, 4 oz | 30 | 0 | 7 |
| Cooked, ½ cup, 2.75 oz | 20 | 0 | 4 |
| **Onions,** Raw: 1 small, 2.5 oz | 30 | 0 | 7 |
| 1 medium, 4 oz | 50 | 0 | 11 |
| 1 large, 5.5 oz | 65 | 0 | 15 |
| 1 jumbo, 16 oz | 190 | 0.5 | 46 |
| Chopped: Raw, ½ cup, 3 oz | 35 | 0 | 8 |
| 1 Tbsp, 0.4 oz | 5 | 0 | 1 |
| Slices: 1 cup, 4 oz | 50 | 0 | 12 |
| 1 medium slice (⅛"), 0.5 oz | 5 | 0 | 1 |
| 1 large slice (¼"), 1.3 oz | 15 | 0 | 4 |
| Dehydrated flakes, ¼ cup, 0.5 oz | 50 | 0 | 12 |
| Rings, breaded & fried, 2 rings | 80 | 5 | 9 |
| Scallions, ½ cup, 2 oz | 15 | 0 | 3 |
| Spring, ½ cup, chopped, 2 oz | 15 | 0 | 3 |
| French's Fried Onions ~ *See Page 112* | | | |
| Blossom/Blooming ~ *See Fast-Foods (Chili's/Outback)* | | | |

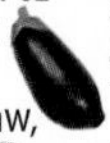

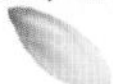

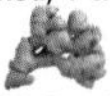

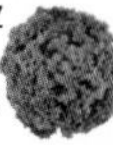

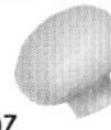

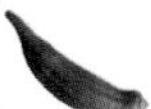

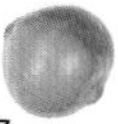

| Vegetables (Cont) | C | F | Cb |
|---|---|---|---|
| **Parsley,** chopped, ½ cup, 1 oz | 10 | 0 | 2 |
| **Parsnip:** 1 medium, 4 oz | 85 | 0 | 20 |
| Cooked, ½ cup slices, 2.75 oz | 55 | 0 | 13 |
| **Peas:** Green, raw, ¼ cup, 1.5 oz | 30 | 0 | 5 |
| With pods, 0.5 lb | 70 | 0 | 13 |
| Snow Peas, 10 pods, 1.2 oz | 15 | 0 | 3 |
| Split: Dry, hulled, 1 oz | 100 | 0.5 | 17 |
| Cooked, 1 cup, 7 oz | 230 | 1 | 42 |
| **Peppers:** Sweet, 1 medium, 4.2 oz | 30 | 0 | 7 |
| Bell: 1 medium, 4.2 oz | 30 | 0 | 7 |
| ½ cup, chopped, raw, 2.5 oz | 20 | 0 | 5 |
| 2 rings (5" diam. x ¼" thick) | 3 | 0 | 1 |
| Chili: Green/Red, 1.5 oz | 20 | 0 | 5 |
| Habanero, 1 only, 0.3 oz | 10 | 0 | 2 |
| **Pigeon Peas,** cooked, ½ cup, 3 oz | 95 | 1 | 17 |
| **Pimientos,** 3 medium, 3.5 oz | 25 | 0 | 5 |
| **Poi,** ½ cup, 4.2 oz | 135 | 0 | 33 |
| **Potatoes:** Raw (with skin) | | | |
| 1 Baby, 2 oz | 45 | 0 | 10 |
| 1 Small, 6 oz | 135 | 0 | 30 |
| 1 Medium, 8 oz | 180 | 0 | 40 |
| 1 Large, 12 oz | 270 | 0 | 60 |
| 1 Extra large, 16 oz | 360 | 0 | 80 |
| **Baked** (no added fat), large, 10 oz (raw wt): | | | |
| **Plain:** With skin, 7 oz (ckd wt) | 185 | 0 | 42 |
| Without skin, 5.5 oz (ckd wt) | 145 | 0 | 34 |
| With Skin/Toppings: | | | |
| + 2 tsp fat | 270 | 8 | 58 |
| + Sour Cream & Chives, 2 T. | 320 | 6 | 60 |
| + Plain Yogurt, 2 Tbsp | 260 | 1 | 60 |
| + Grated Cheese, 1 oz | 370 | 9 | 58 |
| **Mashed:** | | | |
| With milk plus fat, ½ cup, 4 oz | 120 | 4.5 | 18 |
| KFC Style without gravy, 4 oz | 90 | 3 | 15 |
| Loaded (fat/cream/cheese/bacon): | | | |
| Side serving, 6 oz | 180 | 9 | 22 |
| Large serving, 12 oz | 360 | 18 | 44 |
| **Potato Skins** (Baked with cheese topping), | | | |
| ½ whole, 4 oz | 240 | 13 | 22 |
| **French Fries:** Small serving, 2.6 oz | 250 | 13 | 30 |
| Medium serving, 4 oz | 380 | 20 | 47 |
| Frozen, uncooked, 18 fries, 4 oz | 165 | 5.5 | 28 |
| Oven-heated, 18 fries, 4 oz | 165 | 5.5 | 28 |
| Take-Out, 1 cup, 5 oz | 440 | 25 | 60 |
| McDonald's ~ *See Page 215* | | | |
| **Fried,** 18 pieces, 4 oz | 165 | 5.5 | 28 |
| **Au Gratin,** ½ c., 4.3 oz | 160 | 9 | 14 |
| **Pancakes,** 2 small, 2 oz | 120 | 6.5 | 12 |
| **Puffs,** fried, 4 puffs, 1 oz | 55 | 2.5 | 8 |
| **Scalloped,** 1 cup, 8.5 oz | 220 | 9 | 26 |
| Ore-Ida Frozen Potatoe ~ *See Page 161* | | | |

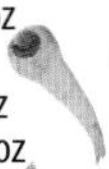

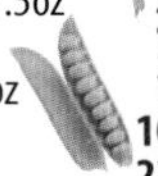

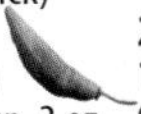

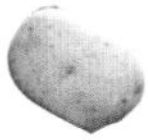

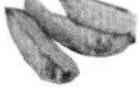

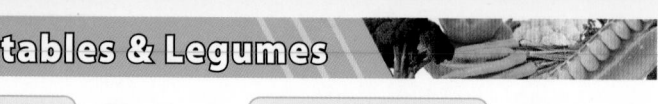

## Vegetables (Cont)

| | C | F | Cb |
|---|---|---|---|
| **Potato Salad,** ½ cup, 4.5 oz | 180 | 10 | 14 |
| **Pumpkin:** | | | |
| Raw, 1" cubes, 1 cup, 4 oz 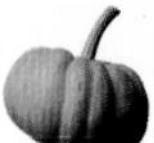 | 30 | 0 | 7 |
| Cooked: | | | |
| Baked, without fat, 4 oz | 90 | 7 | 9 |
| Mashed: 1 scoop, 2 oz | 10 | 0 | 2 |
| ½ cup, 4⅓ oz | 25 | 0 | 6 |
| Pumpkin Flowers, 1 cup, 1.2 oz | 5 | 0 | 1 |
| **Purslane:** Cooked, ½ cup, 2 oz | 10 | 0 | 1 |
| Raw, 1" cubes, 1 cup, 1.5 oz | 5 | 0 | 1.5 |
| **Radicchio:** 2 leaves, 0.5 oz | 5 | 0 | 1 |
| Shredded, 1 cup, 1.5 oz 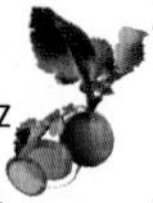 | 20 | 0 | 4 |
| **Radishes:** 1 small | 0 | 0 | 0 |
| 10 medium/5 large, 1.6 oz | 5 | 0 | 1 |
| ½ cup (slices), 2 oz | 10 | 0 | 2 |
| **Rhubarb,** raw, ½ cup, 2 oz | 15 | 0 | 3 |
| **Rutabaga,** ckd, ½ c., (cubes), 3 oz | 30 | 0 | 7 |
| **Salsify,** ckd, ½ c., (slices), 2.5 oz | 50 | 0 | 11 |
| **Sauerkraut,** ½ cup, 2.5 oz 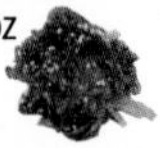 | 15 | 0 | 3 |
| **Seaweed:** Dried, 1 oz | 5 | 0 | 2 |
| Soaked, drained, 1 oz | 15 | 0 | 4 |
| Nori/Laver, dried, 6 sheets, 0.5 oz | 35 | 0 | 5 |
| **Shallots,** 1 Tbsp, (Chopped) ,0.5 oz 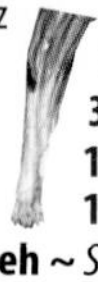 | 5 | 0 | 1 |
| **Sorrel,** raw, ½ cup, 4 oz | 20 | 0 | 4 |
| **Soybeans:** Dry, ½ cup, 3.3 oz | 390 | 18 | 28 |
| Mature, dry, 1 oz | 120 | 5.5 | 9 |
| Cooked, ½ cup, 3 oz | 150 | 7.5 | 8 |
| **Soy Products/Tofu/Tempeh ~** See Page 156) | | | |
| **Spinach:** Cooked, ½ cup, 3 oz | 20 | 0 | 4 |
| Creamed, average, ½ cup, 4.5 oz | 190 | 15 | 8 |
| Raw: 3 leaves/1 cup, 1 oz 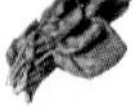 | 7 | 0 | 1 |
| 1 Bunch, 12 oz | 80 | 1.5 | 12 |
| **Squash:** | | | |
| Summer: Raw: ½ cup, 2.5 oz | 10 | 0 | 2 |
| Cooked, ½ cup slices, 3 oz 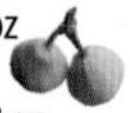 | 15 | 0 | 3 |
| **Winter,** cooked: | | | |
| Acorn: ½ cup cubes, 3.5² oz | 35 | 0 | 9 |
| ½ medium (10 oz raw weight) | 115 | 0 | 30 |
| Butternut: ½ cup, (cubes), 3.5 oz | 40 | 0 | 10 |
| ¼ medium (9 oz raw weight) | 115 | 0 | 30 |
| Spaghetti, ½ cup, 1.75 oz | 15 | 0 | 3 |
| **Succotash,** cooked, ½ cup,3.3 oz | 110 | 1 | 23 |
| **Sweetcorn ~** See Corn | | | |
| **Sweet Potatoes:** 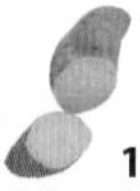 | | | |
| Cooked with skin (w/o fat), | | | |
| 1 medium, 4 oz | 105 | 0 | 24 |
| Without skin, mashed, ½ c., 5.5 oz | 125 | 0 | 29 |

## Vegetables (Cont)

| | C | F | Cb |
|---|---|---|---|
| **Swiss Chard,** cooked, chopped, 1 c., 6 oz | 35 | 0 | 7 |
| **Taro,** cooked, ½ cup, 2.3 oz | 95 | 0 | 23 |
| **Tomatoes:** 1 small (2¼" diam.), 3 oz | 15 | 0 | 3 |
| 1 medium (2¾" diameter), 5 oz | 25 | 0 | 5 |
| 1 large (3½" diameter), 8 oz 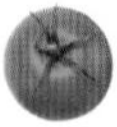 | 40 | 0.5 | 9 |
| 1 extra lge (3" diam.), 12 oz | 60 | 0.5 | 14 |
| Chopped, 1 cup, 6.5 oz | 35 | 0.5 | 7 |
| **Tomatillo,** 1 medium, 1.2 oz | 10 | 0 | 2 |
| **Turnip:** Cooked, ½ cup, 2.75 oz 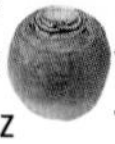 | 15 | 0 | 4 |
| Greens, cooked, ½ cup, 2.5 oz | 15 | 0 | 3 |
| **Water Chestnuts:** 5-6 nuts, 1 oz | 56 | 0.5 | 13 |
| ½ cup, (slices), 2.25 oz, raw | 60 | 0 | 15 |
| Canned, 1 oz | 15 | 0 | 3 |
| **Watercress,** 10 sprigs, 1 oz 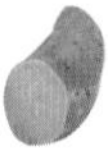 | 3 | 0 | 0.5 |
| **Yams:** Cooked, ½ cup, 2.5 oz | 80 | 0 | 19 |
| Baked: 1 medium (6") 8 oz | 265 | 0.5 | 63 |
| 1 large (9") 12 oz | 400 | 0.5 | 94 |
| **Yardlong Bean,** 1 pod, 0.5 oz | 5 | 0 | 1 |
| **Yucca Root,** ½ cup, 3.5 oz 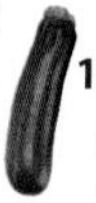 | 165 | 0.5 | 39 |
| **Zucchini:** 1 medium, 7 oz, raw | 30 | 0.5 | 7 |
| Cooked, ½ cup, (slices), 3 oz | 15 | 0 | 4 |

## Frozen Vegetables

| | C | F | Cb |
|---|---|---|---|
| **Birds Eye:** 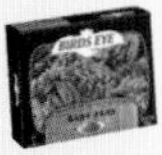 | | | |
| **Baby Varieties:** | | | |
| Peas, ⅔ cup, 3 oz | 70 | 0 | 12 |
| Gold & White Corn, ⅔ cup, 3.2 oz | 100 | 1 | 20 |
| **Steamfresh:** | | | |
| **Pure & Simple:** Brocc. Florets, 2.9 oz | 30 | 0 | 5 |
| Sweet Peas, 3.1 oz | 70 | 0 | 12 |
| **Pure & Simple Premium:** | | | |
| Brussels Sprouts, 2.9 oz | 45 | 0 | 8 |
| Gold & White Corn, ⅔ cup | 80 | 1 | 16 |
| Blends, Brocc. & Cauliflower, 3.1 oz | 30 | 0 | 4 |
| **Lightly Sauced:** | | | |
| Broccoli with Cheese Sauce, 1 cup | 60 | 2 | 7 |
| Rstd Red Pot. w/ Garl. Butter Sauce, | | | |
| 1¼ cups, cooked | 190 | 7 | 30 |

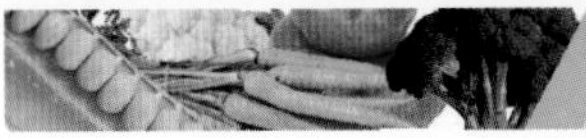

## Frozen Vegetables (Cont)

| | C | F | Cb |
|---|---|---|---|
| **Green Giant:** | | | |
| **Just for One,** | | | |
| Broccoli & Cheese Sauce, 4.25 oz | **40** | 1 | 7 |
| **Vegetables:** Asparagus Cuts, ¾ cup | **20** | 0 | 4 |
| Corn: Nibblers, 1 mini ear, 2 oz | **70** | 0.5 | 14 |
| Extra Sweet Niblets: ⅔ cup | **70** | 1 | 13 |
| In Butter Sauce, ¾ cup | **80** | 1.5 | 15 |
| Shoepeg, w/o sauce, ½ cup | **80** | 0.5 | 17 |
| Honey-Glazed Carrots, 1 cup | **90** | 3 | 15 |
| Spinach, without sauce, ¾cup, | **20** | 0 | 3 |
| **Rice & Vegetables:** *Per ½ Package, Prepared* | | | |
| Cheesy Rice & Broccoli | **150** | 2.5 | 28 |
| Rice Medley | **125** | 2 | 24 |
| Rice Pilaf | **105** | 1.5 | 20 |
| White & Wild Rice | **140** | 3 | 25 |
| **Steamers:** Brocc. & Cheese Sauce, 1 c. | **45** | 1.5 | 7 |
| Brocc, Crts, Cauli., w/ Chse Sce, 1 c. | **45** | 1 | 8 |
| Buttery Rice & Vegetables, 2 cups | **180** | 2 | 37 |
| Garden Vegetable Medley, 1¼ cup | **80** | 1 | 17 |
| **Valley Fresh Steamers,** | | | |
| Rstd Red Potatoes, ½ cup prepared | **80** | 1 | 16 |
| **Ore-Ida:** | | | |
| **Fries:** *Per 3 oz* | | | |
| Classic: Golden Crinkles | **120** | 3.5 | 20 |
| Golden; Shoestring, av. | **125** | 3.5 | 21 |
| Steak | **110** | 3 | 19 |
| Extra Crispy Easy, Crinkles; Golden | **180** | 8 | 25 |
| Extra Crispy: Fast Food Fries | **160** | 6 | 23 |
| Golden Crinkles | **170** | 7 | 24 |
| Seasoned Crinkles | **150** | 6 | 22 |
| Premium: Cottage; Country, av. | **130** | 4.5 | 21 |
| Crispers | **220** | 13 | 23 |
| Golden Twirls | **160** | 6 | 24 |
| Pixie Crinkles; Texas Crispers, av. | **145** | 6 | 21 |
| **Hash Browns:** Golden Patties (1) | **170** | 8 | 15 |
| Potatoes O'Brien, ¾ cup, 3 oz | **60** | 0 | 14 |
| Southern Style, ⅔ cup, 3 oz | **70** | 0 | 16 |
| Toaster Patties (1), 3.65 oz | **220** | 12 | 25 |
| **Onion Rings:** Gourmet, 2.7 oz | **180** | 8 | 25 |
| Onion Ringers (6), 3 oz | **180** | 10 | 21 |
| **Steam n' Mash:** Cut Russet, ¾ cup | **80** | 0 | 17 |
| Cut Sweet Potatoes, 3.3 oz | **90** | 0 | 20 |
| Garlic Seasoned Potatoes, ¾ cup | **110** | 4 | 17 |
| **Tater Tots:** 10 pieces, 3 oz | **170** | 8 | 20 |
| ABC (7), 3 oz | **160** | 8 | 22 |
| Extra Crispy, 9 pieces, 3 oz | **170** | 9 | 20 |

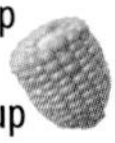

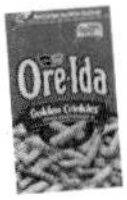


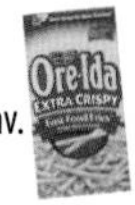


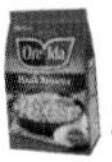

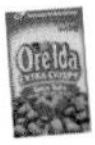


Updated Nutrition Data ~ www.CalorieKing.com
Persons with Diabetes ~ See Disclaimer (Page 22)

## Canned/Bottled

| | C | F | Cb |
|---|---|---|---|
| *Solids & Liquid* | | | |
| **Artichoke Hearts** *(Fanci Foods):* | | | |
| Plain, 1 oz (1) | **8** | 0 | 1 |
| Marinated, ¼ bottle, 1 oz | **25** | 1.5 | 2 |
| **Asparagus:** Drained, 3 spears | **10** | 0 | 1.5 |
| Pieces, ½ cup, 4.3 oz | **25** | 0.5 | 3 |
| **Bamboo Shoots,** 1 cup, 4.5 oz | **25** | 0 | 4 |
| **Bean Salad,** ½ cup, 4.35 oz | **90** | 0 | 20 |
| **Beans:** Green, ½ cup, 2.5 oz | **15** | 0 | 3 |
| Baked Beans, ½ cup, 4.5 oz | **120** | 0.5 | 27 |
| Butter Beans, ½ c., 4.5 oz | **90** | 0 | 16 |
| Italian, ½ cup, 4.5 oz | **30** | 0 | 6 |
| Kidney Beans, ½ cup 3.5 oz | **105** | 0.5 | 19 |
| Lima Beans, ½ cup, 4.5 oz | **80** | 0 | 15 |
| Pinto Beans, ½ cup, 4.5 oz | **105** | 1 | 18 |
| **Beets:** Sliced, ½ cup, 3 oz | **25** | 0 | 6 |
| Crinkle/Pickled *(Del Monte)* ½ c. | **80** | 0 | 20 |
| **Carrots:** Sliced, ½ cup, 2.5 oz | **20** | 0 | 4 |
| Honey Glazed *(Del Monte)* ½ cup | **75** | 0 | 18 |
| **Corn:** Kernels, ½ cup, 4.5 oz | **80** | 0.5 | 18 |
| Creamed style, ½ cup, 4.5 oz | **90** | 0.5 | 23 |
| **Garbanzo/Chick Peas,** ½ c., 4.2 oz | **145** | 1.5 | 27 |
| **Green Chilies,** diced, 2 Tbsp, 1 oz | **6** | 0 | 1.5 |
| **Hearts of Palm,** (1), 1.2 oz | **7** | 0 | 1 |
| **Mushrooms:** ½ cup, 2.5 oz | **20** | 0 | 4 |
| In Butter Sauce, 2 oz | **20** | 1 | 2 |
| **Onions:** Cocktail (1) | **0** | 0 | 0 |
| Pickled, 1 medium, 0.5 oz | **10** | 0 | 2 |
| **French's Fried Onions** ~ *See Page 112* | | | |
| **Peas,** ½ cup, 3 oz | **60** | 0.5 | 10 |
| **Peppers:** Hot Chili, Jalapeno, (1), 1 oz | **5** | 0 | 1 |
| Sweet, undrained, 2.5 oz | **13** | 0 | 3 |
| Jalapeno, with liquid, ½ cup chopped | **20** | 0.5 | 3 |
| Fried, drained, 2 Tbsp, 1 oz | **60** | 5 | 3 |
| **Salsa,** average all types, 2 Tbsp | **10** | 0 | 2 |
| **Sauerkraut,** drained, 1 cup, 5 oz | **25** | 0 | 6 |
| **Spinach,** ½ cup, 3.5 oz | **25** | 0.5 | 3.5 |
| **Succotash:** Cream Style, ½ cup | **100** | 0.5 | 23 |
| w/ whole kernels, undrained, ½ cup | **80** | 0.5 | 18 |
| **Sweetcorn** ~ *See Corn* | | | |
| **Sweet Potato,** ½ cup, 3.5 oz | **90** | 0 | 24 |
| **Tomatoes:** Sundr.: Natural, 5-6 pces | **20** | 0 | 5 |
| In Oil, drained, 6 pieces,0.5 oz | **40** | 2.5 | 4 |
| **Tomato Products** ~ *See Page 144* | | | |
| **Vegetables,** mixed, ½ cup, 4 oz | **45** | 0 | 8 |
| **Yams:** In Light Syrup, ½ cup, 4 oz | **105** | 0 | 25 |
| Candied, ½ cup, 5 oz | **170** | 0 | 46 |
| **Zucchini,** in Tomato Sauce, ½ c., 4 oz | **30** | 0 | 8 |

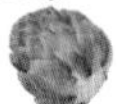

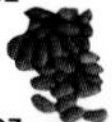

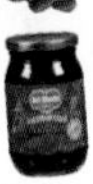

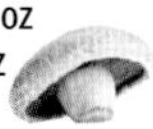

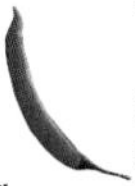

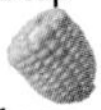

## Quick Guide | C | F | Cb

**Yogurt:** *Average All Brands: Per 8 oz Container*

| | C | F | Cb |
|---|---|---|---|
| **Plain Yogurt:** Whole | 140 | 8 | 10 |
| Low-Fat | 145 | 3.5 | 16 |
| Fat-Free | 125 | 0.5 | 17 |
| **Fruit Flavored:** Whole, 8 oz | 225 | 8 | 32 |
| Low-Fat | 230 | 3 | 43 |
| Fat-Free, regular | 215 | 0.5 | 43 |
| Fat-Free, no sugar added | 80 | 0 | 15 |

**Yogurt Parfait/Deli Cups**
**With Fruit Pieces:** (⅔ Yogurt + ⅓ Fruit)

| | C | F | Cb |
|---|---|---|---|
| Small, 8 oz cup | 140 | 3 | 20 |
| Large, 12 oz cup | 210 | 4.5 | 30 |

**With Fruit + Granola:**

| | C | F | Cb |
|---|---|---|---|
| Small, 8 oz cup (+ ¾ oz Granola) | 235 | 7 | 30 |
| Large, 12 oz cup (+ 1½ oz Granola) | 400 | 13 | 58 |

## Yogurt ~ Brands | C | F | Cb

**Alta Dena:** *Per 8 oz*

| | C | F | Cb |
|---|---|---|---|
| **Low-Fat:** Plain | 170 | 4.5 | 20 |
| All Natural, average all flavors | 215 | 2 | 41 |
| **Non-Fat:** Plain | 110 | 0 | 16 |
| Fruit, average all flavors | 185 | 0 | 38 |
| Vanilla | 160 | 0 | 30 |
| **Amande:** Plain, 8 oz | 170 | 9 | 19 |
| Vanilla, 8 oz | 220 | 8 | 25 |
| Fruit Flavors, average, 6 oz | 150 | 6 | 23 |
| **Axelrod:** Fat free: Plain, 8 oz | 140 | 0 | 21 |
| Fruit flavors, av. all, 6 oz | 90 | 0 | 17 |
| Low Fat, Plain, 8 oz | 160 | 2.5 | 20 |
| **Blue Bunny,** Light, fruit, av. 6 oz | 85 | 0 | 14 |

**Brown Cow:** *Per 6 oz Ctn*
**Cream Top:**

| | C | F | Cb |
|---|---|---|---|
| Smooth & Creamy: Plain | 130 | 7 | 9 |
| Coffee; Vanilla; Maple, av | 165 | 7 | 21 |
| Fruit On The Bottom: Apricot Mango | 170 | 6 | 23 |
| Cherry-Vanilla | 180 | 6 | 28 |
| Low Fat, Fruit flavors, average | 150 | 2 | 26 |

**Cabot:** *Per 8 oz*

| | C | F | Cb |
|---|---|---|---|
| **Non-Fat,** Plain | 110 | 0 | 18 |
| **Greek Style:** Plain | 290 | 23 | 12 |
| Plain, Lowfat (2%) | 150 | 5 | 11 |
| Strawberry, Lowfat | 220 | 4 | 33 |

**Cascade Fresh:**

| | C | F | Cb |
|---|---|---|---|
| Low-Fat, all flavors, 6 oz | 140 | 2 | 23 |
| Fat-Free, all flavors, 6 oz | 110 | 0 | 20 |
| Whole Milk: Plain, 8 oz | 170 | 8 | 12 |
| Vanilla, 8 oz | 200 | 7 | 24 |

**Chobani Greek Yogurt:** *Per 6 oz* | C | F | Cb

| | C | F | Cb |
|---|---|---|---|
| Non-Fat: Plain | 100 | 0 | 7 |
| Fruit flavors, average | 140 | 0 | 21 |
| Low-Fat (2%): Plain | 130 | 3.5 | 7 |
| Fruit flavors, av. | 160 | 3 | 19 |

**Dannon:**
**Activia Yogurt:** *Per 4 Pack, 4 oz ctn*

| | C | F | Cb |
|---|---|---|---|
| Vanilla (1) | 120 | 2 | 22 |
| Light (1), av. all flavors | 70 | 0 | 13 |
| Fiber (1), av. all flavors | 110 | 2 | 19 |
| Desserts, average | 145 | 4 | 22 |
| Parfait, average all flavors, 6 oz | 220 | 3 | 42 |

**All Natural:** *Per 6 oz ctn*

| | C | F | Cb |
|---|---|---|---|
| Average all flavors | 150 | 2.5 | 25 |
| Low-Fat, Plain | 100 | 2.5 | 12 |
| Non-Fat, Plain | 80 | 0 | 12 |
| **Danimals:** Crush Cups, all flav., 4 oz | 110 | 1.5 | 19 |
| Smoothies, average, 3.1 fl.oz | 70 | 0.5 | 15 |

**Fruit On The Bottom,**

| | C | F | Cb |
|---|---|---|---|
| average, 6 oz | 150 | 1.5 | 29 |
| **Light & Fit:** All flav., 6 oz | 80 | 0 | 16 |
| Quarts, all flavors, 8 oz serving | 110 | 0 | 21 |

**Carb & Sugar Control,**

| | C | F | Cb |
|---|---|---|---|
| average all flavors, 4 oz cup | 50 | 1.5 | 3 |

**Greek** ~ *See Oikos*
**Emmi:** *Per 6 oz container*

| | C | F | Cb |
|---|---|---|---|
| **Swiss:** Plain, lowfat | 170 | 2.5 | 10 |
| Average other flavors | 170 | 3 | 27 |

**Fage:**

| | C | F | Cb |
|---|---|---|---|
| **Total Classic:** Plain, single size, 7 oz | 270 | 29 | 6 |
| Fruit Flavors, 5.3 oz | 210 | 12 | 17 |
| Honey, 5.3 oz | 260 | 12 | 28 |
| **Total 0%:** Plain, single size, 5.3 oz | 120 | 0 | 17 |
| Fruit Flavors, average, 5.3 oz | 120 | 0 | 18 |
| Honey, 5.3 oz | 170 | 0 | 30 |
| **Total 2%:** Plain, 5.3 oz | 190 | 2.5 | 29 |
| Fruit Flavors, av., 5.3 oz | 140 | 2.5 | 17 |
| Honey, 5.3 oz | 140 | 2.5 | 18 |

**Fresh & Easy:**

| | C | F | Cb |
|---|---|---|---|
| Greek, Vanilla, 6 oz | 230 | 14 | 20 |
| Lowfat, av., 6 oz ctn | 140 | 1.5 | 28 |
| Nonfat, average all flavors, 6 oz ctn | 140 | 0 | 29 |

**Horizon Organic:** *Per 8 oz serving*
**Cream-on-Top,** Whole Milk:

| | C | F | Cb |
|---|---|---|---|
| Plain | 160 | 7 | 14 |
| Vanilla | 220 | 6 | 32 |
| **Fat Free:** Plain | 80 | 0 | 12 |
| Vanilla | 160 | 0 | 33 |
| **Yogurt Tuberz (1),** all flavors | 60 | 0.5 | 11 |

## Brands (Cont)

| | C | F | Cb |
|---|---|---|---|
| **Jewel:** 6 oz Carton | | | |
| **Blended Low Fat:** Av. all flavors | 150 | 1.5 | 30 |
| Light, average all flavors | 110 | 0 | 20 |
| Fruit On The Bottom, av. | 180 | 2 | 33 |
| Fat-Free, Plain | 90 | 0 | 14 |
| **32 oz Tubs:** Per 8 oz | | | |
| Lowfat, average fruit flav. | 205 | 2 | 39 |
| Plain, Non-Fat | 120 | 0 | 18 |
| **Kemps:** 'Light' 80 Cals, av., 6 oz | 80 | 0 | 16 |
| **Yo-J Drink,** all flavors, 8.3 fl.oz | 150 | 0 | 34 |
| **Kirkland,** Low-Fat, | | | |
| Blueberry; Peach; Strawberry, 6 oz | 180 | 1.5 | 36 |
| **Kroger:** Per 6 oz carton | | | |
| **Blended,** all flavors | 190 | 2 | 35 |
| **Carb Master,** av. all flav. | 80 | 1.5 | 4 |
| **Fruit On The Bottom,** | | | |
| average all flavors | 170 | 2 | 30 |
| **Lite,** average all flavors | 80 | 0 | 13 |
| **La Yogurt:** Per 6 oz ctn | | | |
| **Probiotic,** Low Fat: Orig., av. all. | 150 | 2.5 | 27 |
| **Rich & Creamy,** average all flavors | 185 | 2 | 35 |
| **Sabor Latino:** | | | |
| Dulche De Leche, 6 oz | 190 | 1.5 | 36 |
| Fruit Flavors, av., 6 oz | 190 | 1.5 | 37 |
| **LALA:** Per 6 oz Carton | | | |
| **Blended,** Fruit Flavors, av. all | 150 | 3 | 27 |
| **Smoothies,** Berry Flavors, | | | |
| 8.1 fl.oz | 170 | 3 | 31 |
| **Lucerne:** Per 6 oz ctn | | | |
| **Low-Fat,** average all var. | 170 | 2 | 32 |
| **Fat-Free:** Plain | 80 | 0 | 13 |
| Light Fat-Free, fruit, 6 oz | 90 | 0 | 17 |
| **Mountain High:** Per 8 oz | | | |
| **Original Style:** Plain | 180 | 8 | 17 |
| Strawb./Vanilla, average | 210 | 7 | 28 |
| **Low-Fat:** Plain | 140 | 2.5 | 18 |
| Rasp./Strawb./Vanilla, average | 175 | 2.5 | 29 |
| **Fat-Free:** Plain | 120 | 0 | 18 |
| Strawberry; Vanilla, average | 160 | 0 | 30 |
| **Nancy's:** Per 8 oz Carton | | | |
| **Nonfat:** | | | |
| Fruit On The Top: Cherry; Peach, av. | 145 | 0.5 | 26 |
| Raspberry; Strawberry, av. | 165 | 0 | 31 |
| **Whole Milk:** With Honey | 170 | 8 | 17 |
| With Fruit on Top, average | 230 | 5 | 41 |
| **Low Fat:** Plain; Lemon | 150 | 3 | 16 |
| Average other flavors | 175 | 3 | 27 |
| **Organic Soy Cultured:** Plain, 6 oz | 150 | 3 | 25 |
| Berry flavors, average | 140 | 3.5 | 24 |
| **O Organics,** Low-Fat, av., 6 oz | 140 | 2.5 | 23 |

| | C | F | Cb |
|---|---|---|---|
| **Oikos:** | | | |
| **Dannon Greek:** Per 5.3 oz Unless Indicated | | | |
| Traditional, Fruit Flavors | 160 | 4.5 | 18 |
| Nonfat: Plain | 80 | 0 | 6 |
| Fruit flavors, average | 125 | 0 | 20 |
| Quarts, Vanilla, 8 oz | 190 | 0 | 29 |
| **Stonyfield Greek:** Per 5.3 oz Unless Indicated | | | |
| Nonfat: Honey Fig | 110 | 0 | 14 |
| Average fruit flavors | 120 | 0 | 18 |
| **Publix:** Fat-Free, Plain, 8 oz | 140 | 0 | 23 |
| Swiss Style, Low-Fat, 8 oz | 240 | 2.5 | 41 |
| **Ralphs** ~ Same as Kroger | | | |
| **Roberts:** Per 6 oz Ctn | | | |
| Low-Fat, average all flavors | 165 | 1.5 | 32 |
| Fat-Free, all flavors | 90 | 0 | 15 |
| **Silk Live! (Soy):** | | | |
| **32 oz Ctn,** Plain, 8 oz serving | 150 | 4 | 22 |
| **6 oz Cup:** Fruit flavors, average | 150 | 3 | 24 |
| Vanilla | 150 | 3 | 24 |
| **So Delicious (Dairy/Soy Free):** | | | |
| **Cultured Coconut Milk:** Plain, 6 oz | 130 | 7 | 16 |
| Chocolate, 4 oz | 110 | 3.5 | 20 |
| Pina Colada; Raspb. av., 6 oz | 150 | 6 | 25 |
| Vanilla, 6 oz | 140 | 6 | 24 |
| **Stater Bros:** Per 6 oz Ctn | | | |
| Plain | 105 | 1.5 | 14 |
| Fruit on the Bottom, av all flavors | 170 | 1.5 | 34 |
| Blended Low-Fat, av. all flavors | 155 | 1.5 | 29 |
| 32 oz Tubs: Non-Fat, Plain, 8 oz | 120 | 0 | 18 |
| Low Fat, 8 oz | 140 | 2 | 19 |
| **Stonyfield Organic:** | | | |
| **Organic Activia,** 4-Pack, | | | |
| Strawberry; Vanilla, av, 4 oz | 90 | 1 | 16 |
| **Smooth & Creamy:** Per 6 oz | | | |
| Whole Milk, av. all flavors | 170 | 6 | 23 |
| Low Fat, average all flavors | 130 | 2 | 22 |
| Fat Free, average all flavors | 100 | 0 | 22 |
| **Fruit On Bottom:** Per 6 oz | | | |
| Whole Milk: Choc. U'ground | 220 | 5 | 37 |
| Strawb. & Cream | 150 | 6 | 20 |
| Low Fat, average all flavors | 125 | 2 | 21 |
| Fat Free: Choc Underground | 150 | 0 | 30 |
| average other flavors | 115 | 0 | 22 |
| **Fruit On Bottom,** av all flav., 6 oz | 170 | 2.5 | 29 |
| **Trader Joe's:** | | | |
| **French Village:** Non-Fat, all flav., 6 oz | 130 | 0 | 24 |
| 32 oz Containers: Plain, 8 oz | 120 | 0 | 17 |
| Vanilla, 8 oz | 180 | 0 | 34 |
| **Greek Style:** Plain, 8 oz | 260 | 18 | 14 |
| Apricot Mango; Honey, av., 8 oz | 300 | 15 | 28 |

*continued next page*

## Brands (Cont)

| | C | F | Cb |
|---|---|---|---|
| **Trader Joe's (Cont):** | | | |
| **Greek Style (Cont.)** | | | |
| Non-Fat: Plain, 8 oz | 120 | 0 | 7 |
| Blueb.; Honey 5.3 oz | 120 | 0 | 16 |
| Vanilla, 5.3 oz | 130 | 0 | 20 |
| With Fiber: Plain, 5.3 oz | 80 | 0 | 8 |
| Peach | 110 | 0 | 8 |
| **Low-Fat,** Pre-Stirred, Fruit, 8 oz | 220 | 3 | 40 |
| **Low-Fat:** With Almonds/Granola: | | | |
| Pomegranate, 4.6 oz | 140 | 2.5 | 27 |
| Vanilla, 4.6 oz | 160 | 7 | 20 |
| **Organic Lowfat,** | | | |
| Fruit flavors, av., 6 oz | 140 | 2.5 | 23 |
| **Rich & Creamy,** average, 4 oz | 140 | 6 | 19 |
| **Soy,** Peach; Strawberry, av., 6 oz | 160 | 3.5 | 29 |
| **Squishers,** Org., low fat, 1 tube, 2 oz | 60 | 1 | 10 |
| **Voskos,** Greek, nonfat, Vanilla, 5.3 oz | 130 | 0 | 20 |
| **Wallaby Organic,** Blended, | | | |
| Low-Fat, average all flavors, 6 oz | 150 | 2.5 | 26 |
| **Weight Watchers,** | | | |
| av. all flavors, 6 oz ctn | 100 | 0.5 | 17 |
| **Whole Foods (365):** | | | |
| Non-Fat, Plain, 6 oz | 90 | 0 | 13 |
| Fruit flavors, average 6 oz | 145 | 0 | 30 |
| Vanilla, 6 oz | 130 | 0 | 23 |
| **Whole Soy:** Plain, 6 oz | 150 | 4.5 | 19 |
| Average all flavors, 6 oz | 170 | 3.5 | 33 |
| **YoCrunch:** | | | |
| **Cookies & Candy Crunch:** *Per 6 oz Container:* | | | |
| Strawberry: W/ Nestle Crunch pcs | 200 | 4.5 | 36 |
| With Oreo Cookie pieces | 180 | 3 | 34 |
| Vanilla, with pieces, av. all varieties | 195 | 4 | 34 |
| **Fruit Parfait,** w/Granola, all flavors | 170 | 1.5 | 35 |
| **Nonfat Greek,** w/Granola, av all flav | 175 | 1.5 | 33 |
| **100 Calorie,** av. all flavors, 3¾ oz | 100 | 1.5 | 19 |
| **Yoplait:** | | | |
| **Original:** *6 oz Ctn* | | | |
| 99% Fat-Free, av. all flav. | 170 | 1.5 | 33 |
| Light, Fat Free, Fruit Flavors, all | 100 | 0 | 19 |
| Thick & Creamy, average all flav. | 180 | 2.5 | 31 |
| Large 2lb Carton: Nat., Plain, 8 oz | 130 | 0 | 19 |
| 99% Fat-Free, av., 8 oz | 210 | 1.5 | 42 |
| Light, Fat-Free, av., 8 oz | 140 | 0 | 27 |
| **Greek:** Plain, 6 oz | 120 | 0 | 12 |
| Fruit Flavors, av., 6 oz | 160 | 0 | 25 |
| Honey Vanilla, 6 oz | 150 | 0 | 22 |

## Brands (Cont)

| | C | F | Cb |
|---|---|---|---|
| **Yoplait (Cont):** | | | |
| **Fiber One,** average all flavors, 4 oz | 50 | 0 | 13 |
| **Delights,** av. all flavors, 4 oz | 100 | 1.5 | 17 |
| **Whips!:** Chocolate flavors, | | | |
| 4 oz cup | 160 | 4 | 25 |
| Fruit flavors, 4 oz cup | 140 | 2.5 | 25 |
| **Yo-Plus,** av. all flav., 4 oz | 110 | 1.5 | 21 |
| **Yoplait Kids,** all flav., 4 oz cup | 90 | 1 | 17 |
| **Go-Gurt!,** all flavors, 2.25 oz tube | 70 | 0.5 | 13 |
| **Splitz,** av. all flavors, 3.25 oz ctn | 90 | 1 | 17 |
| **Trix,** Fruit Flavors, av. all, 4 oz cup | 100 | 0.5 | 20 |

## Yogurt Drinks & Probiotics

| | C | F | Cb |
|---|---|---|---|
| **BioKult,** | | | |
| Cultured, all flav. | | | |
| 2.1 oz bottle | 35 | 0 | 8 |
| **Cacique,** Yonique, | | | |
| av. all flav., 7 fl.oz | 200 | 1.5 | 35 |
| **Dannon:** Activia, all flavors, 7 fl oz | 160 | 3 | 27 |
| Danimals, all flav., 3.1 fl.oz | 70 | 0.5 | 15 |
| DanActive, | | | |
| average all flav., 3.1 fl.oz | 80 | 1.5 | 13 |
| Dan-o-nino, all flav., 3.1 fl.oz | 70 | 0.5 | 15 |
| **Danone** *(Canada),* | | | |
| Danacol, av. all flavors, 80 ml | 35 | 1 | 4 |
| **Glen Oaks,** av. all flavors, 8 fl.oz | 190 | 3.5 | 35 |
| **Good Belly:** *Per 2.7 fl.oz Bottle* | | | |
| **Probiotics:** BigShot, all flavors | 60 | 1 | 11 |
| Plus, average all flavors | 50 | 0 | 12 |
| **Kemps,** Yo-J Drink, | | | |
| all flavors, 8 fl. oz | 150 | 0 | 34 |
| **LaLa,** Yogurt Smoothies, | | | |
| average all flavors, 8.1 fl.oz | 130 | 2 | 24 |
| **Lifeway,** Kefir Smoothie (Probiotic), | | | |
| 8 fl.oz | 140 | 2 | 20 |
| **Ralphs,** | | | |
| Smoothies, av., 7 fl.oz | 200 | 2.5 | 37 |
| **Stonyfield Organic:** | | | |
| **Super Smoothies:** Av. all flav, 10 oz | 230 | 3 | 40 |
| 4-pack, average all flavors, 6 oz | 140 | 2 | 22 |
| **Oikos,** 4-pack, av. all flavors, 6 oz | 155 | 2 | 26 |
| **Trader Joe's,** | | | |
| Lowfat Smoothies, fruit flav., 6 fl.oz | 140 | 2 | 23 |
| **Wildwood,** | | | |
| Probiotic, av., 8 fl.oz | 185 | 2.5 | 32 |
| **Yakult,** 2.7 fl.oz bottle | 50 | 0 | 12 |
| **Yoplait,** Frozen Smoothies, | | | |
| all flavors, ½ pouch, 8 fl.oz prep'd | 110 | 1.5 | 19 |

## Cafeteria-Style Foods  C  F  Cb

*Average All Preparations:*

| | C | F | Cb |
|---|---|---|---|
| Beef Stroganoff, 5 oz | 195 | 13 | 7 |
| Beef Stroganoff with 4 oz noodles | 350 | 14 | 36 |
| Chicken Lasagna, 1 piece | 300 | 11 | 32 |
| Chicken Chop Suey with 4 oz rice | 245 | 4 | 37 |
| Deep Dish Burrito, 7 oz | 265 | 13 | 20 |
| Grnd Beef Casserole, 2 scps, 6 oz | 245 | 13 | 17 |
| Italian Meat Sce for Spaghetti, 5 oz | 150 | 9 | 9 |
| with 5 oz Spaghetti | 350 | 10 | 49 |
| Lasagna, 1 piece | 275 | 11 | 25 |
| Meatloaf, 3 oz | 205 | 13 | 4 |
| Ranch Beans, 2 scoops, 6 oz | 350 | 11 | 45 |
| Red Beans & Rice, 7 oz | 280 | 9 | 37 |
| Scalloped Potato/Ham, 2 scps, 6 oz | 160 | 6 | 20 |
| Stuffed Shells in Sauce (1) | 105 | 3 | 17 |
| Swedish Meatballs (3) | 205 | 12 | 9 |
| Sweet & Sour Pork/Rice, 9 oz | 240 | 3 | 40 |
| Swiss Steak w/ Mushr. Gravy, 6 oz | 280 | 11 | 4 |
| Tator Tot Casserole, 2 scoops, 6 oz | 260 | 15 | 20 |
| Tenderloin Tips/Mushr. Gravy, 5 oz | 210 | 13 | 3 |
| with 5 oz noodles | 395 | 15 | 38 |
| Tuna Noodle Casserole, 2 scps, 6 oz | 180 | 6 | 17 |
| Turkey Tetrazzini, 2 scoops, 6 oz | 195 | 7 | 17 |
| Vegetable Lasagna, 1 piece | 250 | 13 | 21 |

### Croissants

| | C | F | Cb |
|---|---|---|---|
| **Unfilled,** medium 1.5 oz | 180 | 10 | 21 |
| **Filled:** With Ham (2 oz), garnish | 280 | 14 | 24 |
| With Ham (2 oz), Cheese (2 oz) | 470 | 30 | 20 |
| With Chick (2 oz), Cheese (2 oz) | 470 | 30 | 20 |
| With Turkey/Ham/Cheese (2 oz ea.) | 580 | 36 | 20 |
| Au Bon Pain: Ham & Cheese | 390 | 21 | 35 |
| Spinach & Cheese | 290 | 17 | 28 |

7-Eleven ~ See Page 236

### Bagels

| | C | F | Cb |
|---|---|---|---|
| **Plain:** Large, 4 oz (without filling) | 320 | 2 | 65 |
| With 2 oz Cream Cheese | 500 | 27 | 54 |
| With 2 oz Lox (Smoked Salmon) | 400 | 4 | 65 |

**Also see Bagels Section ~** *Page 54*
**Fast-Foods Restaurants ~** *Page 175*
**Au Bon Pain ~** *Page 179*
**Bruegger's ~** *Page 185*
**Einstein Bros Bagels ~** *Page 199*

## Sandwiches  C  F  Cb

*No Spreads Unless Indicated:*
*(Includes 2 Slices Bread ~ 3 oz)*

| | C | F | Cb |
|---|---|---|---|
| BLT (5 strips Bacon, 2 Tbsp Mayo) | 600 | 40 | 46 |
| Breaded Chicken & Garnish | 540 | 28 | 46 |
| Chicken Salad with Mayo., 5 oz | 580 | 30 | 49 |
| Chopped Liver, Egg, Mayonnaise | 630 | 25 | 44 |
| Corned Beef with Mustard, 5 oz | 560 | 28 | 44 |
| Egg Salad with Mayonnaise | 570 | 29 | 49 |
| Egg Salad Club w/ Bacon & Mayo. | 780 | 53 | 49 |
| Grilled Cheese (3 oz) | 540 | 30 | 44 |
| Ham (4 oz); Cheese (4 oz), & Mayo. | 910 | 56 | 44 |
| Lobster Salad (4 oz) w/ Mayonnaise | 530 | 25 | 45 |
| Overstuffed Tuna Salad (7 oz) | 870 | 39 | 75 |
| Philadelphia Cheese Steak Sandwich | 550 | 23 | 42 |
| Reuben (6 oz Beef/Pastrami, | | | |
| 2 oz Cheese, 2 Tbsp Dressing) | 920 | 60 | 28 |
| Roast Beef (4 oz) with Mustard | 460 | 12 | 45 |
| Roast Pork (4 oz) with Apple Sauce | 500 | 16 | 55 |
| Shrimp Salad Club w/ Bacon & Mayo | 800 | 57 | 48 |
| Sloppy Joe with Sauce (7 oz) | 600 | 30 | 45 |
| Steak Sandwich (5 oz cooked) | 680 | 32 | 41 |
| Triple Cheese Melt (4 oz) | 720 | 45 | 46 |
| Tuna Salad (5 oz) with Mayonnaise | 610 | 30 | 49 |
| Turkey Breast (5 oz) w/ Mayonnaise | 460 | 18 | 44 |
| Turkey Breast (5 oz) w/ Mustard | 360 | 7 | 44 |
| Turkey Club with Bacon, Mayonnaise | 830 | 38 | 31 |
| Vegetarian with Avocado & Cheese | 820 | 49 | 72 |

**7-Eleven ~** *Page 236*
**Schlotzsky's ~** *Page 237*
**Subway ~** *Page 245*

### Wraps & Roll-Ups  C  F  Cb

*Average All Types*
**Meat/Chicken/Fish/Veggie:**

| | C | F | Cb |
|---|---|---|---|
| Small, approximately 9 oz | 500 | 25 | 48 |
| Regular, approximately 15 oz | 830 | 40 | 80 |
| Large, approximately 22 oz | 1400 | 70 | 134 |

**Fast-Foods Restaurants ~** *Page 175*
**Au Bon Pain ~** *Page 179*
**Sonic Drive-In ~** *Page 241*
**Subway ~** *Page 245*
**WAWA ~** *Page 254*

---

Updated Nutrition Data ~ www.CalorieKing.com
Persons with Diabetes ~ See Disclaimer (Page 22)

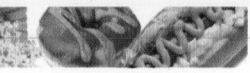

## Fair & Carnival Foods

| | C | F | Cb |
|---|---|---|---|
| **Mexican:** | | | |
| Burrito with Bean/Beef, 17 oz | 1100 | 41 | 104 |
| Carne Asada, 14.5 oz | 820 | 44 | 58 |
| Chicken Taco, 3.3 oz | 210 | 12 | 16 |
| Fish Taco, 5 oz | 270 | 13 | 31 |
| Nachos with Cheese, 9" plate | 860 | 59 | 70 |
| Tamale (1), 3.5 oz | 180 | 8 | 21 |
| Taquito, 5 oz | 370 | 17 | 43 |
| **Greek:** | | | |
| Baklava, 2" square | 245 | 13 | 32 |
| Falafel, 11.6 oz | 660 | 27 | 85 |
| Greek Salad, 14 oz | 520 | 48 | 17 |
| Gyro, 7.5", 12 oz | 680 | 40 | 55 |
| Spanakopita, 8 oz | 200 | 7.5 | 23 |
| **Italian:** | | | |
| Garlic Bread, ½ loaf, 10 oz | 1135 | 40 | 147 |
| Pizza Bread, Pepperoni, ½ loaf, 12 oz | 1115 | 32 | 151 |
| Pizza on a Stick, 1 piece | 535 | 28 | 55 |
| **Personal Pizza:** 7" | | | |
| Cheese (1) | 670 | 24 | 80 |
| Pepperoni (1) | 795 | 35 | 80 |
| Ham & Pineapple (1) | 800 | 31 | 87 |
| **Low Carb:** | | | |
| Beef Patty, wrapped in lettuce, 4 oz | 480 | 33 | 0 |
| **Sandwiches:** Per 7½" Roll | | | |
| Ham, 11 oz | 645 | 39 | 47 |
| Hot Pastrami, 9 oz | 760 | 17 | 62 |
| Roast Beef, 11 oz | 620 | 36 | 46 |
| Philadelphia Cheese Steak, 13 oz | 680 | 36 | 49 |
| Tuna, 12 oz | 830 | 60 | 46 |
| Turkey, 11 oz | 665 | 24 | 65 |
| Veggie, 11 oz | 490 | 23 | 49 |
| **Oriental:** | | | |
| **Fried Egg Roll,** 6 oz | 400 | 19 | 44 |
| **Rice Bowl:** Beef, 6" Bowl | 880 | 13 | 136 |
| Chicken, 6" Bowl | 870 | 15 | 135 |
| **Hamburgers:** | | | |
| ⅓ Pound Burger, 7.5 oz | 670 | 41 | 26 |
| Cheeseburger, 6 oz | 550 | 36 | 25 |
| **Hot Dogs/Franks:** With Bun | | | |
| **Hot Dog:** Regular, (1) | 215 | 14 | 28 |
| With Chili, 6 oz | 450 | 32 | 32 |
| With Chili & Cheese, 7.3 oz | 500 | 36 | 31 |
| ⅓ Pound Hot Dog | 550 | 41 | 31 |
| Foot Long Hot Dog | 470 | 26 | 41 |
| **Corn Dog:** Regular, 4 oz | 250 | 14 | 23 |
| Jumbo, 6 oz | 375 | 21 | 36 |
| **Jumbo Franks with Bun,** | | | |
| Bratwurst; Sausage; Kielbasa, av. | 800 | 60 | 28 |

## Fair & Carnival Foods (Cont)

| | C | F | Cb |
|---|---|---|---|
| **Barbeque:** Weights with Bone | | | |
| Chicken, 15 oz | 740 | 24 | 34 |
| Corn Cob, 8" (1), 16 oz | 200 | 1 | 42 |
| Pork Ribs, 18 oz | 1360 | 68 | 21 |
| Smoked Turkey Legs (w/ skin), 19 oz | 1135 | 54 | 0 |
| **Beef Stew over Rice,** 2 cups | 440 | 14 | 61 |
| **Butter Balls:** | | | |
| **Deep-fried:** 1 Ball | 115 | 10 | 6 |
| 4 Balls | 460 | 38 | 24 |
| **Burrito,** with Bean/Beef, 17 oz | 1110 | 41 | 104 |
| **Cheese Curds,** | | | |
| Breaded & Fried, | | | |
| (Culver's), 6.7 oz | 670 | 38 | 54 |
| **Potatoes & Fries:** | | | |
| Australian Battered Potato, 12 oz | 1290 | 66 | 155 |
| Baked Potato, 14 oz | 435 | 0.5 | 100 |
| **Fries:** French, 7 oz | 560 | 24 | 70 |
| Cheese Fries, 10 oz | 645 | 38 | 62 |
| Chili Fries, 10 oz | 700 | 36 | 83 |
| Curly Fries, 7 oz | 620 | 30 | 78 |
| Tasti Chips, 40 chips, 6.5 oz | 780 | 33 | 117 |
| Sweet Potato, 14 oz | 405 | 0.5 | 97 |
| Ranch Dip, 3 oz | 165 | 14 | 9 |
| **Finger Foods:** | | | |
| Artichoke: Steamed, 6 pieces | 65 | 0 | 16 |
| Fried, 9 pieces | 250 | 14 | 24 |
| Chicken Nuggets (6) | 340 | 17 | 26 |
| Chicken Strips (4), 4.5 oz | 445 | 21 | 33 |
| Finger Steaks (2), 4 oz | 400 | 20 | 26 |
| Mushrooms, Fried, 10-12 pieces | 395 | 26 | 34 |
| Onion Rings, 3 rings | 310 | 13 | 40 |
| Onion Flower | 1320 | 72 | 140 |
| Shrimp, Fried, 10-12 pieces, 5 oz | 555 | 30 | 36 |
| Sweet Potato Strips, Fried, 4 pces | 750 | 30 | 106 |
| Zucchini, Fried, 4 slices | 620 | 40 | 42 |
| **Salads/Sides:** | | | |
| Chili, 1 cup | 280 | 11 | 24 |
| Cole Slaw, 5 oz | 350 | 21 | 37 |
| Pickle, whole (6") | 30 | 0 | 8 |
| Potato Salad, 5 oz | 290 | 15 | 35 |
| **Candied Apple,** 7 oz | 330 | 0 | 80 |
| **Cotton Candy:** Small, 1 oz | 110 | 0 | 27 |
| Large, 2.25 oz | 250 | 0 | 62 |
| Family Size, 5.5 oz | 610 | 0 | 151 |
| **Popcorn:** | | | |
| Plain: Small, 3 oz | 450 | 24 | 48 |
| Large, 6 oz | 900 | 48 | 96 |
| Kettle Corn: Small, 5 oz | 600 | 15 | 110 |
| Large, 10 oz | 1200 | 30 | 220 |

# Eating Out – Fair ◇ Stadium

## Fair & Carnival Foods (Cont)

| Cakes, Donuts, Cookies: | C | F | Cb |
|---|---|---|---|
| **Funnel Cake:** Plain (1) | 760 | 44 | 80 |
| Toppings: Apple Cinn., 2 oz | 85 | 3 | 36 |
| Cinn. & Sugar, 2 tsp | 40 | 0 | 10 |
| Strawberry & Cream, 2 oz | 70 | 0 | 16 |
| Cheesecake on a Stick, 6 oz | 655 | 47 | 56 |
| Churro (1), 9", 1.6 oz | 170 | 8 | 22 |
| Cobbler, 5 oz | 350 | 10 | 62 |
| Cream Puff, 4.3 oz | 500 | 43 | 22 |
| Donuts, Jumbo Twist, (1), 7.5 oz | 905 | 49 | 109 |
| Fried Snicker Bar, 5 oz | 445 | 29 | 42 |
| Fried Twinkie, 1 | 420 | 34 | 45 |
| Fudge, 1.5 oz | 200 | 11 | 25 |
| Key Lime Pie Bar, 6 oz | 635 | 40 | 59 |
| Puff-on-a-Stick (4), 8.6 oz | 995 | 86 | 44 |
| Soft Pretzel, 4.5 oz | 340 | 2 | 70 |
| Strawberry Crepe, 4.3 oz | 280 | 14 | 36 |
| Sweet Martha Cookie (1), 3/4 oz | 90 | 4 | 14 |
| Regular Cone, 9 cookies | 810 | 36 | 126 |
| Twinkie Dog (Sundae) | 500 | 14 | 89 |
| Fried Dough/FryBread: | | | |
| Plain: 7", 3.7 oz | 390 | 19 | 47 |
| 9", 4¾ oz | 510 | 25 | 61 |
| Toppings: Cinnamon Sugar, 2 tsp | 40 | 0 | 10 |
| Butterscotch; Caramel, 2 Tbsp | 115 | 0 | 29 |
| Chocolate, Fat-Free, 2 Tbsp | 100 | 0 | 23 |
| Hot Fudge, average, 2 Tbsp | 110 | 4 | 22 |
| Pineapple, Strawberry, 2 Tbsp | 100 | 0 | 26 |
| Cheese Powder, 2 tsp | 70 | 3 | 2 |
| Honey, 1 Tbsp, ¾ oz | 65 | 0 | 17 |
| Ice Cream & Frozen Treats: | | | |
| Dippin' Dots Ice Cream: Small, 4 oz | 150 | 7 | 17 |
| Medium, 8 oz | 305 | 14 | 35 |
| Frozen Banana, chocolate coated, 5 oz | 240 | 4 | 53 |
| Frozen Yogurt in sugar cone, 14 oz | 475 | 2 | 94 |
| Ice Cream: Small, sugar cone, 10 oz | 775 | 42 | 83 |
| Large, sugar cone, 14 oz | 935 | 54 | 96 |
| Sherbet, 8 oz | 270 | 4 | 59 |
| Snow Cone (includes 3 oz syrup) | 270 | 0 | 68 |
| Strawberry, Choc. Dipped, 1 piece | 125 | 7 | 15 |
| Drinks, Slushies: | | | |
| Horchata, 16 fl.oz | 280 | 8 | 50 |
| Lemonade, 18 fl.oz | 210 | 0 | 52 |
| Orange Julius, 20 fl.oz | 490 | 10 | 96 |
| Strawberry Julius, 20 fl.oz | 430 | 0 | 98 |
| Icee, 16 fl.oz | 235 | 0 | 59 |
| Malt/Shake, 16 fl.oz | 690 | 33 | 85 |
| Slushies, 16 fl.oz | 260 | 0 | 65 |
| Soft Frozen Lemonade, 12 fl.oz | 300 | 0 | 78 |
| **Smoothies,** Berry Flavors, 16 fl.oz | 350 | 1 | 80 |

## Stadium Foods

| Sandwiches: | C | F | Cb |
|---|---|---|---|
| Bacon Burger, 8.3 oz | 470 | 25 | 34 |
| Cheeseburger, 8.3 oz | 450 | 23 | 33 |
| Chicken Sandwich: W/Cheese, 8.3 oz | 510 | 29 | 40 |
| Without Cheese, 7.7 oz | 460 | 25 | 40 |
| With Bacon, 8.3 oz | 530 | 31 | 41 |
| Hamburger, 7.8 oz | 400 | 19 | 33 |
| Polish Sausage S'wich, 7 oz | 565 | 33 | 46 |
| **French Fries,** 6.4 oz | 470 | 34 | 39 |
| **Fruit Cup,** 6 oz | 80 | 0 | 20 |
| Hot Dogs: | | | |
| Chili Dog, 7.7 oz | 520 | 29 | 45 |
| Hot Dog, 6.4 oz | 465 | 21 | 50 |
| Jumbo Dog, 6 oz | 440 | 25 | 38 |
| Kraut Dog with Sauerkraut , 7.8 oz | 490 | 27 | 41 |
| **Nachos,** 40 chips w/4 oz cheese | 1100 | 59 | 132 |
| **Individual Pan Pizza (6"):** *Per 10 oz Pizza* | | | |
| BBQ Chicken | 630 | 24 | 71 |
| Cheese | 630 | 27 | 71 |
| Pepperoni | 660 | 30 | 70 |
| Snacks: | | | |
| Brownie, 2.5" x 4.5" | 360 | 18 | 44 |
| Cheese Sauce, 1.25 oz | 100 | 8 | 4 |
| Cheetos, 2.75 oz package | 440 | 28 | 42 |
| Chocolate Chip Cookie, 2.3 oz | 280 | 12 | 40 |
| Churro (1), 10", 2.1 oz | 210 | 10 | 26 |
| Doritos, Nacho, 2.75 oz package | 390 | 20 | 48 |
| King Size Candy: Butterfinger, 3.75 oz | 485 | 18 | 75 |
| Nestle Crunch, 2.75 oz | 390 | 21 | 85 |
| Lays Chips, 2.75 oz package | 440 | 28 | 42 |
| Peanuts in shell, 8 oz | 930 | 80 | 24 |
| **Popcorn:** Small (9 cup size) | 575 | 35 | 56 |
| Large (15 cup size) | 950 | 58 | 93 |
| **Red Vines,** 5 oz box | 495 | 0 | 121 |
| **Snow Cone,** (includes 3 oz syrup) | 270 | 0 | 68 |
| **Soft Pretzel:** Reg., 5.5 oz | 490 | 3.5 | 101 |
| Giant, 8 oz | 710 | 5 | 147 |
| **Beverages:** Orange Juice, 12 fl.oz | 180 | 0 | 2 |
| Beer: Heineken, 16 fl.oz | 200 | 0 | 16 |
| Light Miller, 16 fl.oz | 125 | 0 | 4 |
| Miller Draft, 16 fl.oz | 195 | 0 | 17 |
| Jack Daniels Punch, 12 fl.oz | 235 | 0 | 34 |
| Wine, White, 9 fl.oz | 190 | 0 | 6 |
| Soda (with ½ ice), average: 20 fl.oz | 160 | 0 | 40 |
| 32 fl.oz | 260 | 0 | 65 |
| Starbuck's, Coffee Frapp., 9.5 fl.oz bottle | 200 | 3 | 37 |

## Chinese & Asian Dishes

**Appetizers:** | C | F | Cb
---|---|---|---
**Crab Cake,** 2¼ oz | 125 | 10 | 1
**Dumplings:** Pork, steamed, (1) | 80 | 4.5 | 5
Pork, fried, (1) | 90 | 6 | 5
Vegetable, steamed, (1) | 35 | 1 | 5
**Egg Rolls,** mini, 3 rolls | 100 | 3 | 11
**Spring Roll:** | | |
Small, 1.5 oz | 85 | 4 | 9
Medium, 3 oz | 170 | 8 | 17
Large, 5 oz | 290 | 15 | 29
**Wonton,** 1 only | 75 | 4 | 5
**Soup:** Egg Flower, bowl 12 oz | 90 | 2 | 16
Hot & Sour Soup, bowl 12 oz | 110 | 3.5 | 14
**Rice:** Plain, 1 cup (½ Pint), 6.5 oz | 320 | 2 | 66
2 cups (1 Pint), 13 oz | 640 | 4 | 132
Fried: 1 cup, 5 oz | 365 | 11 | 55
Large dish, 16 oz | 950 | 28 | 67
**Noodles,** Chinese Egg, ckd, 1 cup | 200 | 4 | 37

*Entrees & Mains: Per Serving*

| | C | F | Cb
---|---|---|---
Almond Chicken, 6 oz | 270 | 10 | 21
BBQ Pork, 5.5oz | 440 | 23 | 15
Beef in Black Bean Sauce, 8.5 oz | 390 | 17 | 17
Broccoli Beef, 6 oz | 370 | 21 | 13
Chicken & Broccoli, 5.5 oz | 160 | 8 | 10
Chicken Skewers, 3 oz | 210 | 9 | 18
Chop Suey: | | |
Chicken, 5 oz | 140 | 9 | 2
Pork, 5 oz | 170 | 12 | 3
Chow Mein, Beef/Chicken, 8 oz | 390 | 12 | 59
Crab Puff/Rangoon, 1 dumpling | 190 | 11 | 13
Crispy Fried Chicken, 8 oz | 485 | 33 | 12
Egg Drop Soup: With Noodles, 1 cup | 110 | 3 | 16
Without Noodles, 1 cup | 60 | 3 | 4
Egg Foo Yung with Sauce, 1 cup | 270 | 15 | 16
Kung Pao Chicken, 5.5 oz | 240 | 15 | 12
Lemon Chicken, 5 oz | 525 | 21 | 57
Lo Mein (stir-fried), 8 oz | 705 | 42 | 49
Omelet, Chicken/Shrimp, 16 oz | 990 | 82 | 10
Orange Chicken, 5.5 oz | 500 | 27 | 42
Steamed Whole Fish, | | |
½ Sockeye Salmon | 646 | 36 | 23
Sweet & Sour: | | |
Fish, 20 oz | 1160 | 58 | 106
Pork, 5.5 oz | 400 | 23 | 35
Vegetable Combination, w/ oil, 6 oz | 367 | 5 | 66
Vegetables, Steamed, w/o oil, 6 oz | 137 | 1 | 29
**Sauces:** Mandarin Sauce 1.5 oz | 70 | 0 | 17
Potsticker Sauce 1.5 oz | 35 | 0 | 8
**Bubble Tea,** average, 12 fl oz | 280 | 0.5 | 68
**Fortune Cookie,** each | 32 | 0.5 | 7

## Cajun & Creole

| | C | F | Cb
---|---|---|---
Alligator, cooked, 4 oz | 160 | 2 | 0
Baked Herb Chicken, 1 serving | 850 | 53 | 2
Bouillabaisse | 400 | 15 | 10
Cajun Fried Turkey, 1 serving | 630 | 25 | 0
Cocktail Sauce, 2 Tbsp | 30 | 0 | 6
Couche-couche, ½ cup | 80 | 0 | 17
Crawfish Bisque, 1 serving | 500 | 10 | 10
Crawfish, cooked, 2 oz | 45 | 0.5 | 0
Creole Jambalaya, | | |
1 serving | 550 | 30 | 15
Frog Legs, steamed (2) | 45 | 0 | 0
Guinea Fowl, flesh, 4 oz, cooked | 160 | 4 | 0
Hogshead Cheese, ¼ cup | 80 | 5.5 | 0
Jambalaya, Shrimp & Crabmeat | 520 | 14 | 12
Red Beans & Rice, 1 serving | 400 | 17 | 52
Roasted Quail, w/ Bacon on Toast | 550 | 25 | 15
Remoulade Sauce, 2 Tbsp, 1 oz | 110 | 11 | 2
Shrimp Creole, 1 serving | 450 | 20 | 10
Stuffed Smothered Steak, | | |
with 1 cup Rice | 890 | 50 | 50
Turtle, cooked, 3 oz | 120 | 3 | 0

## Cuban

| | C | F | Cb
---|---|---|---
Bl. Beans w/ Rice (Moros con Cristianos) | 510 | 22 | 76
Black-Eyed Pea Fritters (Bollitos de Carita) | 80 | 5 | 6
Casserole Corn Tamale | 445 | 20 | 55
Chicken w/ Yellow Rice (Arroz con Pollo) | 925 | 49 | 87
Cuban Bread (Pan Cubano) | 80 | 1.5 | 15
Donuts in Syrup (Bunuelos), | 170 | 5 | 10
with Melado | 100 | 5 | 10
Grilled Plantains | 145 | 0 | 40
Gypsy's Arm Cake (Brazo Gitano) | 260 | 18 | 42
Roast Pork S'wich (Pan con Lechon) | 640 | 30 | 62
Seasoned Beef with Olives & Raisins | | |
(Picadillo) | 435 | 36 | 10
Shredded Beef (Ropa Vieja) | 550 | 35 | 10
Taro Root Mash (Pure de Malanga) | 315 | 3 | 69
Yuca with Citrus Garlic Dressing | | |
(Yuca con Mojo) | 190 | 9 | 25

## French Foods

| | C | F | Cb
---|---|---|---
Blanquette d'Agneau (Lamb Stew) | 800 | 30 | 17
Brioche, 1 cake | 280 | 14 | 34
Bouillabaisse | 400 | 15 | 10
Coq au Vin | 800 | 30 | 16
Coquilles St. Jacques | 320 | 13 | 36
Crème Brulée, 1 serving | 460 | 40 | 21

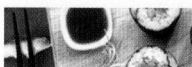 

## French Foods (Cont)

| | C | F | Cb |
|---|---|---|---|
| Baguette, 3 slices, 2.2 oz | 150 | 1 | 35 |
| Creme Caramel (Caramel Custard) | 260 | 10 | 38 |
| Crepe Suzette, 1x6" crepe with sauce | 220 | 10 | 13 |
| Duck a l'Orange | 780 | 35 | 47 |
| Escargot (Snails), in garlic butter (6) | 200 | 10 | 4 |
| Frog Legs, fried, 4 medium pairs | 400 | 20 | 10 |
| Lamb Noisettes, fried, 2 chops | 500 | 40 | 1 |
| Potage Creme Crecy (Carrot Soup) | 360 | 18 | 14 |
| Salade Nicoise (Tuna/Olives/Vegs) | 450 | 13 | 14 |
| Veal Cordon Bleu (Veal/Ham) | 650 | 25 | 18 |
| Vichyssoise (Potato /Leek Soup), 1 c. | 200 | 9 | 15 |

**Baguette & French Stick** ~ Page 54
**Croissants** ~ Pages 135, 165

## German

| | C | F | Cb |
|---|---|---|---|
| **Beef:** Goulash with Veggies | 520 | 20 | 46 |
| Weiner Schnitzel, 1 medium | 750 | 35 | 38 |
| **Chicken:** Fried, Viennese-style | 530 | 20 | 28 |
| Livers with Apple/Onion, 6 oz | 460 | 28 | 10 |
| **Herring,** Pickled: Rollmops, 4 oz | 260 | 16 | 3 |
| With Sour Cream, 4 oz | 310 | 20 | 3 |
| **Sausage:** Bratwurst, grilled, 6 oz | 450 | 37 | 2 |
| Hot Sausage Curry | 300 | 7 | 6 |
| **Pork:** Sauerbraten (Pot Roast) | 650 | 35 | 15 |
| **Cake:** Black Forest, 1 slice | 380 | 16 | 30 |
| Bavarian Bread Dumpling, 3 small | 330 | 10 | 28 |
| Kugelhupf Cake, 1 large slice, 4 oz | 400 | 23 | 40 |
| **Torte:** Linzer (Almond/Raspb. Jam) | 430 | 18 | 58 |
| Sacher (Chocolate/Apricot Jam) | 260 | 12 | 23 |

## Greek

| | C | F | Cb |
|---|---|---|---|
| Baklava Pastry: Small | 240 | 13 | 32 |
| Large, 3¾ oz | 400 | 21 | 45 |
| Calamari, deep fried, 1 cup | 300 | 13 | 17 |
| Chicken Kebob Plate | 345 | 13 | 8 |
| Dolmades (Stuffed Grape Leaves), | | | |
| 2 rolls, 6 oz | 200 | 5 | 13 |
| Galactobureko, 1 only | | | |
| (Filo, Custard, Pastry in Syrup) | 360 | 15 | 48 |
| Greek Chicken Salad | 400 | 18 | 9 |
| Gyros: 6" Pita, 8 oz | 475 | 32 | 35 |
| 7½" Pita, 12 oz | 680 | 40 | 55 |
| Hummus & Pita, 4 oz | 260 | 12 | 30 |
| Kataifi, (Filo, Nut, Pastry in Syrup) | 350 | 11 | 56 |
| Moussaka: Small serving, 8 oz | 350 | 22 | 22 |
| Large serving, 16 oz | 700 | 44 | 44 |
| Soup, Avgolemono (Egg Lem. Soup | | | |
| with Chicken & Rice), 1 cup | 85 | 6 | 5 |
| Souvlaki (Lamb), each, 2 oz | 120 | 6 | 1 |

## Greek (Cont)

| | C | F | Cb |
|---|---|---|---|
| Stuffed Tomatoes, 2 | 250 | 12 | 17 |
| Taramosalata, 1 T., 0.5 oz | 40 | 3 | 2 |
| Tyropita (Filo/Egg/Cheese Pastry) | 350 | 26 | 31 |

**Daphne's Greek Cafe** ~ See Fast-Foods Section

## Hawaiian

| | C | F | Cb |
|---|---|---|---|
| Ahi Tuna, grilled w/o fat, (6 oz fillet) | 220 | 2 | 0 |
| Chicken Long Rice, 1 cup, 7 oz | 240 | 14 | 12 |
| Gyoza, 1 only | 55 | 2 | 6 |
| Haupia (Coconut Pudd.), 1 pce (4"x 2½) | 120 | 6 | 17 |
| Hawaiian Sweet Bread, ½" sl., 2 oz | 180 | 4.5 | 29 |
| Kalua: Chicken, 4 oz | 280 | 16 | 0 |
| Pork, 4 oz | 350 | 24 | 0 |
| Kim Chee (pickled cabbage), ½ c., 4 oz | 20 | 0 | 5 |
| Kulolo (Taro Pudding), 1 slice | 125 | 5 | 19 |
| Lau Lau: | | | |
| Chicken (1) 7 oz | 280 | 21 | 3 |
| Pork (1) 7 oz | 320 | 26 | 5 |
| Loco Moco (rice/burger/egg/gravy) | 650 | 27 | 63 |
| Lomi Salmon, ¼ cup, 4 oz | 20 | 1 | 2 |
| Malasadas (Donut), 2 oz | 240 | 13 | 26 |
| Manapua (Char Siu Pork Bun), 2.3 oz | 180 | 8 | 25 |
| Poi (mashed cooked taro), 1 c., 8.5 oz | 270 | 0.5 | 65 |
| Poke, average all types, 3 oz | 90 | 1 | 0 |
| Portuguese Sausage, 2 oz | 180 | 15 | 2 |
| Potato Salad, ½ cup, 5 oz | 170 | 10 | 17 |
| Shave Ice (Matsumoto), | | | |
| all flavors: | | | |
| With Icecream, 1 large | 300 | 4 | 64 |
| With Beans, 1 large | 290 | 0 | 72 |
| **Spam Musubi:** | | | |
| With Regular Spam | 265 | 11 | 34 |
| (4 oz rice+1.3 oz Spam/7-Eleven Hawaii) | | | |
| Homemade: w/ Lite Spam (50% less fat) | 220 | 5 | 34 |
| Taro Pancake Mix, ⅓ cup (makes 2) | 140 | 2 | 26 |
| **Plate Lunches:** | | | |
| **Chicken Katsu,** (9 oz:) With Rice | 1110 | 48 | 108 |
| + Macaroni Salad, ¾ cup | 1360 | 68 | 123 |
| or Tossed Salad + Fr. Dress. (2 T.) | 1240 | 61 | 111 |
| **Hamburger,** (5 oz): With Rice | 710 | 24 | 81 |
| Gravy + Macaroni Salad | 1135 | 49 | 112 |
| **MahiMahi,** (7 oz): With Rice | 650 | 12 | 90 |
| + Macaroni Salad + Tartar Sce | 1150 | 58 | 109 |
| or Macaroni Salad, w/o Tartar ce | 935 | 34 | 108 |
| or Tossed Salad + Fr. Dress. (3 T.) | 815 | 27 | 96 |
| or Tossed Salad, without dressing | 670 | 12 | 93 |
| **Teri Beef,** (5 oz): With 2 scps Rice | 790 | 23 | 94 |
| + Macaroni Salad, ¾ cup | 1095 | 47 | 113 |
| or Tossed Salad, without dressing | 800 | 23 | 95 |

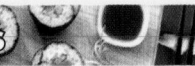

## Indian & Pakistani | C | F | Cb

*Per Serving, Meat dishes allow 4 oz meat/serving*

| | C | F | Cb |
|---|---|---|---|
| Aloo Samosa, each | 155 | 12 | 12 |
| Alu Gosht Kari (Meat/Potato Curry) | 600 | 40 | 23 |
| Chicken Korma | 500 | 35 | 6 |
| Chicken Pilaf (Murgh Biriyani) | 700 | 53 | 50 |
| Chicken Tikka | 260 | 16 | 2 |
| Chicken Vindaloo | 400 | 20 | 8 |
| Chapati/Roti, 7" diameter, 1 piece | 60 | 0.5 | 11 |
| Dahl (Lentil Puree): 1 cup, without oil | 230 | 1 | 37 |
| 1 Tbsp Tadka (oil topping) | 120 | 13 | 0 |
| Dhakla (Lentil Dish), 1" square, 1 oz | 105 | 5 | 13 |
| Dhansak, ½ cup | 105 | 3.5 | 11 |
| Gosht Kari (Meat Curry/Tomato/Pot.) | 460 | 25 | 17 |
| Lamb Pilaf | 520 | 35 | 40 |
| Lassi (Sweet or Mango), 1 cup, 8 oz | 160 | 4 | 24 |
| Masala Gosht (Beef/Tomato/Gravy) | 400 | 25 | 18 |
| Mulligatawney Soup, average | 300 | 15 | 8 |
| Murgh Tikka, 1 cup | 300 | 4 | 7 |
| Naan Flatbread, ½, 2 oz | 160 | 3.5 | 29 |
| Pappadum, 1 large/2 small | 50 | 3 | 5 |
| Pesrattu (Lentil Crepe), 9", 2.6 oz | 130 | 5 | 15 |
| Pork Vindaloo Curry, without Rice | 620 | 47 | 3 |
| Rajmah (Kidney Bean Curry), 1 cup | 225 | 5 | 35 |
| Rogan Josh (Lamb/Yogurt Sauce), without Rice/Potatoes | 500 | 30 | 3 |
| Shahi Korma (Braised Lamb) | 430 | 28 | 3 |
| **Tandoori Chicken:** Breast | 260 | 13 | 5 |
| Leg/Thigh portion | 300 | 17 | 6 |

## Italian Dishes | C | F | Cb

**Entrees:**

| | C | F | Cb |
|---|---|---|---|
| Baked Ziti: Small | 370 | 27 | 32 |
| Regular | 575 | 42 | 49 |
| Breadstick (1), 2 oz | 120 | 2.5 | 25 |
| Broccoli Fettucine Alfredo, regular | 815 | 23 | 125 |
| Bruschetta, 2 slices | 380 | 17 | 53 |
| Calzones, average, all types | 840 | 34 | 101 |
| Cannelloni, 1 tube, 6 oz | 280 | 15 | 18 |
| Cheese Breadstick (1), 2.4 oz | 180 | 8 | 20 |
| Cheese Ravioli with Sauce | 495 | 17 | 65 |
| Chicken Alfredo | 775 | 29 | 82 |
| Chicken Parmigiana, 11 oz | 520 | 22 | 16 |
| Chicken Scallopine, dinner | 1110 | 71 | 68 |
| Eggplant Parmigiana | 900 | 39 | 78 |
| Fettucine Alfredo: Lunch, 9 oz | 885 | 65 | 63 |
| Dinner, 15 oz | 1475 | 108 | 104 |
| Linquine & Seafood, dinner | 1130 | 71 | 79 |
| Manicotti Formaggio | 800 | 38 | 57 |
| Meat Lasagne: Small, 10 oz | 440 | 23 | 39 |
| Large, 16 oz | 700 | 36 | 60 |
| Meat Ravioli | 725 | 22 | 102 |
| Minestrone Soup, 1 bowl | 110 | 2 | 18 |
| Penne Rustica: Lunch | 1300 | 71 | 76 |
| Dinner | 1540 | 80 | 101 |
| Ravioli, over-stuffed, av. | 990 | 67 | 57 |

**Spaghetti & Meatballs:**

| | C | F | Cb |
|---|---|---|---|
| With Tomato Sauce: Kids | 500 | 20 | 58 |
| Medium/Lunch | 1080 | 63 | 89 |
| Large/Dinner | 1430 | 81 | 119 |
| With Meat Sauce: Kids | 550 | 25 | 56 |
| Medium/Lunch | 1300 | 79 | 84 |
| Large/Dinner | 1700 | 103 | 110 |
| Veal Marsala, dinner | 1320 | 66 | 132 |
| Veal Parmigiana, dinner | 1270 | 65 | 116 |
| Vegetable Primavera | 610 | 8 | 116 |

**Macaroni & Cheese** ~ *Page 133*

**Panini Sandwich:**

| | C | F | Cb |
|---|---|---|---|
| Chicken, 16 oz | 900 | 38 | 81 |
| Meats, average, 18 oz | 940 | 39 | 81 |
| Vegetarian, 15 oz | 750 | 31 | 83 |

**Pizza: Ready-To-Eat** ~ *Page 135*
**Gourmet Deep Dish (Gino's East)** ~ *Page 202*

**Salad,**

| | C | F | Cb |
|---|---|---|---|
| Caprese , 11 oz | 445 | 34 | 10 |

**Desserts:**

| | C | F | Cb |
|---|---|---|---|
| Gelato: Vanilla (Milk Base), ½ c. | 200 | 15 | 18 |
| Choc. Hazelnut (Milk), ½ cup | 370 | 29 | 26 |
| Water Base, ½ cup | 100 | 0 | 25 |
| Lemon Ice | 180 | 0 | 45 |
| Tiramisu, 1 piece, 5 oz | 400 | 29 | 30 |

**For more listings** ~ *See Fast-Foods Section*

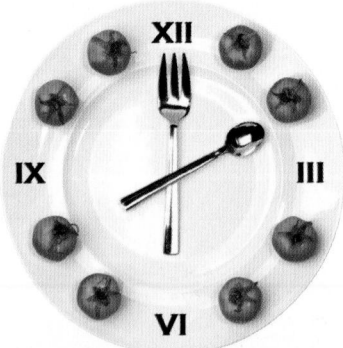

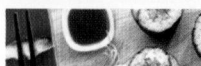 

| Japanese | C | F | Cb |
|---|---|---|---|
| **Sushi Rice:** Cooked, 1 Tbsp | 25 | 0 | 5 |
| 1 cup, 5.25 oz | 380 | 3 | 82 |
| **Sushi (Maki) Rolls:** *Per Piece* | | | |
| Average all types (California Rolls; Cream Cheese with Crab; Eel; Salmon; Shrimp; Tuna; Yellowtail; Vegetable) | | | |
| Small (1⅛" diam. x 1⅛" high), 0.8 oz | 25 | 0.5 | 3.5 |
| Med. (1¾" diam. x 1¾" high), 1.6 oz | 50 | 1 | 7 |
| Large (2¼" diam. x ⅞" high), 2 oz | 60 | 1.5 | 9 |
| **Sushi Packs:** *Per Pack* | | | |
| Average all types: 6 large pieces | 370 | 5 | 55 |
| 9 medium pieces | 360 | 6 | 60 |
| 12 small pieces | 265 | 3 | 45 |
| Futomaki (thick roll), 6 pieces | 380 | 5 | 72 |
| Hand Roll (Cone), 4 oz | 120 | 2 | 18 |
| Inari (rice filled soybean pocket), 4 pces | 420 | 9 | 73 |
| **Sushi-Nigiri,** (fish on rice), average all types, 1 piece | 70 | 0.5 | 12 |
| **Sushi Plate:** Assorted: 6 pieces | 420 | 3 | 36 |
| Combination (Sushi & Sushi Rolls) 2 Sushi + 6 small & 3 med. rolls | 400 | 7 | 72 |
| **Sashimi:**(Sl. Raw Seafood/Beef) | | | |
| Ika (Squid), 4 oz | 105 | 2 | 0 |
| Hamachi (Yellowtail), 4 oz | 165 | 6 | 0 |
| Maguro (Yellowfin Tuna), 4 oz | 120 | 1 | 0 |
| Niku (Beef), 5 oz | 200 | 10 | 0 |
| Saba (Mackerel), 4 oz | 160 | 7 | 0 |
| Suzuki (Sea Bass), 4 oz | 110 | 0.5 | 0 |
| Tako (Octopus), 4 oz | 95 | 1 | 0 |
| **Dipping Sauces:** Average, 2 Tbsp | 30 | 0 | 7 |
| Ginger Vinegar Dressing, 2 Tbsp | 20 | 0 | 5 |
| **Edamame:** (young green soybeans): | | | |
| Boiled beans (no pods), 4 oz | 160 | 7 | 12 |
| Steamed (in pods), 4 oz | 60 | 3 | 5 |
| **Katsu-don,** Pork with Rice | 1100 | 39 | 141 |
| **Miso Soup,** with Tofu pieces, 1 cup | 85 | 3 | 11 |
| **Seaweed Salad,** 1.5 oz | 20 | 2 | 0 |
| **Sukiyaki,** (Beef/Tofu/Veg.), 8 oz | 400 | 24 | 32 |
| **Tempura:** | | | |
| 3 large shrimp & veggies | 320 | 18 | 25 |
| 1 shrimp only | 60 | 4 | 3 |
| **Teppan Yaki,** (Steak, Seafood & Veggies), 10 oz serving | 470 | 30 | 15 |
| **Teriyaki:** Beef, 4 oz | 350 | 25 | 4 |
| Chicken, 4 oz | 260 | 9 | 7 |
| Salmon, medium, 6 oz | 270 | 8 | 3 |
| **Sake Wine,** (16% alcohol), 3 fl.oz | 115 | 0 | 7 |
| **Yakatori,** 1 skewer, 2.5 oz | 140 | 5 | 1 |

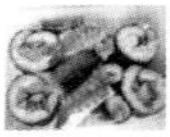

| Kosher/Deli Foods | C | F | Cb |
|---|---|---|---|
| Bagel/Bialy, 1 small, 2 oz | 160 | 2 | 32 |
| Beiglach (Cheese Knish) | 350 | 17 | 35 |
| **Blintzes:** Average, 1 only | 120 | 1 | 25 |
| With Sour Cream & Preserves | 370 | 10 | 30 |
| **Borscht:** (Without Sour Cream): 1 cup | 85 | 3 | 14 |
| Diet/Reduced Calorie, 1 cup | 30 | 1 | 7 |
| **Cabbage Roll,** (meat/rice), 5 oz | 170 | 6 | 21 |
| **Chicken Broth:** 1 cup | 80 | 8 | 0 |
| With vegetables | 100 | 8 | 5 |
| With noodles | 150 | 9 | 16 |
| Lowfat, plain, 1 cup | 25 | 1 | 0 |
| **Cholent,** 1 medium serving, 1 cup | 350 | 16 | 48 |
| **Chopped Liver:** 1 serving, 3 oz | 110 | 6 | 5 |
| With Egg Salad, ¼ cup | 100 | 7 | 3 |
| **Farfel,** dry, ½ cup | 90 | 0.5 | 21 |
| **Gefilte Fish Balls:** Regular, med., 2 oz | 55 | 2 | 4 |
| With Jelled Broth | 80 | 2 | 6 |
| Cocktail size, 1 oz | 30 | 1 | 2 |
| Sweet, medium, 2 oz | 65 | 2 | 4 |
| With Jelled Broth | 95 | 2 | 9 |
| **Hallah,** (Yeast Bread), 1 slice, 1 oz | 85 | 2 | 14 |
| **Herring:** Smoked, 2 oz | 120 | 8 | 0 |
| In Sour Cream, 2 oz | 150 | 10 | 0 |
| **Kasha,** cooked, ½ cup | 100 | 0.5 | 20 |
| **Kipfel (Vanilla/Almdond Cookie),** 1 pce | 60 | 2 | 7 |
| **Knaidlach ~** *See Matzo Balls* | | | |
| **Knish:** Kasha/Potato, 1 only | 130 | 4 | 22 |
| Cheese, 1 only | 350 | 17 | 35 |
| **Kreplach,** beef, 1 piece | 40 | 1 | 6 |
| **Kugel,** potato/noodle, 1 serving | 300 | 20 | 25 |
| **Latkes,** (Potato Pancake), 2 oz | 200 | 11 | 22 |
| 3 Latkes with Sour Cran Apple Sce | 750 | 25 | 95 |
| **Lochshen: Plain,** 1 cup | 130 | 2 | 26 |
| Pudding, 1 cup | 380 | 13 | 48 |
| **Lox (Smoked Salmon),** 2 oz | 65 | 2 | 0 |
| **Mandelbrot,** (Almond Bread), 1 slice, ¼" thick | 45 | 2 | 5 |
| **Matzo,** 1 oz board | 110 | 0.5 | 21 |
| **Matzo Balls:** 2 small, or 1 large, 2" | 90 | 3 | 12 |
| Extra large ball, 3" | 180 | 6 | 24 |
| **Matzo Ball Soup:** | | | |
| Cup with 2 small or 1 large ball | 150 | 5 | 27 |
| Bowl with Chicken & Noodles | 325 | 13 | 34 |
| Jerry's Deli, large bowl | 560 | 17 | 56 |
| **New York Cheesecake,** 4 oz | 350 | 24 | 26 |
| **Pierogi,** potato/cheese, 1 piece | 90 | 4 | 11 |
| **Reuben S'wich,** w/ ½ lb Corned Beef | 920 | 60 | 28 |
| **Schmaltz,** (Rend'd Chicken Fat), 1 T. | 90 | 10 | 0 |

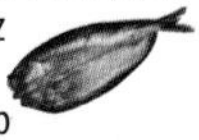

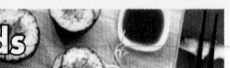

# Restaurant & International Foods

## Korean Food

| | C | F | Cb |
|---|---|---|---|
| Bibimbab (Veggies & Beef on Rice), 1 cup | 565 | 15 | 89 |
| Bulgogi (Barbeque Beef), 3.5 oz | 325 | 12 | 15 |
| Galbi (Short Ribs), 16 oz | 975 | 61 | 16 |
| Gujeolpan (Pancake with Meat & Vegetables), 1 cup w/ 1 pancake | 340 | 11 | 39 |
| Japchae (Noodle w/ Veggies & Meat), 1¼ cup | 365 | 19 | 34 |

**Sides:**

| | C | F | Cb |
|---|---|---|---|
| Kimchee (Cabbage Relish), ½ cup | 30 | 0 | 6 |
| Namool (Assorted Veggies), 1 cup | 125 | 6.5 | 9 |

**Soups:** *Per Serving*

| | C | F | Cb |
|---|---|---|---|
| Muguk (Radish & Chive Soup), 6 oz | 105 | 7 | 6 |
| Samgyetang (Ginseng Chkn Soup): | | | |
|   Without Chicken Skin, 1 cup | 520 | 11 | 60 |
|   With Chicken Skin, 1 cup | 725 | 35 | 60 |
| Yuk Gae Jang (Spicy Beef Soup), 1¼ cup | 180 | 13 | 5 |

## Lebanese/Middle East

| | C | F | Cb |
|---|---|---|---|
| Baba Ghannouj, 2 Tbsp, 1 oz | 70 | 6 | 2 |
| Baklava (Pastry, Nuts, Syrup), 1 pastry, 1¾ oz | 245 | 18 | 18 |
| Cabbage Rolls (Cabb. Leaf, Meat, Rice), 1 roll, 3 oz | 100 | 3 | 12 |
| Cous Cous (Semolina, Milk, Fruit, Nuts), 1 serving | 400 | 21 | 43 |
| Felafel (Chick Pea Fritter), Fried, 1 medium, 1 oz | 60 | 4 | 4 |
| Hummus, ¼ cup, 2.2 oz | 105 | 3 | 5 |
| Fried Kibbi (Wheat, Meat Pinenuts), 1 piece, 3 oz | 180 | 8 | 15 |
| Kafta (Ground Lamb, Ssge on Skewer), 1 skewer, 1½ oz | 85 | 5 | 2 |
| Kibbeh Naye (raw Lamb, Bulgur & Spice) 1 cup, 9 oz | 450 | 18 | 28 |
| Lebanese Omelet, 1 serving, 4 oz (Egg, Spinach, Pinenuts, Onion) | 200 | 12 | 13 |
| Pilaf (Rice, Onion, Raisins, Apr., Spice) 1 cup | 400 | 11 | 60 |
| Shawourma (Spit-Roast Beef), 4 oz serving | 280 | 15 | 2 |
| Shish Kabob, 1 stick, 2½ oz | 130 | 7 | 2 |
| Spinach Pie, 1 piece, 3½ oz | 290 | 21 | 20 |
| Sweet Almond Sanbusak, (Pastry, Almonds, Spices), 1 pce | 200 | 15 | 11 |
| Tabouli, 1 serving, 4 oz | 125 | 7 | 13 |
| Tahini Sauce, average, 1 Tbsp | 90 | 8 | 2 |

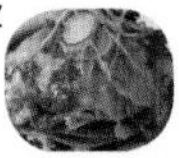

## Mexican

| | C | F | Cb |
|---|---|---|---|
| **Burritos** *(Taco Bell):* Bean | 370 | 10 | 56 |
|   Supreme Beef | 420 | 16 | 53 |
| Chili, plain, ¼ cup | 90 | 6 | 8 |
| Chili con Carne: With Beans, 1 cup | 310 | 17 | 15 |
|   Without Beans, 1 cup | 370 | 28 | 10 |
| Chimichangas, Beef, 5 oz | 400 | 19 | 43 |
| Chorizo Sausage, 2 oz | 265 | 23 | 0 |
| Churros, 1½ oz | 150 | 8 | 18 |
| Corn Chips, ½ cup, 1 oz | 160 | 10 | 17 |
| Costillas Ribs, 6 oz | 675 | 52 | 0 |
| Enchilada, average | 330 | 10 | 49 |
| Fajitas, Chicken | 200 | 7 | 20 |
| Guacamole, average, 2 Tbsp, 1 oz | 45 | 4 | 2 |
| **Horchata:** *(Don Jose),* 1 c. 8 fl. oz | 140 | 4 | 25 |
|   *Cacique,* 1 pint bottle, 16 fl. oz | 320 | 7 | 62 |
| Margarita, with 1½ oz Tequila | 160 | 0 | 6 |
| Masa (Pre-mixed for Tamales), 1 oz | 80 | 5 | 9 |
| Menudo, ½ cup | 55 | 1.5 | 10 |
| **Nachos:** *(Del Taco),* Regular, 4 oz | 370 | 22 | 28 |
|   Macho Nachos, 17 oz | 1000 | 56 | 94 |
|   *Taco Bell:* BellGrande®, 10.75 oz | 770 | 42 | 79 |
|   Supreme®, 6.75 oz | 440 | 25 | 42 |
| **Nachos:** With cheese, peppers, 1 portion, 6-8 nachos, 7 oz | 600 | 33 | 60 |
|   W/ cheese, beans, beef, peppers, 1 portion, 6-8 nachos, 9 oz | 570 | 31 | 56 |
| Nopal Cactus Salad, 1 serving | 130 | 9 | 11 |
| **Papas Fritas**, (1), 6 oz | 325 | 18 | 40 |
| **Piloncillo:** (Brown Sugar) | | | |
|   1 T., 0.46 oz | 50 | 0 | 13 |
|   Cone, small, 3″, 3 oz | 325 | 0 | 81 |
| **Quesadilla,** Cheese | 490 | 28 | 39 |
| Queso Fresco, ¼ cup | 80 | 4.5 | 8 |
| Refried Beans, ¾ cup, 6 oz | 160 | 3 | 26 |
| **Rice Pudding** *(Arroz Con Leche),* 4 oz | 140 | 3 | 24 |
| **Soup,** Black Bean, 1 bowl | 200 | 3 | 34 |
| **Tacos** *(Taco Bell):* | | | |
|   Crunchy: Regular | 170 | 10 | 12 |
|     Supreme | 200 | 12 | 15 |
|   Soft: Crispy Potato | 270 | 13 | 31 |
|     Grilled Steak | 250 | 14 | 19 |
| Taco Salad with Salsa | 840 | 52 | 85 |
| Taco Sauce, average, ¼ cup | 15 | 0 | 3 |
| Taco Shell, regular | 50 | 2 | 8 |
| Tamales, Beef/Chicken, av. 4½ oz | 250 | 11 | 27 |
| Taquitos, Beef & Cheese, 4½ oz | 330 | 15 | 36 |
| Tostada *(Taco Bell)* | 250 | 10 | 29 |
| Tortilla, Corn, 6″ diameter | 70 | 1 | 14 |
| Tortilla Chips, 1 oz | 150 | 8 | 18 |

Extra Listings of Mexican Dishes ~ Fast-Foods Section (Taco Bell, Del Taco)

**Canned Bean/Chili Products** ~*See Page 111*

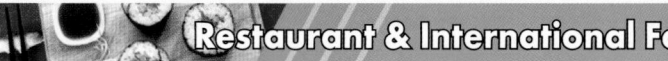

## Mexican (Cont)

| | C | F | Cb |
|---|---|---|---|
| **Breads:** Bolillos, 1 roll, 3½ oz | 240 | 4 | 42 |
| Telera, 2 oz | 150 | 1.5 | 19 |
| Mexican Cornbread, 4" square | 210 | 11 | 19 |
| **Cakes, Cookies, Pastries:** | | | |
| Banderilla (Pastry Puff), 1 shell | 140 | 10 | 8 |
| Bigotes, 7" | 570 | 22 | 44 |
| Calvos, 2½ oz | 320 | 18 | 38 |
| Capirotada (Bread Pudding), 10 oz | 810 | 38 | 107 |
| Cinnamon Cookies, 2 | 125 | 8 | 13 |
| Cocadas, 1 oz | 120 | 6 | 15 |
| Cortadillo, 1 cookie, 1.9 oz | 300 | 11 | 48 |
| Concha (All Colors): | | | |
| Small (3" diameter), 2½ oz | 250 | 8 | 38 |
| Medium (4" diameter), 3½ oz | 350 | 11 | 53 |
| Large (5" diameter), 5½ oz | 550 | 18 | 84 |
| Cream Puff with Custard, 4¼ oz | 255 | 14 | 25 |
| Cuerno, 2 oz | 200 | 4.5 | 34 |
| Cuerno Fine, 2¾ oz | 330 | 17 | 40 |
| Donut, large, 4", 3½ oz | 440 | 21 | 58 |
| Elotes, 3½ oz | 450 | 24 | 51 |
| Empanadas (Average all types): | | | |
| Small, 2 oz | 230 | 10 | 28 |
| Regular, 3 oz | 300 | 14 | 42 |
| Fiesta Cookie (1), 2¼ oz | 280 | 8 | 47 |
| Galletas Mixtas (1), 1 oz | 100 | 2.5 | 16 |
| Guayaba, 3¼ oz | 360 | 14 | 53 |
| Jelly Roll (1), 3¼ oz | 240 | 4 | 46 |
| Mantecadites, 4½ oz | 670 | 42 | 64 |
| Mini Pound Cake, 1 slice, 3 oz | 260 | 12 | 33 |
| Mini Cupcake (1), 1¾ oz | 180 | 8 | 25 |
| Muffins/Nino Enbuelto, large, 6 oz | 465 | 11 | 48 |
| Nuez, 3¼ oz | 380 | 17 | 52 |
| Ojo De Buey, 4 oz | 360 | 15 | 55 |
| Oreja (Elephant Ear), 3 oz | 310 | 15 | 38 |
| Pan Dulce), 1 bun | 330 | 10 | 45 |
| Panquecitos, 2½ oz | 260 | 11 | 36 |
| Piedras, 4 oz | 470 | 15 | 76 |
| Polvorones (1), 3 oz | 370 | 18 | 48 |
| Puerquitos, 5 oz | 600 | 24 | 88 |
| Rebanadas, 3½ oz | 390 | 18 | 51 |
| Roles De Canela (Cinn. Roll), 4½ oz | 490 | 15 | 81 |
| Roscas, 2¾ oz | 360 | 18 | 44 |
| Semitas, 3 oz | 300 | 10 | 46 |
| Sopapillas (flaky pastry puffs): 1 piece | 100 | 7 | 10 |
| With Honey & Cream | 200 | 14 | 18 |
| Strawberry Crema Roll (⅙), 2½ oz | 240 | 5 | 45 |

**Extra Food Listings** ~ *See CalorieKing.com*

## Polish

| | C | F | Cb |
|---|---|---|---|
| Cabbage Rolls with Sour Cream, 2 sm. | 220 | 10 | 30 |
| Chicken Casserole w/ Mushrooms, 1 c. | 520 | 27 | 5 |
| Kielbasa (Sausages, Onions, fried), 2 large | 350 | 28 | 2 |
| Meatballs in Sour Cream, 3 x 1½" balls | 300 | 16 | 11 |
| Pierogi, Fruit/Vegetables, 3" ball | 80 | 2 | 15 |
| Pork Goulash (Pork/Vegetable Stew) | 550 | 21 | 38 |
| Pot Roast with Vegetables | 630 | 21 | 28 |

## Soul Foods

| | C | F | Cb |
|---|---|---|---|
| Breakfast Sausage, fried, 2 patties | 250 | 17 | 0 |
| Brunswick Stew, 1 cup, 8.5 oz | 320 | 14 | 19 |
| Cornbread, homemade, 3 oz | 200 | 7.5 | 28 |
| Fatback, raw, 0.25 oz | 60 | 6.5 | 0 |
| Ham Hock | 90 | 6.5 | 2 |
| Hog Maw | 45 | 2.5 | 0 |
| Hominy, cooked, ¾ cup | 110 | 0.5 | 25 |
| Hush Puppies, 5 pieces | 260 | 12 | 35 |
| Kale, cooked, ½ cup | 20 | 0.5 | 4 |
| Oxtail | 70 | 3.5 | 0 |
| Pig's Ear, ¼ ear | 50 | 3 | 0 |
| Pig's Foot, ½ foot | 70 | 4.5 | 0 |
| Pig's Tail, ⅓ tail | 115 | 10 | 0 |
| Poke Salad, cooked, ½ cup | 16 | 0.5 | 3 |
| Pork Brains | 40 | 2.5 | 0 |
| Pork Chitterlings, simmered, 3 oz | 260 | 25 | 0 |
| Pork Cracklings, 0.5 oz | 80 | 6 | 0 |
| Pork Neck Bones | 65 | 4 | 0 |
| Pork Skin, 1 cup | 70 | 4.5 | 0 |
| Pork Tongue, ⅓ tongue | 75 | 5.5 | 0 |
| Possum | 65 | 3 | 0 |
| Sousemeat | 60 | 4.5 | 0 |
| Succotash, ½ cup | 80 | 1 | 17 |
| Sweet Potato Pie, ⅛ of 9" pie | 250 | 12 | 34 |
| Tripe, 2 oz | 55 | 2 | 0 |
| Vienna Sausage, 2 small | 90 | 8 | 1 |
| 1 small | 45 | 4 | 0.5 |

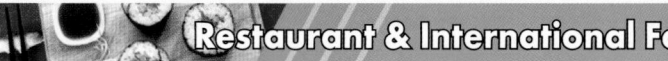

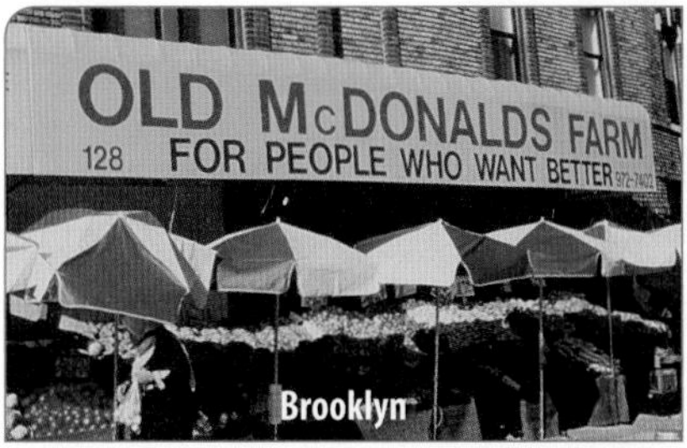

OLD McDONALDS FARM
128
FOR PEOPLE WHO WANT BETTER

**Brooklyn**

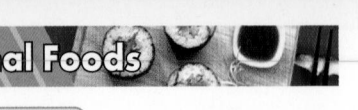

## Restaurant & International Foods

### Spanish

| | C | F | Cb |
|---|---|---|---|
| Arroz Abanda (Fish with Rice) | 340 | 8 | 31 |
| Arroz Con Pollo (Rice/Chicken Salad) | 500 | 23 | 50 |
| Clams Marinara, 8 clams | 330 | 16 | 22 |
| Cochifrito (Lamb with Lemon/Garlic) | 650 | 25 | 5 |
| Cochinillo Asado, 2 sl. (Rst Suckling Pig) | 300 | 15 | 3 |
| Cocido Madrileno | | | |
| (Madrid-Style Boiled Dinner) | 450 | 27 | 18 |
| Flan de Leche (Caramel Custard) | 325 | 9 | 52 |
| Fritadera de Ternera (Sauteed Veal) | 450 | 27 | 2 |
| Gazpacho, 1 bowl | 60 | 0 | 15 |
| Mole Poblano, ½ cup | 205 | 14 | 16 |
| Paella a la Valenciana | | | |
| (Chicken & Shellfish Rice) | 900 | 42 | 70 |
| Pollo a la Espanola (Chicken) | 475 | 30 | 4 |
| Ternera al Jerez (Veal with Sherry) | 660 | 29 | 6 |
| Zarzuela (Fish & Shellfish Medley) | 530 | 27 | 40 |

### Thai Foods

| | C | F | Cb |
|---|---|---|---|
| **Appetizers:** Satay Pork, 1 oz | 100 | 4 | 2 |
| Spring Roll, 1¼ oz | 110 | 6 | 13 |
| **Soups Tom Yam (Hot & Sour):** | | | |
| Spicy Shrimp/Seafood: 1 cup | 100 | 4 | 6 |
| 1 bowl | 160 | 7 | 10 |
| Vegetarian, 1 cup | 50 | 0 | 11 |
| **Curries:** Chicken with Ginger, 1 c. | 390 | 34 | 4 |
| Thick Red Curry withBeef, 1 cup | 600 | 50 | 7 |
| Thai Chicken Curry, 1 cup | 340 | 23 | 4 |
| Massaman Curry, 1 cup | 680 | 57 | 8 |
| Green Curry with Pork, 1 cup | 480 | 44 | 5 |
| **Pad Thai,** large serving, 18 oz | 990 | 38 | 125 |
| **Fish:** Steamed with Spicy Thai Sce | 450 | 8 | 46 |
| Crispy Fried, 5 oz | 290 | 15 | 9 |
| **Spicy Chicken,** stir-fry | 450 | 22 | 14 |
| **Spicy Garlic Tofu,** stir-fry | 340 | 18 | 18 |
| **Sticky Thai Rice:** Plain 1 cup, 6 oz | 170 | 0.5 | 36 |
| With Coconut & Sesame Seeds, 1 c. | 880 | 28 | 120 |
| **Stir-fried Rice Noodles,** 1 c. 5.5 oz | 270 | 9 | 40 |
| **Stir-fried Vegetables,** 1 cup | 100 | 3 | 18 |
| **Salads:** Green Papaya Salad | 160 | 0 | 40 |
| Spicy Prawn, 9 shrimp | 170 | 3 | 15 |
| Thai Chicken, 1 serving | 330 | 9 | 17 |
| Thai Beef Salad, 1 serving | 260 | 9 | 15 |
| Thai Noodle, 1 serving | 410 | 13 | 45 |
| **Satay Chicken & Peanut Sauce,** | | | |
| 1 satay stick | 390 | 24 | 20 |
| **Sauce,** Peanut Satay, ½ c., 4 oz | 160 | 10 | 13 |

### Vietnamese

| | C | F | Cb |
|---|---|---|---|
| Banh Cuon (Steam Rice w/ Pork), 1 roll | 105 | 7 | 8 |
| Bo Nuong (Beef Satay), 2 sticks | 265 | 9 | 4 |
| Bo Xao Dau Phong | | | |
| (Ginger Beef with Onion, Fish Sce) | 750 | 30 | 10 |
| Ca Chien Gung (Whole Snapper/Ginger) | 600 | 16 | 6 |
| Canh Chay (Vegetable/Tofu Soup) | 80 | 3 | 13 |
| Cari Chicken, 1 cup | 475 | 29 | 16 |
| Cari Chicken w/ Rice Noodle, | | | |
| cup curry & cup cooked noodles | 660 | 29 | 60 |
| Cari Chicken, w/ Steamed Rice, | | | |
| cup curry & cup rice | 650 | 29 | 55 |
| Cuu Xao Lan (Curried Lamb, | | | |
| Veggies in Coconut) | 900 | 40 | 80 |
| Ga Chien (Crisp Chick + Plum Sauce) | 900 | 40 | 105 |
| Ga Nuong (Chicken Satay + Sauce) | 240 | 10 | 4 |
| Ga Xao Rau (Marinated Chicken | | | |
| Braised with Vegetables) | 800 | 26 | 100 |
| Gio Lua (Lean Pork Pie), ⅙ of pie | 245 | 12 | 0 |
| Goi Cuon (Cold Spring Rolls), 1 roll | 60 | 1 | 7 |
| Rau Cai Xao Chay (Stir Fried Veges) | 400 | 15 | 65 |
| Thit Bo Vien (Beef Balls), 6 balls | 225 | 14 | 2 |
| Thit Heo Goi Baup Cai | | | |
| (Spicy Cabb. Rolls with Pork), 1roll | 200 | 7 | 11 |
| **Soup:** *Per Bowl, ½ Cup* | | | |
| Bun Bo Hue (Hot & Spicy Soup): | | | |
| Without Pork Feet | 340 | 9 | 35 |
| With Pork Feet | 830 | 45 | 35 |
| Chicken & Rice Noodle Soup | 400 | 3 | 55 |
| Pho Bo (Beef Noodle Soup) | 410 | 7 | 59 |
| Pho Ga (Chicken Noodle Soup) | 460 | 6 | 58 |
| Pho Tai (Rare Beef & Noodle Soup) | 440 | 7 | 73 |
| **Salad,** Goi Du Du, | | | |
| (Green Papaya), ½ cup | 155 | 3 | 29 |
| **Sauce,** Nuoc Cham (Hot Sauce) | 5 | 0 | 1 |

### Gourmet & Miscellaneous

| | C | F | Cb |
|---|---|---|---|
| **Ants Eggs/Larvae,** 1 Tbsp | 20 | 0 | 0 |
| **Ants,** chocolate coated, 3 Tbsp | 140 | 7 | 2 |
| **Bee Maggots,** canned, 3 Tbsp | 65 | 2 | 0 |
| **Caviar,** black/red, 1 Tbsp | 40 | 3 | 0 |
| **Caterpillars,** canned, 2 oz | 60 | 2 | 0 |
| **Frog Legs,** fried, 1 pair (large) | 125 | 7 | 0 |
| **Haggis,** boiled, 4 oz | 350 | 24 | 22 |
| **Locusts,** roasted, 1 oz | 35 | 1 | 0 |
| **Silkworms,** raw, 1 oz | 60 | 2 | 0 |
| **Snails in garlic butter,** 6 large | 200 | 10 | 4 |
| **Snake,** roasted, 4 oz | 160 | 6 | 0 |

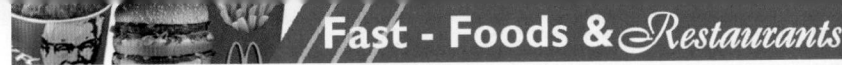

# Fast - Foods & Restaurants

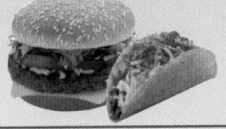

©2012
Allan Borushek

**For More Restaurants & Full Nutritional Data ~ See CalorieKing.com**

# Fast - Foods & Restaurants

## A&W® (Dec '11)

| Burgers: | C | F | Cb |
|---|---|---|---|
| Hamburger | 380 | 19 | 33 |
| Cheeseburger | 420 | 21 | 37 |
| Double Cheeseburger | 680 | 38 | 44 |
| Bacon Cheeseburger | 530 | 30 | 39 |
| Bacon Double Cheeseburger | 760 | 45 | 45 |
| Papa Burger | 690 | 39 | 44 |
| Papa Single Burger | 470 | 25 | 38 |
| *Sandwiches:* Crispy Chicken | 550 | 25 | 52 |
| Grilled Chicken | 400 | 15 | 31 |
| *Chicken Strips:* 3 pieces | 500 | 29 | 32 |
| *Hot Dogs:* Plain | 310 | 19 | 23 |
| Coney Chili Dog | 340 | 20 | 26 |
| Coney Chili Cheese Dog | 380 | 23 | 28 |
| *Corn Dog Nuggets:* 5 pieces | 180 | 8 | 20 |
| 8 pieces | 280 | 13 | 32 |
| **Fries/Sides:** | | | |
| **French Fries:** Small/Kids, 2½ oz | 200 | 8 | 28 |
| Regular, 4 oz | 310 | 12 | 45 |
| Large, 5½ oz | 430 | 17 | 61 |
| **Cheese Fries:** 6 oz | 390 | 18 | 50 |
| Chili Cheese Fries, 7 oz | 410 | 17 | 52 |
| **Cheese Curds,** Breaded/Fried, 5 oz | 570 | 40 | 27 |
| **Onion Rings:** Reg., Breaded, 4 oz | 350 | 16 | 45 |
| Large, 5½ oz | 480 | 27 | 62 |
| **Dipping Sauces:** BBQ, 1 oz | 40 | 0 | 10 |
| Honey Mustard, 1 oz | 100 | 6 | 12 |
| Ranch, 1 oz | 160 | 17 | 2 |
| *Desserts:* Per Small Serving | | | |
| **Polar Swirl:** M&M/Oreo, average | 700 | 25 | 107 |
| Reese's | 740 | 31 | 97 |
| **Sundaes:** Choc.; Caramel; Fudge, av. | 340 | 9 | 55 |
| Strawberry | 300 | 8 | 47 |
| **Soft Serve,** Vanilla cone, 5½ oz | 260 | 7 | 41 |
| *Milkshakes:* Strawb., Small, 16 fl.oz | 670 | 29 | 90 |
| Chocolate; Vanilla, average: | | | |
| Small, 16 fl.oz | 710 | 30 | 100 |
| Medium, 20 fl.oz | 890 | 38 | 123 |
| **Floats:** | | | |
| **A&W Root Beer:** 20 oz | 350 | 5 | 77 |
| Large, 32 fl.oz | 640 | 10 | 136 |
| Diet, 20 oz | 170 | 5 | 30 |
| *Freeze,* A&W Root Beer, 16 oz | 370 | 8 | 68 |
| **Sodas:** | | | |
| **Pepsi:** Small, 16 fl.oz | 200 | 0 | 56 |
| Regular, 20 fl.oz | 250 | 0 | 70 |
| **A&W Root Beer:** Reg., 20 fl.oz | 270 | 0 | 72 |
| Diet, 20 fl.oz | 0 | 0 | 0 |
| *Tea,* Lipton Raspberry: Small, 16 fl.oz | 160 | 0 | 42 |
| Regular, 20 fl.oz | 200 | 0 | 52 |

## Applebee's® (Dec '11)

| Appetizers: As Served | C | F | Cb |
|---|---|---|---|
| **Classic Wings:** Classic Buffalo | 710 | 49 | 8 |
| Honey BBQ | 790 | 35 | 59 |
| Hot Buffalo | 720 | 49 | 9 |
| **Boneless Wings:** Classic | 1160 | 69 | 66 |
| Honey BBQ | 1240 | 55 | 117 |
| Hot Buffalo | 1170 | 69 | 67 |
| Dips: Bleu Cheese | 240 | 26 | 0.5 |
| Ranch | 200 | 21 | 1 |
| Chili Cheese Nachos | 1680 | 107 | 134 |
| Crunchy Onion Rings | 1290 | 56 | 181 |
| Mozzarella Sticks (9) | 940 | 48 | 84 |
| **Quesadillas:** Cheese Grande | 1130 | 87 | 85 |
| Chicken Grande | 1290 | 90 | 90 |
| *Chicken:* Includes Standard Sides | | | |
| Chicken Fried Chicken | 1230 | 59 | 112 |
| Chicken Tenders: Basket | 1020 | 60 | 85 |
| Platter | 1320 | 78 | 107 |
| Crispy Orange Chicken | 1520 | 53 | 208 |
| Fiesta Lime Chicken | 1160 | 67 | 94 |
| Margherita Chicken | 800 | 30 | 67 |
| *Pasta:* As Served | | | |
| Chicken Broccoli Alfredo | 1350 | 72 | 111 |
| Shrimp Fettuccine Alfredo | 1430 | 81 | 113 |
| Three-Cheese Chicken Penne | 1460 | 75 | 127 |
| *Realburgers:* Without Fries | | | |
| Bacon Cheddar Cheeseburger | 970 | 60 | 51 |
| Cowboy Burger | 1180 | 70 | 77 |
| Fire Pit Bacon Burger | 1100 | 73 | 53 |
| Quesadilla Burger | 1240 | 103 | 44 |
| Steakhouse Burger with A1 Sauce | 1250 | 84 | 68 |
| *Ribs:* Includes Standard Sides | | | |
| Applebees Riblets: Basket | 1180 | 55 | 109 |
| Platter | 1820 | 87 | 162 |
| *Sandwiches:* Without Sides | | | |
| Applebees Reuben | 1140 | 81 | 49 |
| Blackened Tilapia | 740 | 42 | 54 |
| Oriental Chicken Rollup | 1160 | 60 | 121 |
| Slow Simmered Beef | 980 | 50 | 101 |
| *Sizzling Entrees:* Includes Sides | | | |
| Asian Shrimp | 850 | 33 | 118 |
| Bourbon Street Steak | 760 | 44 | 35 |
| Chicken with Spicy Queso Blanco | 570 | 22 | 40 |
| Steak & Cheese | 1050 | 65 | 49 |
| **Skillet Fajitas:** Chicken | 1370 | 52 | 149 |
| Combo | 1470 | 67 | 151 |
| Shrimp | 1400 | 65 | 151 |
| Steak | 1410 | 55 | 152 |

## Applebees® cont... (Dec '11)

*Under 550 Calories: Includes Sides*

| | C | F | Cb |
|---|---|---|---|
| Asiago Peppercorn Steak | 380 | 14 | 25 |
| Grilled Dijon Chicken & Portobello | 470 | 16 | 30 |
| Grilled Shrimp & Island Rice | 370 | 4.5 | 56 |
| Signature Sirloin w Garlic Shrimp | 500 | 21 | 31 |
| Teriyaki Chicken Pasta | 450 | 8 | 73 |
| Teriyaki Shrimp Pasta | 440 | 8 | 74 |

*Seafood: As Served*

| | | | |
|---|---|---|---|
| Cajun Lime Tilapia | 350 | 5 | 43 |
| Double Crunch Shrimp | 1280 | 69 | 133 |
| Garlic Herb Salmon | 690 | 29 | 61 |
| Hand-Battered Fish & Chips | 1570 | 106 | 108 |
| Spicy P'apple Glazed Shrimp & Spin. | 310 | 5 | 48 |

*Sliders: Without Sides*

| | | | |
|---|---|---|---|
| BBQ Pulled Pork | 1030 | 48 | 90 |
| Cheeseburger | 1270 | 82 | 82 |
| French Dip | 840 | 49 | 75 |

*Steaks & Toppers: Without Sides*

| | | | |
|---|---|---|---|
| House Sirloin, 9 oz | 310 | 13 | 0 |
| New York Strip, 12 oz | 590 | 39 | 0 |
| Ribeye, 12 oz | 670 | 47 | 3 |
| Shrimp 'N Parmesan Sirloin | 660 | 42 | 4 |
| Steak Combos: With Fried Shrimp | 650 | 34 | 37 |
| With Grilled Shrimp | 540 | 36 | 2 |
| With Honey BBQ Chicken | 600 | 15 | 37 |
| Toppers: Baked Potato | 430 | 28 | 42 |
| Garlic Mashed Potatoes | 330 | 18 | 38 |
| Sauteed Garlic Mushrooms | 130 | 12 | 4 |

*Salads: Regular, Without Dressing Unless Indicated*

| | | | |
|---|---|---|---|
| Apple Walnut Chicken | 470 | 22 | 18 |
| Grilled Shrimp 'N Spinach | 680 | 51 | 20 |
| Oriental Grilled Chicken w/ Dressing | 1290 | 79 | 92 |
| Paradise Chicken | 340 | 4 | 35 |
| Santa Fe Chicken | 870 | 56 | 52 |
| Steak & Potato | 380 | 12 | 32 |

*Sides: As Served*

| | | | |
|---|---|---|---|
| Chili bowl | 370 | 28 | 16 |
| Loaded Baked Potato | 500 | 35 | 42 |
| Loaded Mashed Potatoes | 550 | 42 | 41 |

*Soups: Per Bowl*

| | | | |
|---|---|---|---|
| Clam Chowder | 350 | 24 | 22 |
| French Onion | 260 | 14 | 16 |
| Tomato Basil Soup | 250 | 14 | 28 |

*Desserts: As Served*

| | | | |
|---|---|---|---|
| Maple Butter Blondie | 1110 | 63 | 115 |
| Shooters: Chocolate Mousse | 450 | 31 | 42 |
| Hot Fudge Sundae | 350 | 18 | 43 |
| Triple Chocolate Meltdown | 820 | 48 | 97 |

## Arby's® (Dec '11)

*Sandwiches:*

| | C | F | Cb |
|---|---|---|---|
| Beef 'n Cheddar: Classic | 450 | 21 | 43 |
| Mid | 550 | 28 | 43 |
| Max | 680 | 37 | 46 |
| Roast Beef: Classic, 3 oz Beef | 360 | 14 | 37 |
| Mid, 5 oz Beef | 470 | 22 | 38 |
| Ultimate Angus: | | | |
| Angus Three Cheese & Bacon | 660 | 33 | 46 |
| Angus Cool Deli | 640 | 35 | 47 |
| Chicken: | | | |
| Chicken Bacon & Swiss: Crispy | 600 | 28 | 53 |
| Roasted | 470 | 19 | 43 |
| Chicken Fillet: Crispy | 530 | 25 | 52 |
| Roast | 400 | 16 | 40 |
| Cravin: Crispy Chicken | 500 | 21 | 53 |
| Roast Chicken | 370 | 12 | 42 |
| Roast Chicken Club | 460 | 18 | 41 |

*Chicken:*

| | | | |
|---|---|---|---|
| Prime Cuts: Chicken Tenders (3) | 360 | 17 | 31 |
| Chicken Tenders (5) | 610 | 28 | 52 |

*Market Fresh Sandwiches:*

| | | | |
|---|---|---|---|
| Reuben | 700 | 32 | 64 |
| Roast Turkey & Swiss | 710 | 28 | 78 |
| Roast Turkey, Ranch & Bacon | 810 | 36 | 78 |
| Wraps: Roast Turkey & Swiss | 500 | 24 | 42 |
| Roast Turkey, Ranch & Bacon | 600 | 32 | 42 |

*Optional/Regional Items:*

| | | | |
|---|---|---|---|
| Homestyle Fries: Small | 360 | 16 | 52 |
| Medium | 480 | 21 | 69 |
| Large | 610 | 26 | 86 |
| Loaded Potato Bites: 5 Bites | 350 | 21 | 32 |
| 8 Bites | 570 | 34 | 51 |
| Melts: Arby's | 390 | 16 | 39 |
| Ham & Swiss | 300 | 8 | 37 |
| Toasted Subs: Classic Italian | 590 | 37 | 47 |
| Turkey Bacon Club | 480 | 21 | 47 |

*Regular Combos: Includes Medium Curly Fries Plus 15¾ oz Pepsi, Without Ice*

| | | | |
|---|---|---|---|
| Beef 'n Cheddar Sandwich | 1230 | 52 | 166 |
| Chicken Bacon & Swiss Crispy | 1380 | 58 | 178 |
| Corned Beef Reuben Sandwich | 1480 | 63 | 187 |
| Pecan Grilled Chicken Salad S'wich | 1530 | 65 | 208 |
| Roast Turkey & Swiss Sandwich | 1490 | 59 | 201 |

*Sides & Sidekickers:*

| | | | |
|---|---|---|---|
| Curly Fries: Small, 4½ oz | 450 | 24 | 55 |
| Medium, 6 oz | 600 | 31 | 74 |
| Large, 7 oz | 710 | 37 | 87 |
| Mozzarella Sticks, regular, 4 sticks | 440 | 23 | 39 |
| Potato Cakes: 3 Cakes | 390 | 23 | 42 |
| 4 Cakes | 510 | 30 | 57 |

*Continued Next Page ...*

## Arby's® cont... (Dec '11)

| | C | F | Cb |
|---|---|---|---|
| **Market Fresh Chopped Salads:** *Without Dressing* | | | |
| Chopped Farmhouse Chicken: | | | |
| Crispy | 430 | 24 | 30 |
| Roasted | 250 | 13 | 11 |
| **Dressings:** *Per 1.5 oz packet* | | | |
| Balsamic Vinaigrette | 130 | 12 | 5 |
| Buttermilk Ranch | 210 | 23 | 2 |
| Dijon Honey Mustard | 180 | 16 | 8 |
| **Kids Meals:** Curly Fries, 2¾ oz | 270 | 14 | 33 |
| Homestyle Fries, 2.76 oz | 270 | 14 | 33 |
| Jr Rst Beef Sandwich | 210 | 8 | 24 |
| Jr Turkey & Cheese Sandwich | 200 | 5 | 24 |
| Macaroni & Cheese | 170 | 5 | 25 |
| Prime Cut Chicken Tenders (2), 3 oz | 240 | 11 | 21 |
| **Breakfast:** *Per Serving* | | | |
| **Biscuits:** Bacon, Egg & Cheese | 450 | 26 | 34 |
| Ham, Egg & Cheese | 420 | 22 | 34 |
| Sausage, Egg & Cheese | 590 | 42 | 35 |
| **Croissants:** | | | |
| Bacon, Egg & Cheese | 390 | 24 | 24 |
| Ham, Egg & Cheese | 360 | 20 | 24 |
| Sausage, Egg & Cheese | 530 | 40 | 24 |
| **Sourdoughs:** | | | |
| Bacon, Egg & Cheese | 490 | 22 | 46 |
| Ham, Egg & Cheese | 440 | 17 | 45 |
| Sausage, Egg & Cheese | 660 | 41 | 46 |
| **Wraps:** | | | |
| Bacon, Egg & Cheese | 560 | 29 | 45 |
| Ham, Egg & Cheese | 520 | 24 | 45 |
| Sausage, Egg & Cheese | 690 | 43 | 45 |
| **Sauces:** | | | |
| Arby's, ½ oz | 15 | 0 | 3 |
| Bronco Berry, 1½ oz | 90 | 0 | 22 |
| Cheddar Cheese, 1½ oz | 50 | 3.5 | 4 |
| Horsey, ½ oz | 50 | 5 | 3 |
| Marinara, 1½ oz | 35 | 1.5 | 5 |
| **Dipping Sauces:** | | | |
| Au Jus, 3 oz | 50 | 2 | 8 |
| Ranch, 1½ oz | 160 | 16 | 2 |
| **Desserts:** | | | |
| **Turnovers:** Apple with Icing | 440 | 18 | 68 |
| Cherry Turnover with Icing | 440 | 18 | 67 |
| **Shakes:** *Per 17 fl. oz* | | | |
| Chocolate | 570 | 15 | 97 |
| Vanilla | 480 | 15 | 74 |
| **Drinks:** *Per Small, 16 fl.oz Cup* | | | |
| Mountain Dew | 200 | 0 | 54 |
| Pepsi | 180 | 0 | 49 |

## Arthur Treachers®
*See CalorieKing.com*

## Atlanta Bread Co® (Dec '11)

| **Sandwiches:** | C | F | Cb |
|---|---|---|---|
| Chicken Salad on Sourdough | 440 | 19 | 42 |
| Honey Maple Ham on Honey Wheat | 410 | 5 | 64 |
| Tuna Salad on French | 630 | 33 | 57 |
| Turkey on Nine Grain | 370 | 6 | 50 |
| Veggie on Nine Grain | 500 | 25 | 52 |
| **Signature Sandwiches:** *On Focaccia Unless Indicated* | | | |
| ABC Special on French Baguette | 750 | 38 | 57 |
| Bella Chicken | 610 | 38 | 34 |
| California Avocado | 930 | 50 | 98 |
| Chicken Waldorf | 450 | 29 | 26 |
| NY Hot Pastrami on Rye | 660 | 29 | 59 |
| Turkey Bacon Rustica | 960 | 56 | 62 |
| **Paninis:** Chicken Pesto | 710 | 26 | 80 |
| Chicken Cordon Bleu | 670 | 19 | 80 |
| Cubano | 650 | 19 | 80 |
| Italian Vegetarian | 570 | 16 | 84 |
| Turkey Club | 710 | 24 | 81 |
| **Salads:** *Without Dressing* | | | |
| Caesar | 150 | 9 | 7 |
| Balsamic Bleu Salad | 330 | 18 | 35 |
| Chopstix Chicken Salad | 240 | 10 | 22 |
| Greek Salad | 240 | 16 | 15 |
| House Salad | 90 | 2 | 13 |
| Salsa Fresca Salmon Salad | 560 | 29 | 40 |
| **Soups:** *Per 1¼ Cup* | | | |
| Baja Chicken Enchilada | 330 | 19 | 23 |
| Broccoli Cheese | 250 | 17 | 14 |
| Chicken & Sausage Gumbo | 190 | 6 | 24 |
| Chili, Beef/Frontier, average | 290 | 10 | 30 |
| Homestyle Chicken & Dumpling | 400 | 34 | 17 |
| Tomato Fennel & Dill | 290 | 23 | 18 |
| Wisconsin Cheese | 290 | 15 | 24 |

*For Complete Menu & Data ~ see CalorieKing.com*

## Au Bon Pain® (Dec '11)

| **Bagels:** *Per Bagel* | C | F | Cb |
|---|---|---|---|
| Asiago Cheese | 370 | 8 | 57 |
| Cinnamon Crisp | 410 | 7 | 77 |
| Everything | 320 | 4 | 60 |
| Jalapeno Double Cheddar | 340 | 10 | 53 |
| Honey 9 Grain | 350 | 4 | 69 |
| **Cream Cheese Spreads:** *Per 2 oz* | | | |
| Lite Cream Cheese | 120 | 9 | 5 |
| Honey Pecan, 2½ oz | 200 | 16 | 10 |
| Vegetable | 170 | 16 | 3 |

*Continued Next Page ...*

## Au Bon Pain® cont... (Dec'11)

| Breakfast Sandwiches: | C | F | Cb |
|---|---|---|---|
| **Egg on a Bagel:** | 430 | 12 | 58 |
| With Bacon | 510 | 18 | 58 |
| With Bacon & Cheese | 600 | 25 | 59 |
| With Cheese | 510 | 18 | 59 |
| Smkd. Salmon & Wasabi/On. Dill | 430 | 12 | 62 |
| *Cafe Sandwiches:* | | | |
| Arizona Chicken | 720 | 29 | 62 |
| Caprese | 680 | 32 | 65 |
| Chicken Pesto | 660 | 24 | 66 |
| Lobster Salad | | | |
| Mozzarella Chicken | 690 | 24 | 66 |
| Pastrami | 590 | 23 | 52 |
| Spicy Tuna | 490 | 16 | 60 |
| *Hot Sandwiches and Melts:* | | | |
| Baked Turkey | 750 | 28 | 79 |
| Eggplant & Mozzarella | 640 | 27 | 74 |
| Steakhouse on Ciabatta | 590 | 18 | 72 |
| *Wraps:* Chicken Caesar Asiago | 640 | 32 | 49 |
| Mediterranean Wrap | 630 | 34 | 61 |
| Southwest Tuna | 800 | 46 | 54 |
| Thai Peanut Chicken | 560 | 17 | 68 |
| *Harvest Rice Bowls:* | | | |
| Angus Steak Teriyaki | 660 | 18 | 101 |
| with Brown Rice | 620 | 19 | 86 |
| Mayan Chicken | 550 | 11 | 87 |
| with Brown Rice | 510 | 13 | 72 |
| *Breads: Per Piece* | | | |
| Artisan Honey Baguette, 4¾ oz | 340 | 5 | 66 |
| Bread Bowl , 9¼ oz | 620 | 3 | 123 |
| Focaccia, 4½ oz | 360 | 7 | 62 |
| Rosemary Garlic Bread Stick, 2 oz | 190 | 5 | 31 |
| *Soups: Per Medium 12 oz Bowl* | | | |
| Baked Stuffed Potato | 380 | 22 | 32 |
| Carrot Ginger | 140 | 5 | 24 |
| Chicken Gumbo | 190 | 9 | 22 |
| Corn & Green Chili Bisque | 290 | 17 | 29 |
| Cream of Chicken & Wild Rice | 250 | 15 | 24 |
| Italian Wedding | 190 | 10 | 16 |
| Southern Black-Eyed Pea | 190 | 2 | 31 |
| Tomato Florentine | 140 | 3 | 20 |
| Vegetarian Chili | 240 | 3 | 43 |
| Wild Mushroom Bisque | 200 | 10 | 24 |
| *Salads: Without Dressing* | | | |
| Asian Chicken | 260 | 7 | 25 |
| Caesar Asiago Salad, 6 oz | 220 | 12 | 18 |
| Chef's Salad, 9 oz | 260 | 15 | 8 |

## Au Bon Pain® cont... (Dec'11)

| Salads (Cont): Without Dressing | C | F | Cb |
|---|---|---|---|
| Mandarin Sesame Chicken, 9¾ oz | 310 | 11 | 31 |
| Mediterranean Chicken, 10¼ oz | 290 | 16 | 12 |
| Thai Peanut Chicken, 10½ oz | 200 | 5 | 18 |
| Tuna Garden, 12 oz | 270 | 13 | 19 |
| Turkey Cobb, 11½ oz | 330 | 18 | 16 |
| *Dressing:* Caesar, 2 oz | 270 | 28 | 4 |
| Hazelnut Vinaigrette, 2 oz | 270 | 25 | 11 |
| Sesame Ginger, 2 oz | 230 | 20 | 12 |
| *Bakery: Per Item* | | | |
| **Brownie,** Choc Chip, 4 oz | 440 | 21 | 62 |
| **Cookies:** English Toffee, 1½ oz | 250 | 14 | 27 |
| Shortbread, 2¼ oz | 340 | 20 | 37 |
| **Croissants:** *Per Croissant, Filled* | | | |
| Almond | 600 | 38 | 55 |
| Apple | 280 | 11 | 44 |
| Chocolate | 440 | 22 | 58 |
| Raspberry Cheese | 370 | 17 | 46 |
| Strawberry Cheese | 420 | 22 | 47 |
| Sweet Cheese | 400 | 19 | 49 |
| **Desserts:** Banana Cupcake | 350 | 16 | 44 |
| Creme de Fleur | 500 | 25 | 56 |
| Lemon Pound Cake, 4.3 oz | 490 | 25 | 63 |
| Marble Pound Cake, 4.1 oz | 420 | 23 | 50 |
| Red Velvet Cupcake, 3.1 oz | 400 | 22 | 46 |
| **Muffins:** Blueberry | 490 | 17 | 74 |
| Carrot/Cranberry Walnut | 550 | 26 | 69 |
| Low-Fat Triple Berry | 300 | 3 | 65 |
| Raisin Bran | 480 | 11 | 85 |
| *Beverages:* Caffe Latte, 16 fl.oz | 250 | 14 | 21 |
| Hot Chocolate, 16 fl.oz | 460 | 15 | 74 |
| Peach Iced Tea, 22 fl.oz | 240 | 0 | 61 |
| Coffee Blast, 16 fl.oz | 440 | 21 | 71 |
| Strawberry Smoothie, 16 fl.oz | 310 | 1 | 66 |

*For Complete Nutritional Data ~ see CalorieKing.com*

## Auntie Anne's® (Dec'11)

| Pretzels: With Butter | C | F | Cb |
|---|---|---|---|
| Almond | 390 | 6 | 74 |
| Cinnamon Sugar | 470 | 12 | 84 |
| Garlic | 350 | 5 | 65 |
| Jalapeno | 330 | 5 | 63 |
| Original | 340 | 5 | 63 |
| Original Stix, 6 sticks | 340 | 5 | 65 |
| Sesame | 400 | 10 | 67 |
| Sour Cream & Onion | 360 | 5 | 68 |

*Continued Next Page ...*

# Fast - Foods & *Restaurants*

## Auntie Anne's® cont... (Dec '11)

**Pretzels:** *Without Butter*

| | C | F | Cb |
|---|---|---|---|
| Almond Pretzel | 350 | 2 | 74 |
| Cinnamon Sugar | 380 | 1 | 84 |
| Garlic Pretzel | 310 | 1 | 65 |
| Jalapeno | 300 | 1 | 63 |
| Original | 310 | 1 | 65 |
| Original Stix, 6 sticks | 310 | 1 | 65 |
| Sesame | 360 | 6 | 67 |

**Dipping Sauces:**

| | C | F | Cb |
|---|---|---|---|
| Caramel Dip, 1½ oz | 130 | 3 | 23 |
| Cheese Sce; Hot Salsa Cheese, av., 1 oz | 95 | 7 | 3 |
| Cream Cheese, 1¼ oz | 80 | 6 | 1 |
| Heated Marinara Sauce, 2 oz | 45 | 1 | 7 |
| Sweet Glaze, 1½ oz | 130 | 0 | 32 |
| Sweet Mustard, 1¼ oz | 60 | 2 | 10 |

**Beverages:** *Per Serving*

| | C | F | Cb |
|---|---|---|---|
| **Auntie Anne's Lemonade,** 21 fl.oz | 260 | 0 | 66 |
| **Dutch Ice (20 fl.oz):** Blue Raspberry | 240 | 0 | 62 |
| Kiwi-Banana | 220 | 0 | 53 |
| Lemonade | 300 | 0 | 76 |
| Mocha | 390 | 12 | 73 |
| Pina Colada | 300 | 0 | 73 |
| Strawberry | 230 | 0 | 58 |
| Wild Cherry | 280 | 0 | 69 |
| **Dutch Smoothie:** *Per 20 fl.oz* | | | |
| Blue Raspberry | 440 | 15 | 72 |
| Kiwi-Banana | 420 | 15 | 66 |
| Lemonade | 470 | 15 | 81 |
| Mocha | 540 | 22 | 79 |
| Pina Colada | 470 | 15 | 79 |
| Strawberry | 430 | 15 | 69 |

## Back Yard Burgers® (Dec '11)

**Burgers:**

| | C | F | Cb |
|---|---|---|---|
| American Cheeseburger ⅓ lb | 730 | 44 | 47 |
| Back Yard Burger ⅓ lb | 680 | 39 | 47 |
| Black Jack | 780 | 49 | 48 |
| Bleu Cheeseburger: ⅓ lb | 780 | 47 | 47 |
| ⅔ lb | 1270 | 86 | 47 |
| Cheddar Cheeseburger: ⅓ lb | 790 | 48 | 47 |
| ⅔ lb | 1290 | 88 | 47 |
| Jr Burger | 530 | 27 | 47 |
| Mushroom Swiss | 790 | 49 | 45 |
| Pepper Jack, ⅓ lb | 740 | 45 | 47 |
| Swiss Cheeseburger: ⅓ lb | 790 | 48 | 47 |
| ⅔ lb | 1290 | 88 | 47 |

**Chicken Sandwiches:**

| | C | F | Cb |
|---|---|---|---|
| Blackened Chicken | 540 | 24 | 53 |
| Crispy Chicken | 590 | 26 | 65 |
| Grilled Chicken | 350 | 4.5 | 47 |
| Hawaiian Chicken | 450 | 11 | 59 |

## Back Yard Burgers® (Dec '11)

**Specialities:**

| | C | F | Cb |
|---|---|---|---|
| Big Dog | 500 | 33 | 32 |
| Bak-Pak: Chicken Tender Meal | 1110 | 71 | 91 |
| Dog | 320 | 18 | 29 |
| Chicken Tender Meal | 1260 | 79 | 102 |
| Chili Cheese Big Dog | 630 | 44 | 34 |
| Garden Veggie Burger | 400 | 8 | 57 |

**Sides:** *Per Serving*

| | C | F | Cb |
|---|---|---|---|
| Chili | 150 | 9 | 8 |
| **Seasoned Fries:** Regular, 6 oz | 640 | 45 | 58 |
| Large, 9 oz | 960 | 68 | 87 |

**Salads:** *Without Dressing*

| | C | F | Cb |
|---|---|---|---|
| Blackened Chicken | 330 | 15 | 25 |
| Fried Chicken | 410 | 19 | 41 |
| Garden Fresh | 100 | 2 | 20 |
| Grilled Chicken | 220 | 4 | 23 |
| Side Salad | 30 | 0 | 6 |

**Dressings:** *Per Serving*

| | C | F | Cb |
|---|---|---|---|
| Bleu Cheese | 220 | 24 | 1 |
| Honey Mustard | 240 | 23 | 7 |
| Ranch | 150 | 15 | 2 |

**Desserts:** *Per Serving*

| | C | F | Cb |
|---|---|---|---|
| **Cobblers:** Apple | 360 | 14 | 59 |
| Blackberry | 290 | 8 | 51 |
| Cherry | 350 | 12 | 59 |
| Peach | 330 | 11 | 56 |
| **Shakes:** *Per 12 fl.oz* | | | |
| Chocolate; Strawberry, average | 630 | 29 | 83 |
| Vanilla | 620 | 28 | 83 |

## Baja Fresh® (Dec '11)

**Burritos:** *As Served*

| | C | F | Cb |
|---|---|---|---|
| Baja Burrito: With Chicken | 790 | 38 | 65 |
| With Steak | 850 | 46 | 67 |
| Bare Burrito: With Charbroiled Chkn | 640 | 7 | 97 |
| Veggie and Cheese | 580 | 10 | 101 |
| Bean & Cheese Burrito: With Chicken | 970 | 35 | 96 |
| With Steak | 1030 | 43 | 97 |
| No Meat (Vegetarian) | 840 | 33 | 96 |
| Burrito Mexicano: With Chicken | 790 | 13 | 117 |
| With Steak | 860 | 21 | 118 |
| Burrito Ultimo: With Chicken | 880 | 36 | 84 |
| With Steak | 950 | 44 | 85 |
| Grilled Veggie | 800 | 33 | 94 |

**Fajitas:** *As Served, Without Tortilla Chips*

| | C | F | Cb |
|---|---|---|---|
| Chicken with Corn Tortillas | 860 | 24 | 105 |
| Chicken with Flour Tortillas | 1140 | 33 | 147 |

*Continued Next Page ...*

## Baja Fresh® cont... (Dec'11)

| | C | F | Cb |
|---|---|---|---|
| **Nachos:** *As Served* | | | |
| With Charbroiled Chicken | 2020 | 110 | 164 |
| With Charbroiled Steak | 2120 | 118 | 163 |
| With Cheese | 1890 | 108 | 163 |
| **Quesadillas:** *As Served* | | | |
| With Charbroiled Chicken | 1330 | 80 | 84 |
| With Charbroiled Steak | 1430 | 87 | 84 |
| With Cheese | 1200 | 78 | 84 |
| Vegetarian | 1260 | 78 | 96 |
| **Tacos:** *As Served* | | | |
| Baja Fish Taco, Fried | 250 | 13 | 27 |
| Grilled Mahi Mahi Taco | 230 | 9 | 26 |
| Original Baja Style Taco: W/ Chicken | 210 | 5 | 28 |
| With Charbroiled Shrimp | 200 | 5 | 28 |
| **Salads:** *As Served, Without Dressing* | | | |
| **Baja Ensalada:** | | | |
| With Charbroiled Chicken | 310 | 7 | 18 |
| With Charbroiled Shrimp | 230 | 6 | 18 |
| With Charbroiled Steak | 450 | 18 | 18 |
| **Tostada:** Charbroiled Fish | 1130 | 55 | 99 |
| Charbroiled Shrimp | 1120 | 55 | 99 |
| Charbroiled Steak | 1230 | 63 | 98 |
| Savory Pork Carnitas | 1180 | 62 | 100 |

*For Complete Nutritional Data ~ see CalorieKing.com*

## Baskin Robbins® (Dec'11)

| | C | F | Cb |
|---|---|---|---|
| **Ice Creams:** *Per 4 oz Scoop* | | | |
| **Classic Flavors:** Cherries Jubilee | 240 | 12 | 30 |
| Chocolate | 260 | 14 | 33 |
| Jamoca Almond Fudge | 270 | 15 | 31 |
| Mint Chocolate Chip | 260 | 16 | 28 |
| Old Fashioned Butter Pecan | 280 | 18 | 25 |
| Oreo Cookies 'n Cream | 280 | 15 | 32 |
| Pralines 'n Cream | 280 | 14 | 35 |
| Rainbow Sherbet | 160 | 2 | 33 |
| Reese's P'nut Butter Cup | 300 | 18 | 31 |
| Vanilla | 260 | 16 | 27 |
| Very Berry Strawberry | 220 | 11 | 28 |
| World Class Chocolate | 280 | 16 | 31 |
| **Premium Churned:** *Per 2½ oz Scoop* | | | |
| Light: Aloha Brownie | 150 | 5 | 26 |
| Cappuccino | 140 | 5 | 20 |
| Mint Oreo | 150 | 4.5 | 26 |
| **Frozen Yogurt,** Fat-Free Van., 4 oz | 150 | 0 | 32 |
| **Sorbets:** *Per 4 oz Scoop* | | | |
| Lemon; Pink Grapefruit, average | 130 | 0 | 34 |

## Baskin Robbins® cont... (Dec'11)

| | C | F | Cb |
|---|---|---|---|
| **Sundaes:** | | | |
| **Classic :** Banana Royale, 11.3 oz | 620 | 28 | 87 |
| Banana Split, 20 oz | 1010 | 34 | 173 |
| Brownie, 10.68 oz | 920 | 47 | 119 |
| **Premium Sundaes:** | | | |
| Choc. Chip Cookie Dough, 11.9 oz | 990 | 43 | 138 |
| Reese's P'nut Butter Cup, 12.13 oz | 1220 | 80 | 109 |
| **Soft Serve:** | | | |
| **Parfaits:** *Per Regular 15 oz Size* | | | |
| Oreo | 740 | 27 | 114 |
| Reeses | 990 | 63 | 86 |
| Strawberry 'n Almonds | 600 | 27 | 76 |
| **'31 Below' Mix-In:** *Per 16 oz Medium Cup* | | | |
| Butterfinger | 840 | 32 | 127 |
| Chocolate Chip Cookie Dough | 860 | 30 | 132 |
| Heath | 940 | 43 | 121 |
| Made with M&M's | 1050 | 41 | 151 |
| Oreo | 750 | 28 | 110 |
| Reese's Peanut Butter Cup | 880 | 40 | 115 |
| **Cups:** Vanilla: Kid's, 3 oz cup | 130 | 4.5 | 18 |
| Regular, 6 oz cup | 250 | 9 | 37 |
| Large, 9 oz cup | 380 | 14 | 55 |
| **Cake Bites:** Chocolate Mint, 3 oz | 330 | 20 | 33 |
| Double Chocolate, 3 oz | 310 | 18 | 35 |
| Praline Caramel, 3.1 oz | 360 | 22 | 39 |
| Vanilla Blondie, 3.1 oz | 350 | 22 | 35 |
| **Beverages:** | | | |
| **Freezes with Orange Sherbet:** | | | |
| Small | 370 | 4 | 82 |
| Medium | 510 | 5 | 112 |
| **Cappuccino Blast:** *Per Medium, 24 fl.oz* | | | |
| Original, without cream | 480 | 19 | 72 |
| Mocha, without cream | 610 | 19 | 104 |
| **Fruit Blast:** *Per Medium, 24 fl.oz* | | | |
| Peach Passion Fruit | 370 | 0.5 | 94 |
| Strawberry Citrus | 330 | 0 | 83 |
| Wild Mango | 470 | 1.5 | 116 |
| **Milk Shakes:** *Per Medium, 24 fl.oz* | | | |
| Choc Chip Cookie Dough | 1030 | 42 | 137 |
| Vanilla | 980 | 45 | 125 |
| Chocolate with Vanilla Ice Cream | 990 | 44 | 131 |
| Strawberry w/ Strawb. Ice Cream | 770 | 31 | 105 |
| **Smoothie:** *Per Medium, 24 fl.oz* | | | |
| Mango | 620 | 2 | 148 |
| Peach Passion Banana | 540 | 1 | 131 |
| **Cones:** Cake | 25 | 0 | 5 |
| Sugar | 45 | 0.5 | 9 |
| Waffle | 160 | 4 | 28 |

*For Complete Nutritional Data ~ see CalorieKing.com*

## Big Apple Bagels® (Dec'11)

*Bagels:*

| | C | F | Cb |
|---|---|---|---|
| All types, average, 5 oz | 340 | 2 | 68 |
| ½ bagel, 2½ oz | 170 | 1 | 34 |

*Choice Bagels: Per Bagel*

| | C | F | Cb |
|---|---|---|---|
| Blueberry Cobbler | 390 | 8 | 70 |
| Cheddar Nacho | 350 | 6 | 60 |
| Cinnamon Apple Pie | 385 | 8 | 68 |
| Cinnamon Bun | 400 | 8 | 70 |
| Cinnamon Danish | 395 | 8 | 72 |
| French Toast | 370 | 4 | 74 |
| Quiche Lorraine | 355 | 8 | 54 |
| Strawberry White Chocolate | 365 | 4 | 72 |
| Swiss Melt | 370 | 8 | 58 |
| White Chocolate Swirl | 395 | 8 | 70 |

*Cream Cheese: Per 2 Tbsp , 1 oz*

| | C | F | Cb |
|---|---|---|---|
| Plain | 90 | 9 | 2 |
| Plain, Lite | 60 | 4.5 | 3 |
| Other varieties, average | 90 | 8 | 2 |
| Whipped: Classic Plain | 70 | 7 | 1 |
| Brown Sugar Cinnamon | 70 | 5 | 5 |
| Reduced-Fat Spring Veggie | 60 | 5 | 2 |

*My Favorite Muffin: Per Jumbo, 5¾ oz*

| | C | F | Cb |
|---|---|---|---|
| **Regular:** Blueberry | 505 | 24 | 66 |
| Chocolate Chip | 635 | 33 | 81 |
| Cinnamon Swirl Cheesecake | 640 | 33 | 84 |
| Pumpkin Spice | 545 | 24 | 78 |
| **Fat Free:** Blueberry | 325 | 0 | 78 |
| Chocolate Marble | 375 | 0 | 87 |
| Cinnamon Bun | 505 | 0 | 126 |

*Sandwiches:*

| | C | F | Cb |
|---|---|---|---|
| Big Apple Club | 795 | 37 | 75 |
| Classic Reuben, Overstuffed | 960 | 43 | 57 |
| Grilled Chicken Bruschetta Pizzaah | 345 | 21 | 24 |
| Morning Classic | 485 | 11 | 73 |
| Roast Beef Parmesan Grinder | 585 | 15 | 76 |

*For Complete Nutritional Data ~ see CalorieKing.com*

## Biggby Coffee® (Dec'11)

*Hot Drinks: Per Tall, 16 fl.oz, W/o Sugar Unless Indicated*

| | C | F | Cb |
|---|---|---|---|
| **Caffe Latte:** With 2% Milk | 175 | 7 | 16 |
| With Non-Fat Milk | 115 | 0 | 16 |
| With Soy | 160 | 5 | 19 |
| **Cappuccino:** With 2% Milk | 105 | 4 | 10 |
| With Non-Fat Milk | 70 | 0 | 9.5 |
| With Soy | 95 | 3 | 11 |
| **Chai Latte:** With 2% Milk | 315 | 8 | 51 |
| With Non-Fat Milk | 255 | 0 | 51 |
| **Cocoa Carmella:** *With Sugar* | | | |
| With 2% Milk | 325 | 9 | 51 |
| With Whipped Cream | 405 | 15 | 55 |
| **Mocha Mocha:** *With Sugar* | | | |
| With 2% Milk | 295 | 8 | 48 |
| With Whipped Cream | 375 | 14 | 50 |

## Biggby Coffee® cont... (Dec'11)

*Cold Drinks: Per Tall, 16 fl.oz*

| | C | F | Cb |
|---|---|---|---|
| **Creme Freeze:** Banana | 395 | 5.5 | 86 |
| Berry Fruizen-T w/ Whipped Crm | 465 | 10 | 90 |

*Frozen Lattes: With Whipped Cream & Sugar*

| | C | F | Cb |
|---|---|---|---|
| Caramel Marvel | 480 | 16 | 80 |
| Irish Cream | 460 | 15 | 78 |

*For Complete Menu & Data ~ see CalorieKing.com*

## Blimpie® (Dec'11)

*Cold Deli Subs: Per 6" Sub on White, Includes Dressing*

| | C | F | Cb |
|---|---|---|---|
| Blimpie Best, with Provolone | 450 | 17 | 49 |
| BLT, without Cheese | 430 | 22 | 43 |
| Club, with Swiss | 410 | 13 | 49 |
| Cuban, with Swiss | 410 | 11 | 43 |
| Ham & Swiss Cheese | 420 | 14 | 49 |
| Roast Beef & Provolone | 430 | 14 | 46 |
| Tuna without Cheese | 470 | 21 | 43 |
| Turkey & Provolone | 410 | 13 | 49 |
| **Wraps:** Chicken Caesar | 560 | 24 | 56 |
| Southwestern | 530 | 22 | 61 |

*Hot Deli Subs: Per 6" Sub on White*

| | C | F | Cb |
|---|---|---|---|
| Meatball, with Provolone | 580 | 31 | 50 |
| Pastrami, with Swiss | 430 | 16 | 42 |
| VegiMax, with Provolone | 520 | 20 | 56 |

*Salads: Regular, Without Dressing*

| | C | F | Cb |
|---|---|---|---|
| Buffalo Chicken | 220 | 9 | 10 |
| Garden | 30 | 0 | 6 |
| Tuna Salad | 270 | 19 | 6 |
| Ultimate Club | 260 | 14 | 10 |

*Dressings & Sauces: Per 1½ oz*

| | C | F | Cb |
|---|---|---|---|
| Creamy Caesar | 210 | 21 | 2 |
| Creamy Italian | 180 | 18 | 4 |

*Soups: Per 8½ oz Serving*

| | C | F | Cb |
|---|---|---|---|
| Chicken Noodle | 130 | 4 | 18 |
| Cream of Broccoli with Cheese | 250 | 19 | 13 |
| Harvest Vegetable | 100 | 1 | 19 |
| Minestrone | 90 | 3 | 14 |
| New England Clam Chowder | 170 | 3 | 28 |

*Desserts:*

| | C | F | Cb |
|---|---|---|---|
| Brownie | 230 | 10 | 28 |
| Cookies: Oatmeal Raisin | 180 | 7 | 27 |
| Sugar | 320 | 16 | 42 |

*For Complete Nutritional Data ~ see CalorieKing.com*

Updated Nutrition Data ~ www.CalorieKing.com
Persons with Diabetes ~ See Disclaimer (Page 22)

## Bob Evans® (Dec '11)

| Breakfast: | C | F | Cb |
|---|---|---|---|
| **Biscuit Bowls:** Sausage, 19 oz | 975 | 59 | 76 |
| Spinach, Bacon & Tomato, 18½ oz | 1015 | 60 | 79 |
| Sausage Biscuit, 19 oz | 975 | 59 | 76 |
| **Hotcakes:** *Without Topping* | | | |
| Buttermilk (1) | 330 | 8 | 58 |
| Cranberry Multigrain (1) | 330 | 4 | 68 |
| **Loaded Hash Browns,** 6½ oz | 525 | 24 | 56 |
| **Omelets:** Border Scramble | 635 | 46 | 14 |
| With Egg Lites | 415 | 24 | 13 |
| Farmer's Market | 640 | 45 | 14 |
| Western | 530 | 36 | 8 |
| **Pot Roast Hash,** 14½ oz | 750 | 49 | 32 |
| **Sunshine Skillet,** 11½ oz | 420 | 24 | 33 |
| *Starters:* | | | |
| Breaded Garlic Mushrooms, 11 oz | 460 | 18 | 63 |
| Country Fair Cheese Bites | 950 | 66 | 49 |
| Fried Green Tomatoes | 765 | 45 | 85 |
| Garden Salad, without dressing | 90 | 1 | 9 |
| *Soup: Per Bowl* | | | |
| Beef Vegetable | 160 | 3 | 23 |
| Cheddar Baked Potato | 330 | 19 | 26 |
| Farm Festival Bean | 200 | 3 | 28 |
| Tomato Basil | 405 | 31 | 23 |
| **Dinners:** *Without Sides Unless Indicated* | | | |
| **Beef:** Country Fried with Gravy | 565 | 37 | 41 |
| Open-Faced Roast Beef Sandwich | 470 | 24 | 21 |
| Pot Roast Stroganoff, 24 oz | 815 | 43 | 65 |
| Spaghetti with Meat Sce, 21½ oz | 785 | 35 | 87 |
| **Chicken:** Chicken & Brocc. Alfredo | 860 | 46 | 61 |
| Chicken-N-Noodles: Deep-Dish | 700 | 31 | 75 |
| Slow Roasted, 13½ oz | 225 | 5 | 31 |
| Chicken Parmesan, w/ sauce, 27 oz | 1145 | 53 | 100 |
| Chicken Pot Pie, slow roasted | 860 | 56 | 63 |
| Garlic Butter Grilled Chkn Breast | 160 | 4 | 1 |
| **Fish:** Garlic Butter Salmon, 8 oz | 255 | 9 | 1 |
| Potato-Crusted Flounder, 5 oz | 175 | 7 | 9 |
| Wildfire Salmon, 8½ oz | 310 | 9 | 15 |
| **Turkey:** Slow-Roasted, 3½ oz | 115 | 4 | 3 |
| Turkey & Dressing, 16½ oz | 645 | 31 | 53 |
| *Fit From The Farm:* | | | |
| **Breakfast:** Blueb. Ban. French Toast | 345 | 6 | 44 |
| Fresh Fruit Plate, w/ Low Fat Yogurt | 355 | 2 | 84 |
| Veggie Omelet w/ Fruit/Toast/Jelly | 310 | 6 | 43 |
| **Dinners:** *Includes Menu-Listed Sides, Condiments* | | | |
| Chicken, Spin. & Tom. Pasta, 12 oz | 355 | 13 | 38 |
| Grilled Chicken Breast, 19½ oz | 425 | 8 | 58 |
| Potato Crusted Flounder, 20½ oz | 455 | 12 | 67 |
| **Salad:** Apple Cranberry Spinach, | | | |
| with reduced fat raspb. dressing | 380 | 15 | 48 |

## Bob Evans® cont... (Dec '11)

| Sandwiches & Burgers: | C | F | Cb |
|---|---|---|---|
| **Big Farm Burgers:** Cheeseburger | 830 | 50 | 51 |
| Bacon Cheeseburger | 900 | 58 | 51 |
| Hamburger | 725 | 42 | 50 |
| Smokehouse Burger | 1200 | 82 | 64 |
| **Sandwiches:** Knife & Fork Meatloaf | 775 | 42 | 62 |
| Pot Roast | 640 | 32 | 52 |
| Turkey Bacon Melt | 570 | 27 | 49 |
| Turkey Club Wrap | 695 | 34 | 58 |
| **Farm-Grill Sandwiches:** | | | |
| Chicken, Fried | 540 | 16 | 61 |
| Grilled | 405 | 7 | 48 |
| Chicken Club: Fried | 675 | 29 | 60 |
| Grilled | 545 | 20 | 48 |
| *Salads: Large, Without Dressing* | | | |
| Cobb, 14½ oz | 515 | 31 | 10 |
| Blue Cheese Dressing, 3 oz | 410 | 44 | 5 |
| Cranberry Pecan Chicken, 14 oz | 630 | 36 | 33 |
| Heritage Chef, 12½ oz | 400 | 24 | 11 |
| Buttermilk Ranch Dressing, 3 oz | 290 | 29 | 3 |
| Southwest Chipotle Chicken | 1085 | 70 | 71 |
| Sweet Italian Dressing, 3 oz | 255 | 23 | 12 |
| Wildfire Grilled Chicken, 13½ oz | 390 | 13 | 37 |
| *Side Dishes:* Coleslaw, 3½ oz | 210 | 14 | 19 |
| Baked Potato, Plain, 10 oz | 200 | 0 | 50 |
| Bread & Celery Dressing, 6 oz | 300 | 19 | 29 |
| French Fries, 7 oz | 500 | 21 | 71 |
| Hash Browns, 4½ oz | 325 | 8 | 53 |
| Home Fries, 5 oz | 165 | 6 | 24 |
| Loaded Baked Potato, 12 oz | 395 | 16 | 53 |
| Macaroni & Cheese, 7 oz | 305 | 15 | 29 |
| Mashed Potatoes, 5½ oz | 190 | 7 | 16 |
| Sweet Potato Fries, 5 oz | 465 | 29 | 49 |
| *Gravy:* Beef, 2¼ oz | 20 | 1 | 2 |
| Chicken Roasted, 2 oz | 50 | 4 | 3 |
| Country, 3 oz | 55 | 2 | 18 |
| *Sauces:* Hollandaise, 1 oz | 25 | 1 | 3 |
| Wildfire BBQ, 1 oz | 60 | 0 | 15 |
| *Kid's Menu:* French Fries, 4½ oz | 320 | 13 | 46 |
| Fried Chicken Strips (1), 1½ oz | 135 | 8 | 10 |
| Mac & Cheese, 7 oz | 300 | 9 | 45 |
| Mini Cheeseburger (1) | 275 | 15 | 21 |
| Plenty-O-Pancakes, | | | |
| Plain, without Topping, 11½ oz | 710 | 18 | 130 |
| Smiley Face Potatoes, 3 oz | 270 | 16 | 29 |
| Sundae, Fudge Blast, 4 oz | 215 | 9 | 31 |
| *Dessert:* French Silk Pie, 5½ oz sl. | 660 | 44 | 60 |
| Peach Cobbler, 8 oz | 400 | 13 | 65 |
| Peanut Butter Brownie Bites (8) | 1025 | 49 | 134 |

## Bojangles® (Dec'11)

**Cajun & Southern Style Chicken Dinners:** *With Dirty Rice, Cajun Pintos & Buttermilk Biscuit*

| | C | F | Cb |
|---|---|---|---|
| 1 Breast Dinner | 1010 | 46 | 89 |
| 2 Piece Dinner (Leg & Thigh) | 1160 | 61 | 98 |
| 3 Piece Dinner (Leg & 2 Thighs) | 1530 | 87 | 110 |
| 3 Wing Dinner | 1160 | 59 | 107 |

*Sandwiches:*

| | C | F | Cb |
|---|---|---|---|
| Cajun Club | 645 | 39 | 44 |
| Cajun Filet: Without Mayonnaisse | 495 | 27 | 43 |
| With Mayonnaise | 555 | 34 | 43 |
| Grilled Chicken: Without Mayo | 365 | 15 | 33 |
| With Mayonnaise | 425 | 22 | 33 |
| Club | 515 | 27 | 34 |

*Biscuit:: Plain*

| | C | F | Cb |
|---|---|---|---|
| Biscuit:: Plain | 185 | 14 | 33 |
| Bacon, Egg & Cheese | 485 | 37 | 35 |
| Cajun Filet | 425 | 28 | 45 |
| Country Ham | 255 | 18 | 33 |
| Egg & Cheese | 445 | 34 | 35 |
| Gravy Biscuits | 290 | 20 | 43 |
| Sausage | 335 | 27 | 33 |
| Steak | 455 | 35 | 44 |

**Fixins':** *Per Individual Serve Unless Indicated*

| | C | F | Cb |
|---|---|---|---|
| Bo-Tato Rounds, medium | 350 | 22 | 35 |
| Cajun Pintos | 115 | 0 | 20 |
| Cole Slaw | 250 | 20 | 18 |
| Dirty Rice | 165 | 6 | 24 |
| Macaroni & Cheese | 290 | 7 | 33 |
| Mashed Potatoes 'N Gravy | 130 | 6 | 21 |
| Picnic Grits | 230 | 2 | 47 |
| Seasoned Fries, medium size | 300 | 20 | 27 |
| *Sweet Biscuits:* Bo Berry (1) | 375 | 15 | 55 |
| Cinnamon (1) | 240 | 14 | 51 |

*For Complete Nutritional Data ~ see CalorieKing.com*

## Boston Market® (Dec'11)

*Sandwiches:*

| | C | F | Cb |
|---|---|---|---|
| All White Rotisserie Chicken Salad | 1050 | 64 | 87 |
| Roasted Turkey Carver: | | | |
| Full, with Swiss Cheese | 790 | 35 | 66 |
| Half, with Swiss Cheese | 395 | 18 | 33 |
| Rotisserie Chicken Carver: Full | 820 | 36 | 66 |
| Half | 410 | 18 | 33 |
| Turkey BLT | 1030 | 57 | 89 |

**Individual Meals:** *Without Sides*

| | C | F | Cb |
|---|---|---|---|
| Beef Brisket, 4 oz | 230 | 13 | 0 |
| Half Rotisserie Chicken, 12 oz | 640 | 33 | 2 |
| Meatloaf, 7½ oz | 480 | 36 | 21 |

## Boston Market® cont... (Dec'11)

*Salads:* Includes Dressing

| | C | F | Cb |
|---|---|---|---|
| Caesar: With Chicken, 13.5 oz | 660 | 43 | 31 |
| Without Chicken, 9.7 oz | 560 | 42 | 31 |
| Mediterranean: Full, 15 oz | 640 | 44 | 27 |
| Half, 7.5 oz | 320 | 22 | 14 |
| Southwest Santa Fe: Full, 17.8 oz | 740 | 46 | 50 |
| Half, 8.9 oz | 370 | 23 | 25 |

*Sides:*

| | C | F | Cb |
|---|---|---|---|
| Cinnamon-Apples, 5 oz | 210 | 3 | 47 |
| Creamed Spinach, 6¾ oz | 280 | 23 | 12 |
| Fresh Steamed Vegetables, 4¾ oz | 60 | 2 | 8 |
| Fresh Vegetable Stuffing, 4¾ oz | 190 | 8 | 25 |
| Garlic Dill New Potatoes, 5½ oz | 140 | 3 | 24 |
| Gravy: Beef, 3 oz | 35 | 1.5 | 4 |
| Poultry, 4 oz | 50 | 1 | 8 |
| Green Beans, 3 oz | 60 | 3.5 | 7 |
| Macaroni & Cheese, 7¾ oz | 300 | 11 | 35 |
| Mashed Potatoes, 7¾ oz | 270 | 11 | 36 |
| Sweet Corn, 6¼ oz | 170 | 4 | 37 |
| Sweet Potato Casserole, 7 oz | 460 | 16 | 77 |

*Soups:*

| | C | F | Cb |
|---|---|---|---|
| Chicken Noodle, 14 oz | 240 | 8 | 23 |
| Chicken Tortilla: W/ Toppings, 12.8 oz | 410 | 25 | 30 |
| Without Toppings, 10.8 oz | 160 | 8 | 13 |

*Desserts:*

| | C | F | Cb |
|---|---|---|---|
| Apple Pie, 5¾ oz | 580 | 30 | 74 |
| Chocolate Cake, 5 oz | 580 | 34 | 67 |
| Chocolate Brownie, 4.7 oz | 470 | 19 | 74 |

*For Complete Nutritional Data ~ see CalorieKing.com*

## Boston's Gourmet Pizza® (Dec'11)

*Starters:* Per Order

| | C | F | Cb |
|---|---|---|---|
| Cactus Cut Potatoes with Dip, 16 oz | 1170 | 70 | 113 |
| Oven Roasted Wings, Cajun, 15 oz | 360 | 57 | 21 |

*Burgers & Sandwiches:*

| | C | F | Cb |
|---|---|---|---|
| **Burgers:** Bacon Cheeseburger | 1240 | 92 | 45 |
| Boston Cheeseburger | 1110 | 74 | 59 |
| **Sandwiches:** | | | |
| Beef Dip with Horseradish | 1170 | 61 | 92 |
| Boston's Cheesesteak | 1300 | 69 | 95 |
| Double Decker Club | 780 | 33 | 57 |
| Gr. Chipotle Chicken w/o Bacon | 530 | 24 | 40 |
| The Reuben | 750 | 37 | 54 |

## Boston's Pizza® cont... (Dec '11)

*Pizzas (Medium): Per Slice*

| | C | F | Cb |
|---|---|---|---|
| Basic Cheese | 150 | 3.5 | 22 |
| BLT | 300 | 15 | 24 |
| Chicken Parmesan | 220 | 7 | 25 |
| Double Meat & Peppers | 250 | 10 | 26 |
| Hawaiian | 180 | 4 | 25 |
| Pepperoni | 190 | 7 | 22 |
| Sicilian | 220 | 8 | 30 |
| Tropical Chicken | 300 | 14 | 26 |
| Tuscan | 265 | 10 | 30 |

*Pastas: Full Order, Without Garlic Bread*

| | | | |
|---|---|---|---|
| Chicken Milano | 1700 | 54 | 236 |
| Fettuccini with Alfredo Sauce | 1490 | 52 | 222 |

*Salads: Meal Size, Includes Dressing*

| | | | |
|---|---|---|---|
| Caesar, 11.3 oz | 570 | 32 | 43 |
| Spinach & Cranberry, 15½ oz | 810 | 66 | 44 |

*Desserts: With Ice Cream & Sauce*

| | | | |
|---|---|---|---|
| Apple Crisp, 12 oz | 960 | 42 | 140 |
| Choc.Brownie Addiction, 14 oz | 1450 | 70 | 188 |

*For Complete Nutritional Data ~ see CalorieKing.com*

## Braum's® (Dec '11)

*Frozen Yogurt: Per ½ Cup*

| | | | |
|---|---|---|---|
| Chocolate Peanut Butter Cup | 180 | 10 | 19 |
| Average Fruit Flavors | 130 | 5 | 19 |

*Ice Cream: Per ½ Cup*

| | | | |
|---|---|---|---|
| **Carb Watch:** Chocolate Chip | 180 | 10 | 17 |
| Other flavors, average | 155 | 11 | 17 |
| **Light,** average all varieties | 130 | 4 | 19 |
| **Premium:** Peanut Butter Cup | 190 | 12 | 18 |
| Other flavors, average | 150 | 6 | 18 |

*For Complete Nutritional Data ~ see CalorieKing.com*

## Bruegger's Bagels® (Dec '11)

*Bagels:*

| | | | |
|---|---|---|---|
| Chocolate Chip, 4.1 oz | 330 | 3.5 | 65 |
| Jalapeno Cheddar, 5.5 oz | 450 | 9 | 75 |
| Plain, 4.1 oz | 300 | 2 | 61 |
| Sourdough, 4.1 oz | 290 | 2 | 56 |
| Whole Wheat, 4.1 oz | 310 | 3.5 | 61 |

*Breakfast S'wiches: On Plain Bagel*

| | | | |
|---|---|---|---|
| Egg & Cheese | 430 | 18 | 63 |
| With Bacon | 500 | 24 | 64 |
| Smoked Salmon | 460 | 10 | 66 |
| Spinach & Cheddar Omelet | 500 | 16 | 63 |
| Western | 890 | 58 | 66 |

## Bruegger's Bagels® cont.. (Dec '11)

| | C | F | Cb |
|---|---|---|---|

*Deli Sandwiches: On Plain Bagel Unless Indicated*

| | | | |
|---|---|---|---|
| BLT on Hearty White Bread | 720 | 42 | 62 |
| Chicken Breast | 550 | 6 | 81 |
| Garden Veggie | 360 | 2 | 72 |
| Ham On Honey Wheat Bread | 540 | 16 | 64 |

*Hot Paninis: On Hearty White Unless Indicated*

| | | | |
|---|---|---|---|
| Four Cheese & Tomato | 630 | 29 | 66 |
| Ham & Cheddar on Honey Wheat | 610 | 17 | 72 |
| Tuna & Cheddar Melt (Honey Wheat) | 970 | 61 | 57 |
| Turkey Toscana | 650 | 28 | 58 |

*Signature & Classic Sandwiches:*

| | | | |
|---|---|---|---|
| Herby Turkey/Sesame Bagel | 530 | 14 | 73 |
| Leonardo da Veggie/Plain Softwich | 560 | 15 | 76 |
| Roma Roast Bef on Hearty White | 770 | 44 | 62 |
| Tarragon Chicken Salad/White Bread | 750 | 37 | 75 |
| Thai Peanut Chicken/Plain Bagel | 580 | 11 | 91 |
| Turkey Chipotle Club/Honey Wheat Bread | 540 | 18 | 60 |

*Cafe Salads: With Dressing*

| | | | |
|---|---|---|---|
| Classic Cobb, w/ Red Wine Vinaig. | 280 | 16 | 9 |
| Chicken Caesar, with Caesar Dress. | 240 | 12 | 15 |
| Harvest Chicken, w/ Strawb. Vinaig. | 260 | 9 | 30 |
| Mandarin Medley, w/ Bals. Vinaig. | 250 | 14 | 13 |
| Sesame Chicken, w/ Asian Dress. | 340 | 20 | 22 |
| Cookies, average, 3 oz | 390 | 18 | 51 |
| Dessert Bars: Seven Layer, 4.7 oz | 650 | 43 | 58 |
| Chocolate Chunk Brownie, 2½ oz | 310 | 18 | 38 |
| Toffee Almond, 3.1 oz | 400 | 19 | 53 |

*For Complete Menu & Data ~ see CalorieKing.com*

## Burgerville® (Dec '11)

*Burgers:*

| | | | |
|---|---|---|---|
| Original Hamburger | 320 | 17 | 30 |
| Cheeseburger | 380 | 20 | 30 |
| Double Beef Cheeseburger | 450 | 27 | 30 |
| Half Pound Colossal Cheeseburger | 750 | 45 | 43 |
| Tillamook Cheeseburger | 640 | 39 | 42 |

*Sandwiches: Crispy Chicken*

| | | | |
|---|---|---|---|
| Crispy Chicken | 490 | 24 | 50 |
| Deluxe Crispy Chicken | 630 | 59 | 72 |
| Turkey Club | 590 | 38 | 33 |
| French Fries, regular, 5 oz | 360 | 15 | 52 |

*For Complete Menu & Data ~ see CalorieKing.com*

## Burger King® (Dec '11)

| | C | F | Cb |
|---|---|---|---|
| ***Flame Broiled Whoppers:*** *With Standard Sides* | | | |
| Whopper | 670 | 40 | 51 |
| Double Whopper | 900 | 57 | 51 |
| Mustard Whopper | 530 | 23 | 52 |
| Texas Triple Whopper | 1270 | 86 | 50 |
| Triple Whopper | 1140 | 75 | 51 |
| Whopper JR. | 340 | 19 | 28 |
| ***Flame Broiled Burgers:*** *With Standard Toppings* | | | |
| BK Stackers: Single | 380 | 22 | 28 |
| Double | 500 | 31 | 28 |
| Triple | 650 | 43 | 29 |
| Cheeseburger | 300 | 14 | 28 |
| Double Cheeseburger | 450 | 26 | 29 |
| Hamburger | 260 | 10 | 28 |
| Mushroom & Swiss | 410 | 27 | 27 |
| ***Chicken & Fish Sandwiches:*** *With Standard Toppings* | | | |
| BK Big Fish | 590 | 31 | 57 |
| Original Chicken | 630 | 39 | 46 |
| Spicy Chick'N Crisp | 460 | 30 | 34 |
| TenderCrisp Chicken | 750 | 45 | 58 |
| TenderGrill Chicken on Ciabatta | 470 | 18 | 40 |
| **BK Chicken Fries:** *Without Sauce:* | | | |
| 6 pieces | 250 | 15 | 16 |
| 9 pieces | 380 | 22 | 24 |
| **Chicken Tenders:** | | | |
| 4 pieces | 190 | 11 | 10 |
| 8 pieces | 380 | 22 | 20 |
| ***Dipping Sauces:*** *Per 1 oz* | | | |
| BBQ; Sweet & Sour, average | 45 | 0 | 11 |
| Buffalo | 80 | 8 | 2 |
| Honey Mustard | 90 | 6 | 8 |
| Ranch; Zesty Onion, average | 145 | 15 | 2 |
| *Sides:* | | | |
| **French Fries:** Salted | | | |
| Small, 4¼ oz | 340 | 17 | 44 |
| Medium, 5¾ oz | 440 | 22 | 56 |
| Large, 7 oz | 540 | 27 | 69 |
| **Onion Rings:** | | | |
| Small (15) | 310 | 17 | 36 |
| Medium (20) | 400 | 21 | 47 |
| Large (24) | 490 | 26 | 57 |
| **Fresh Apple Fries,** w/ Sauce | 70 | 0.5 | 16 |
| ***Salads:*** *W/o Dressing or Croutons* | | | |
| **Garden:** With TenderCrisp Chicken | 410 | 22 | 28 |
| With TenderGrill Chicken | 230 | 7 | 9 |
| **Dressings:** | | | |
| Ken's Creamy Caesar, 2 oz | 210 | 21 | 4 |
| Ken's Fat Free Ranch, 2 oz | 60 | 0 | 15 |

## Burger King® cont... (Dec '11)

*Breakfast:*

| | C | F | Cb |
|---|---|---|---|
| **Biscuits:** Bacon, Egg & Cheese | 420 | 25 | 34 |
| Ham, Egg & Cheese | 420 | 22 | 33 |
| Sausage, Egg & Cheese | 570 | 37 | 34 |
| **Blueberry Biscuits,** with Icing (4) | 390 | 15 | 57 |
| **Burritos:** *Includes Salsa* | | | |
| Bacon, Egg & Cheese | 300 | 16 | 24 |
| Potato, Egg & Cheese | 320 | 17 | 29 |
| **Cheesy Bacon BK Wrapper** | 380 | 24 | 28 |
| **Croissan'wich:** Bacon Egg & Chse | 360 | 19 | 26 |
| Egg & Cheese | 320 | 16 | 26 |
| Ham Egg & Cheese | 350 | 17 | 27 |
| **Double Croissan'wich:** | | | |
| Double Bacon, Egg & Dble Cheese | 440 | 25 | 27 |
| Ham, Bacon, Egg & Dble Cheese | 440 | 24 | 28 |
| Ham, Sausage, Egg & Dble Chse | 570 | 35 | 28 |
| Dble Sausage, Egg & Dble Cheese | 700 | 49 | 29 |
| **Hash Browns:** Small, 2.95 oz | 250 | 16 | 24 |
| Medium, 5.95 oz | 500 | 33 | 48 |
| Large, 7.9 oz | 670 | 44 | 65 |
| **Hot Oatmeal:** Original | 140 | 3.5 | 23 |
| Fruit Topped Maple & Brn. Sugar Flavor | 270 | 4 | 55 |
| **Platters:** 2 Biscuits & Sausage Gravy | 680 | 35 | 76 |
| Breakfast, 10.6 oz | 810 | 54 | 57 |
| Fr. Toast Sticks w/ bacon & syrup | 550 | 22 | 79 |
| With Sausages | 670 | 33 | 80 |
| Pancake, with Sausage & Syrup | 500 | 19 | 77 |
| Ultimate Breakfast, 17.17 oz | 1310 | 72 | 134 |
| ***Desserts/Pies:*** Dutch Apple Pie | 320 | 14 | 46 |
| Hershey's Sundae Pie | 300 | 18 | 31 |
| *Shakes:* | | | |
| **Chocolate:** Small, 12 fl.oz | 420 | 8 | 81 |
| Medium, 16 fl.oz | 690 | 18 | 121 |
| Large, 24 fl.oz oz | 900 | 21 | 163 |
| **Vanilla:** Small, 12 fl.oz | 400 | 7 | 75 |
| Medium, 16 fl.oz | 660 | 17 | 114 |
| Large, 24 fl.oz | 850 | 20 | 152 |
| *Beverages:* | | | |
| **Coca Cola Classic:** Value, 16 fl. oz | 140 | 0 | 39 |
| Small, 20 fl. oz | 190 | 0 | 51 |
| Medium, 30 fl.oz | 290 | 0 | 77 |

*For Complete Nutritional Data ~ see CalorieKing.com*

Updated Nutrition Data ~ www.CalorieKing.com
Persons with Diabetes ~ See Disclaimer (Page 22)

## California Pizza Kitchen
*~ See CalorieKing.com*

## Captain D's Seafood® (Dec'11)

*Dinners/Platters: Includes Cole Slaw, French Fries & Hush Puppies*

| | C | F | Cb |
|---|---|---|---|
| Bite Size Shrimp Dinner | 1140 | 61 | 120 |
| Catfish Feast | 995 | 57 | 88 |
| Clam Platter, ½ lb | 1450 | 87 | 133 |
| Country Style Fish Dinner | 1070 | 59 | 97 |
| Deluxe Seafood Platter | 1610 | 94 | 138 |
| Fried Flounder | 1530 | 93 | 115 |
| Oyster Dinner | 1000 | 58 | 100 |
| Ultimate Premium Shrimp Platter | 1290 | 65 | 141 |
| *Salads:* | | | |
| Fried Chicken Salad | 235 | 12 | 21 |
| Side Salad | 20 | 0 | 3 |
| Wild Alaskan Salmon Salad | 175 | 1 | 8 |
| *Sides:* | | | |
| Baked Potato, plain | 240 | 0 | 54 |
| Broccoli, 3.5 oz | 40 | 1 | 5 |
| Macaroni & Cheese, 4 oz | 160 | 7 | 17 |
| *Dessert,* Cheesecake w/ Strawb. | 430 | 26 | 45 |

## Caribou Coffee® (Dec'11)

*Without Whipped Cream Unless Indicated*

*Classic Hot Coffee Beverages: Per Medium*

| | | | |
|---|---|---|---|
| Coffee Of The Day, with 2% Milk | 20 | 0.5 | 1 |
| Espresso, 1 medium, 3 shots, 6 fl.oz | 0 | 0 | 0 |
| Breve | 510 | 45 | 17 |
| Cappuccino, with 2% Milk | 70 | 3 | 6 |
| Latte, with 2% Milk | 200 | 8 | 19 |
| Macchiato, with 2% Milk, 6 fl.oz | 20 | 1 | 1 |
| *Hot Chocolate: Per Medium, With Whipped Cream* | | | |
| Berry Mocha | 570 | 31 | 67 |
| Mint Cond. Milk Choc., 2% Milk | 580 | 31 | 68 |
| *Cold Beverages: Per Medium* | | | |
| Iced Americano | 5 | 0 | 0 |
| Iced Coffee, Cold Pressed | 5 | 0 | 0 |
| Iced Latte, with 2% Milk | 150 | 6 | 14 |
| Iced Mocha , Milk Choc., 2% Milk | 350 | 11 | 51 |
| *Coolers: Per Medium With Whipped Cream* | | | |
| Caramel | 500 | 16 | 88 |
| Coffee | 420 | 17 | 67 |
| Espresso | 370 | 16 | 57 |
| *Smoothies: Per Medium* | | | |
| Passion Fruit Green Tea | 290 | 0 | 70 |
| Pom-a-Mango | 350 | 0.5 | 85 |
| Strawberry Banana, 22 fl.oz | 350 | 0 | 84 |
| *Snowdrift: Per Medium With Milk Chocolate* | | | |
| Cookies & Cream, with 2% Milk | 630 | 18 | 103 |
| Mint,  with 2% Milk | 510 | 13 | 84 |

*For Complete Menu & Data ~ see CalorieKing.com*

## Carl's Jr.® (Dec'11)

| *Charbroiled Burgers:* | C | F | Cb |
|---|---|---|---|
| Big Hamburger | 490 | 18 | 59 |
| Famous Star with Cheese | 680 | 39 | 57 |
| Kid's Hamburger | 280 | 10 | 34 |
| Super Star with Cheese | 940 | 59 | 59 |
| The Big Carl | 930 | 58 | 55 |
| The Six Dollar Burger: Original | 910 | 54 | 63 |
| Guacamole Bacon | 1060 | 72 | 55 |
| Jalapeno | 950 | 63 | 55 |
| Low-Carb | 570 | 43 | 9 |
| Portobello Mushroom | 880 | 53 | 56 |
| Steakhouse | 1060 | 67 | 69 |
| Western Bacon | 1030 | 55 | 81 |
| *Chicken Sandwiches:* | | | |
| Charbroiled: Bacon Swiss | 770 | 42 | 60 |
| BBQ Chicken | 390 | 7 | 50 |
| Chicken Club | 580 | 29 | 45 |
| Santa Fe Chicken | 630 | 35 | 46 |
| Spicy Chicken Sandwich | 460 | 26 | 47 |
| *Chicken Tenders,* hand breaded, | | | |
| 5 pieces, without sauce | 560 | 31 | 24 |
| *Chicken Stars,* 6 pieces, w/o sce | 260 | 16 | 18 |
| *Fish:* With Chips | 710 | 38 | 69 |
| Carl's Catch Fish Sandwich | 700 | 37 | 73 |
| *Breakfast:* Bacon & Egg Burrito | 560 | 32 | 37 |
| Breakfast Burger | 810 | 42 | 69 |
| French Toast Dips, 5 pcs, w/o syrup | 460 | 21 | 60 |
| Hash Brown Nuggets, 4 oz | 350 | 23 | 32 |
| Loaded Breakfast Burrito | 780 | 48 | 51 |
| Sourdough Breakfast Sandwich | 450 | 21 | 38 |
| Steak & Egg Burrito | 650 | 36 | 42 |
| Sunrise Croissant Sandwich | 590 | 44 | 28 |
| *Fries:* Chili Cheese | 820 | 46 | 81 |
| CrissCut Fries, 5 oz | 450 | 29 | 42 |
| Natural Cut: Small, 4¼ oz | 310 | 15 | 40 |
| Medium, 6 oz | 430 | 21 | 56 |
| Large, 6½ oz | 470 | 23 | 61 |
| *Onion Rings,* 4½ oz | 530 | 28 | 61 |
| *Salads: Without Dressing or Croutons* | | | |
| Cranb. Apple Walnut Gr. Chicken | 320 | 11 | 29 |
| Original Grilled Chicken | 270 | 9 | 23 |
| *Dressings: Per 2 oz Package* | | | |
| Blue Cheese | 320 | 34 | 1 |
| House | 220 | 22 | 3 |
| Low-Fat Balsamic | 35 | 1.5 | 5 |
| *Shakes:* Vanilla; Choc.; Strawb. av. | 700 | 34 | 85 |
| Oreo | 720 | 38 | 79 |
| Malts, average all flavors | 770 | 35 | 100 |

# Fast - Foods & Restaurants

## Carvel® (Dec'11)

*Ice Creams: Per Small, 7½ oz*
*Dashers: Per Small 12 oz*

| | C | F | Cb |
|---|---|---|---|
| Mint Chocolate Chip | 770 | 42 | 95 |
| Peanut Butter Cup | 1060 | 60 | 95 |
| Strawberry Shortcake | 580 | 29 | 74 |
| **Novelties:** Brown Bonnet | 390 | 23 | 43 |
| Deluxe Flying Saucer with Sprinkles | 350 | 16 | 49 |
| Flying Saucer, Chocolate | 230 | 10 | 33 |
| *Classic Sundaes: Small* | | | |
| Caramel | 700 | 36 | 84 |
| Hot Fudge | 540 | 30 | 60 |
| Strawberry | 610 | 34 | 67 |
| *Beverages:* | | | |
| **Blended Drinks:** *Per Small, 16 fl.oz* | | | |
| Arctic Blender: Cookie Dough | 920 | 40 | 126 |
| Fried Ice Cream | 670 | 31 | 85 |
| Peanut Butter | 870 | 33 | 88 |
| Carvelanche: Butterfinger | 730 | 38 | 92 |
| M&M; Reese's, average | 755 | 39 | 87 |
| **Smoothies,** av. all flav.,16 fl.oz | 315 | 0 | 78 |
| **Thick Shake,** Strawberry | 600 | 31 | 70 |
| **Thick ShakeFloats:** Chocolate | 790 | 34 | 109 |
| Strawberry | 750 | 39 | 85 |
| Vanilla | 810 | 39 | 102 |

## Checkers®

**Same Menu & Data as Rally's ~ See Page 231**

## Cheesecake Factory® (Dec'11)

*10" Cheesecake: Per Slice*

| | C | F | Cb |
|---|---|---|---|
| Chocolate Raspberry Truffle | 1070 | n/a | 103 |
| Original: With Strawberries | 750 | n/a | 72 |
| Low Carb | 540 | n/a | 41 |
| Reeses P.B. Chocolate Cake | 1560 | n/a | 170 |
| *Small Plates & Snacks: Per Dish, As Served* | | | |
| Crispy Crab Bites | 360 | n/a | 11 |
| Sausage & Ricotta Flatbread | 460 | n/a | 35 |
| Vietnamese Tacos | 950 | n/a | 155 |
| *GlamBurgers & Sandwiches: Without Sides* | | | |
| Chicken Almond Salad | 1530 | n/a | 83 |
| Factory Burger | 780 | n/a | 64 |
| Portabella/Turkey Burger | 1265 | n/a | 60 |
| *Specialties: Per Dish, As Served* | | | |
| Famous Factory Meatloaf | 1810 | n/a | 127 |
| Lemon-Herb Roasted Chicken | 2100 | n/a | 72 |
| White Chicken Chile | 585 | n/a | 35 |
| *Salads: As Served, Includes Dressing* | | | |
| Herb-Crusted Salmon | 770 | n/a | 22 |
| Santa Fe Salad | 1700 | n/a | 97 |
| Skinnyliciouos Spicy Chicken | 440 | n/a | 42 |

## Charley's Grilled Subs® (Dec'11)

*Subs: Regular 7¾" Includes Standard Toppings, Without Sauce or Dressings Unless Indicated*

| | C | F | Cb |
|---|---|---|---|
| BBQ Cheddar, with Sauce | 580 | 20 | 68 |
| Bacon 3 Cheese Steak | 635 | 32 | 54 |
| Buffalo Chicken, with Sauce | 530 | 16 | 60 |
| Chicken Bacon Club | 570 | 25 | 53 |
| Chicken Cordon Blue | 570 | 18 | 54 |
| Chicken Teriyaki with Sauce | 520 | 16 | 58 |
| Italian Deli | 585 | 25 | 53 |
| Mushroom Swiss Steak | 520 | 19 | 57 |
| Philly Cheesesteak | 520 | 19 | 56 |
| Philly Chicken | 515 | 16 | 58 |
| Philly Ham & Swiss | 515 | 15 | 59 |
| Philly Steak Deluxe | 525 | 19 | 58 |
| Philly Veggie | 450 | 15 | 62 |
| Sicilian Steak | 640 | 31 | 54 |
| Turkey Cheddar Melt | 470 | 12 | 53 |
| Ultimate Club | 560 | 23 | 54 |
| *Salads: Cheese/Dressings not included* | | | |
| Chicken, Teriyaki; Buffalo, average | 210 | 7 | 13 |
| Fresh Garden Salad | 60 | 2 | 9 |
| Grilled Steak Salad | 210 | 10 | 10 |
| *Dressings,* Italian/Ranch, av., 1 oz | 150 | 16 | 1 |
| *Mayo,* 1 Tbsp., ½ oz | 100 | 11 | 0 |
| *Original Lemonade,* 8fl.oz | 85 | 0 | 20 |

**For Complete Menu & Data ~ see CalorieKing.com**

## Chevys Fresh Mex® (Dec'11)

*Sizzling Fajitas: As Served*

| | C | F | Cb |
|---|---|---|---|
| Original Famous Chicken | 930 | 32 | 95 |
| Sizzling Steak | 1030 | 46 | 94 |
| *Mesquite Grilled Tacos: As Served* | | | |
| Chicken | 1050 | 35 | 125 |
| Fish | 1060 | 39 | 125 |
| Steak | 1110 | 44 | 124 |
| *Fresh Mex Specialties: As Served* | | | |
| Chili Verde | 1030 | 44 | 113 |
| Crispy Chicken Flautas | 1510 | 76 | 156 |
| Red Chile Pork Taquitos | 1350 | 69 | 136 |
| *Signature Enchiladas: As Served* | | | |
| Chicken Mole | 950 | 51 | 84 |
| Chipotle Chicken | 1070 | 64 | 87 |
| Shrimp & Crab | 1360 | 97 | 87 |
| *Grande Salads: With Dressing Unless Indicated* | | | |
| Grilled Chicken Caesar | 860 | 69 | 32 |
| Grilled Fajita | 1585 | 128 | 70 |
| Santa Fe Chopped, w/o Dressing | 670 | 39 | 30 |
| Tostada without Dressing | 1680 | 115 | 105 |
| *Soup,* Tortilla, 1 bowl | 390 | 17 | 35 |
| *Tamalito,* Sweet Corn, (2) | 190 | 7 | 29 |
| *Tortilla,* El Machino, (2) | 140 | 4 | 22 |

Updated Nutrition Data ~ www.CalorieKing.com
Persons with Diabetes ~ See Disclaimer (Page 22)

## Chick-fil-A® (Dec'11)

| Chick-fil-A Sandwiches: W/o Sauce | C | F | Cb |
|---|---|---|---|
| Chargrilled Chicken | 290 | 4 | 36 |
| Chargrilled Chicken Club | 410 | 12 | 37 |
| Chicken Salad | 490 | 19 | 55 |
| *Cool Wraps: Without Dressing* | | | |
| Chargrilled Chicken | 410 | 12 | 50 |
| Chicken Caesar | 460 | 15 | 47 |
| Spicy Chicken | 410 | 12 | 48 |
| *Breakfast:* | | | |
| **Biscuits:** Chicken | 440 | 20 | 47 |
| Bacon, Egg & Cheese | 500 | 27 | 44 |
| Sausage Biscuit | 590 | 39 | 43 |
| **Burritos:** Chicken | 450 | 20 | 43 |
| Sausage | 510 | 28 | 40 |
| Chick-n-Minis, 1 box, 3 pieces | 280 | 10 | 30 |
| Chicken, Egg & Cheese Bagel | 490 | 20 | 49 |
| Cinnamon Cluster | 430 | 17 | 63 |
| Hash Browns, 2.7 oz | 270 | 18 | 25 |
| Oatmeal: Multigrain w/ toppings | 280 | 11 | 44 |
| Without toppings | 120 | 2.5 | 21 |
| Chargrilled Chicken & Fruit | 220 | 6 | 22 |
| Chargrilled Chicken Garden | 180 | 6 | 11 |
| Chick-n-Strips | 460 | 22 | 26 |
| Southwest Chargrilled Chicken | 240 | 9 | 18 |
| *Salad Dressings, Sauces & Condiments:* | | | |
| Garlic & Butter Croutons, ½ oz | 60 | 2 | 9 |
| Harvest Nut Granola, salad portion | 60 | 3 | 8 |
| Honey Rstd Sunfl. Knls, salad portion | 90 | 7 | 4 |
| Tortilla Strips,½ oz | 80 | 4 | 8 |
| **Dressings:** Blue Cheese, 1 oz | 160 | 16 | 1 |
| Buttermilk Ranch; Caesar, 1 oz | 160 | 17 | 1 |
| Light Italian, 1 oz | 15 | 1 | 2 |
| Thousand Island, 1 oz | 150 | 14 | 5 |
| **Sauces:** BBQ; Honey Mustard, 1 oz | 45 | 0 | 11 |
| Buffalo, ¾ oz | 10 | 0 | 1 |
| Buttermilk Ranch, ¾ oz | 110 | 12 | 1 |
| Chick-fil-A, 1 oz | 140 | 13 | 6 |
| Honey Roasted BBQ, ½ oz | 60 | 5 | 2 |
| *Sides:* Carrot & Raisin Salad, 9 oz | 390 | 18 | 60 |
| Chicken Salad Cup, 6 oz | 350 | 22 | 9 |
| Cole Slaw, 10½ oz | 580 | 50 | 31 |
| Side Salad w/o Crtons or Dress., 4 oz | 70 | 4.5 | 5 |
| **Waffle Potato Fries:** Small | 300 | 16 | 36 |
| Medium | 390 | 21 | 47 |
| Large | 520 | 27 | 62 |
| Desserts: | | | |
| Cheesecake, 3¼ oz | 310 | 23 | 22 |
| Fudge Nut Brownie, 3oz | 370 | 19 | 45 |
| Lemon Pie, 1 slice, 4¼ oz | 360 | 13 | 58 |
| **Icedream Cone,** w/o Toppings | 170 | 4 | 31 |
| *Milkshake,* Chocolate, 18¼ oz | 750 | 28 | 113 |

## Chili's® (Dec'11)

| Appetizers: As Served | C | F | Cb |
|---|---|---|---|
| Bottomless Tostada Chips w/ Salsa | 1020 | 51 | 125 |
| Crispy Onion Str. & Jalap. Stack/Ranch | 1050 | 81 | 71 |
| Classic Nachos: Beef (12) | 1720 | 108 | 86 |
| Chicken (12) | 1670 | 103 | 83 |
| Skillet Queso with Tostada Chips | 1710 | 101 | 147 |
| Sthwestern Eggrolls w/ Avoc. Ranch | 780 | 41 | 81 |
| Triple Dipper: Big Mouth Bites w/ Ranch | 850 | 58 | 51 |
| Boneless Buffalo Wings, w/ Dress. | 810 | 54 | 43 |
| Chicken Crispers w/out Dressing | 340 | 15 | 21 |
| Hot Spin. & Artichoke Dip with Chips | 1290 | 77 | 128 |
| *Burgers: As Served, On white Bun with Fries* | | | |
| Big Mouth Bites with Ranch | 2120 | 133 | 163 |
| Classic Bacon Burger | 1570 | 91 | 125 |
| Jalapeno Smokehouse with Ranch | 2210 | 144 | 136 |
| *Chicken, Seafood & Pasta: As Served* | | | |
| **Cajun Pasta:** | | | |
| With Grilled Chicken | 1500 | 76 | 124 |
| With Shrimp | 1480 | 81 | 125 |
| **Chicken:** | | | |
| Chkn Crispers w/ Hon. Mustard | 1350 | 68 | 129 |
| Margarita Grilled Chicken | 550 | 14 | 62 |
| Monterey Chicken | 890 | 48 | 51 |
| *Southwest Grill:* | | | |
| **Fajitas:** *Without Tortillas & Condiments* | | | |
| Beef | 390 | 14 | 27 |
| Chicken | 360 | 10 | 24 |
| Trio | 530 | 20 | 30 |
| + Condiments only (1) | 230 | 19 | 7 |
| + Flour Tortillas only (3) | 390 | 10 | 63 |
| **Quesadillas:** *As Served* | | | |
| Bacon Ranch Chicken | 1650 | 107 | 96 |
| Bacon Ranch Steak | 1680 | 111 | 98 |
| **Steaks:** *As Served* | | | |
| Classic Sirloin, 8 oz | 1010 | 60 | 59 |
| Country-Fried Steak | 1270 | 71 | 120 |
| Flame-Grilled Ribeye, 12 oz | 1570 | 116 | 57 |
| *In-House Slow Smoked Ribs: Full Rack, As Served* | | | |
| Original | 2170 | 123 | 137 |
| Memphis Dry Rub | 1990 | 111 | 137 |
| Shiner Bock BBQ | 2310 | 123 | 168 |
| *Salads: Large, Includes Dressing* | | | |
| Boneless Buffalo Chicken | 990 | 68 | 48 |
| Carribean with Grilled Shrimp | 620 | 31 | 66 |
| Quesadilla Explosion | 1400 | 89 | 90 |
| *Sweet Endings: Per Slice* | | | |
| Cheesecake | 710 | 42 | 68 |
| Chocolate Chip Paradise Pie | 1250 | 64 | 163 |
| Molten Chocolate Cake | 1020 | 46 | 144 |

*For Complete Menu & Data ~ see CalorieKing.com*

## Chipotle® (Dec'11)

| Breads: | C | F | Cb |
|---|---|---|---|
| Crispy Taco Shells (3) | 180 | 6 | 27 |
| Flour Tortillas (Burrito), (1) | 290 | 9 | 44 |
| Flour Tortillas (Taco), (3) | 270 | 8 | 39 |
| *Meal Components:* | | | |
| Barbacoa, 4 oz | 170 | 7 | 2 |
| Black Beans, 4 oz | 120 | 1 | 23 |
| Carnitas, 4 oz | 190 | 8 | 1 |
| Cheese, 1 oz | 100 | 9 | 0 |
| Chicken, 4 oz | 190 | 6.5 | 1 |
| Cilantro-Lime Rice, 3 oz | 130 | 3 | 23 |
| Lettuce, 1 oz | 5 | 0 | 0 |
| Pinto Beans, 4 oz | 120 | 1 | 22 |
| Steak, 4 oz | 190 | 7 | 2 |
| *Condiments:* | | | |
| Salsa: Corn, 3½ oz | 80 | 1.5 | 15 |
| Green Tomatillo, 2 oz | 15 | 0 | 3 |
| Red Tomatillo, 2 oz | 40 | 1 | 8 |
| Tomato, 3½ oz | 20 | 0 | 4 |
| Sour Cream, 2 oz | 120 | 10 | 2 |
| Vinaigrette, 2 fl.oz | 260 | 25 | 12 |
| *Extras:* Chips, serving, 4 oz | 570 | 27 | 73 |
| Guacamole, 3½ oz | 150 | 13 | 8 |

## Chuck E. Cheese® (Dec'11)

| Appetizers: *Includes Condiments* | C | F | Cb |
|---|---|---|---|
| Buffalo Wings (12) | 900 | 60 | 48 |
| Italian Bread Stick (1) | 175 | 9 | 18 |
| Mozzarella Stick (1) | 95 | 6 | 6 |
| *Pizzas: Per Medium Slice* | | | |
| BBQ Chicken | 185 | 6 | 24 |
| Cheese | 155 | 5 | 21 |
| Super Combo | 185 | 8 | 22 |
| Veggie Combo | 160 | 6 | 22 |
| *Oven Baked Sandwiches:* | | | |
| Ham & Cheese | 685 | 27 | 79 |
| Italian Sub | 790 | 39 | 78 |
| Roasted Chicken Ciabatta | 715 | 28 | 80 |
| *French Fries:* | | | |
| With Ketchup & Ranch: 4 oz | 420 | 20 | 55 |
| 8 oz | 840 | 40 | 110 |
| *Hot Dog,* with Mustard & Relish | 310 | 19 | 35 |
| *Desserts:* Apple Dessert Pizza, 1 sl. | 190 | 5 | 33 |
| Chocolate Cake (8"), 1 slice | 290 | 13 | 41 |
| Cinnamon Stick, w/ Toppings (1) | 70 | 2 | 11 |

## Church's Chicken® (Dec'11)

| Chicken: *Per Serving* | C | F | Cb |
|---|---|---|---|
| **Original:** Breast, 1 piece | 200 | 11 | 3 |
| Leg, 1 piece | 110 | 6 | 3 |
| Thigh, 1 piece | 330 | 23 | 8 |
| Wing, 1 piece | 300 | 18 | 7 |
| **Spicy:** Breast, 1 piece | 320 | 20 | 12 |
| Leg, 1 piece | 180 | 11 | 8 |
| Thigh, 1 piece | 480 | 35 | 20 |
| Wing, 1 piece | 430 | 27 | 17 |
| **Tender Strips:** 1 piece | 120 | 6 | 6 |
| Spicy, 1 piece | 140 | 7 | 7 |
| *Sides: Per Regular Serving* | | | |
| Cajun Rice, 6 oz | 130 | 7 | 16 |
| Cole Slaw, 4.15 oz | 155 | 10 | 15 |
| Corn on the Cob (1) | 140 | 3 | 24 |
| French Fries, 3½ oz | 280 | 12 | 40 |
| Honey Butter Biscuits (1), 2.1 oz | 240 | 12 | 28 |
| Jalapeno Cheese Bombers (4), 2.8 oz | 160 | 8 | 20 |
| Macaroni & Cheese, 6 oz | 190 | 7 | 24 |
| Mashed Potatoes & Gravy, 6 oz | 110 | 2 | 21 |
| Okra, 3½ oz | 300 | 19 | 31 |
| *Sauces: Per Packet* | | | |
| BBQ; Sweet & Sour | 25 | 0 | 6 |
| Creamy Jalapeno | 80 | 9 | 1 |
| Honey Mustard | 90 | 9 | 3 |
| Ketchup | 15 | 0 | 4 |
| Ranch | 100 | 10 | 1 |

## Cici's Pizza® (Dec'11)

| Buffet: *Per ⅒ of 12" Pizza* | C | F | Cb |
|---|---|---|---|
| Alfredo | 120 | 3.5 | 18 |
| Bar-B-Que | 150 | 2.5 | 25 |
| Beef | 150 | 4 | 20 |
| Cheese | 150 | 4 | 19 |
| Ham & Pineapple | 150 | 3.5 | 21 |
| Pepperoni & Jalapeno | 150 | 4.5 | 20 |
| Sausage | 140 | 5 | 20 |
| Spinach Alfredo | 120 | 3.5 | 19 |
| Zesty Ham & Cheddar | 120 | 4 | 19 |
| *To-Go: Per ⅒ of 15" Pizza* | | | |
| Alfredo | 170 | 6 | 23 |
| Bar-B-Que | 240 | 6 | 36 |
| Beef | 190 | 8 | 24 |
| Pepperoni & Jalapeno | 210 | 7 | 24 |
| Sausage | 220 | 8 | 25 |
| Spinach Alfredo | 170 | 6 | 23 |
| Zesty Ham & Cheddar | 160 | 7 | 23 |
| Zesty Pepperoni | 170 | 9 | 23 |

Updated Nutrition Data ~ www.CalorieKing.com
Persons with Diabetes ~ See Disclaimer (Page 22)

## Cinnabon® (Dec '11)

| | C | F | Cb |
|---|---|---|---|
| **Baked Goods:** Cinnabon Bites (6) | 620 | 24 | 88 |
| Caramel Pecanbon (1) | 1080 | 50 | 147 |
| Bites (6) | 800 | 39 | 100 |
| Classic Cinnabon (1) | 880 | 36 | 127 |
| Stix (5) | 390 | 21 | 46 |
| **Sweet Roll Icing,** Frosting Cup, 1.4 oz | 180 | 11 | 20 |

## Claim Jumper® (Dec '11)

| | C | F | Cb |
|---|---|---|---|
| **Appetizers:** As Served | | | |
| Southwest Eggrolls | 1165 | 50 | 114 |
| Three Cheese Potatocakes (3) | 1140 | 73 | 90 |
| **Burgers & Sandwiches:** Without Sides | | | |
| Grilled Cobb Sandwich | 1210 | 78 | 78 |
| Widow Maker Burger | 1150 | 65 | 79 |
| **Meals:** Per Whole Dish, Unless Indicated | | | |
| **Favorites:** Country Fried Steak | 2030 | 107 | 189 |
| Giant Stuffed Baker | 990 | 34 | 118 |
| Meatloaf & Mashed Potatoes | 1300 | 75 | 117 |
| **Pasta/Pizza:** | | | |
| Grilled Chicken Pasta | 1400 | 94 | 93 |
| Margherita Pizza | 1095 | 54 | 104 |
| **Specialties:** Without Sides | | | |
| BBQ Baby Back Pork Ribs, Full Rack | 1745 | 111 | 111 |
| Roasted Tri-Tip | 800 | 47 | 19 |
| **Seafood:** Fish & Chips with Sauce | 1405 | 69 | 148 |
| Lobster Tail Dinner | 595 | 46 | 16 |
| **Entree Salads:** Without Dressing Or Bread | | | |
| Californian Citrus Chkn, Charbrolied | 1480 | 71 | 139 |
| Seared Ahi Spinach | 570 | 30 | 28 |
| **Soups:** Per Bowl | | | |
| Potato Cheddar | 710 | 61 | 31 |
| New England Clam Chowder | 525 | 45 | 23 |
| **Desserts:** Choc. Motherlode Cake | 2770 | 144 | 340 |
| Lemon Bar Brulee | 860 | 40 | 113 |
| *For Complete Menu & Data ~ see CalorieKing.com* | | | |

## Coldstone Creamery® (Dec '11)

| | C | F | Cb |
|---|---|---|---|
| **Ice Creams:** | | | |
| **Amaretto:** Like it | 330 | 20 | 33 |
| Love it | 530 | 31 | 53 |
| Gotta have it | 790 | 47 | 80 |
| **Sorbet:** Average all flavors | | | |
| Like it | 155 | 0 | 38 |
| Love it | 250 | 0 | 62 |
| Gotta have it | 370 | 0 | 93 |

## Cosi® (Dec '11)

| | C | F | Cb |
|---|---|---|---|
| **Flatbread Pizza:** Individual | | | |
| Original Crust: Margherita | 740 | 27 | 90 |
| Pepperoni | 850 | 37 | 90 |
| Traditional Cheese | 710 | 24 | 90 |

## Cosi® cont... (Dec '11)

| | C | F | Cb |
|---|---|---|---|
| **Melts:** With Rustic Bread | | | |
| Chicken TBM | 695 | 31 | 49 |
| Pesto Chicken | 640 | 27 | 48 |
| Steakhouse Gorgonzola | 750 | 47 | 49 |
| Tuna Melt | 860 | 40 | 52 |
| **Sandwiches:** With Rustic Bread | | | |
| Buffalo Bleu | 565 | 25 | 47 |
| Fire Roasted Veggie | 330 | 9 | 51 |
| Italiano | 780 | 42 | 49 |
| TBM | 595 | 35 | 47 |
| **Soup:** Per 5 oz Bowl, w/o Flatbread | | | |
| Pollo e Pasta | 70 | 2 | 7 |
| Tomato Basil Aurora | 205 | 18 | 9 |
| **Salads:** Includes Dressing | | | |
| Cosi Cobb, 14 oz | 720 | 55 | 18 |
| Greek Salad, 14 oz | 515 | 47 | 19 |
| Signature Salad, 12.8 oz | 620 | 45 | 46 |
| Tuscan Steak, 14.9 oz | 540 | 34 | 27 |

## Costco Food Court® (Dec '11)

| | C | F | Cb |
|---|---|---|---|
| **Pizza:** Per Slice | | | |
| Combo, 11oz | 680 | 29 | 72 |
| Cheese, 10 oz | 700 | 28 | 70 |
| Pepperoni , 9 oz | 620 | 24 | 68 |
| **Dogs,** average, 8¼ oz | 570 | 33 | 46 |
| **Salad:** Chicken Caesar, 20½ oz, with dressing | 670 | 40 | 35 |
| **Meals:** Carne Asada Bake, 14½ oz | 740 | 26 | 78 |
| Cheese Burger Fry Combo | 860 | 45 | 72 |
| Chicken Asada Bake, 12¾ oz | 770 | 25 | 78 |
| Chicken Bake 12¾ oz | 770 | 25 | 78 |
| Ital. Sausage Sandwich, 12½ oz | 700 | 42 | 46 |
| **Beverages:** Hot Latte, 9½ fl oz | 190 | 5 | 24 |
| Hot Mocha, 11¼ fl oz | 310 | 9 | 45 |
| Mocha Freeze, 16¼ fl .oz | 320 | 7 | 49 |
| Latte Freeze, 15½ fl.oz | 240 | 7 | 32 |
| **Smoothie,** Fruit Smoothie, 16 fl.oz | 290 | 0 | 72 |
| **Desserts:** Ice cream Bar, 8 oz | 870 | 65 | 60 |
| Berry Sundae, 12¼ oz | 410 | 0 | 87 |
| Pistachio Gelato, 7¾ oz | 480 | 13 | 82 |
| Yogurt, 12 oz | 390 | 0 | 82 |

## Cousins Subs® (Dec '11)

| | C | F | Cb |
|---|---|---|---|
| **Subs:** Per 7½" With Italian Bread | | | |
| BLT with Mayo | 590 | 38 | 47 |
| Cheese Steak | 505 | 19 | 49 |
| Chicken Cheddar Deluxe w/ Mayo | 670 | 39 | 51 |
| Club with Mayo | 645 | 35 | 51 |
| Double Cheese Steak | 745 | 36 | 49 |
| Garden Provolone | 550 | 29 | 51 |
| Italian Special with Dressing | 815 | 51 | 50 |
| Philly Cheese Steak with Sauce | 530 | 19 | 55 |

*Continued Next Page ...*

# Fast - Foods & Restaurants

## Cousins Subs® cont... (Dec '11)

### 7½" Subs (cont)

| | C | F | Cb |
|---|---|---|---|
| Roast Beef with Mayo | 605 | 30 | 50 |
| Tuna with Mayo Blend | 670 | 40 | 49 |
| Turkey Breast with Mayo | 530 | 28 | 50 |

### Better Bunch, 7½ Mini Subs: W/o Mayo & Cheese

| | C | F | Cb |
|---|---|---|---|
| Club | 370 | 5 | 51 |
| Garden | 265 | 2 | 50 |
| Ham; Turkey Breast, average | 330 | 3.5 | 50 |
| *French Fries:* Small, 2¾ oz | 250 | 13 | 30 |
| Medium, 4 oz | 365 | 19 | 43 |
| Large, 5¼ oz | 485 | 25 | 57 |

### Salads: Without Dressing

| | | | |
|---|---|---|---|
| Chef Salad | 325 | 14 | 25 |
| Italian | 405 | 24 | 24 |
| Tuna Salad | 625 | 46 | 23 |

*For Complete Nutritional Data ~ see CalorieKing.com*

## Culver's® (Dec '11)

### Butter Burgers:

| | C | F | Cb |
|---|---|---|---|
| Original: Single; Kids | 345 | 15 | 36 |
| Double | 485 | 23 | 37 |
| Triple | 620 | 31 | 38 |
| Cheddar with Bacon, Single | 540 | 32 | 31 |
| Cheese: Single | 425 | 21 | 38 |
| Double | 625 | 35 | 39 |
| Culver's Bacon Deluxe: Single | 595 | 39 | 35 |
| Double | 790 | 53 | 35 |
| Culver's Deluxe: Single | 515 | 32 | 35 |
| Double | 710 | 46 | 35 |
| Mushroom & Swiss, Single | 430 | 23 | 33 |
| Sourdough Melt, Single | 415 | 20 | 33 |
| *Corn Dog,* Kids | 260 | 14 | 26 |
| *Chicken Tenders,* 4 pieces | 440 | 20 | 32 |
| *Hot Dog:* Regular (1) | 465 | 26 | 47 |
| Kids (1) | 440 | 26 | 39 |

### Sides:

| | | | |
|---|---|---|---|
| **Crinkle Cut Fries:** Kids | 275 | 12 | 38 |
| Regular | 385 | 17 | 53 |
| Large | 495 | 22 | 68 |
| **Chili Cheddar Fries,** 8¾ oz | 605 | 29 | 72 |
| **Mashed Potatoes,** with Gravy | 140 | 2 | 26 |
| **Wisconsin Cheese Curds,** 6½ oz | 670 | 38 | 54 |
| *Sandwiches:* Beef Pot Roast | 365 | 16 | 33 |
| Crispy Chicken Filet | 580 | 34 | 50 |
| Flame Roasted Chicken | 310 | 8 | 36 |
| Grilled Reuben Melt | 590 | 30 | 42 |
| North Atlantic Cod Filet | 665 | 40 | 47 |
| Pork Tenderloin (Breaded) | 600 | 29 | 63 |
| Shaved Prime Rib | 505 | 28 | 35 |
| Turkey Sourdough BLT | 560 | 31 | 36 |

## Culver's® cont... (Dec '11)

### Dinner Plates: Per Serving

| | C | F | Cb |
|---|---|---|---|
| Beef Pot Roast | 745 | 36 | 73 |
| Butterfly Jumbo Shrimp, 6 pieces | 1320 | 67 | 152 |
| Chopped Steak | 850 | 49 | 63 |
| Fried Chicken: 2 pieces | 1790 | 99 | 141 |
| 4 Pieces | 2220 | 121 | 159 |
| North Atlantic Cod, Fried, 2 pieces | 1865 | 121 | 136 |

### Salads: Without Dressing

| | | | |
|---|---|---|---|
| Chicken Cashew w/ Flame Rstd Chkn | 445 | 24 | 19 |
| Classic Caesar w/ Flame Roasted Chkn | 340 | 16 | 14 |
| Garden Fresco | 230 | 10 | 19 |
| Side Caesar | 55 | 2 | 5 |
| Side Salad | 60 | 2 | 6 |

### Desserts:

| | | | |
|---|---|---|---|
| **Frozen Custard:** Chocolate, 1 scoop | 295 | 14 | 35 |
| Vanilla, 1 scoop | 310 | 18 | 30 |
| **Concrete Mixers:** *Per Medium* | | | |
| Chocolate | 995 | 49 | 122 |
| Turtle | 1155 | 71 | 114 |
| *Sundaes:* Per 2 Scoops | | | |
| Banana Split | 1085 | 64 | 115 |
| Fudge Pecan | 980 | 62 | 94 |
| *Beverages:* Choc. Malt, medium | 970 | 45 | 122 |
| Chocolate Shake, medium | 910 | 44 | 114 |
| Root Beer Float, medium | 550 | 18 | 90 |

## D'Angelo's® (Dec '11)

**Sandwiches:** *Based on Honey Wheat Bread with Standard Toppings*

### Subs: Per Medium Size

| | C | F | Cb |
|---|---|---|---|
| Cheeseburger | 870 | 40 | 67 |
| Chicken Stir Fry | 740 | 19 | 78 |
| Classic Veggie | 650 | 24 | 80 |
| Roast Beef | 490 | 8 | 67 |
| Turkey Breast | 500 | 5 | 65 |

### Pokkets: Per Plain Pokket With Standard Toppings

| | | | |
|---|---|---|---|
| Cheeseburger | 530 | 24 | 39 |
| Caesar Salad | 650 | 39 | 57 |
| Lobster | 510 | 25 | 38 |
| Steak & Cheese | 530 | 24 | 37 |

### Wraps: Per Small White Wrap with Standard Toppings

| | | | |
|---|---|---|---|
| Buffalo Chicken Salad | 830 | 45 | 66 |
| Caesar Salad | 790 | 48 | 72 |
| Chicken Caesar Salad | 930 | 51 | 74 |
| Chicken Cobb | 1070 | 66 | 71 |
| Greek | 810 | 54 | 60 |
| Turkey Club | 660 | 30 | 52 |
| *Grilled Quesadillas:* Number 9 | 370 | 19 | 31 |
| Chicken Stir Fry | 350 | 14 | 32 |
| Veggie | 280 | 13 | 33 |

### Salads: Entree Size, Includes Pokket Bread

| | | | |
|---|---|---|---|
| Caesar with dressing | 800 | 53 | 62 |
| Chicken Caesar with dressing | 940 | 56 | 64 |

*For Complete Menu & Data ~ see CalorieKing.com*

## Dairy Queen® (Dec '11)

*Burgers & Sandwiches:*

| | C | F | Cb |
|---|---|---|---|
| **GrillBurgers:** | | | |
| Bacon Cheese, ¼ lb | 630 | 37 | 44 |
| ½ lb Burger | 710 | 44 | 43 |
| ½ lb Flame Thrower | 1010 | 73 | 41 |
| Bacon Doublel Cheeseburger | 720 | 41 | 34 |
| Cheeseburger | 400 | 18 | 34 |
| Hamburger | 350 | 14 | 33 |
| Double | 540 | 26 | 33 |
| **Sandwiches:** Crispy Chicken | 560 | 27 | 47 |
| Grilled Chicken | 370 | 16 | 32 |
| *Baskets:* | | | |
| Chkn Strips: 4 piece with Gravy | 1360 | 63 | 103 |
| 6 piece, with Country Gravy | 1640 | 74 | 121 |
| Iron Grilled Chicken Quesadilla | 1210 | 60 | 115 |
| *Hot Dogs:* Beef | 290 | 17 | 22 |
| With Chili & Cheese | 380 | 24 | 23 |
| *Salads: With Dressing* | | | |
| Crispy Chicken | 510 | 24 | 30 |
| Grilled Chicken | 330 | 16 | 14 |
| *Sides:* | | | |
| **DQ French Fries,** Regular, 4 oz | 310 | 13 | 43 |
| **DQ Onion Rings,** Regular, 4 oz | 360 | 16 | 47 |
| *Desserts: Per Medium* | | | |
| **Blizzard Treats:** Banana Cream Pie | 770 | 28 | 117 |
| Butterfinger | 740 | 26 | 114 |
| Cappuccino Heath | 870 | 9 | 122 |
| Cookie Dough | 1020 | 40 | 148 |
| Oreo Cookies | 680 | 25 | 100 |
| Reese's Peanut Butter Cups | 760 | 31 | 101 |
| Strawberry CheeseQuake | 690 | 28 | 92 |
| **DQ Blizzard Cakes (10"):** *Per ⅒ Cake* | | | |
| Oreo | 760 | 33 | 104 |
| Reese's Peanut Butter Cup | 730 | 34 | 93 |
| Strawberry CheeseQuake | 610 | 27 | 79 |
| **DQ Dipped Cones:** *Per Medium Cone* | | | |
| Butterscotch | 470 | 21 | 62 |
| Chocolate | 470 | 22 | 61 |
| **DQ Sundaes:** *Per Medium, 8¼ oz* | | | |
| Caramel | 430 | 11 | 74 |
| Hot Fudge | 440 | 15 | 67 |
| Strawberry | 350 | 10 | 56 |
| *Malts: Per Medium, With Whipped Topping* | | | |
| Caramel | 840 | 26 | 134 |
| Chocolate | 800 | 27 | 130 |
| Strawberry | 710 | 24 | 107 |
| *Moo Latte: Per Medium, With Whipped Topping* | | | |
| Cappuccino | 570 | 19 | 84 |
| French Vanilla | 630 | 19 | 101 |
| Mocha | 660 | 25 | 96 |

*For Complete Nutritional Data ~ see CalorieKing.com*

## Daphne's Greek Cafe® (Dec '11)

*Starters:*

| | C | F | Cb |
|---|---|---|---|
| Original Hummus & Original Pita | 330 | 17 | 37 |
| Fire Feta & Original Pita | 335 | 19 | 31 |
| *Pita Sandwiches: Without Fries, Rice or Salad* | | | |
| Crispy Shrimp | 430 | 23 | 39 |
| **Fire Roasted Vegetables** | 380 | 20 | 33 |
| Fresh Carved Gyros | 665 | 46 | 42 |
| Grilled Chicken | 480 | 18 | 33 |
| *Plates: Without Sides, Pita Bread or Tzatziki* | | | |
| **Mix & Match:** *Choose any Two* | | | |
| Falafel | 200 | 15 | 14 |
| Fresh-Carved Gyros | 300 | 25 | 7 |
| Grilled Chicken Kabob | 160 | 4 | 3 |
| Grilled Steak Kabob | 220 | 11 | 9 |
| Grilled Salmon | 330 | 19 | 0 |
| *Classic Greek Salads: Without Dressing* | | | |
| Crispy Shrimp | 360 | 16 | 20 |
| Falafel | 650 | 42 | 54 |
| Grilled Chicken | 365 | 11 | 14 |
| *Dressings:* Classic Greek | 105 | 12 | 2 |
| Lite Greek | 60 | 6 | 2 |
| *Sides:* Fire Roasted Vegetables | 60 | 4 | 0 |
| Fries | 270 | 12 | 37 |
| Muligrain Pita Chips | 170 | 4.5 | 27 |
| Original Pita Bread | 230 | 8 | 28 |
| Seasoned Rice Pilaf | 240 | 5 | 45 |
| Tabouli Salad | 80 | 1 | 17 |

## Davanni's® (Dec '11)

*Half Hoagies: Includes 6" White Bun, Cheese, Salad, Butter, Dressing, Mayo & Sauce*

| | C | F | Cb |
|---|---|---|---|
| Assorted | 490 | 30 | 39 |
| BLT | 645 | 44 | 40 |
| Chicken & Bacon with Honey Mustard | 530 | 24 | 47 |
| Chicken Parmigiana | 485 | 18 | 41 |
| Club | 495 | 27 | 40 |
| Italian Sausage | 620 | 38 | 46 |
| Pastrami | 540 | 27 | 40 |
| Southwestern Chicken | 565 | 28 | 44 |
| Three Cheese | 525 | 33 | 39 |
| Tuna Melt | 645 | 44 | 42 |
| Turkey | 455 | 24 | 39 |
| Turkey Bacon Chipotle | 565 | 33 | 39 |
| Veggie | 445 | 24 | 43 |
| *Calzones:* Sausage, Peppers & On. | 920 | 50 | 83 |
| Pepperoni Sausage | 960 | 56 | 80 |
| *Pizzas: Per Slice* | | | |
| **5 Meat:** Thin Crust | 520 | 33 | 20 |
| Traditional Crust | 565 | 33 | 30 |
| Solo, Thin Crust | 1115 | 69 | 47 |
| **The Works:** Thin Crust | 285 | 16 | 19 |
| Traditional Crust | 330 | 16 | 29 |
| **Veggie:** Thin Crust | 240 | 12 | 19 |
| Traditional Crust | 285 | 12 | 29 |

# Fast - Foods & *Restaurants*

## Del Taco® (Dec '11)

| Breakfast: | C | F | Cb |
|---|---|---|---|
| Breakfast Burrito | 280 | 13 | 28 |
| Bacon & Egg Quesadilla | 430 | 20 | 37 |
| Egg & Cheese Burrito | 400 | 17 | 22 |
| Steak & Egg Burrito | 520 | 23 | 22 |
| Hash Brown Sticks (5) | 215 | 15 | 18 |
| *Burgers:* Cheeseburger | 430 | 22 | 40 |
| Double Del Cheeseburger | 720 | 48 | 40 |
| Triple Del Cheeseburger | 950 | 66 | 40 |
| **Burritos:** | | | |
| Del Beef | 470 | 19 | 24 |
| Del Classic Chicken | 475 | 31 | 23 |
| Deluxe Combo | 515 | 17 | 50 |
| Deluxe Del Beef | 475 | 21 | 26 |
| Half Pound Red/Green, average | 440 | 9 | 54 |
| Macho Beef | 1010 | 44 | 82 |
| Macho Chicken | 920 | 32 | 109 |
| Macho Combo | 990 | 36 | 110 |
| Shredded Beef Combo | 500 | 20 | 47 |
| Spicy Chicken; Veggie Works, av. | 615 | 14 | 83 |
| *Nachos:* 4 oz | 370 | 22 | 28 |
| Del, 7¼ oz | 440 | 23 | 45 |
| **Quesadillas:** | | | |
| Cheddar; Spicy Jack | 480 | 25 | 37 |
| Chicken Cheddar; Spicy Jack Chicken | 570 | 30 | 40 |
| *Tacos:* Big Fat Chicken | 330 | 14 | 34 |
| Big Fat Steak | 390 | 18 | 33 |
| Chicken Del Carbon | 150 | 4 | 19 |
| Chicken, Soft | 220 | 12 | 16 |
| Classic | 200 | 12 | 10 |
| Crispy Fish | 300 | 17 | 29 |
| Macho | 300 | 17 | 16 |
| Steak Taco Del Carbon | 210 | 8 | 18 |
| *Salad,* Deluxe Taco Salad | 845 | 47 | 69 |
| *Sides:* Chips & Salsa, 3 oz | 140 | 8 | 15 |
| **Fries:** Small, 5 oz | 260 | 15 | 28 |
| Macho, 10 oz | 515 | 30 | 56 |
| Chili Cheese, 10½ oz | 550 | 32 | 42 |
| Deluxe Chili Cheese, 12 oz | 590 | 35 | 44 |
| **Nachos,** Macho, 17 oz | 1000 | 56 | 94 |
| *Premium Shakes: Per 16 oz* | | | |
| Chocolate | 560 | 11 | 105 |
| Strawberry | 520 | 10 | 95 |
| Vanilla | 520 | 11 | 94 |

## Denny's® (Dec '11)

| Breakfast: *Without Sides* | C | F | Cb |
|---|---|---|---|
| **Favorites:** Banana Pecan Pancake, 17 oz | 780 | 15 | 55 |
| Country Fried Steak & Eggs, 11 oz | 660 | 43 | 29 |
| Moons Over My Hammy, 13 oz | 760 | 41 | 51 |
| Sthwest Steak Burrito w/ Hash | 1120 | 63 | 101 |
| T-Bone Steak & Eggs, 16 oz | 780 | 36 | 4 |
| **Omelettes:** Fit Fare, 16 oz | 390 | 18 | 25 |
| Ultimate, 12 oz | 620 | 48 | 8 |
| Veggie-Cheese, 13 oz | 460 | 33 | 9 |
| Western, 16 oz | 700 | 46 | 32 |
| **Scrambles:** Heartland, 21 oz | 1160 | 63 | 110 |
| Meat Lovers, 21 oz | 1140 | 63 | 94 |
| **Skillets:** Prime Rib, 21 oz | 850 | 46 | 64 |
| Santa Fe, 14 oz | 710 | 52 | 30 |
| Ultimate, 15 oz | 740 | 56 | 34 |
| **Slams:** All American, 10 oz | 800 | 68 | 5 |
| Fit Slam, 15 oz | 390 | 12 | 46 |
| French Toast, 15 oz | 780 | 58 | 35 |
| Lumberjack, 15 oz | 960 | 50 | 80 |
| **Sides:** Buttermilk Biscuit (1) | 190 | 9 | 24 |
| English Muffin, w/o Margarine, (1) | 130 | 1 | 25 |
| Hash Browns, 5 oz | 210 | 12 | 26 |
| Oatmeal, with milk, 13 oz | 370 | 5 | 74 |
| *Pancakes: Without Margarine, Syrup or Toppings* | | | |
| Buttermilk, 2 cakes | 330 | 4 | 67 |
| Hearty Wheat, 2 cakes | 310 | 1.5 | 64 |
| Toppings: Caramel, 1.5 oz | 190 | 1 | 44 |
| Cherry, 2 oz | 55 | 0 | 14 |
| Chocolate, 1.5 oz | 100 | 0 | 9 |
| Fudge, 1.5 oz | 150 | 6 | 23 |
| *Burgers & Sandwiches: Without Sides* | | | |
| **Burgers:** | | | |
| Bacon Cheddar, 15 oz | 880 | 49 | 45 |
| Bacon Slamburger, 15 oz | 1010 | 58 | 47 |
| Chkn Ranch Melt, w/o dress, 13 oz | 910 | 52 | 76 |
| Double Cheeseburger, 23 oz | 1400 | 87 | 49 |
| Mushroom Swiss, 18 oz | 860 | 48 | 41 |
| Prime Rib Philly Melt, 13 oz | 670 | 36 | 52 |
| Spicy Buffalo Chicken Melt, 15 oz | 860 | 48 | 76 |
| Veggie Burger with dressing | 540 | 13 | 76 |
| **Sandwiches:** BLT, 7 oz | 520 | 35 | 35 |
| Chkn Avoc. w/ Fit Fare Veges, 15 oz | 520 | 16 | 48 |
| Club, 11 oz | 630 | 33 | 55 |
| Hickory Grilled Chkn w/ dressing | 900 | 47 | 67 |
| The Super Bird, 11 oz | 610 | 29 | 54 |

Updated Nutrition Data ~ www.CalorieKing.com
Persons with Diabetes ~ See Disclaimer (Page 22)

## Denny's® cont... (Dec '11)

| *Let's Get Cheesy:* | C | F | Cb |
|---|---|---|---|
| Big Chse Ctry Fried Steak & Eggs, 18 oz | 1210 | 84 | 53 |
| Cheese Please Omelette, 16 oz | 800 | 57 | 34 |
| Cheesy Breakfast Sampler, 13 oz | 710 | 50 | 29 |
| Mac'n Chse Big Daddy Patty Melt, 21 oz | 1690 | 99 | 126 |
| Say Cheese Sizzlin' Skillet, 22 oz | 1120 | 84 | 41 |
| Winner Winner Cheesy Dinner, 22 oz | 1520 | 101 | 77 |

| *Dinners:* | | | |
|---|---|---|---|
| **American Classics:** *With Bread, Without Sides* | | | |
| Chicken Strips, 10 oz | 760 | 29 | 84 |
| Lemon Pepper Tilapia, 13 oz | 800 | 35 | 59 |
| Mushroom Swiss Steak, | | | |
| with Toppings & Gravy, 16 oz | 1080 | 75 | 34 |
| T-Bone Steak: 12 oz | 820 | 35 | 24 |
| With Breaded Shrimp, 13 oz | 900 | 54 | 27 |
| With Shrimp Skewer, 12 oz | 1000 | 59 | 47 |
| Tilapia Ranchero, 14 oz | 630 | 27 | 60 |

| *Sides (Dinner):* | | | |
|---|---|---|---|
| Coleslaw, 5 oz | 260 | 22 | 15 |
| Garlic Bread, 2 pieces | 170 | 9 | 21 |
| Golden Fried Shrimp, 6 pieces | 190 | 8 | 20 |
| Mashed Potatoes, 4 oz | 100 | 3 | 55 |
| Red Skinned Potatoes, 4 oz | 210 | 7 | 27 |

| *Soups: Without Bread* | | | |
|---|---|---|---|
| Chicken Noodle, 12 oz | 140 | 4 | 35 |
| Clam Chowder, 12 oz | 270 | 17 | 24 |
| Vegetable Beef, 12 oz | 140 | 5 | 17 |

| *Salads: Without Dressing or Bread* | | | |
|---|---|---|---|
| Chicken Strip Deluxe, 18 oz | 590 | 29 | 43 |
| Cranberry Apple Chicken, 13 oz | 370 | 12 | 32 |
| Grilled Chicken Deluxe, 17 oz | 340 | 13 | 13 |

| *Dressings: Per 1 oz* | | | |
|---|---|---|---|
| Bleu Cheese | 110 | 11 | 1 |
| Caesar | 100 | 10 | 0 |
| French | 75 | 5 | 8 |
| Honey Mustard | 160 | 15 | 5 |
| Ranch | 130 | 14 | 0 |

| *Desserts:* | | | |
|---|---|---|---|
| Apple Pie, 7 oz | 480 | 22 | 67 |
| Banana Split, 15 oz | 810 | 31 | 125 |
| Caramel Apple Crisp, 13 oz | 740 | 21 | 134 |
| Coconut Cream Pie, 7 oz | 630 | 39 | 65 |
| Hot Fudge Brownie a` la Mode, 9 oz | 830 | 37 | 122 |
| NY Style Cheesecake, 5 oz | 510 | 34 | 43 |
| Oreo Blender Blaster, 14 oz | 890 | 44 | 113 |

| *Beverages:* | | | |
|---|---|---|---|
| Flav. Cappuccino; Hot Choc., 8 fl.oz | 100 | 2 | 28 |
| Milkshakes, Van/Choc, 12 fl.oz | 560 | 26 | 76 |

*For Complete Nutritional Data ~ see CalorieKing.com*

## Dippin' Dots® (Dec '11)

| *Flavored Ices:* | C | F | Cb |
|---|---|---|---|
| All flavors, ½ cup, 3 oz | 90 | 0 | 23 |
| *Frozen Yogurt,* | | | |
| Strawberry Cheesecake, ½ cup | 100 | 0 | 21 |
| *Ice Cream: Per ½ Cup* | | | |
| Banana Split | 170 | 10 | 16 |
| Chocolate Chip Cookie dough | 215 | 11 | 26 |
| Peanut Butter Chip | 165 | 10 | 15 |
| Strawberry | 170 | 10 | 16 |
| **Fat-Free,** Fudge, no sugar added | 90 | 0 | 18 |
| **Red.-Fat,** Vanilla, no sugar added | 125 | 6 | 13 |

## Donato's Pizza®(Dec '11)

| *Thin Crust Pizza: ¼ Large Pizza* | C | F | Cb |
|---|---|---|---|
| Chicken Vegy Medley | 495 | 20 | 51 |
| Classic Trio | 675 | 37 | 52 |
| Founder's Favorite | 700 | 38 | 52 |
| Hawaiian | 590 | 27 | 56 |

| *Thicker Crust Pizza: ¼ Large Pizza* | | | |
|---|---|---|---|
| Founder's Favorite | 770 | 36 | 70 |
| Mariachi Beef | 710 | 30 | 73 |
| Mariachi Chicken | 700 | 28 | 74 |
| Pepperoni | 710 | 32 | 69 |
| Serious Cheese | 700 | 30 | 69 |
| The Works | 760 | 35 | 74 |
| Vegy | 620 | 22 | 75 |

| *No Dough Pizza: Individual* | | | |
|---|---|---|---|
| Chicken Vegy Medley | 495 | 29 | 20 |
| Classic Trio | 530 | 37 | 18 |
| Founder's Favorite | 560 | 38 | 18 |
| Hawaiian | 435 | 26 | 22 |
| Mariachi Beef | 530 | 34 | 23 |
| Mariachi Chicken | 495 | 30 | 21 |
| Pepperoni | 500 | 35 | 17 |
| Pepperoni Zinger | 585 | 42 | 17 |
| Serious Cheese | 455 | 31 | 17 |
| Serious Meat | 655 | 46 | 19 |
| The Works | 545 | 37 | 21 |
| *Stromboli:* 3 Meat | 690 | 31 | 67 |
| Cheese | 695 | 31 | 66 |
| Deluxe | 615 | 25 | 68 |
| Pepperoni | 715 | 34 | 67 |
| Vegy | 605 | 24 | 69 |

| *Desserts:* | | | |
|---|---|---|---|
| Apple Timpano, 2 slices | 405 | 9 | 72 |
| Cinnamon Timpano, 2 slices | 525 | 22 | 73 |

*For Complete Nutritional Data ~ see CalorieKing.com*

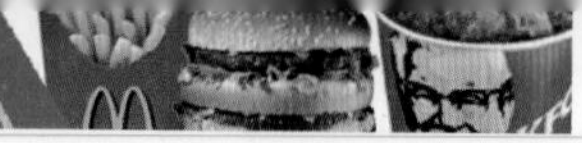

## Domino's® (Dec '11)

| | C | F | Cb |
|---|---|---|---|
| **12" Hand-Tossed:** *Per Slice, ⅛ Pizza, Includes Cheese* | | | |
| Beef | 225 | 10 | 25 |
| Cheese Only | 210 | 8 | 25 |
| Green Peppers, Onion & Mushroom | 185 | 6.5 | 25 |
| Ham | 195 | 7 | 25 |
| Ham & Pineapple | 200 | 6.5 | 26 |
| Pepperoni | 215 | 9 | 25 |
| Pepperoni & Sausage | 240 | 11 | 26 |
| Sausage | 230 | 10 | 26 |
| Wisconsin 6 Cheese | 250 | 12 | 25 |
| **14" Thin Crust:** *Per Slice, ⅛ Pizza, Includes Cheese* | | | |
| Beef | 250 | 14 | 19 |
| Cheese Only | 230 | 12 | 20 |
| Green Pepper Onion & Mushroom | 200 | 10 | 19 |
| Ham | 215 | 10 | 19 |
| Ham & Pineapple | 220 | 10 | 21 |
| Pepperoni | 240 | 13 | 19 |
| Pepperoni & Sausage | 275 | 16 | 20 |
| Sausage | 260 | 15 | 21 |
| **12" Deep Dish:** *Per Slice, ⅛ Pizza, Includes Cheese* | | | |
| Beef | 270 | 13 | 28 |
| Cheese Only | 260 | 12 | 29 |
| Green Pepper Onion & Mushroom | 230 | 10 | 28 |
| Ham | 240 | 10 | 28 |
| Ham & Pineapple | 245 | 10 | 28 |
| Pepperoni | 260 | 12 | 28 |
| Pepperoni & Sausage | 285 | 14 | 29 |
| Sausage | 275 | 13 | 29 |
| **12" Feast Hand-Tossed:** *Per Slice, ⅛ Pizza* | | | |
| America's Favorite Feast | 250 | 12 | 27 |
| Bacon Cheeseburger Feast | 270 | 13 | 26 |
| Deluxe Feast | 230 | 10 | 27 |
| ExtravaganZZa Feast | 290 | 14 | 28 |
| MeatZZa Feast | 280 | 14 | 27 |
| Ultimate Pepperoni | 260 | 13 | 25 |
| **14" Feast Hand Tossed:** *Per Slice, ⅛ Pizza* | | | |
| America's Favorite Feast | 350 | 17 | 36 |
| Bacon Cheeseburger Feast | 380 | 19 | 36 |
| Deluxe Feast | 320 | 14 | 36 |
| ExtravaganZZa Feast | 390 | 19 | 37 |
| MeatZZa Feast | 380 | 19 | 36 |
| Ultimate Pepperoni | 360 | 18 | 34 |
| Wisconsin 6 Cheese | 340 | 16 | 34 |
| **12" Feast Deep Dish:** *Per Slice, ⅛ Pizza* | | | |
| America's Favorite Feast | 280 | 14 | 29 |
| Bacon Cheeseburger Feast | 300 | 15 | 28 |
| Deluxe Feast | 260 | 12 | 29 |
| ExtravaganZZa Feast | 320 | 16 | 30 |
| MeatZZA Feast | 310 | 16 | 29 |
| Ultimate Pepperoni | 290 | 15 | 27 |

## Domino's® cont... (Dec '11)

| | C | F | Cb |
|---|---|---|---|
| **Oven Baked Sandwiches:** | | | |
| Buffalo Chicken with Blue Cheese | 830 | 41 | 74 |
| Chicken Bacon Ranch | 870 | 45 | 72 |
| Chicken Parm | 750 | 30 | 73 |
| Italian | 820 | 41 | 70 |
| Italian Sausage & Peppers | 860 | 45 | 74 |
| Mediterranean Veggie | 680 | 29 | 72 |
| Philly Cheese Steak | 690 | 28 | 70 |
| Sweet & Spicy Chicken Habanero | 800 | 32 | 83 |
| **BreadBowl Pasta:** *Per ½ Bowl* | | | |
| Chicken Alfredo, 10¾ oz | 700 | 26 | 93 |
| Chicken Carbonara, 11¾ oz | 740 | 28 | 94 |
| Italian Sausage Marinara, 12 oz | 730 | 27 | 78 |
| Mac-N-Cheese | 730 | 28 | 95 |
| Pasta Primavera, 11 oz | 670 | 24 | 94 |
| **Salads:** *Per Servings* | | | |
| Garden Fresh | 70 | 3.5 | 5 |
| Grilled Chicken Caesar | 90 | 3.5 | 5 |
| **Salad Dressings & Condiments:** *Per 1½ oz Package* | | | |
| Blue Cheese | 230 | 24 | 2 |
| Buttermilk Ranch | 230 | 24 | 2 |
| Creamy Caesar | 210 | 21 | 2 |
| Golden Italian | 210 | 22 | 2 |
| Light Italian | 20 | 1 | 3 |
| **Bread Side Items:** | | | |
| **Breadsticks:** 1 stick, without sauce | 110 | 6 | 11 |
| 8 sticks, without sauce | 880 | 48 | 88 |
| **Cheesy Bread:** | | | |
| 1 stick, without sauce | 120 | 6 | 11 |
| 8 sticks, without sauce | 960 | 48 | 88 |
| **Bread Dipping Sauces:** *Per Container* | | | |
| Garlic | 250 | 28 | 0 |
| Marinara | 25 | 0 | 5 |
| **Cinna Stix:** | | | |
| 1 stick, without icing | 120 | 6 | 14 |
| 8 sticks, without icing | 960 | 48 | 112 |
| **Sweet Icing,** Dipper Cup | 250 | 2.5 | 57 |
| **Chicken Side Items:** | | | |
| **Buffalo Wings:** | | | |
| Barbecue, 4 wings, without sauce | 250 | 13 | 14 |
| Hot, 4 wings, without sauce | 200 | 13 | 5 |
| **Chicken Dipping Sauces:** *Per 1½ oz Container* | | | |
| Blue Cheese | 240 | 25 | 2 |
| Hot | 50 | 4.5 | 3 |
| Ranch | 200 | 21 | 2 |
| **Dessert,** Chocolate Lava Crunch Cake | 350 | 17 | 47 |

Updated Nutrition Data ~ www.CalorieKing.com
Persons with Diabetes ~ See Disclaimer (Page 22)

## Don Pablos® (Dec '11)

*Appetizers: Per Serving, Includes Garnish*

| | C | F | Cb |
|---|---|---|---|
| Don's Wings: 4 Wings | 875 | 67 | 17 |
| Boneless, 3 strips | 625 | 48 | 28 |
| Flautas, 2 pieces | 190 | 12 | 13 |
| Taquitos, 2 pieces | 210 | 15 | 9 |
| The Don's Sampler, ¼ plate | 495 | 29 | 35 |
| Nachos: Acapulco Beef, 3 chips | 460 | 29 | 23 |
| Acapulco Chicken, 3 chips | 430 | 27 | 23 |
| Quesadillas, Mesquite Grilled: | | | |
| Chicken, small, 2 wedges | 415 | 25 | 31 |
| Steak, small, 2 wedges | 430 | 27 | 27 |

*Don's Dips: Per 2 fl. oz , Without Chips*

| | C | F | Cb |
|---|---|---|---|
| Bowls: Queso Blanco | 180 | 15 | 2 |
| Prairie Fire Bean | 120 | 7 | 9 |

*Entrees: Per Order, Without Optional Beans*

| | C | F | Cb |
|---|---|---|---|
| **Burritos:** Chicken | 1180 | 58 | 105 |
| Fajita Steak | 1145 | 52 | 102 |
| **Carnitas:** Pork | 985 | 34 | 120 |
| Cold Set, Side | 160 | 11 | 18 |
| **Chimichangas:** Chicken | 1110 | 61 | 91 |
| Spicy Beef De Oro | 1475 | 80 | 112 |
| **Classic Fajitas:** *With Onions, Peppers & 3x7" Fajitas* | | | |
| Combo - Steak & Chicken | 625 | 31 | 47 |
| Mesquite-Grilled: Chicken | 570 | 27 | 58 |
| Steak | 680 | 36 | 36 |
| **Fajita Fixin's:** 7" Flour Tortilla (1) | 125 | 4 | 20 |
| Combo Cheese Toppings, 1 oz | 110 | 8 | 0 |
| Corn Tortillas (1) | 60 | 1 | 12 |
| Guacamole, #30 scoop | 70 | 6 | 4 |
| Sour Cream, #30 scoop | 80 | 8 | 2 |
| **Enchiladas:** Cadillac: Chicken | 1090 | 48 | 87 |
| Steak | 1155 | 57 | 88 |
| **Tacos:** Buffalo Chicken Trio | 1155 | 59 | 117 |
| Chipotle Pork Trio | 925 | 41 | 92 |
| Fried: Chicken Trio | 1050 | 48 | 116 |
| Fish | 1135 | 58 | 100 |
| Shrimp | 860 | 42 | 98 |
| Grilled: Chicken Trio | 1115 | 45 | 129 |
| Fish | 990 | 57 | 71 |
| Shrimp | 740 | 45 | 69 |

*Fresh Salads: Includes Dressing*

| | C | F | Cb |
|---|---|---|---|
| Caesar: With Chicken | 1285 | 76 | 114 |
| With Steak | 1360 | 82 | 99 |
| Southwest: With Buffalo Sauce | 950 | 57 | 73 |
| With Chipotle-Honey BBQ Sce | 1215 | 67 | 118 |

*Sides:*

| | C | F | Cb |
|---|---|---|---|
| Mexican Rice, 3 oz | 120 | 2 | 23 |
| Refritos, 5 oz | 215 | 7 | 27 |
| Seasoned Vegetables, 6 oz | 110 | 5 | 16 |

## Dunkin Donuts® (Dec '11)

| | C | F | Cb |
|---|---|---|---|
| *Donuts:* Apple 'n Spice | 270 | 14 | 32 |
| Bavarian Kreme | 270 | 15 | 31 |
| Boston Kreme | 310 | 16 | 39 |
| Bow Tie Donut | 310 | 15 | 39 |
| Chocolate Frosted | 270 | 15 | 31 |
| Chocolate Kreme Filled | 370 | 21 | 42 |
| French Cruller | 250 | 20 | 18 |
| Jelly Filled | 290 | 14 | 36 |
| Old Fashioned Cake | 320 | 22 | 33 |
| Powdered Cake | 340 | 22 | 38 |
| Strawberry Frosted | 280 | 15 | 32 |
| Sugar Raised | 230 | 14 | 22 |
| Vanilla Kreme Filled | 380 | 23 | 42 |
| **Sticks:** Plain Cake | 330 | 18 | 36 |
| Cinnamon Cake | 350 | 18 | 44 |
| Glazed: Cake | 370 | 18 | 48 |
| Chocolate Cake | 390 | 25 | 40 |
| Jelly | 420 | 18 | 60 |
| Powdered Cake | 360 | 18 | 43 |
| *Munchkins:* Plain Cake (4) | 240 | 14 | 24 |
| Blueberry | 330 | 3 | 65 |
| Glazed, average all varieties (4) | 280 | 16 | 28 |
| Jelly Filled (5) | 400 | 20 | 45 |
| Powdered Cake (4) | 240 | 14 | 28 |
| Sugared (5) | 300 | 18 | 30 |
| *Danish:* Apple Cheese | 330 | 16 | 41 |
| Cheese | 330 | 17 | 39 |
| Strawberry Cheese | 320 | 16 | 40 |
| *Muffins:* Chocolate Chip | 610 | 23 | 92 |
| Blueberry | 500 | 16 | 83 |
| Reduced Fat | 450 | 15 | 82 |
| Coffee Cake | 650 | 27 | 95 |
| Corn | 510 | 18 | 80 |
| Honey Bran Raisin | 490 | 15 | 82 |
| *Bagels:* Plain; Salt | 320 | 2.5 | 65 |
| Cinnamon Raisin | 330 | 3.5 | 65 |
| Everything | 350 | 4.5 | 66 |
| Multigrain | 390 | 8 | 65 |
| Onion; Wheat, average | 315 | 3 | 62 |
| Sesame | 360 | 6 | 63 |
| Sour Cream & Onion | 330 | 2.5 | 66 |
| *Wake Up Wrap:* | | | |
| Bacon, Egg & Cheese | 210 | 12 | 14 |
| Egg & Cheese | 180 | 11 | 14 |
| Egg White Turkey Sausage | 150 | 5 | 14 |
| Egg White Veggie | 150 | 6 | 14 |
| Ham, Egg & Cheese | 200 | 11 | 14 |
| Sausage, Egg & Cheese | 290 | 20 | 14 |

*Continued Next Page ...*

## Dunkin Donuts® cont... (Dec '11)

### Breakfast Sandwiches:

| | C | F | Cb |
|---|---|---|---|
| Big N Toasty | 580 | 35 | 41 |
| **Bagels:** Egg & Cheese | 480 | 15 | 66 |
| Bacon, Egg & Cheese | 530 | 19 | 66 |
| Ham, Egg & Cheese | 510 | 16 | 66 |
| Sausage, Egg & Cheese | 690 | 35 | 66 |
| **Biscuits:** Bacon, Egg & Cheese | 490 | 30 | 35 |
| Sausage, Egg & Cheese | 650 | 46 | 36 |
| **Croissant:** Bacon, Egg & Cheese | 530 | 33 | 38 |
| Ham, Egg & Cheese | 510 | 31 | 38 |
| Sausage, Egg & Cheese | 690 | 48 | 39 |
| **English Muffin:** | | | |
| Bacon, Egg & Cheese | 370 | 18 | 34 |
| Ham, Egg & Cheese | 360 | 16 | 34 |
| Sausage, Egg & Cheese | 530 | 34 | 34 |

### Dunkin' Deli:

| | C | F | Cb |
|---|---|---|---|
| **Breadsticks:** | | | |
| Cheeseburger Stuffed (1) | 200 | 6 | 28 |
| Pepperoni & Cheese Stuffed (1) | 210 | 7 | 27 |
| **Salads:** Caesar, 7.3 oz | 320 | 29 | 11 |
| Chicken Caesar, 10.4 oz | 440 | 33 | 11 |
| Garden, 12.3 oz | 180 | 6 | 21 |
| **Sandwiches:** Chicken Bruschetta | 580 | 26 | 49 |
| Chipotle Chicken | 600 | 25 | 50 |
| Pastrami Supreme | 750 | 39 | 51 |
| Pressed Cuban | 680 | 33 | 50 |
| Steak & Cheese | 470 | 16 | 50 |
| Toasted Italian | 560 | 25 | 52 |
| Tuna Melt | 770 | 30 | 57 |
| Turkey and Bacon Club | 440 | 13 | 51 |
| Turkey & Cheese | 450 | 13 | 52 |
| **Croissants:** Chicken Salad | 560 | 37 | 38 |
| Tuna Melt Croissant | 630 | 40 | 42 |
| English Muffin: Chicken Salad | 400 | 23 | 33 |
| **Soup:** Broccoli Cheddar Soup, 8 oz | 190 | 11 | 14 |
| Chicken Noodle Soup, 8 oz | 130 | 3 | 19 |

### Beverages:

| | C | F | Cb |
|---|---|---|---|
| **Cappuccino,** without sugar, 10 fl.oz | 80 | 4 | 7 |
| **Coolatta:** | | | |
| Coffee: With Skim Milk, 16 fl.oz | 200 | 0 | 48 |
| With Cream, 16 fl.oz | 400 | 23 | 49 |
| With Milk, 16 fl.oz | 240 | 4 | 50 |
| Strawberry Fruit, 16 fl.oz | 310 | 0 | 75 |
| Tropicana Orange, 16 fl.oz | 230 | 0 | 57 |
| **Hot Chocolate:** Small, 10 fl.oz | 220 | 7 | 39 |
| White, 1 medium, 14 fl.oz | 340 | 12 | 56 |
| **Iced Coffee,** 16 fl.oz | 10 | 0 | 2 |
| **Flavored Coffee:** Caramel, 10 fl.oz | 10 | 0 | 2 |
| Toasted Almond, 10 fl.oz | 10 | 0 | 1 |

## Eat 'N Park® (Dec '11)

### Breakfast:

| | C | F | Cb |
|---|---|---|---|
| Fruit Cup | 60 | 0.5 | 15 |
| Hash Browns | 200 | 8 | 28 |
| Home Fries | 210 | 12 | 24 |
| Oatmeal with Milk | 200 | 4 | 33 |
| **Omelette:** Cheese | 390 | 30 | 2 |
| Ham & Cheese | 535 | 35 | 4 |
| Veggie | 415 | 30 | 8 |
| Western | 345 | 21 | 7 |
| **Pancakes,** Buttermilk: Plain (1) | 75 | 1 | 15 |
| Blueberry (1) | 85 | 1 | 16 |
| **Waffles:** Belgian (1) | 280 | 12 | 35 |
| Strawberry (1) | 375 | 18 | 48 |

### Appetizers:

| | C | F | Cb |
|---|---|---|---|
| Buffalo Chicken Tenders (5) | 535 | 26 | 29 |
| Fried Cheese Sticks | 535 | 36 | 26 |
| Grilled Chicken Quesadillas | 905 | 55 | 51 |
| Onion Rings Basket | 365 | 24 | 34 |

### Burgers:

| | C | F | Cb |
|---|---|---|---|
| **Black Angus:** American Grill | 610 | 37 | 31 |
| BBQ Bacon Cheddar | 865 | 53 | 53 |
| Mushroom & Onion | 710 | 41 | 45 |
| Superburger | 1085 | 73 | 28 |
| **Classic:** Black Angus | 420 | 21 | 22 |
| Bacon Cheeseburger | 535 | 31 | 22 |
| Cheeseburger | 465 | 25 | 22 |
| Garden Burger | 290 | 5 | 43 |
| **Original,** Superburger | 565 | 38 | 27 |

### Sandwiches: With Menu Board Standard Add-Ins

| | C | F | Cb |
|---|---|---|---|
| BLT | 490 | 15 | 66 |
| Buffalo Chicken Wrap | 835 | 48 | 61 |
| Chargrilled Chicken | 320 | 6 | 32 |
| Grilled Cheese | 725 | 39 | 65 |
| Hot Turkey | 500 | 9 | 71 |
| Santa Fe Turkey & Bacon | 880 | 60 | 45 |
| Shredded Pot Roast | 530 | 31 | 28 |
| Turkey Club | 835 | 50 | 52 |
| Whale of a Cod Fish | 880 | 41 | 76 |

### Dinners: Without Sides

| | C | F | Cb |
|---|---|---|---|
| Baked Lemon Sole, 2 fillets | 385 | 20 | 11 |
| Chargrilled Chicken, 2 pieces | 350 | 9 | 0 |
| Chicken Fillets (5) | 530 | 26 | 28 |
| **Chicken Parmigiana:** | | | |
| W/ Marinara Sauce & Parm. Cheese | 960 | 37 | 100 |
| W/ Meat Sauce & Mozz. Cheese | 985 | 40 | 95 |
| Chicken Stir-Fry | 390 | 8 | 47 |
| Cod Floridian, 2 fillets | 240 | 3 | 8 |
| Spaghetti Marinara | 695 | 9 | 129 |
| Spaghetti with Meat Sauce | 830 | 16 | 145 |
| T Bone Steak | 575 | 39 | 1 |

## Eat 'N Park® cont... (Dec '11)

### Salads: *Without Dressing*

| | C | F | Cb |
|---|---|---|---|
| Buffalo Chicken Salad | 610 | 35 | 42 |
| Chicken Fajita | 410 | 15 | 29 |
| Garden Salad | 95 | 3 | 15 |
| Grilled Chicken | 445 | 19 | 30 |
| Grilled Chicken Portobella | 320 | 11 | 23 |

### Dressings: *Per 2 oz*

| | C | F | Cb |
|---|---|---|---|
| Bleu Cheese | 245 | 25 | 3 |
| French Fat Free | 75 | 0 | 18 |
| Italian Fat Free | 20 | 0 | 5 |
| House Ranch | 215 | 21 | 4 |
| Thousand Island | 190 | 19 | 4 |

### Desserts:

| | C | F | Cb |
|---|---|---|---|
| Grilled Stickies a la Mode | 725 | 39 | 81 |
| Ice Cream, 2 scoops | 230 | 12 | 27 |

### Pies: *Per Slice*

| | C | F | Cb |
|---|---|---|---|
| Apple | 525 | 27 | 67 |
| Cherry | 520 | 28 | 63 |
| Peachberry | 390 | 19 | 51 |
| Strawberry | 295 | 12 | 45 |

## Edo Japan® (Dec '11)

### Meals: *Per Bento Box w/o Teriyaki*

| | C | F | Cb |
|---|---|---|---|
| Beef Yakisoba, 20¼ oz | 830 | 30 | 102 |
| Chicken Yakisoba, 20½ oz | 800 | 25 | 102 |
| Seafood Grill, 23 oz | 860 | 16 | 129 |
| Sizzling Shrimp, 22 oz | 800 | 16 | 122 |
| Sukiyaki Beef, 20¼ oz | 900 | 28 | 120 |

### Specialties: *Without Teriyaki Sauce*

| | C | F | Cb |
|---|---|---|---|
| Curry Chicken Bowl, 13¼ oz | 500 | 21 | 27 |
| Hawaiian Chicken, 15½ oz | 590 | 12 | 85 |
| Seafood Grill, 17¾ oz | 570 | 4 | 89 |
| Sukiyaki Beef, 14¾ oz | 610 | 16 | 80 |
| Teriyaki Chicken, 15 oz | 580 | 12 | 80 |

## Einstein Bros® (Dec '11)

### Bagels:

| | C | F | Cb |
|---|---|---|---|
| **Classics,** Plain; Honey Whole Wheat | 260 | 1 | 56 |
| **Gourmet Bagels:** Dutch Apple | 350 | 7 | 66 |
| Green Chile | 350 | 8 | 58 |
| Power Bagel | 310 | 5 | 61 |
| Six-Cheese | 330 | 6 | 56 |
| Spinach Florentine | 340 | 8 | 57 |
| **Pizza Bagels:** Cheese | 400 | 11 | 59 |
| Pepperoni | 450 | 15 | 59 |
| **Signature Flavors:** Asiago Cheese | 310 | 5 | 56 |
| Blueberry | 300 | 1 | 65 |
| Chocolate Chip | 290 | 2.5 | 58 |
| Cinnamon Sugar | 290 | 2.5 | 63 |
| Egg | 300 | 5 | 54 |
| Everything | 270 | 2 | 56 |
| Garlic | 270 | 2.5 | 56 |
| Onion | 270 | 1 | 59 |
| Poppy | 280 | 3 | 56 |
| Potato | 270 | 4 | 52 |
| Sesame | 280 | 3 | 56 |

### Bagel Dogs: *With Cheddar Cheese*

| | C | F | Cb |
|---|---|---|---|
| Original | 540 | 27 | 56 |
| Asiago | 550 | 28 | 56 |

### Paninis:

| | C | F | Cb |
|---|---|---|---|
| **Lunch:** Italian Chicken | 750 | 39 | 50 |
| Turkey Club | 680 | 37 | 50 |
| **Breakfast, Egg:** W/ Spinach & Bacon | 720 | 43 | 50 |
| With Southwest Turkey Sausage | 600 | 27 | 49 |

### Sandwiches:

| | C | F | Cb |
|---|---|---|---|
| **Egg:** With Bacon & Cheddar | 550 | 23 | 58 |
| With Ham & Swiss | 550 | 20 | 59 |
| With Turkey Sausage & Cheddar | 580 | 24 | 59 |
| With Spinach, Mushroom & Swiss | 560 | 24 | 61 |
| *Wraps:* California Chicken | 710 | 35 | 64 |
| Chipotle Turkey | 670 | 30 | 71 |
| **Breakfast, Egg:** Santa Fe | 720 | 37 | 60 |
| Spicy Elmo | 720 | 40 | 56 |

### Cream Cheese: *Per 1¼ oz, Schmear*

| | C | F | Cb |
|---|---|---|---|
| Reduced Fat: Blueberry | 120 | 9 | 11 |
| Garlic Herb/Garden Veggie | 110 | 9 | 5 |
| Honey Almond; Strawberry, av. | 120 | 9 | 10 |
| Plain; Sun Dried Tomato & Basil | 110 | 9 | 4 |
| Onion and Chive | 120 | 11 | 5 |
| Smoked Salmon | 110 | 11 | 4 |

### Salads: *With Dressing*

| | C | F | Cb |
|---|---|---|---|
| Bros Bistro, 10 oz | 810 | 68 | 35 |
| Bros Bistro with Chicken, 15 oz | 950 | 71 | 36 |
| Chipotle, 12 oz | 520 | 37 | 37 |
| Chicken Chipotle, 16 oz | 660 | 41 | 38 |
| Caesar Salad with Chicken, 14 oz | 740 | 59 | 20 |

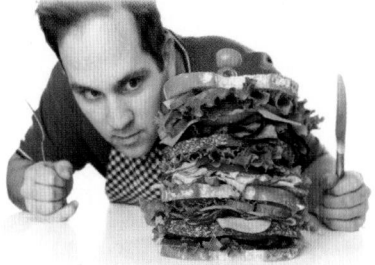

## El Pollo Loco® (Dec'11)

### Brand Nuevo Burritos:

| | C | F | Cb |
|---|---|---|---|
| BRC, 7.6 oz | 425 | 12 | 64 |
| El Traditional, 14.7 oz | 785 | 31 | 86 |
| The Poblano, 18.6 oz | 900 | 39 | 91 |

### Chicken Meals: Without Sides

| | | | |
|---|---|---|---|
| 2 piece, 1 Wing & 1 Breast | 315 | 14 | 0 |
| 4 piece, 2 Wings & 2 Breasts | 630 | 27 | 1 |

### Flame-Grilled Chicken: Skin On

| | | | |
|---|---|---|---|
| Breast | 225 | 9 | 0 |
| Leg | 85 | 4 | 0 |
| Thigh | 215 | 14 | 0 |
| Wing | 90 | 5 | 0 |

### Bowls: The Original Pollo, 18.1 oz

| | | | |
|---|---|---|---|
| The Original Pollo, 18.1 oz | 605 | 10 | 87 |
| Ultimate Pollo, 24.2 oz | 960 | 34 | 92 |

### Loco Value Menu:

| | | | |
|---|---|---|---|
| Crunchy Chicken Taco | 190 | 8 | 16 |
| Flan, 5.1 oz | 265 | 12 | 34 |
| Taco al Carbon | 160 | 6 | 18 |

### Soup:

| | | | |
|---|---|---|---|
| Chicken Tortilla w/ Tortilla Strips: | | | |
| Regular, 10.8 oz | 215 | 9 | 18 |
| Large, 23.6 oz | 455 | 19 | 39 |

### Salads:

| | | | |
|---|---|---|---|
| Chicken Tostada w/o dress., 17.3 oz | 860 | 42 | 77 |
| Grilled Chkn, w/out dress., 10.3 oz | 245 | 8 | 19 |

### Dressings: Per Packet

| | | | |
|---|---|---|---|
| Creamy Cilantro, 3 oz | 440 | 46 | 3 |
| Light Creamy Cilantro, 2 oz | 70 | 5 | 6 |
| Light Italian, 2 oz | 20 | 1 | 2 |
| Ranch, 2 oz | 230 | 24 | 2 |
| Thousand Island, 2 oz | 220 | 21 | 6 |

### Condiments: Per 1½ oz

| | | | |
|---|---|---|---|
| Guacamole | 70 | 6 | 3 |
| Salsa: Avocado | 35 | 3.5 | 2 |
| House | 10 | 0 | 2 |
| Pico de Gallo | 15 | 1 | 1 |

### Sides:

| | | | |
|---|---|---|---|
| Corn Cobbette, 6.2 oz | 160 | 5 | 25 |
| Flame Grilled Corn, 4 oz | 125 | 5 | 21 |
| French Fries, 3.8 oz | 330 | 17 | 40 |
| Fresh Vegetables, 4.1 oz | 60 | 3 | 8 |
| Macaroni & Cheese, 5½ oz | 255 | 15 | 22 |
| Mashed Potatoes with Gravy, 6 oz | 125 | 2 | 25 |
| Pinto Beans, 6 oz | 195 | 4 | 29 |
| Spanish Rice, 4½ oz | 170 | 2.5 | 32 |
| Sweet Corn Cake, 3.7 oz | 250 | 10 | 36 |
| Sweet Potato Fries, 3.6 oz | 325 | 20 | 34 |

*For Complete Nutritional Data ~ see CalorieKing.com*

## Fatburger® (Dec'11)

### Burgers: Without Extras

| | C | F | Cb |
|---|---|---|---|
| Baby Fat | 400 | 21 | 37 |
| Fatburger | 590 | 31 | 46 |
| Kingburger | 850 | 41 | 69 |
| Turkeyburger | 480 | 21 | 50 |
| Veggieburger | 510 | 20 | 60 |

### Sandwiches: Without Extras

| | | | |
|---|---|---|---|
| Crispy Chicken | 560 | 27 | 53 |
| Grilled Chicken | 430 | 14 | 42 |
| Fish | 560 | 31 | 55 |

### Sides and Fries:

| | | | |
|---|---|---|---|
| Fries: Fat Fries; Skinny Fries, av. | 385 | 17 | 53 |
| With Chili, average | 485 | 23 | 57 |
| With Chili & Cheese, average | 595 | 32 | 58 |
| Sides: American Cheese, 1 slice | 70 | 5 | 1 |
| Cheddar Cheese, 1 slice | 110 | 9 | 1 |
| Chili Cup | 200 | 11 | 10 |
| with Cheese & Onions | 320 | 20 | 12 |
| Mayonnaise | 90 | 10 | 1 |
| Onion Rings | 540 | 29 | 64 |
| Relish | 20 | 0 | 5 |

### Shakes: Chocolate

| | | | |
|---|---|---|---|
| Chocolate | 910 | 45 | 115 |
| Cookies & Ice Cream | 1180 | 59 | 163 |
| Maui Banana | 940 | 44 | 126 |
| Peanut Butter | 950 | 53 | 114 |
| Strawberry; Vanilla, average | 885 | 44 | 112 |

*For Complete Nutritional Data ~ see CalorieKing.com*

## Fazoli's® (Dec'11)

### Fresh Made Pasta: Per Serving

| | C | F | Cb |
|---|---|---|---|
| Chicken Carbonara, 17.8 oz | 790 | 26 | 87 |
| Classic Sampler Platter, 21.6 oz | 890 | 25 | 122 |
| Fettuccine with Alfredo, 17.8 oz | 800 | 26 | 108 |
| Ravioli with Meat Sauce, 13.1oz | 570 | 21 | 70 |
| Spaghetti with Marinara, 18.2 oz | 560 | 2.5 | 111 |
| Tortellini & Sun Dried Tom. Rustico | 850 | 46 | 81 |
| Ultimate Sampler Platter, 30 oz | 1150 | 29 | 166 |

### Oven-Baked Pasta: Per Serving

| | | | |
|---|---|---|---|
| Chicken Broccoli Penne, 21.3 oz | 900 | 40 | 76 |
| Chicken Parmigano, 21.3 oz | 920 | 32 | 106 |
| Baked Spaghetti, 15½ oz | 640 | 22 | 80 |
| With Meatballs, 18.8 oz | 890 | 39 | 86 |
| Penne with Creamy Basil Chkn, 18.8 oz | 970 | 51 | 73 |
| Rigatoni Romano, 17.3 oz | 880 | 44 | 76 |
| Tortellini Robusto, 17.4 oz | 1000 | 49 | 79 |
| Twice-Baked Lasagna, 18.4 oz | 700 | 39 | 47 |

*Continued next page...*

## Fazoli's® cont... (Dec '11)

*Pizzas: Per Slice*

| | C | F | Cb |
|---|---|---|---|
| Cheese, 4 oz | 290 | 12 | 32 |
| Pepperoni, 4.2 oz | 300 | 13 | 32 |

*Oven Baked Submarinos:*

| | | | |
|---|---|---|---|
| Club Italiano, 13 oz | 800 | 38 | 71 |
| Fazoli's Original, 12.8 oz | 880 | 49 | 70 |
| Smoked Turkey Basil, 12.8 oz | 750 | 37 | 68 |
| Ultimate M'ball Smasher, 13.7 oz | 1070 | 65 | 76 |

*Salads: With Dressing Unless Indicated*

| | | | |
|---|---|---|---|
| Cherry Almond Chicken | 480 | 25 | 38 |
| Country Caesar | 780 | 51 | 48 |
| Fazoli's Italian House | 600 | 45 | 16 |
| Pasa Ranch Italia | 770 | 50 | 44 |
| Side, Chopped, without dressing | 60 | 3.5 | 5 |

*Salad Dressing: Per 1.5 oz*

| | | | |
|---|---|---|---|
| Caesar | 230 | 25 | 1 |
| Italian | 160 | 14 | 7 |
| Fat Free | 25 | 0 | 6 |
| Honey French | 220 | 18 | 14 |
| Ranch | 220 | 24 | 2 |
| Lite Ranch | 120 | 12 | 2 |

*For Complete Nutritional Data ~ see CalorieKing.com*

## Firehouse Subs® (Dec '11)

| | C | F | Cb |
|---|---|---|---|

*Subs: Per Medium White Sub, With Standard Toppings and Dressings*

| | | | |
|---|---|---|---|
| Chicken Salad | 820 | 48 | 60 |
| Engine Company | 700 | 36 | 57 |
| Engineer | 690 | 35 | 61 |
| Ham | 730 | 36 | 70 |
| Hero | 770 | 37 | 65 |
| Hook & Ladder | 700 | 36 | 64 |
| Italian | 910 | 57 | 65 |
| Meatball | 820 | 50 | 60 |
| Roast Beef | 710 | 36 | 54 |
| Tuna | 1000 | 68 | 67 |
| Turkey | 670 | 34 | 58 |
| Veggie | 720 | 45 | 60 |
| *Chili* | 340 | 17 | 25 |

*Salads: Without Dressing*

| | | | |
|---|---|---|---|
| Chief's Salad: With Chicken | 370 | 18 | 17 |
| With Chicken Salad | 490 | 29 | 20 |
| With Tuna | 670 | 48 | 27 |
| With Ham | 410 | 17 | 31 |
| With Turkey | 350 | 15 | 19 |

*Desserts:* Brownie (1) | 490 | 20 | 80 |
| Chocolate Chip Cookie | 290 | 14 | 52 |

## Five Guys® (Dec '11)

*Burgers:*

| | C | F | Cb |
|---|---|---|---|
| Bacon Burger | 780 | 50 | 39 |
| Bacon Cheeseburger | 920 | 62 | 40 |
| Cheeseburger | 840 | 55 | 40 |
| Hamburger | 700 | 43 | 39 |
| Little: Bacon Burger | 560 | 33 | 39 |
| Bacon Cheeseburger | 630 | 39 | 40 |
| Cheeseburger | 550 | 32 | 40 |
| Hamburger | 480 | 26 | 39 |

*Dogs:*

| | | | |
|---|---|---|---|
| Bacon Dog | 625 | 42 | 40 |
| Bacon Cheese Dog | 695 | 48 | 41 |
| Cheese Dog | 615 | 41 | 41 |
| Hot Dog | 545 | 35 | 40 |
| *Fries:* Regular 8½ oz | 620 | 30 | 78 |
| ½ Regular Order | 310 | 15 | 39 |

## Freshens® (Dec '11)

| | C | F | Cb |
|---|---|---|---|

*Smoothies: 100% Juice (21 fl.oz)*

**Blended Fruit Classics:**

| | | | |
|---|---|---|---|
| Caribbean Craze; Maui Mango | 290 | 0 | 73 |
| Citrus Mango | 490 | 7 | 108 |
| Jamaican Jammer | 350 | 0 | 77 |
| Orange Sunrise | 360 | 3 | 82 |
| Peach Sunset | 270 | 0 | 67 |
| Strawberry Kiwi | 320 | 0 | 81 |
| Strawberry Squeeze | 310 | 0 | 68 |
| Tropical Pineapple | 310 | 4 | 97 |
| **High Protein:** Peanut Butter | 540 | 12 | 84 |
| Strawberry & Cream | 370 | 1 | 75 |
| **Low Calorie:** *No Sugar Added* | | | |
| Average all flavors | 80 | 0 | 50 |

(Note: Carbs include 1¼ oz Erythritol Sweetener)

| | | | |
|---|---|---|---|
| **Rainforest Energy:** Acai Energy | 320 | 3 | 71 |
| Brazillian Energy | 290 | 0 | 73 |
| Mangosteen | 320 | 0 | 89 |
| **Fro-Yo Blasts:** Cookie Dough | 570 | 7 | 112 |
| Oreo Overload | 430 | 3.5 | 83 |
| *Indulgent Shakes:* Chocolate | 530 | 4 | 103 |
| Oreo Cream | 610 | 7 | 115 |
| Strawberry | 490 | 4 | 94 |

*Breakfast:*

| | | | |
|---|---|---|---|
| **Crepes:** Denver | 460 | 24 | 26 |
| Steak & Eggs | 480 | 26 | 25 |
| Wake Up | 420 | 22 | 23 |
| *Savory Golden Crepes:* Fajita Chkn | 500 | 13 | 58 |
| Fajita steak | 530 | 19 | 59 |
| Honey Mustard Chicken | 470 | 15 | 46 |
| Philly Cheese Chicken | 610 | 25 | 54 |
| *Dessert Crepes:* Caramel Apple | 590 | 15 | 104 |
| Cheesecake Supreme | 510 | 20 | 69 |

## Godfather's Pizza® (Dec'11)

*Golden Pizza: Per Slice*

| | C | F | Cb |
|---|---|---|---|
| Cheese: Medium, ⅛ pizza | 220 | 8 | 25 |
| Large, ⅒ pizza | 250 | 9 | 28 |
| Combo: Medium, ⅛ pizza | 290 | 13 | 27 |
| Large, ⅒ pizza | 330 | 15 | 30 |
| Super Combo: Medium, ⅛ pizza | 320 | 15 | 28 |
| Large, ⅒ pizza | 370 | 18 | 31 |

*Original Pizza:*

| | C | F | Cb |
|---|---|---|---|
| Cheese: Mini, ¼ pizza | 150 | 4 | 20 |
| Medium, ⅛ pizza | 260 | 7 | 34 |
| Jumbo, 1/12 pizza | 350 | 10 | 44 |
| Combo: Mini, ¼ pizza | 200 | 8 | 21 |
| Medium, ⅛ pizza | 350 | 14 | 36 |
| Jumbo, 1/12 pizza | 480 | 20 | 47 |
| Super Combo: Mini, ¼ pizza | 220 | 9 | 22 |
| Medium, ⅛ pizza | 350 | 14 | 36 |
| Jumbo, 1/12 pizza | 520 | 23 | 48 |

*Thin Pizza:*

| | C | F | Cb |
|---|---|---|---|
| Cheese: Medium, ⅛ pizza | 170 | 8 | 15 |
| Large, ⅒ pizza | 210 | 10 | 17 |
| Combo: Medium, ⅛ pizza | 240 | 13 | 17 |
| Large, ⅒ pizza | 280 | 16 | 20 |
| Super Combo: Medium, ⅛ pizza | 290 | 16 | 19 |
| Large, ⅒ pizza | 330 | 19 | 20 |

*Calzones: Per Medium Calzone*

| | C | F | Cb |
|---|---|---|---|
| Cheese | 1660 | 51 | 200 |
| Combo | 1450 | 40 | 199 |
| Pepperoni | 1410 | 39 | 195 |

*Sides:*

| | C | F | Cb |
|---|---|---|---|
| Breadstick (1) | 110 | 2 | 20 |
| Cheesestick,1 piece, ⅙ | 130 | 3.5 | 18 |
| Garlic Toast: 1 piece | 150 | 9 | 15 |
| With Cheese, 1 piece | 210 | 12 | 16 |
| Hot Wings, breaded, 1 wing | 45 | 3 | 1 |
| Potato Wedges, 4 oz | 175 | 8 | 24 |

## Gold Star Chili® (Dec'11)

*Meals:*

| | C | F | Cb |
|---|---|---|---|
| **Bowls:** Low Carb Coney, 10½ oz | 570 | 47 | 7 |
| Veggie Chili, 9 oz | 160 | 2 | 29 |
| **Coney:** 5¼ oz | 285 | 14 | 30 |
| Cheese Coney, 5½ oz | 345 | 18 | 31 |
| **Chili:** 8 oz | 215 | 12 | 8 |
| Tex Mex, 8 oz | 210 | 9 | 17 |
| Chili Cheese Nachos, 8½ oz | 410 | 25 | 30 |
| **Regular:** 2-Way | 420 | 11 | 58 |
| 3-Way | 650 | 30 | 59 |
| 4-Way | 665 | 30 | 63 |
| 5-Way | 735 | 30 | 76 |
| **Super,** 5-Way | 1140 | 51 | 109 |

## Gold Star Chili® cont... (Dec'11)

*Sandwiches:*

| | C | F | Cb |
|---|---|---|---|
| Chili | 210 | 5 | 32 |
| Chili Cheese | 290 | 12 | 30 |

*Salads: Without Dressing*

| | C | F | Cb |
|---|---|---|---|
| Cafe: 8 oz | 160 | 10 | 15 |
| With Crispy Chicken | 310 | 15 | 24 |
| With Grilled Chicken, 10½ oz | 250 | 12 | 15 |
| Caesar Salad, 6 oz | 130 | 6 | 12 |
| With Crispy Chicken, 8½ oz | 280 | 11 | 22 |
| With Grilled Chicken, 8½ oz | 210 | 8 | 12 |
| South of the Border Chili, 16¾ oz | 640 | 39 | 55 |

*Sides:* Fries, 5 oz

| | C | F | Cb |
|---|---|---|---|
| *Sides:* Fries, 5 oz | 365 | 19 | 44 |
| Chili Cheese, 9½ oz | 595 | 36 | 46 |
| Garlic Bread: With Cheese, 2½ oz | 270 | 18 | 19 |
| Without Cheese, 2 oz | 215 | 13 | 19 |

## Golden Corral® (Dec'11)

*Breakfast:*

| | C | F | Cb |
|---|---|---|---|
| Bacon & Cheese Quiche, 1 slice | 290 | 21 | 15 |
| Corned Beef Hash, 1 cup | 440 | 28 | 26 |
| Creamed Chipped Beef, 1 cup | 320 | 18 | 20 |
| French Toast, 1 slice | 200 | 6 | 29 |
| Hash Brown Casserole, 1 cup | 260 | 10 | 28 |
| Sausage Links (1) | 120 | 11 | 1 |
| Sausage Patties (1) | 100 | 9 | 0 |

*Meals: Without Sides*

**Hot Buffet:**

| | C | F | Cb |
|---|---|---|---|
| Awesome Pot Roast, 3 oz | 100 | 4.5 | 5 |
| Baked Fish w/ Shrimp & Sce, 3 oz | 160 | 10 | 2 |
| Baked Florentine Fish, 1 piece | 180 | 12 | 2 |
| BBQ: Chicken Leg Quarter, 1 pce | 490 | 22 | 21 |
| Pork, 3 oz | 170 | 8 | 5 |
| Bone-In Breaded Catfish, 3 oz | 210 | 14 | 7 |
| Bourbon Street Chicken, 3 oz | 170 | 9 | 4 |
| Breaded Scallops (10) | 140 | 6 | 13 |
| Coconut Shrimp (5) | 200 | 12 | 16 |
| Crab Cakes (1) | 180 | 15 | 8 |
| Hickory Bourbon Chkn Tenders (1) | 140 | 2 | 17 |
| Meatloaf,1 slice | 220 | 11 | 11 |
| Sirloin Steak, 4½ oz | 230 | 9 | 1 |

*Salad Buffet: Per ½ Cup Unless Indicated*

| | C | F | Cb |
|---|---|---|---|
| Coleslaw | 110 | 9 | 6 |
| **Salads:** Caesar, w/out dress., 1 cup | 110 | 8 | 8 |
| Cajun Potato | 230 | 17 | 15 |
| Chicken | 240 | 20 | 3 |
| Seafood | 140 | 10 | 9 |
| Spinach Bacon , 1 cup | 120 | 9 | 4 |
| Tuna | 190 | 13 | 5 |

*Dressings:* Balsamic Vinaig., 2 T.

| | C | F | Cb |
|---|---|---|---|
| *Dressings:* Balsamic Vinaig., 2 T. | 20 | 0 | 5 |
| Caesar, 2 Tbsp | 150 | 15 | 2 |
| Ranch, 2 Tbsp | 110 | 12 | 2 |

## (The) Great American Bagel Co (Dec '11)

| Bagels: | C | F | Cb |
|---|---|---|---|
| Asiago Cheese | 520 | 16 | 72 |
| Cheddar Herb | 390 | 8 | 66 |
| Cinnamon Raisin | 380 | 3.5 | 76 |
| Jalapeno Cheddar | 370 | 7 | 63 |
| Plain | 360 | 4 | 71 |
| Spinach Tomazzo | 640 | 20 | 86 |
| Swiss Everything | 470 | 10 | 77 |
| Tomazzo | 520 | 13 | 77 |
| *Paninis: On Regular Baguette* | | | |
| Chicken Pesto | 770 | 35 | 70 |
| Ham & Swiss | 600 | 26 | 58 |
| Philly Beef | 920 | 40 | 92 |
| Turkey Club | 680 | 29 | 67 |
| *Sandwiches:* BLT | 550 | 17 | 72 |
| Chicken Parmigiana | 740 | 22 | 81 |
| Ham | 460 | 9 | 71 |
| Roast Beef | 465 | 9 | 71 |
| Turkey | 435 | 5 | 72 |
| *Cream Cheese Filling: Per 1 oz* | | | |
| Apple Cinn; Blueberry; | 60 | 5 | 4 |
| Chocolate Chip; Caramel Apple, av | 70 | 4 | 8 |
| Scallion; Spinach; Strawberry, av. | 55 | 5 | 1 |
| *Pastries:* | | | |
| **Cookies:** Chocolate Chunk, 4 oz | 110 | 3.5 | 19 |
| Oatmeal Raisin, 4 oz | 120 | 5 | 18 |
| **Muffins:** Blueberry, 4¼ oz | 430 | 16 | 64 |
| Banana Nut, 4¼ oz | 430 | 18 | 61 |

## Green Burrito (Dec '11)

| *Burritos:* Bean & Cheese | 780 | 36 | 94 |
|---|---|---|---|
| Grilled Chicken | 880 | 46 | 81 |
| The Green Burrito with Steak | 850 | 32 | 109 |
| *Specialties:* | | | |
| **Super Nachos:** Chicken | 920 | 48 | 93 |
| Ground Beef | 1060 | 61 | 95 |
| **Taco Salad:** Chicken | 780 | 44 | 66 |
| Ground Beef | 920 | 56 | 69 |
| Steak | 810 | 46 | 69 |
| *Tacos:* Fish with 2 Tortillas | 320 | 15 | 36 |
| **Hard Shell:** Chicken; Steak, av. | 195 | 9 | 15 |
| Ground Beef | 240 | 14 | 15 |
| **Soft Shell:** Chicken | 200 | 7 | 17 |
| Ground Beef | 250 | 13 | 18 |
| *Sides:* Chips, 2 oz | 300 | 17 | 35 |
| Chips & Cheese, 5 oz | 700 | 42 | 62 |
| Guacamole, 1½ oz | 60 | 5 | 3 |
| Pinto Beans & Cheese, small, 7.8oz | 300 | 15 | 40 |
| Rice, small, 6 oz | 290 | 9 | 50 |
| Sour Cream, 1½ oz | 50 | 3.5 | 3 |

## (The) Great Steak & Potato Company (Dec '11)

| Breakfast Sandwiches: | C | F | Cb |
|---|---|---|---|
| Bacon, Egg & Cheese, 7.6 oz | 600 | 36 | 39 |
| Egg and Cheese, 7 oz | 500 | 29 | 39 |
| Ham and Cheese, 5½ oz | 430 | 22 | 41 |
| Ham, Egg and Cheese, 9 oz | 570 | 32 | 42 |
| Sausage, Egg and Cheese, 9 oz | 700 | 47 | 39 |
| Steak, Egg & Cheese, 10 oz | 600 | 34 | 40 |
| *Breakfast Potatoes,* | | | |
| Deluxe/Fresh Cut, average | 385 | 23 | 43 |
| *Sandwiches: 7"* | | | |
| Bacon Cheddar Cheesesteak, 12.2 oz | 720 | 32 | 62 |
| Buffalo Chicken Philly, 13.8 oz | 660 | 24 | 65 |
| Chicagoland Cheesesteak, 13.3 oz | 680 | 29 | 63 |
| Chicken Bacon Ranch, 15.2 oz | 990 | 56 | 66 |
| Chicken Cordon Bleu, 13.4 oz | 580 | 16 | 78 |
| Great Steak Cheesesteak, 13.6 oz | 740 | 37 | 62 |
| Gyro, 11.9 oz | 580 | 30 | 52 |
| Ham Delight/Explosion, av., 14 oz | 710 | 34 | 71 |
| Pastrami, 13.3 oz | 790 | 41 | 65 |
| Pepper Steak, 15.17 oz | 880 | 50 | 67 |
| Philly Cheesesteak, 11.8 oz | 650 | 26 | 62 |
| Reuben, 11.9 z | 690 | 33 | 61 |
| Super Steak Cheesesteak, 15 oz | 750 | 37 | 64 |
| Veggie Delight, 11.7 oz | 510 | 19 | 64 |
| *Baked Potatoes:* | | | |
| **The Great Potato:** Chicken, 12½ oz | 500 | 22 | 37 |
| Ham, 12.3 oz | 420 | 16 | 43 |
| Steak, 13 oz | 520 | 26 | 37 |
| Turkey, 12.3 oz | 390 | 13 | 39 |
| The King, 8.4 oz | 490 | 29 | 31 |
| *Fries:* | | | |
| **Great Fry:** Kids, 6¼ oz | 270 | 13 | 36 |
| Regular, 10¼ oz | 440 | 20 | 60 |
| Large, 12½ oz | 540 | 25 | 72 |
| Coney Island Fry, regular, 12.7 oz | 570 | 30 | 61 |
| King Fry, regular, 11.4 oz | 630 | 39 | 52 |
| Nacho Fry, regular, 11.8 oz | 510 | 27 | 53 |
| *Salads: Without Dressing* | | | |
| Chef Salad, 16 oz | 260 | 11 | 15 |
| Great Salad: Grilled Chicken, 19 oz | 380 | 18 | 18 |
| Grilled Steak, 19.4 oz | 400 | 23 | 18 |
| Wedge: Grilled Chicken, 14.8 oz | 270 | 12 | 11 |
| Grilled Steak, 15.3 oz | 290 | 16 | 11 |
| Salad Dressings: Ranch, 1 oz | 170 | 18 | 1 |
| Thousand Island, 1 oz | 130 | 12 | 4 |

**203**

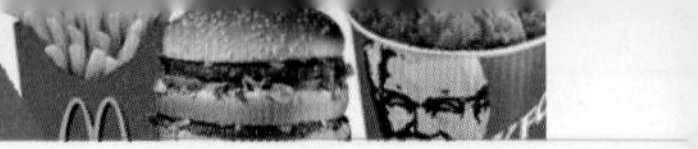

## Haagen-Dazs® (Dec'11)

*Ice Cream: Per ½ Cup*

| | C | F | Cb |
|---|---|---|---|
| Amaretto Almond Crunch | 270 | 17 | 24 |
| Bananas Foster | 240 | 13 | 27 |
| Banana Split | 280 | 16 | 31 |
| Butter Pecan | 310 | 23 | 21 |
| Caramel Cone | 320 | 19 | 32 |
| Cherry Vanilla | 240 | 15 | 23 |
| Chocolate | 260 | 17 | 22 |
| Chocolate Chip Cookie Dough | 310 | 20 | 29 |
| Chocolate Chocolate Chip | 300 | 20 | 26 |
| Chocolate Peanut Butter | 360 | 24 | 27 |
| Coffee | 270 | 18 | 21 |
| Cookies & Cream | 270 | 17 | 23 |
| Creme Brulee | 280 | 19 | 23 |
| Dark Chocolate | 260 | 17 | 21 |
| Dulce de Leche | 290 | 17 | 28 |
| Mango | 250 | 14 | 28 |
| Pineapple Coconut | 230 | 13 | 25 |
| Pistachio | 290 | 20 | 22 |
| Rum Raisin | 270 | 17 | 22 |
| Vanilla Bean | 290 | 18 | 26 |
| **Five:** Caramel | 240 | 11 | 29 |
| Average other flavors | 215 | 11 | 24 |

*Frozen Yogurt: Per ½ Cup*

| | C | F | Cb |
|---|---|---|---|
| Coffee | 200 | 4.5 | 31 |
| Dulce de Leche | 190 | 2.5 | 35 |
| Peach | 170 | 2 | 31 |
| Vanilla Raspberry Swirl | 170 | 2.5 | 32 |
| Wildberry | 180 | 2 | 34 |

*Sorbet: Per ½ Cup*

| | C | F | Cb |
|---|---|---|---|
| Blackberry Cabernet | 100 | 0 | 26 |
| Raspberry; Zesty Lemon | 120 | 0 | 30 |
| Strawberry | 130 | 0 | 31 |

*Ice Cream Bars ~ See Page 109*

## Hardee's® (Dec'11)

*Burgers:*

| | C | F | Cb |
|---|---|---|---|
| Big Shef, 7½ oz | 660 | 46 | 36 |
| Cheeseburger: Regular, 4½ oz | 350 | 19 | 32 |
| Double, 7¼ oz | 530 | 32 | 34 |
| Hamburger, regular, 4½ oz | 310 | 15 | 32 |
| Thickburger: Original, ⅓ lb | 770 | 48 | 53 |
| Bacon Cheese, ⅓ lb | 850 | 57 | 49 |
| Little Thick Cheeseburger, 6 oz | 450 | 23 | 38 |
| Low-Carb, ⅓ lb | 420 | 32 | 5 |
| Monster, ⅔ lb | 1320 | 95 | 46 |
| Mushroom 'N' Swiss, ⅓ lb | 650 | 36 | 47 |
| Six Dollar, ½ lb | 930 | 59 | 57 |
| Steakhouse, ⅓ lb | 1010 | 66 | 68 |

## Hardee's® cont... (Dec'11)

*Breaded Chicken Tenders: W/o Sauce*

| | C | F | Cb |
|---|---|---|---|
| 3 pieces, 4.5 oz | 260 | 13 | 13 |
| 5 pieces, 7.5 oz | 440 | 21 | 21 |

*Sandwiches:*

| | C | F | Cb |
|---|---|---|---|
| Big Hot Ham 'N' Cheese | 460 | 20 | 40 |
| Chicken: Charbroiled BBQ Chicken | 400 | 6 | 62 |
| Charbroiled Chicken Club | 630 | 32 | 54 |
| Hand Breaded Chicken Fillet | 680 | 37 | 55 |
| Fish, Supreme | 630 | 38 | 51 |

*Sides:*

| | C | F | Cb |
|---|---|---|---|
| Beer Battered Onion Rings, 4.5 oz | 410 | 24 | 45 |
| **Fries:** Small, 4¼ oz | 320 | 14 | 45 |
| Medium, 5¾ oz | 430 | 19 | 60 |
| Large, 6¼ oz | 470 | 21 | 65 |

*Kids Meals: Includes Kid's Fries & Small Drink*

| | C | F | Cb |
|---|---|---|---|
| Breaded Chicken Tenders (2), without sauce | 380 | 18 | 36 |
| Cheeseburger | 560 | 29 | 59 |
| Hamburger | 520 | 25 | 59 |

*Breakfast :*

| | C | F | Cb |
|---|---|---|---|
| **Biscuits:** Bacon, Egg & Cheese | 530 | 36 | 36 |
| Biscuit 'N' Gravy | 530 | 34 | 47 |
| Chicken Fillet | 620 | 37 | 47 |
| Cinnamon 'N' Raisin | 300 | 15 | 40 |
| Country Ham | 440 | 26 | 36 |
| Country Steak | 590 | 40 | 43 |
| Loaded Omelet | 610 | 42 | 36 |
| Made from Scratch | 370 | 23 | 35 |
| Monster | 770 | 55 | 37 |
| Pork Chop 'N' Gravy | 680 | 42 | 48 |
| Sausage | 530 | 38 | 36 |
| Sausage and Egg | 610 | 44 | 36 |
| Smoked Sausage | 620 | 46 | 37 |
| Smoked Sausage w/ Egg & Cheese | 750 | 56 | 38 |
| **Bowl,** Low Carb | 620 | 50 | 6 |
| **Burrito,** Loaded | 760 | 49 | 39 |
| **Sandwiches,** Frisco | 420 | 18 | 39 |
| **Sunrise Croissants:** With Bacon | 450 | 29 | 28 |
| With Ham | 400 | 23 | 27 |
| With Sausage | 550 | 38 | 29 |
| **Sides:** Grits, 5 oz | 110 | 5 | 16 |
| Hash Rounds: Small, 3 oz | 250 | 16 | 25 |
| Medium, 4¼ oz | 390 | 26 | 36 |
| Large, 5¾ oz | 530 | 35 | 49 |

*Continued next page...*

Updated Nutrition Data ~ www.CalorieKing.com
Persons with Diabetes ~ See Disclaimer (Page 22)

## Hardee's® cont... (Dec '11)

*Dessert,*

| | C | F | Cb |
|---|---|---|---|
| Apple Turnover w/o Cinn. Sugar | 270 | 13 | 35 |

*Drinks:*

| | C | F | Cb |
|---|---|---|---|
| **Hot Chocolate** | 150 | 3 | 18 |

**Ice Cream Malts:** *Per 14.6 oz Regular Cup*

| | C | F | Cb |
|---|---|---|---|
| Chocolate | 780 | 35 | 97 |
| Strawberry | 775 | 35 | 98 |
| Vanilla | 710 | 35 | 97 |

**Ice Cream Shakes:** *Per 14 oz Regular Cup*

| | C | F | Cb |
|---|---|---|---|
| Chocolate; Strawberry, average | 700 | 34 | 86 |
| Vanilla | 710 | 33 | 87 |

*For Complete Nutritional Data ~ see CalorieKing.com*

## Hissho Sushi® (Dec '11)

*Starters: Per Serving*

| | C | F | Cb |
|---|---|---|---|
| Edamame, ⅓ order, 3 oz | 105 | 4 | 8 |
| Decopus Salad, 3.5 oz | 150 | 2 | 18 |
| Spring Rolls: Regular (2) | 135 | 2 | 18 |
| Garden (2) | 130 | 3 | 23 |
| Grilled Chicken (2) | 140 | 4 | 19 |
| Ocean Salmon (2) | 150 | 5 | 16 |
| Ocean Tuna (2) | 155 | 4 | 16 |
| Tofu (2) | 125 | 3 | 20 |
| Seaweed Salad, 3.5 oz | 2 | 0 | 0 |

*Sushi: Per Serving, 6 Pieces Unless Indicated*

| | C | F | Cb |
|---|---|---|---|
| **Maki Rolls:** Blazing California | 265 | 2 | 53 |
| Boston | 265 | 2 | 53 |
| California | 275 | 3 | 56 |
| Crab Salad | 270 | 3 | 53 |
| Dynamite: Salmon | 295 | 5 | 51 |
| Shrimp | 285 | 3 | 52 |
| Tuna | 290 | 4 | 49 |
| Yellowtail | 295 | 4 | 51 |
| Healthy: Immitation Crab, 12 pcs | 315 | 0.5 | 68 |
| Cucumber, 12 pieces | 275 | 0.5 | 61 |
| Inari | 285 | 4 | 54 |
| Nippon Favorite: Salmon, 12 pcs | 330 | 2 | 65 |
| Tuna, 12 pieces | 330 | 2 | 64 |
| Philadelphia | 345 | 10 | 56 |
| Snow Crab | 280 | 3 | 56 |
| Sushicado: Salmon, 12 pieces | 510 | 7 | 92 |
| Shrimp | 300 | 3 | 56 |

*Specialty Items: Per Serving, 4 pieces*

| | C | F | Cb |
|---|---|---|---|
| **Rolls:** Alaskan | 245 | 3 | 43 |
| Biggie | 410 | 8 | 74 |
| Caterpillar | 330 | 5 | 60 |
| Colossal: California | 270 | 2 | 57 |
| Dynamite:Salmon | 275 | 4 | 46 |
| Dynamite Shrimp | 265 | 3 | 47 |
| Crying Ocean | 260 | 2 | 48 |
| Crunchy, 6 pieces | 285 | 3 | 53 |

## Hissho Sushi® cont... (Dec '11)

*Specialty Items (Cont): Per Serving*

| | C | F | Cb |
|---|---|---|---|
| **Rolls:** Grande Finale | 280 | 5 | 48 |
| Living Color | 250 | 3 | 43 |
| Mango Tango | 250 | 5 | 37 |
| Salmon Lover | 305 | 8 | 42 |
| Sriracha Party | 450 | 8 | 77 |
| Tempura Shrimp | 255 | 1 | 54 |
| **TNT:** Salmon | 290 | 4 | 52 |
| Shrimp | 280 | 2 | 52 |
| Tuna | 290 | 3 | 50 |
| Wasabi Crunch | 335 | 7 | 53 |

## Heavenly Ham® (Dec '11)

*Meats: Per 3 oz Serving*

| | C | F | Cb |
|---|---|---|---|
| Bone-In Hams: Glazed | 190 | 11 | 4 |
| Fat Removed | 160 | 3 | 4 |
| Boneless Hams: Glazed | 120 | 4 | 4 |
| Fat Removed | 90 | 1 | 4 |

*Classic Sandwiches:*

| | C | F | Cb |
|---|---|---|---|
| Roast Beef | 635 | 36 | 50 |
| Swiss Philly | 700 | 46 | 49 |

*Signature Sandwiches:*

| | C | F | Cb |
|---|---|---|---|
| Paradise Club | 850 | 53 | 65 |
| Smokehouse | 775 | 47 | 54 |
| Turkey Ranch Wrangler | 690 | 39 | 59 |

*Salads: Without Dressing*

| | C | F | Cb |
|---|---|---|---|
| Chicken | 260 | 17 | 14 |
| Taste of Italy | 310 | 20 | 14 |

*Bread:* Croissant

| | C | F | Cb |
|---|---|---|---|
| Croissant | 230 | 12 | 27 |
| French Batard | 210 | 0.5 | 46 |
| Multigrain Batard | 250 | 3.5 | 46 |
| Sliced Wheat Bread | 300 | 5 | 54 |

*Sauces:* BBQ, 1¾ oz

| | C | F | Cb |
|---|---|---|---|
| BBQ, 1¾ oz | 260 | 26 | 4 |
| Mayonnaise, 1 oz | 200 | 24 | 0 |
| Ranch, 1½ oz | 220 | 23 | 2 |
| Sweet Café Spread, 1 oz | 100 | 10 | 4 |
| That Mustard, 1 oz | 150 | 0 | 30 |

## Hot Dog on a Stick® (Dec '11)

*Menu Items:*

| | C | F | Cb |
|---|---|---|---|
| American Cheese on a Stick | 260 | 14 | 22 |
| Beef Hot Dog on a Bun | 470 | 29 | 36 |
| Turkey Hot Dog on a Stick | 250 | 14 | 22 |
| Veggie Dog on a Stick | 220 | 8 | 24 |
| Pepperjack Cheese on a Stick | 240 | 14 | 19 |
| *French Fries,* 4½ oz | 400 | 21 | 49 |
| *Funnel Cake Sticks,* (10) | 210 | 8 | 31 |
| *Lemonade (16 fl.oz):* Original | 150 | 0 | 38 |
| Sugar Free Lemonade | 15 | 0 | 3 |
| Cherry | 210 | 0 | 53 |

# Fast - Foods & Restaurants

## Hungry Howie's Pizza® (Dec '11)

*Counts may vary in Florida.*

*Pizzas: Per Slice*

| | C | F | Cb |
|---|---|---|---|
| Cheese: Small, ⅙ pizza | 160 | 3.5 | 20 |
| Medium, ⅛ pizza | 190 | 5.5 | 23 |
| Large, ¹⁄₁₀ pizza | 210 | 5 | 25 |
| X-Large, ⅛ pizza | 395 | 9 | 42 |
| *Oven Baked Subs: Per ½ Sub* | | | |
| Deluxe Italian | 505 | 18 | 61 |
| Ham & Cheese | 475 | 15 | 61 |
| Steak & Cheese | 490 | 15 | 64 |
| Turkey Club | 555 | 15 | 63 |
| Vegetarian | 530 | 21 | 64 |
| *Sides:* Boneless Wings, 3 pieces | 145 | 5 | 12 |
| Howie Wings, 5 wings | 180 | 13 | 0 |
| *Salads: Per Small Size, Without Dressing* | | | |
| Antipasto | 230 | 15 | 6 |
| Chef | 230 | 13 | 8 |
| Garden | 40 | 0.5 | 7 |
| Greek | 250 | 15 | 16 |
| *Dressings:* Per 1 oz | | | |
| Creamy Italian | 120 | 12 | 2 |
| Greek | 110 | 11 | 2 |
| Ranch | 180 | 19 | 1 |
| Thousand Island | 140 | 14 | 4 |

## In-N-Out Burger® (Dec '11)

*Burgers:*

| | C | F | Cb |
|---|---|---|---|
| Hamburger: With Onion | 390 | 19 | 39 |
| With Mustard/Ketchup, w/o Spread | 310 | 10 | 41 |
| Protein Style w/ Lettuce Wrap, no Bun | 240 | 17 | 11 |
| Cheeseburger: With Onion | 480 | 27 | 39 |
| With Mustard/Ketchup, w/o Spread | 400 | 18 | 41 |
| Protein Style w/ Lettuce Wrap, no Bun | 330 | 25 | 11 |
| Double Double®: With Onion | 670 | 41 | 39 |
| With Mustard/Ketchup, no Spread | 590 | 32 | 41 |
| Protein Style w/ Lettuce Wrap, no Bun | 520 | 39 | 11 |
| *French Fries,* 4½ oz | 395 | 18 | 54 |
| *Drinks:* Milk, 10 fl.oz | 180 | 6 | 18 |
| Coca-Cola®,16 fl.oz | 195 | 0 | 54 |
| Lemonade, 16 fl.oz | 180 | 0 | 40 |
| Root Beer,16 fl.oz | 220 | 0 | 60 |
| **Shakes:** Chocolate, 15 fl.oz | 590 | 29 | 72 |
| Strawberry, 15 fl.oz | 590 | 27 | 81 |

## IHOP® (Dec '11)

*Pancakes:*

| | C | F | Cb |
|---|---|---|---|
| **Buttermilk:** | | | |
| Full Stack (5) without Toppings | 770 | 25 | 115 |
| Short Stack (3) without Toppings | 490 | 18 | 69 |
| Chocolate Chip (4) with Toppings | 720 | 24 | 112 |
| Double Blueberry (4) with Toppings | 800 | 17 | 144 |
| Strawberry Banana (4) with Toppings | 760 | 17 | 137 |
| *Syrup:* Regular, 1 Tbsp | 50 | 0 | 12 |
| Sugar-Free, 1 Tbsp | 10 | 0 | 2 |
| *Whipped Butter/Margarine,* 1 Tbsp | 80 | 9 | 0 |
| *French Toast & Waffles: W/ Toppings Unless Indicated* | | | |
| **French Toast:** Original | 920 | 50 | 88 |
| Cinn-A-Stack | 1120 | 54 | 126 |
| Strawberry Banana | 1060 | 45 | 135 |
| **Waffle,** Belgian, Plain (1) | 360 | 15 | 47 |
| With Butter | 420 | 23 | 47 |
| **Fruit Toppings:** *With Whipped Topping* | | | |
| Blueberry Compote; Strawb., av. | 165 | 2.5 | 37 |
| Cinnamon Apple Compote | 140 | 2.5 | 32 |
| *International Crepe Passport: As Served* | | | |
| Fresh Fruit | 860 | 50 | 69 |
| Nutella | 1100 | 71 | 83 |
| Strawberry Banana Danish | 1000 | 67 | 68 |
| *Savory Crepes:* Chkn Florentine | 880 | 53 | 48 |
| Bacon & Cheddar Stuffed | 1130 | 82 | 43 |
| Garden Stuffed | 1050 | 75 | 51 |
| *Hearty Omelettes: Without Pancakes or Sides* | | | |
| Big Steak | 1220 | 82 | 54 |
| Garden | 840 | 66 | 18 |
| Hearty Ham & Cheese | 870 | 60 | 18 |
| Spinach & Mushroom | 910 | 70 | 24 |
| *Sandwiches & Burgers: Without Sides* | | | |
| Bacon Cheddar Chicken Sandwich | 930 | 61 | 47 |
| Chicken Clubhouse Super Stacker | 1180 | 51 | 55 |
| Patty Melt | 920 | 66 | 42 |
| Philly Cheese Steak Stacker | 780 | 39 | 55 |
| Turkey & Bacon Club Sandwich | 730 | 39 | 50 |
| *Breakfast Combinations: As Served, w/o Syrup* | | | |
| Biscuits & Gravy w/ Country Gravy | 1420 | 95 | 99 |
| Breakfast Sampler | 1180 | 74 | 82 |
| Country Fried Steak & Eggs, with Country Gravy | 1420 | 95 | 99 |
| Split Decision | 1170 | 75 | 80 |
| T-Bone Steak & Eggs, 12 oz | 1250 | 68 | 74 |
| Thick-Cut Bone-In Ham & Eggs | 1170 | 61 | 88 |
| *Hearty Dinner Favorites: As Served* | | | |
| Maui-style Crunchy Shrimp | 720 | 27 | 95 |
| Mediterranean Lemon Chicken | 780 | 41 | 44 |
| Simple & Fit Grilled Tilapia | 490 | 23 | 27 |
| Sirloin Steak Tips | 800 | 40 | 69 |
| T-Bone Steak, 12 oz | 760 | 41 | 40 |

## Jack in the Box® (Dec '11)

| Sandwiches & Burgers: | C | F | Cb |
|---|---|---|---|
| Bacon Ultimate Cheeseburger | 920 | 63 | 45 |
| Hamburger: Original | 290 | 12 | 32 |
| With Cheese | 330 | 15 | 32 |
| Deluxe | 340 | 16 | 33 |
| With Cheese | 420 | 23 | 34 |
| Jumbo Jack: Original | 500 | 27 | 45 |
| With Cheese | 580 | 34 | 45 |
| Junior Bacon Cheeseburger | 400 | 22 | 32 |
| Sirloin Cheeseburger w/ Bacon | 990 | 66 | 52 |
| Sourdough Jack | 660 | 44 | 40 |
| Sourdough Steak Melt | 650 | 38 | 38 |
| Ultimate Cheeseburger | 830 | 57 | 44 |

| Chicken & Fish: | | | |
|---|---|---|---|
| Chicken Sandwich | 410 | 21 | 42 |
| With Bacon | 470 | 25 | 42 |
| Chicken Strips: Crispy (4) | 560 | 24 | 53 |
| Grilled (4) | 250 | 7 | 5 |
| Fish & Chips, small fries, 8½ oz | 710 | 37 | 74 |
| Jack's Spicy Chicken Sandwich | 530 | 21 | 60 |
| With Cheese | 610 | 26 | 61 |
| Sourdough Grilled Chicken Club | 540 | 26 | 38 |

| Breakfast: | | | |
|---|---|---|---|
| Biscuit: Bacon, Egg & Cheese | 430 | 25 | 35 |
| Sausage, Egg & Cheese | 570 | 38 | 36 |
| Breakfast Jack: Regular | 280 | 11 | 30 |
| With Bacon | 310 | 14 | 30 |
| Croissant: Sausage | 570 | 40 | 32 |
| Supreme | 450 | 27 | 32 |
| Sandwiches: Extreme Sausage | 660 | 47 | 32 |
| Sourdough | 410 | 21 | 35 |
| Ultimate | 520 | 25 | 42 |
| Hash Brown Sticks (5) | 280 | 19 | 26 |
| Meaty Burrito, without salsa | 610 | 37 | 38 |

| Snacks & Sides: | | | |
|---|---|---|---|
| Bacon Cheddar Pot. Wedges, 9¼ oz | 680 | 42 | 58 |
| Beef Taco, regular, (1) | 190 | 11 | 17 |
| Chiquita Apple Bites w/ Caramel, med. | 70 | 0 | 17 |
| Egg Rolls, without sauce, (3) | 440 | 22 | 46 |
| Mozzarella Cheese Sticks (3) | 280 | 16 | 22 |
| Mozzarella Cheese Sticks (6) | 560 | 33 | 43 |
| Stuffed Jalapenos, (3) | 220 | 12 | 21 |
| Stuffed Jalapenos, (7) | 510 | 29 | 49 |
| Onion Rings, (8), 4¼ oz | 450 | 28 | 45 |
| Seasoned Curly Fries, med., 4½ oz | 430 | 25 | 46 |

## Jack in the Box® cont... (Dec '11)

| Healthy Choices: | C | F | Cb |
|---|---|---|---|
| Chicken Fajita, without Salsa | 320 | 11 | 33 |
| Chicken Teriyaki Bowl | 580 | 5 | 106 |
| Grilled Chicken Strips, with Teriyaki Dipping Sauce | 310 | 8 | 16 |
| Hamburger Deluxe | 340 | 16 | 33 |

| Salads: No Dressing or Condiments | | | |
|---|---|---|---|
| Chicken Club with Grilled Chicken | 370 | 20 | 13 |
| Side Salad | 20 | 0 | 4 |
| Southwest Chicken, with Grilled Chicken Strips | 350 | 15 | 29 |

| Sauces & Dressings: | | | |
|---|---|---|---|
| Dipping Sauce: Barbecue, 1 oz | 40 | 0 | 10 |
| Buttermilk House, 1 oz | 130 | 13 | 3 |
| Frank's Red Hot Buffalo, 1 oz | 10 | 0 | 2 |
| Sweet & Sour, 1 oz | 45 | 0 | 11 |
| Tartar, 1½ oz | 210 | 22 | 2 |
| Sauce: Mayo-Onion, ½ oz | 90 | 10 | 1 |
| Soy, ¼ oz | 5 | 0 | 1 |
| Taco, ¼ oz | 0 | 0 | 0 |

| Shakes & Desserts: | | | |
|---|---|---|---|
| Chocolate Overload Cake | 300 | 7 | 57 |
| Churros, Mini (5) | 350 | 18 | 42 |
| New York Style Cheesecake | 310 | 17 | 32 |

| Shakes: 16 oz, with Whipped Topping | | | |
|---|---|---|---|
| Chocolate | 800 | 38 | 101 |
| Oreo Cookie | 810 | 43 | 92 |
| Strawberry | 780 | 38 | 95 |
| Vanilla | 700 | 38 | 76 |

*For Complete Nutritional Data ~ see CalorieKing.com*

## Jack's® (Dec '11)

| Sandwiches: Big Bacon Burger | 610 | 41 | 31 |
|---|---|---|---|
| Big Jack Burger | 530 | 33 | 35 |
| Cheeseburger | 380 | 21 | 31 |
| Chicken Fillet Sandwich | 490 | 24 | 40 |
| Double Big Jack Cheese Burger | 850 | 59 | 35 |
| Double Cheeseburger | 540 | 33 | 31 |
| Grilled Chicken Sandwich | 380 | 16 | 32 |
| Hamburger | 340 | 18 | 31 |
| Chicken, Chicken Fingers, 3 pieces | 300 | 14 | 14 |
| Fries, regular | 310 | 13 | 42 |
| Breakfast: Egg & Cheese Biscuit | 360 | 21 | 31 |
| Sausage, Egg & Cheese Biscuit | 520 | 35 | 32 |
| Steak Biscuit | 480 | 28 | 43 |

*For Complete Menu & Data ~ see CalorieKing.com*

## Jamba Juice® (Dec '11)

| | C | F | Cb |
|---|---|---|---|
| *All Fruit:* Original Size, 22 fl.oz | | | |
| Mega Mango | 340 | 0.5 | 85 |
| Peach Perfection; Strawberry Whirl | 300 | 0.5 | 75 |
| Pomegranate Paradise | 340 | 0.5 | 85 |
| *Classics:* Per 16 fl.oz | | | |
| Blackberry Bliss | 230 | 1 | 55 |
| Mango-a-go-go; Aloha Pineapple, av. | 285 | 1 | 66 |
| Peach Pleasure; Pomeg. Pick-Me-Up | 260 | 1 | 61 |
| Strawberry Surf Rider | 300 | 1 | 72 |
| *Creamy Treats:* Per 16 fl oz | | | |
| Chocolate Moo'd | 430 | 4 | 86 |
| Orange Dream Machine | 350 | 1 | 76 |
| Peanut Butter Moo'd | 480 | 10 | 83 |
| *Fruit & Veggie Smoothies:* Per 16 fl.oz | | | |
| Apple & Greens; Berry upBEET, av. | 225 | 1 | 50 |
| Orange Carrot Karma | 180 | 0.5 | 43 |
| *Jamba Light:* Per 16 fl oz | | | |
| Berry Fulfilling | 140 | 0.5 | 29 |
| Mango Mantra; Strawb. Nirvana, av. | 155 | 0 | 33 |
| *Pre Boosted Smoothies:* Per 16 fl.oz | | | |
| Acai Super-Antioxidant | 260 | 4 | 54 |
| Strawbery Energizer | 280 | 1 | 67 |
| The Coldbuster | 250 | 1 | 59 |
| *Probiotic Fruit & Yogurt Blends,* | | | |
| average all flavors, 16 fl.oz | 240 | 0 | 49 |
| *Fresh Squeezed Juices:* Per 12 fl.oz | | | |
| Carrot | 100 | 0.5 | 22 |
| Orange | 170 | 0.5 | 39 |
| *Shots: Single* | | | |
| Matcha Energy Shot-Soymilk, 4 fl.oz | 70 | 0 | 15 |
| Wheatgrass Detox, 1 fl oz | 5 | 0 | 1 |
| *Breakfast:* | | | |
| **Hot Oatmeal:** With Fruit & Brown Sugar | | | |
| Berry Cherry with Pecan | 500 | 15 | 87 |
| Fruit flavors, av | 385 | 4.5 | 81 |
| Plain, brown sugar only | 260 | 4.5 | 52 |
| *California Flat Bread:* Per Flatbread | | | |
| Four Cheesy, 5¾ oz | 420 | 16 | 46 |
| MediterraneaYum, 6 oz | 320 | 8 | 49 |
| Smokehouse Chicken, 6 oz | 390 | 10 | 53 |
| *Baked Goods:* Per Item | | | |
| Berry Agave Bar, 3 oz | 220 | 12 | 26 |
| Muffins: Blueberry Streusel | 400 | 19 | 45 |
| Pumpkin Ginger, reduced fat, | 340 | 8 | 66 |
| Sourdough Parmesan Pretzel, 5 oz | 410 | 10 | 67 |
| *Parfaits:* Per 16 oz | | | |
| Acai/Mango Peach Toppers, average | 480 | 9 | 94 |
| Chunky Strawberry | 570 | 17 | 93 |

## Jersey Mike's Subs® (Dec '11)

| | C | F | Cb |
|---|---|---|---|
| *Cold Subs:* Per Regular, on Wheat, W/out Vinegar, Oil or Mayo Unless Indicated | | | |
| #1 BLT | 570 | 26 | 63 |
| #2 Jersey Shore Favorite | 560 | 18 | 67 |
| #3 American Classic | 560 | 18 | 65 |
| #5 Super Sub | 580 | 19 | 67 |
| #6 Roast Beef & Provolone | 720 | 25 | 64 |
| #7 Turkey Breast & Provolone | 540 | 16 | 64 |
| #8 Club Sub with Mayonnaise | 890 | 52 | 66 |
| #9 Club Supreme w/ Mayonnaise | 940 | 52 | 66 |
| #10 Albacore Tuna | 910 | 59 | 66 |
| #13 Original Italian | 680 | 27 | 68 |
| #14 Veggie | 720 | 33 | 65 |
| *Hot Subs/Cheese Steaks:* Per Regular on Wheat Roll | | | |
| #15 Meatball & Cheese | 890 | 52 | 72 |
| #17 Chicken Philly | 630 | 25 | 65 |
| Steak Philly | 620 | 24 | 64 |
| #43 Chipotle Chicken | 910 | 56 | 68 |
| Chipotle Steak | 900 | 55 | 66 |
| #18 Chicken Parmesan | 650 | 22 | 77 |
| #19 BBQ Beef | 710 | 16 | 83 |
| #20 Pastrami & Swiss | 580 | 18 | 60 |
| #56 Big Kahuna Steak | 670 | 28 | 65 |
| #56 Big Kahuna Chicken | 680 | 29 | 66 |
| *Cold Wraps:* With Flour Tortilla, w/o Vin./Oil or Mayo | | | |
| #1 BLT | 590 | 29 | 60 |
| #2 Jersey Shore Favorite | 580 | 22 | 64 |
| #3 American Classic | 580 | 22 | 63 |
| #5 Super Sub | 600 | 22 | 65 |
| *Salads:* Without Dressing | | | |
| Chef, 16 oz | 240 | 10 | 12 |
| Grilled Chicken Caesar, 12½ oz | 510 | 35 | 11 |
| Tossed, 12 oz | 50 | 0.5 | 11 |
| Tuna, 18 oz | 690 | 60 | 15 |
| *Dressings:* Per 2 Tbsp, 1 oz | | | |
| Caesar | 150 | 15 | 2 |
| Chipotle Mayo | 180 | 20 | 0 |
| Golden Italian | 110 | 11 | 3 |
| Ranch | 120 | 12 | 2 |
| Russian | 160 | 16 | 4 |
| *Condiments:* Oil, regular, 1 oz | 270 | 30 | 0 |
| Mustard, ½ oz | 0 | 0 | 0 |
| *Desserts:* Cookie, Choc Chip, 1½ oz | 200 | 11 | 24 |
| Daves Chocolate Brownie, 4 oz | 440 | 20 | 60 |
| *Drinks:* Mountain Dew, 22 oz | 310 | 0 | 84 |
| Mug Root Beer, 22 oz | 290 | 0 | 79 |
| Tropicana Twister Orange, 22 oz | 360 | 0 | 96 |

## Jimmy John's® (Dec '11)

*Subs: (8")*  | C | F | Cb
*Figures Based on French Bread w/ Standard Toppings & Mayo, Unless Indicated*

| | C | F | Cb |
|---|---|---|---|
| #1 Pepe | 615 | 31 | 50 |
| #2 Big John | 535 | 24 | 49 |
| #3 Totally Tuna without dressing | 650 | 31 | 54 |
| #4 Turkey Tom | 515 | 22 | 50 |
| #5 Vito with Italian Vinaigrette | 600 | 28 | 52 |
| #6 Vegetarian | 580 | 30 | 53 |
| JJBLT | 635 | 35 | 49 |

*Giant Club Sandwiches: Figures Based on French Bread w/ Standard Toppings & Mayo, Unless Indicated*

| | C | F | Cb |
|---|---|---|---|
| #7 Gourmet Smoked Ham | 775 | 32 | 69 |
| #8 Billy | 795 | 34 | 68 |
| #9 Italian Night w/ Mayo & Vinaig. | 950 | 51 | 70 |
| #10 Hunter's | 805 | 35 | 67 |
| #11 Country | 765 | 31 | 69 |
| #12 Beach Club | 730 | 31 | 71 |
| #13 Gourmet Veggie | 775 | 38 | 71 |
| #14 Bootlegger | 685 | 25 | 67 |
| #15 Club Tuna without dressing | 845 | 39 | 72 |
| #16 Club Lulu | 755 | 33 | 67 |
| #17 Ultimate Porker | 760 | 39 | 67 |

*Plain Slims: Figures Based on French Bread without Toppings, Dressing or Mayo*

| | C | F | Cb |
|---|---|---|---|
| Slim 1 Ham & Cheese | 505 | 10 | 66 |
| Slim 2 Roast Beef | 425 | 3 | 64 |
| Slim 3 Tuna Salad | 720 | 31 | 68 |
| Slim 4 Turkey Breast | 400 | 0.5 | 65 |
| Slim 5 Salami Capicola & Cheese | 600 | 20 | 66 |
| Slim 6 Double Provolone | 545 | 16 | 65 |

*Low Carb Options: With Standard Toppings & Mayo, without Bread*

| | C | F | Cb |
|---|---|---|---|
| Hunter's Club Unwich | 470 | 35 | 4 |
| The JJ Gargantuan Unwich | 740 | 54 | 7 |

*Low-Fat Options: W/o Standard Toppings, Dressing or Mayo*

| | C | F | Cb |
|---|---|---|---|
| #4 Turkey Tom | 305 | 0.5 | 48 |
| Slim 4 Turkey Breast | 400 | 0.5 | 65 |

*Sides:*

| | C | F | Cb |
|---|---|---|---|
| **Jimmy Chips:** BBQ, 1 oz | 160 | 9 | 17 |
| Jalapeno, 1 oz | 150 | 7 | 18 |
| Regular, 1 oz | 160 | 8 | 18 |
| Sea Salt & Vinegar, 1 oz | 140 | 8 | 16 |
| Thinny, 1 oz | 130 | 5 | 19 |
| **Pickle:** Spear | 5 | 0 | 1 |
| Whole | 20 | 0 | 4 |
| **Cookies,** Choc Chunk; Oatml Rsn, av. | 420 | 17 | 64 |

## Johnny Rockets® (Dec '11)

*Original Hamburgers:* | C | F | Cb

| | C | F | Cb |
|---|---|---|---|
| Hamburger #12 | 960 | 62 | 60 |
| Original Burger | 870 | 55 | 57 |
| Chili Cheese | 900 | 56 | 52 |
| Patty Melt | 870 | 53 | 52 |
| Rocket: Single | 940 | 61 | 56 |
| Double | 1410 | 98 | 57 |
| Route 66 | 960 | 65 | 50 |
| Smoke House: Single | 1140 | 71 | 70 |
| Double | 1700 | 115 | 70 |
| St Louis | 1060 | 72 | 51 |
| Streamliner | 430 | 11 | 59 |

*Sandwiches:* Chicken Club

| | C | F | Cb |
|---|---|---|---|
| Grilled Breast of Chicken | 580 | 26 | 50 |
| Grilled Cheese on Wheat | 500 | 27 | 48 |
| Philly Cheese Steak with Swiss | 820 | 42 | 56 |
| Tuna Melt on Sourdough | 790 | 48 | 43 |
| Tuna Salad on White | 740 | 48 | 46 |

*Other Favorites:*

| | C | F | Cb |
|---|---|---|---|
| Chicken Club | 730 | 28 | 69 |
| Chicken Tenders, without Sauce | 880 | 56 | 42 |
| Chili Dog | 810 | 53 | 43 |
| Hot Dog, with bun only | 410 | 22 | 34 |
| *Extras:* Bacon, 2 slices, ½ oz | 90 | 7 | 0 |
| Chili, 2 oz | 120 | 10 | 4 |
| Grilled Mushrooms, 2½ oz | 70 | 6 | 2 |
| Grilled Onions, 1 oz | 20 | 0.5 | 3 |

*Starters:*

| | C | F | Cb |
|---|---|---|---|
| Chili Bowl, 9 oz | 610 | 48 | 16 |
| American Fries, 7 oz | 480 | 19 | 69 |
| Cheese Fries, 12 oz | 740 | 38 | 82 |
| Chili Cheese Fries, 14 oz | 890 | 50 | 83 |
| Onion Rings, 9 oz | 880 | 40 | 90 |
| Rocket Wings, Traditional, 9 oz | 660 | 49 | 19 |

*Desserts:* Apple Pie, 7½ oz

| | C | F | Cb |
|---|---|---|---|
| Apple Pie, 7½ oz | 610 | 33 | 73 |
| A la Mode, scoop, 4 oz | 260 | 17 | 24 |
| Super Sundae w/ Hot Fudge, 11 oz | 670 | 37 | 79 |

*Beverages:*

| | C | F | Cb |
|---|---|---|---|
| Root Beer, 22 oz | 280 | 0 | 75 |
| Coke, 22 oz | 240 | 0 | 68 |
| Lemonade, 23 oz | 240 | 0 | 65 |
| Orange, 22 oz | 300 | 0 | 80 |

*Shakes:* Original

| | C | F | Cb |
|---|---|---|---|
| Chocolate, 18.45 oz | 920 | 51 | 105 |
| Strawberry, 17.57 oz | 820 | 50 | 81 |
| Vanilla, 18.35 oz | 890 | 50 | 100 |

## KFC® (Dec '11)

### Original Recipe:

| | C | F | Cb |
|---|---|---|---|
| **Breast:** 1 piece, 5¾ oz | 360 | 21 | 11 |
| without skin or breading, 4 oz | 160 | 3.5 | 2 |
| Drumstick, 1 piece, 1¾ oz | 120 | 7 | 3 |
| Thigh, 1 piece, 3.4 oz | 250 | 17 | 7 |
| Whole Wing, 1 piece, 2 oz | 120 | 7 | 3 |

### Spicy Crispy:

| | C | F | Cb |
|---|---|---|---|
| Breast, 1 piece, 6¼ oz | 420 | 25 | 12 |
| Drumstick, 1 piece, 2 oz | 160 | 10 | 5 |
| Thigh, 1 piece, 4 oz | 360 | 27 | 13 |
| Whole Wing, 1 piece, 1¾ oz | 170 | 12 | 6 |

### Grilled:

| | C | F | Cb |
|---|---|---|---|
| Breast, 4¼ oz | 220 | 7 | 0 |
| Drumstick, 1½ oz | 90 | 4 | 0 |
| Thigh, 2½ oz | 170 | 10 | 0 |
| Whole Wing, 1¼ oz | 80 | 4.5 | 1 |

### Strips & Filets:

| | C | F | Cb |
|---|---|---|---|
| Crispy: 2 Strips, 4 oz | 260 | 14 | 11 |
| 3 Strips, 6 oz | 390 | 21 | 17 |
| Original Filet 3½ oz | 200 | 9 | 8 |

### Popcorn Chicken:

| | C | F | Cb |
|---|---|---|---|
| Kids, 2.85 oz | 260 | 17 | 12 |
| Individual, 4.3 oz | 400 | 26 | 18 |
| Large, 6.15 oz | 560 | 37 | 26 |

### Sandwiches: With Sauce

| | C | F | Cb |
|---|---|---|---|
| Double Down, Original Filet | 610 | 37 | 18 |
| Doublicous, Original Filet | 520 | 25 | 40 |

### KFC Snackers: With Sauce

| | C | F | Cb |
|---|---|---|---|
| Crispy Strip: Original | 310 | 15 | 30 |
| Buffalo | 270 | 9 | 31 |
| Ultimate Cheese | 280 | 11 | 31 |
| Honey BBQ | 210 | 3 | 32 |

### KFC Famous Bowls & Pot Pie:

| | C | F | Cb |
|---|---|---|---|
| Bowls: Snack Size, 6.46 oz | 260 | 13 | 26 |
| Mashed Potato with Gravy, 18½ oz | 680 | 31 | 74 |
| Chicken Pot Pie, 14 oz | 790 | 45 | 66 |

### Value Boxes:

| | C | F | Cb |
|---|---|---|---|
| Drumsticks: Original | 400 | 22 | 37 |
| Extra Crispy | 440 | 25 | 39 |
| Grilled | 380 | 19 | 34 |
| Popcorn Chicken | 680 | 41 | 53 |
| Thighs: Original | 540 | 32 | 42 |
| Extra Crispy | 630 | 39 | 45 |
| Grilled | 460 | 25 | 34 |
| Wings: Fiery | 510 | 28 | 51 |
| Hot | 490 | 27 | 45 |
| HBBQ | 540 | 28 | 58 |

## KFC® cont... (Dec '11)

### Wings: Without Dipping Sauce

| | C | F | Cb |
|---|---|---|---|
| Hot Wings | 70 | 4 | 4 |
| Fiery Buffalo Hot Wings | 70 | 4 | 5 |
| Honey BBQ Hot Wings | 80 | 4 | 8 |

### Salads: Without Dressing or Croutons

| | C | F | Cb |
|---|---|---|---|
| Caesar Side | 40 | 2 | 2 |
| Crispy Chicken BLT | 360 | 19 | 18 |
| Crispy Chicken Caesar | 340 | 18 | 16 |
| House Side Salad | 15 | 0 | 3 |

### Sides: Per Single Portion

| | C | F | Cb |
|---|---|---|---|
| BBQ Baked Beans, 4½ oz | 210 | 1.5 | 41 |
| Biscuit, 2 oz | 180 | 8 | 23 |
| Cole Slaw, 4.2 oz | 150 | 6 | 21 |
| Corn on the Cob (3"), 2½ oz | 70 | 0.5 | 16 |
| Cornbread Muffin, 2 oz | 210 | 9 | 28 |
| Macaroni & Cheese, 4¾ oz | 160 | 7 | 19 |
| Mashed Potatoes with Gravy, 5 oz | 120 | 4 | 19 |
| Potato Wedges, 3.8 oz | 290 | 15 | 35 |

### Dipping Sauces:

| | C | F | Cb |
|---|---|---|---|
| Creamy Ranch, 1 oz | 140 | 15 | 1 |
| Honey BBQ | 40 | 0 | 9 |
| Honey Mustard, 1 oz | 120 | 10 | 6 |
| KFC Signature Sauce | 70 | 5 | 5 |
| Spicy Chipotle | 70 | 3.5 | 8 |
| Sweet & Sour, 1 oz | 45 | 0 | 12 |

### Dressings:

| | C | F | Cb |
|---|---|---|---|
| Original Ranch Fat Free, 1½ oz | 35 | 0 | 8 |
| Creamy Parmesan Caesar, 2 oz | 260 | 26 | 4 |
| Light Italian, 1 oz | 15 | 0.5 | 2 |
| **Croutons,** Parm. Garlic, Pouch (1) | 70 | 3 | 8 |

### Desserts:

**Lil' Buckets Parfait Cups:**

| | C | F | Cb |
|---|---|---|---|
| Chocolate Cream, 4 oz | 280 | 13 | 37 |
| Lemon Creme, 4½ oz | 400 | 13 | 65 |

## Kilwin's® ~ see CalorieKing.com

## Koo Koo Roo® ~ see CalorieKing.com

## Kohr Bros® ~ see CalorieKing.com

## Kolache® ~ see CalorieKing.com

Updated Nutrition Data ~ www.CalorieKing.com
Persons with Diabetes ~ See Disclaimer (Page 22)

## Krispy Kreme® (Dec'11)

| Doughnuts: | C | F | Cb |
|---|---|---|---|
| Apple Fritter | 210 | 14 | 18 |
| Caramel Kreme Crunch | 390 | 20 | 50 |
| Chocolate Iced Glazed Cruller | 260 | 12 | 38 |
| Chocolate Iced Cake | 280 | 15 | 34 |
| Chocolate Iced Custard Filled | 310 | 17 | 36 |
| Chocolate Iced Glazed | 240 | 11 | 33 |
| Chocolate Iced Kreme Filled | 360 | 21 | 40 |
| Chocolate Iced Glazed w/ Sprinkles | 270 | 11 | 41 |
| Cinnamon Apple Filled | 290 | 16 | 33 |
| Cinnamon Bun | 260 | 16 | 28 |
| Cinnamon Twist | 240 | 15 | 23 |
| Dulce de Leche | 300 | 18 | 31 |
| **Glazed:** Chocolate Cake | 300 | 15 | 41 |
| Cinnamon | 200 | 11 | 25 |
| Cruller | 220 | 12 | 27 |
| Kreme Filled | 340 | 20 | 38 |
| Lemon Filled | 290 | 16 | 35 |
| Maple Iced | 230 | 11 | 32 |
| Original | 190 | 11 | 21 |
| Raspberry Filled | 290 | 16 | 36 |
| Sour Cream | 310 | 14 | 43 |
| **Powdered:** Cake | 220 | 11 | 27 |
| Strawberry Filled | 290 | 16 | 33 |
| Sugar | 190 | 11 | 20 |
| Traditional Cake | 190 | 12 | 19 |
| **Doughnut Holes:** Orig. Glazed (4) | 200 | 11 | 26 |
| Glazed Cake, Regular/Choc. (4) | 200 | 10 | 26 |

*Chiller Beverages: Without Whipped Cream Topping*

| Orange You Glad; Very Berry, average, | | | |
|---|---|---|---|
| 12 fl.oz | 175 | 0 | 43 |
| 20 fl.oz | 295 | 0 | 71 |

*Kremey Chillers: Includes Whipped Cream Topping*

| Orange & Kreme: 12 fl.oz | 630 | 28 | 92 |
|---|---|---|---|
| 20 fl.oz | 970 | 40 | 150 |
| Lemon Sherbert: 12 fl.oz | 630 | 28 | 95 |
| 20 fl.oz | 980 | 40 | 155 |
| Choc./Mocha: Average, 12 fl.oz | 670 | 29 | 104 |
| average 20 fl.oz | 1050 | 41 | 171 |
| Lotta Latte: 12 fl.oz | 670 | 28 | 49 |
| 20 fl.oz | 1050 | 40 | 79 |

*For Complete Menu & Data ~ see CalorieKing.com*

## Krystal® (Dec'11)

| Burgers: | C | F | Cb |
|---|---|---|---|
| Big Angus | 550 | 35 | 46 |
| Double, with Bacon & Cheese | 850 | 59 | 48 |
| **Krystal:** Original, Single | 130 | 6 | 20 |
| Double | 290 | 13 | 33 |
| Bacon Cheese | 200 | 11 | 20 |
| Cheese | 160 | 8 | 20 |
| Double Cheese | 350 | 17 | 34 |
| Chik | 300 | 16 | 27 |
| **Pups:** Chili Cheese | 230 | 14 | 16 |
| Corn | 240 | 14 | 22 |
| Plain | 150 | 8 | 15 |

*French Fries:*

| Medium, 4¼ oz | 310 | 13 | 46 |
|---|---|---|---|
| Chili Cheese, 8¼ oz | 570 | 29 | 62 |

*Sides:*

| Large Chili, 12 oz | 300 | 11 | 33 |
|---|---|---|---|
| Chik'n Bites, Small, 3 oz | 200 | 7 | 20 |
| Salad, Crispy Chicken, 11 oz | 370 | 21 | 20 |

*Breakfast Items:*

| **Biscuits:** Bacon, Egg & Cheese | 440 | 24 | 34 |
|---|---|---|---|
| Chik | 400 | 18 | 43 |
| Gravy | 350 | 18 | 41 |
| Plain | 260 | 13 | 32 |
| Sausage | 420 | 28 | 32 |
| **Kryspers:** | 150 | 7 | 19 |
| **Sandwich,** Krystal Sunriser | 200 | 11 | 16 |
| **Scramblers:** Original, with Bacon | 330 | 16 | 27 |
| With Sausage | 420 | 26 | 27 |
| 4-Carb Scramblers: With Bacon | 450 | 31 | 2 |
| With Sausage | 620 | 52 | 3 |

*Desserts:*

| Apple Turnover, fried | 220 | 8 | 34 |
|---|---|---|---|
| Lemon Icebox Pie | 320 | 9 | 56 |

*Drinks: Per 16 fl.oz with ¼ ice*

| Coca-Cola Classic | 120 | 0 | 32 |
|---|---|---|---|
| Diet Coke | 0 | 0 | 0 |
| Sprite | 110 | 0 | 31 |

*For Complete Menu & Data ~ see CalorieKing.com*

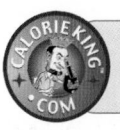

**For Menu Updates,
Check Author's Website
www.CalorieKing.com**

## LaRosa's Pizzeria® (Dec'11)

*Pizzas:*

| | **C** | **F** | **Cb** |
|---|---|---|---|
| **Focaccia Style:** *Per Slice, ⅛ of Medium Pizza* | | | |
| Florentine | 240 | 13 | 24 |
| Roma | 300 | 18 | 23 |
| **Hand Tossed:** *Per Slice, ⅛ of Medium Pizza* | | | |
| Cheese | 230 | 8 | 29 |
| Double Pepperoni | 300 | 14 | 29 |
| Big 4 Meat | 325 | 15 | 29 |
| Big 4 Pick 4 | 280 | 11 | 30 |
| Big 4 Veggie | 240 | 7 | 30 |
| **Pan Crust:** *Per Slice, ⅛ of Medium Pizza* | | | |
| Cheese | 300 | 16 | 30 |
| Double Pepperoni | 370 | 22 | 30 |
| Big 4 Meat | 325 | 15 | 29 |
| Big 4 Pick 4 | 275 | 11 | 30 |
| Big 4 Veggie | 235 | 7 | 30 |
| **Traditional Crust:** *Per Slice, ⅛ of Medium Pizza* | | | |
| Cheese | 200 | 10 | 19 |
| Double Pepperoni | 280 | 16 | 20 |
| Big 4 Meat | 285 | 16 | 20 |
| Big 4 Pick 4 | 240 | 12 | 20 |
| Big 4 Veggie | 200 | 8 | 21 |
| **Calzones:** *Per Calzone, No Dipping Sauce* | | | |
| 3 Meat & 3 Cheese | 1080 | 55 | 102 |
| 3 Veggie & 3 Cheese | 860 | 34 | 105 |
| Cheese & Pepperoni | 960 | 45 | 101 |
| Cheese | 840 | 34 | 101 |
| Philly Cheesesteak | 870 | 39 | 90 |
| Sausage Pelucci | 1040 | 52 | 92 |
| **Pasta Dinner:** *Without Bread, Soup or Salad* | | | |
| Cheese Ravioli | 660 | 26 | 80 |
| Lasagna with Meat Sauce | 735 | 38 | 61 |
| Spaghetti: With Meatballs | 870 | 28 | 119 |
| With Alfredo Sauce | 975 | 50 | 104 |
| With Meat Sauce | 700 | 18 | 104 |
| With Traditional Sauce | 640 | 12 | 113 |
| Ziti Chicken Alfredo | 980 | 42 | 102 |
| Ziti Sausage Pelucci | 765 | 20 | 115 |
| **Appetizers:** *Without Dipping Sauce* | | | |
| Boneless Wings: BBQ (1), 1½ oz | 75 | 3 | 8 |
| Hot (1), 1½ oz | 80 | 5 | 6 |
| Chicken Tenders, 8½ oz | 540 | 31 | 30 |
| Four Taste Sampler, 23½ oz | 1570 | 99 | 82 |
| French Fry Basket with Provolone | 860 | 56 | 73 |
| Mozzarella Cheese Sticks, 6½ oz | 635 | 43 | 36 |
| Onion Twists, Regular, 7¼ oz | 460 | 27 | 48 |

*For Complete Nutritional Data ~ see CalorieKing.com*

## La Salsa Fresh Mexican® (Dec'11)

*Appetizers:*

| | **C** | **F** | **Cb** |
|---|---|---|---|
| Salsa & Chips, 14½ oz | 700 | 32 | 87 |
| With Guacamole, 14½ oz | 970 | 55 | 103 |
| Chips (15), 1.4 oz | 200 | 10 | 25 |
| *Nachos:* | | | |
| **Black Beans:** With Carnitas | 1570 | 83 | 141 |
| With Chicken | 1600 | 83 | 148 |
| With Steak | 1580 | 84 | 142 |
| **Pinto Beans:** With Carnitas | 1560 | 83 | 139 |
| With Chicken | 1590 | 83 | 146 |
| With Steak | 1565 | 84 | 139 |
| *Burritos:* | | | |
| **Black Beans:** With Cheese | 1100 | 48 | 132 |
| With Carnitas | 1205 | 51 | 132 |
| With Chicken | 1240 | 52 | 139 |
| With California Steak | 815 | 35 | 89 |
| **Pinto Beans:** With Cheese | 1070 | 48 | 115 |
| With Carnitas | 1200 | 52 | 122 |
| With Steak | 1175 | 54 | 115 |
| **Baja Fish Burrito** | 875 | 53 | 58 |
| **Overstuffed Grilled Burrito:** | | | |
| With Carnitas | 1200 | 59 | 108 |
| With Chicken | 1260 | 59 | 110 |
| With Steak | 1290 | 66 | 109 |
| **Grande, Black Beans:** | | | |
| With Carnitas | 810 | 34 | 91 |
| With Chicken | 810 | 33 | 93 |
| With Steak | 820 | 35 | 91 |
| *Tacos:* Baja Fish | 395 | 22 | 29 |
| Baja Shrimp | 320 | 19 | 30 |
| Guadalajara Carnitas | 320 | 15 | 30 |
| Mexico City, Chicken | 190 | 3 | 27 |
| *Quesadillas:* *With Chips* | | | |
| **Classic:** Carnitas | 1160 | 68 | 82 |
| Chicken | 1155 | 67 | 83 |
| Steak | 1165 | 69 | 82 |
| **Grande, Pinto Beans:** | | | |
| With Carnitas | 1335 | 71 | 114 |
| With Chicken | 1330 | 71 | 116 |
| With Steak | 1330 | 72 | 115 |
| *Favorites:* *Without Chips* | | | |
| **Stuffed Fajita Quesadilla:** | | | |
| With Carnitas | 855 | 51 | 53 |
| With Chicken | 865 | 52 | 56 |
| With Shrimp | 800 | 49 | 54 |
| With Steak | 885 | 55 | 53 |
| **Fire Roasted Bowls:** | | | |
| **Black Beans:** With Chicken | 730 | 32 | 74 |
| With Steak | 735 | 34 | 73 |
| Without Meat | 630 | 29 | 71 |
| **Pinto Beans:** With Chicken | 730 | 32 | 73 |
| With Steak | 720 | 34 | 70 |
| Without Meat | 620 | 29 | 69 |

## Little Caesars® (Dec '11)

*14" Pizza: Per Slice, 1/8 Pizza*

| | C | F | Cb |
|---|---|---|---|
| **Original Crust:** 3 Meat Treat | 340 | 17 | 32 |
| Hula Hawaiian: With Ham | 280 | 9 | 35 |
| With Canadian Bacon | 280 | 9 | 35 |
| Ultimate Supreme | 310 | 13 | 33 |
| Veggie | 270 | 10 | 32 |
| **Deep Dish:** Just Cheese | 320 | 13 | 38 |
| Pepperoni | 360 | 16 | 38 |
| **Hot-N-Ready:** Just Cheese | 250 | 9 | 32 |
| Pepperoni | 280 | 11 | 32 |

*Baby Pan! Pan!: Per Pan*

| | C | F | Cb |
|---|---|---|---|
| Cheese & Pepperoni | 360 | 18 | 33 |

*Caesar Wings: Per Wing*

| | C | F | Cb |
|---|---|---|---|
| Barbecue | 70 | 4 | 3 |
| Mild/Hot | 50 | 4 | 0 |
| Oven Roasted | 50 | 3.5 | 0 |

*Caesar Dips: Per 1 oz Container Unless Indicated*

| | C | F | Cb |
|---|---|---|---|
| BBQ; Buffalo Ranch | 160 | 17 | 2 |
| Buffalo | 100 | 10 | 2 |
| Buttery Garlic, 1/2 oz | 130 | 14 | 0 |
| Cheezy Jalapeno | 140 | 15 | 2 |
| Ranch | 170 | 18 | 2 |

*Bread: Per Piece*

| | C | F | Cb |
|---|---|---|---|
| Crazy Bread, 1 stick | 100 | 3 | 15 |
| Crazy Sauce, 4 oz | 45 | 0 | 10 |
| Italian Cheese Bread | 130 | 7 | 13 |
| Pepperoni Cheese Bread | 150 | 8 | 13 |

## Lone Star Steakhouse® (Dec '11)

*Appetizers: Per Serving*

| | C | F | Cb |
|---|---|---|---|
| Amarillo Cheese Fries, 31½ oz | 2640 | 153 | 356 |
| Chicken Tenders: 12 oz | 1095 | 66 | 91 |
| Buffalo Style, 14¼ oz | 1195 | 77 | 92 |
| Lone Star Skins, 19 oz | 1310 | 62 | 135 |
| Lone Star Wings, 11 oz | 955 | 62 | 15 |
| Spinach & Artichoke Dip, 10¾ oz | 490 | 40 | 14 |
| Texas Rose, 15½ oz | 1260 | 83 | 108 |

*Meals: Without Sides, Toppings & Sauce*

**Mesquite Grilled Steaks:**

| | C | F | Cb |
|---|---|---|---|
| Cajun Ribeye, 12.7 oz | 815 | 53 | 5 |
| Chopped Steak, 9.6 oz | 710 | 52 | 0 |
| Five Star Filet, 6 oz | 330 | 18 | 2 |
| Garlic Lovers Medallions & Shrimp | 370 | 11 | 0 |
| NY Strip, 9.6 oz | 525 | 28 | 0 |
| Texas Ribeye, 12½ oz | 710 | 40 | 6 |

## Lone Star® cont... (Dec '11)

*Meals (Cont): Without Sides, Toppings & Sauce*

**Mesquite-Grilled Specialties:**

| | C | F | Cb |
|---|---|---|---|
| Baby Back Ribs, 12 oz | 970 | 80 | 0 |
| Grilled Chicken, 3¾ oz | 170 | 4 | 0 |
| Grilled Pork Chops, 16 oz | 1430 | 32 | 0 |

**Seafood:**

| | C | F | Cb |
|---|---|---|---|
| Fried Shrimp Dinner, 11.65 oz | 865 | 40 | 97 |
| King Crab: ½ lb | 100 | 1 | 2 |
| 1lb | 200 | 2 | 4 |
| Lobster tail, 3½ oz | 150 | 1 | 14 |
| Mesquite-Grilled Shrimp Dinner | 230 | 8 | 17 |
| Sweet Bourbon Salmon, 5.36 oz | 310 | 18 | 0 |

*Gourmet Burgers:*

| | C | F | Cb |
|---|---|---|---|
| Lone Star Cheeseburger, 14 oz | 895 | 45 | 50 |
| Swiss & Mushroom, 15.2 oz | 845 | 38 | 53 |

*Soup & Chili: Per 10 oz Bowl*

| | C | F | Cb |
|---|---|---|---|
| Chicken Pot Pie Soup | 50 | 5 | 12 |
| Chili | 345 | 18 | 14 |
| Steak Soup | 65 | 7.5 | 11 |

*Salads: Per Serving, Includes Dressing*

| | C | F | Cb |
|---|---|---|---|
| Dinner, Caesar, 6¼ oz | 145 | 11 | 8 |
| Grilled Chicken Caesar | 480 | 24 | 19 |
| Lettuce Wedge | 395 | 34 | 10 |
| Steakhouse | 710 | 53 | 2 |

*Sides: Per Serving*

| | C | F | Cb |
|---|---|---|---|
| Baked Potatoes: Plain, 8.2 oz | 225 | 0.5 | 50 |
| Jumbo, 13 oz | 330 | 0.5 | 76 |
| Garlic Mashed Potatoes, ½ cup | 130 | 5 | 19 |
| Sauteed Mushrooms | 140 | 9 | 11 |
| Sauteed Onions | 85 | 2.5 | 14 |
| Steak Fries, 8 oz | 610 | 26 | 86 |
| Texas Rice, 8 oz | 100 | 3.5 | 14 |

## Long John Silver's® (Dec '11)

| | C | F | Cb |
|---|---|---|---|

*Sandwiches: Includes Toppings and Condiments*

| | C | F | Cb |
|---|---|---|---|
| Chicken, 6½ oz | 440 | 30 | 47 |
| Fish, 6¼ oz | 470 | 23 | 49 |
| Ultimate Fish, 7 oz | 530 | 27 | 50 |

*Seafood:*

| | C | F | Cb |
|---|---|---|---|
| Battered Fish, 1 piece, 3¼ oz | 260 | 16 | 17 |
| Battered Shrimp, 3 pieces, 1½ oz | 130 | 9 | 8 |
| Breaded Clam Strips, 3 oz | 320 | 19 | 29 |
| Buttered Lobster Bites, snack box, 3¼ oz | 230 | 9 | 24 |

*Continued next page...*

## Long John's® cont... (Dec'11)

*Seafood (Cont):*

| | C | F | Cb |
|---|---|---|---|
| Lobster Stuffed Crab Cake, 2¼ oz | 170 | 9 | 16 |
| Popcorn Shrimp, 1 snack box, 3 oz | 270 | 16 | 23 |
| Shrimp Scampi, 8 pieces | 200 | 13 | 3 |
| *Chicken,* Chicken Strip, 1 piece | 140 | 8 | 9 |

*Freshside Grille: Per Entree Plate, w/ Rice & Vegs*

| | | | |
|---|---|---|---|
| Salmon, 2 filets | 280 | 7 | 27 |
| Shrimp Scampi | 330 | 15 | 29 |
| Tilapia, 1 filet | 250 | 4.5 | 27 |

*Sauces & Condiments:*

**Dipping Sauces:** *Per 1 fl.oz*

| | | | |
|---|---|---|---|
| Cocktail | 25 | 0 | 6 |
| Tartar | 100 | 9 | 4 |
| Louisiana Hot Sauce, 1 tsp | 0 | 0 | 0 |
| Ketchup, 1 packet, ¼ oz | 10 | 0 | 2 |
| Malt Vinegar, ½ oz | 0 | 0 | 0 |

*Sides:*

| | | | |
|---|---|---|---|
| Breaded Mozzarella Sticks (3) | 150 | 9 | 13 |
| Broccoli Cheese Soup, 1 bowl, 7½ oz | 220 | 18 | 8 |
| Cole Slaw, 4 oz | 200 | 15 | 15 |
| Corn Cobbette w. Butter Oil, 3½ oz | 150 | 10 | 14 |
| Crumblies, 1 oz | 170 | 12 | 14 |
| **Fries:** Platter Portion, 3 oz | 230 | 10 | 34 |
| Combo Portion, 4 oz | 310 | 14 | 45 |
| Hushpuppy, 1 pup, 0.8 oz | 60 | 2.5 | 9 |
| Jalapeno Cheddar Bites (5) | 240 | 14 | 23 |
| Rice, 5 oz | 180 | 1 | 37 |
| Vegetable Medley, 4 oz | 50 | 2 | 8 |

*For Complete Menu & Data ~ see CalorieKing.com*

## Macaroni Grill® (Dec'11)

| | C | F | Cb |
|---|---|---|---|

*Tapas & Antipasti: Per Whole Appetizer as Served*

| | | | |
|---|---|---|---|
| Calamari Fritti | 860 | 52 | 58 |
| Goat Cheese peppadew Peppers | 260 | 16 | 21 |
| Mac & Cheese Bites with Dip | 980 | 75 | 44 |
| Spicy Herb-Roasted Mussels | 1240 | 72 | 92 |
| Spicy Ricotta Meatballs | 370 | 25 | 17 |

*Meals: Per Whole Entree, as Served*

**Classics:**
| | | | |
|---|---|---|---|
| Carmela's Chicken | 810 | 30 | 89 |
| Eggplant Parmesan | 950 | 58 | 76 |
| Fettuccine Alfredo, Chicken | 1210 | 69 | 77 |
| Lasagna Bolognese | 720 | 41 | 46 |
| Mama's Trio | 1530 | 91 | 96 |
| Meatballs & Spaghetti: Bolognese | 1190 | 61 | 95 |
| Pomodoro | 960 | 47 | 91 |
| Penne Rustica | 1160 | 48 | 110 |

## Macaroni Grill® cont... (Dec'11)

*Meals (Cont): Per Whole Entree*

| | C | F | Cb |
|---|---|---|---|
| **Fresh Pasta:** Carbonara | 1260 | 68 | 101 |
| Eggplant Quadratini | 910 | 35 | 115 |
| Pasta Di Mare | 1320 | 66 | 118 |
| Pesto Spaghetti | 1140 | 51 | 105 |
| Whole Wheat Fettuccine | 860 | 31 | 90 |
| **Ravioli:** Lobster | 710 | 46 | 39 |
| Mushroom | 900 | 68 | 52 |

*Pizzas & Flatbreads: Per Whole Meal, as Served*

**Flatbread:**
| | | | |
|---|---|---|---|
| Mushroom & Goat Cheese | 1020 | 49 | 103 |
| Roasted Chicken & Arugula | 1160 | 52 | 103 |
| Smoky Shrimp | 1230 | 63 | 97 |

**Pizza:**
| | | | |
|---|---|---|---|
| Italian Sausage | 1100 | 52 | 100 |
| Margherita | 840 | 31 | 101 |
| Primo Pepperoni | 970 | 40 | 99 |

*Principale: Per Whole Entree, as Served*

| | | | |
|---|---|---|---|
| Chicken: Marsala | 810 | 40 | 61 |
| Scallopine | 1180 | 80 | 55 |
| Under a Brick | 1180 | 87 | 23 |
| Florentine Steak & Frites | 1700 | 120 | 65 |
| Grilled King Salmon | 1160 | 73 | 72 |
| Pan-Roasted Pork Chops | 1370 | 93 | 58 |
| Pan-Seared Branzino | 1160 | 67 | 84 |
| Parmesan-Crusted Sole | 1550 | 75 | 99 |
| Pollo Caprese | 550 | 14 | 45 |
| Roasted Chicken Cannelloni | 820 | 48 | 39 |
| Spiedini: Grilled Chicken | 490 | 26 | 24 |
| Grilled Shrimp | 300 | 10 | 22 |
| Veal Saltimbocca | 850 | 56 | 29 |

*Salads: Includes Dressing*

| | | | |
|---|---|---|---|
| Bibb & Blue | 680 | 56 | 22 |
| Caprese | 480 | 41 | 10 |
| Market Chop | 1020 | 72 | 38 |
| Salad Sampler | 1030 | 79 | 38 |
| Warm Spinach & Shrimp | 340 | 11 | 17 |

*Soups: Per 8 oz Bowl*

| | | | |
|---|---|---|---|
| Artichoke | 310 | 24 | 19 |
| Lentil | 440 | 30 | 28 |
| Pomodorina | 240 | 19 | 14 |

*For Complete Nutritional Data ~ see CalorieKing.com*

## McDonald's® (Dec '11)

### Burgers/Sandwiches:

| | C | F | Cb |
|---|---|---|---|
| Angus: Bacon & Cheese | 790 | 39 | 63 |
| Deluxe | 750 | 39 | 61 |
| Mushroom & Swiss | 770 | 40 | 59 |
| Hamburger | 250 | 9 | 31 |
| Cheeseburger | 300 | 12 | 33 |
| Double Cheeseburger | 440 | 23 | 34 |
| Big Mac | 540 | 29 | 45 |
| Big N' Tasty | 460 | 24 | 37 |
| Big N' Tasty with Cheese | 510 | 28 | 38 |
| McDouble | 390 | 19 | 33 |
| Quarter Pounder: Without Cheesse | 410 | 19 | 37 |
| With Cheese | 510 | 26 | 40 |
| Double with Cheese | 740 | 42 | 40 |
| Filet-O-Fish | 380 | 18 | 38 |
| McChicken | 360 | 16 | 40 |
| McRib | 500 | 26 | 44 |
| Southern Style Crispy Chicken | 420 | 19 | 43 |

### Premium Chicken Sandwiches:

| | C | F | Cb |
|---|---|---|---|
| Classic: Crispy Chicken | 510 | 22 | 56 |
| Grilled Chicken | 350 | 9 | 42 |
| Club: Crispy Chicken | 620 | 29 | 57 |
| Grilled Chicken | 460 | 16 | 43 |
| Ranch BLT: Crispy Chicken | 540 | 23 | 56 |
| Grilled Chicken | 380 | 10 | 42 |

### Snack Wraps:

| | C | F | Cb |
|---|---|---|---|
| Angus: Bacon & Cheese | 390 | 21 | 28 |
| Chipotle BBQ Bacon | 400 | 22 | 30 |
| Deluxe | 410 | 25 | 37 |
| Mushroom & Swiss | 430 | 26 | 27 |
| Crispy: Chipotle BBQ | 330 | 15 | 34 |
| Honey Mustard | 330 | 15 | 33 |
| Ranch | 350 | 19 | 31 |
| Grilled: Chipotle BBQ | 250 | 8 | 27 |
| Honey Mustard | 250 | 8 | 27 |
| Ranch | 270 | 12 | 25 |
| Mac | 330 | 19 | 26 |

### French Fries:

| | C | F | Cb |
|---|---|---|---|
| Small, 2½ oz | 230 | 11 | 29 |
| Medium, 4 oz | 380 | 19 | 48 |
| Large, 5½ oz | 500 | 25 | 63 |
| Ketchup, 1 pkg | 15 | 0 | 3 |

### Chicken:

| | C | F | Cb |
|---|---|---|---|
| McNuggets: 4 pieces | 190 | 12 | 12 |
| 6 pieces | 280 | 18 | 18 |
| 10 pieces | 470 | 30 | 30 |
| Strips: 3 pieces | 400 | 24 | 23 |
| 5 pieces | 660 | 40 | 39 |
| Sauces: BBQ/Must./Sweet 'N Sour, 1 oz | 50 | 0 | 12 |
| Creamy Ranch, 1.3 oz | 170 | 18 | 2 |
| Honey, ½ oz | 50 | 0 | 12 |
| Southwestern Chipotle BBQ, 1.3 oz | 60 | 0 | 15 |
| Spicy Buffalo, 1.3 oz | 60 | 6 | 1 |
| Tangy Honey, 1.3 oz | 60 | 2 | 10 |

## McDonald's® cont... (Dec '11)

### Breakfast:

| | C | F | Cb |
|---|---|---|---|
| Big Breakfast: With Regular Biscuit | 740 | 48 | 51 |
| With Hotcakes | 1090 | 56 | 111 |
| **Biscuits:** | | | |
| Bacon Egg & Cheese: Regular | 420 | 23 | 37 |
| With Large Biscuit | 480 | 27 | 43 |
| Sausage with Egg: Regular | 510 | 33 | 36 |
| With Large Biscuit | 570 | 37 | 42 |
| Southern Style Chicken: Regular | 410 | 20 | 41 |
| With Large Biscuit | 470 | 24 | 46 |
| Egg McMuffin, 7.1 oz | 300 | 12 | 30 |
| Fruit & Maple Oatmeal: Regular | 290 | 4.5 | 57 |
| Without sugar, 9.2 oz | 260 | 4.5 | 48 |
| Hash Brown (1), 2 oz | 150 | 9 | 15 |
| Hotcakes: Plain (3) | 350 | 9 | 60 |
| With Margarine (2 pats), no Syrup | 430 | 18 | 60 |
| With Margarine (2 pats), & Syrup (1) | 610 | 18 | 105 |
| McGriddles: Bacon, Egg & Cheese | 420 | 18 | 48 |
| Sausage | 420 | 22 | 44 |
| Sausage, Egg & Cheese | 560 | 32 | 48 |
| McMuffins: Egg | 300 | 12 | 30 |
| Sausage | 370 | 22 | 29 |
| Sausage with Egg | 450 | 27 | 30 |
| McSkillet, Burrito with Sausage | 610 | 36 | 44 |
| Sausage Burrito, 4 oz | 300 | 16 | 26 |

### Happy Meals:

| | C | F | Cb |
|---|---|---|---|
| **With 4 Chicken McNuggets:** | | | |
| + Small Fries + Apple Juice | 520 | 23 | 64 |
| + Small Fries + 1% Low Fat Milk | 520 | 26 | 53 |
| + Apple Dipper/ Dip + 1% Choc Milk | 460 | 16 | 61 |
| **With Hamburger:** | | | |
| + Small Fries + Apple Juice | 580 | 20 | 83 |
| + Small Fries + Sprite (12 oz) | 590 | 20 | 88 |
| + Apple Dippers/Dip + Low-Fat Milk | 450 | 12 | 66 |
| **With Cheeseburger:** | | | |
| + Small Fries & Apple Juice | 630 | 23 | 85 |
| + Small Fries + 1% Low-Fat Milk | 630 | 26 | 74 |
| + Apple Dippers/Dip & 1% Choc Milk | 570 | 16 | 82 |

### Mighty Kids Meals:

| | C | F | Cb |
|---|---|---|---|
| **With 6 Chicken McNuggets:** | | | |
| + Small Fries + Apple Juice | 610 | 29 | 70 |
| + Apple Dippers/Dip + 1% Choc Milk | 550 | 22 | 67 |
| **With Double Cheeseburger:** | | | |
| + Small Fries + Apple Juice | 770 | 34 | 86 |
| + Apple Dippers/Dip + Low-Fat Milk | 640 | 26 | 69 |

*Continued Next Page ...*

## McDonald's® cont... (Dec '11)

### Premium Salads: *Without Dressing*

| | C | F | Cb |
|---|---|---|---|
| **Bacon Ranch:** Without Chicken | 140 | 7 | 10 |
| With Crispy Chicken | 390 | 22 | 24 |
| With Grilled Chicken | 230 | 9 | 10 |
| **Caesar:** Without Chicken | 90 | 4 | 9 |
| With Crispy Chicken | 350 | 18 | 24 |
| With Grilled Chicken | 190 | 5 | 10 |
| **Southwest:** With Crispy Chicken | 450 | 21 | 42 |
| With Grilled Chicken | 290 | 8 | 28 |
| **Fruit & Walnut,** snack size, 1 pkg | 210 | 8 | 31 |
| **Side Salad,** 3 oz | 20 | 0 | 4 |
| **Butter Garlic Croutons,** ½ oz | 60 | 1.5 | 10 |

### Salad Dressings: *Per Package*

| | C | F | Cb |
|---|---|---|---|
| **Newman's Own:** Crmy Caesar, 2 fl.oz | 190 | 18 | 4 |
| Creamy Southwest, 1½ fl.oz | 100 | 6 | 11 |
| Ranch, 2 fl.oz | 170 | 15 | 9 |
| Low-Fat: Balsamic Vinaig., 1½ fl.oz | 35 | 2.5 | 3 |
| Family Recipe Italian, 1½ fl.oz | 50 | 2.5 | 7 |

### Desserts & Cookies:

| | C | F | Cb |
|---|---|---|---|
| **Apple Dippers:** 1 package, 2½ oz | 35 | 0 | 8 |
| With Low-Fat Caramel Dip | 100 | 0.5 | 23 |
| **Baked Hot Apple Pie,** 2.7 oz | 250 | 13 | 32 |
| **Cinnamon Melts,** 4 oz | 460 | 19 | 66 |
| **Cookies:** Chocolate Chip Cookie, (1) | 160 | 8 | 21 |
| McDonaldland Cookies, 2 oz | 260 | 8 | 43 |
| Oatmeal Raisin (1), 1 oz | 150 | 6 | 22 |
| Sugar Cookie (1), 1 oz | 160 | 7 | 21 |
| **Fruit 'n Yogurt Parfait,** 5¼ oz | 160 | 2 | 31 |
| **Ice Cream,** Vanilla Reduced Fat, | | | |
| Cone, 3.2 oz | 150 | 3.5 | 24 |
| **McFlurry:** M&M Candies, 12 fl.oz | 640 | 23 | 95 |
| Oreo Cookies, 12 fl.oz cup | 510 | 17 | 79 |
| **Sundaes:** Hot Caramel, 6.4 oz | 340 | 8 | 60 |
| Hot Fudge, 6.3 oz | 330 | 10 | 54 |
| Strawberry, 6.3 oz | 280 | 6 | 49 |
| Peanuts (for Sundaes), ¼ oz | 45 | 3.5 | 2 |

### McCafe:

| | C | F | Cb |
|---|---|---|---|
| **Shakes:** Chocolate; Strawberry, average, | | | |
| 12 fl.oz cup | 575 | 17 | 93 |
| 16 fl.oz cup | 715 | 20 | 117 |
| 22 fl.oz cup | 870 | 24 | 146 |
| **Vanilla:** 12 fl.oz | 540 | 16 | 88 |
| 16 fl.oz | 680 | 20 | 111 |
| 22 fl.oz | 830 | 24 | 138 |

## McDonald's® cont... (Dec '11)

### McCafe (Cont):
### Hot Coffees:

| | C | F | Cb |
|---|---|---|---|
| **Cappuccino:** | | | |
| Whole Milk: Small, 12 fl oz | 120 | 7 | 9 |
| Medium, 16 fl oz | 140 | 8 | 11 |
| Large, 20 fl oz | 180 | 10 | 13 |
| Nonfat Milk: Small, 12 fl oz | 60 | 0 | 9 |
| Medium, 16 fl oz | 80 | 0 | 12 |
| **Latte:** | | | |
| Whole Milk: Small, 12 fl oz | 150 | 8 | 11 |
| Medium, 16 fl oz | 180 | 10 | 13 |
| Nonfat Milk: Small, 12 fl oz | 90 | 0 | 13 |
| Medium, 16 fl oz | 110 | 0 | 15 |
| **Mocha:** | | | |
| Whole Milk: Small, 12 fl oz | 280 | 11 | 40 |
| Medium, 16 fl oz | 330 | 12 | 48 |
| Nonfat Milk: Small, 12 fl oz | 240 | 5 | 41 |
| Medium, 16 fl oz | 280 | 6 | 50 |

### Iced Coffee: *Regular or Flavors, av.*

| | C | F | Cb |
|---|---|---|---|
| **Premium Roast:** | | | |
| Small, 16 fl.oz | 135 | 5 | 21 |
| Medium, 21 fl.oz | 195 | 8 | 29 |
| Large, 32 fl.oz | 275 | 11 | 43 |
| **Caramel Mocha:** *With Whole Milk* | | | |
| Small, w/ Cream, 12 fl.oz | 260 | 12 | 34 |
| Medium, w/ Cream 16 fl.oz | 310 | 13 | 42 |
| Large, w/ Cream, 20 fl.oz | 390 | 14 | 57 |
| **Iced Tea,** no added sugar | 0 | 0 | 0 |
| **Milk:** 1% Low-Fat, 8 fl.oz | 100 | 2.5 | 12 |
| 1% Chocolate, 8 fl.oz carton | 170 | 3 | 26 |
| **Juice:** Apple Juice, 6.8 fl.oz box | 100 | 0 | 23 |
| Orange Juice: Small, 12 fl.oz | 150 | 0 | 30 |
| Medium, 16 fl.oz | 190 | 0 | 39 |
| Large, 22 fl.oz | 280 | 0 | 58 |

### Sodas: *Without Ice*

| | C | F | Cb |
|---|---|---|---|
| **Coca-Cola or Sprite:** | | | |
| Child, 12 fl.oz cup | 110 | 0 | 28 |
| Small, 16 fl.oz cup | 150 | 0 | 40 |
| Medium, 21 fl.oz cup | 210 | 0 | 58 |
| Large, 32 fl.oz cup | 310 | 0 | 86 |
| **Diet Coke** | 0 | 0 | 0 |
| **Hi-C Orange Lavaburst** | | | |
| Child, 12 fl.oz cup | 120 | 0 | 32 |
| Small, 16 fl.oz cup | 160 | 0 | 44 |
| Medium, 21 fl.oz cup | 240 | 0 | 64 |
| Large, 32 fl.oz cup | 350 | 0 | 94 |
| **Powerade Mountain Blast:** | | | |
| Child, 12 fl.oz | 70 | 0 | 20 |
| Small, 16 fl.oz | 100 | 0 | 27 |
| Medium, 21 fl.oz | 150 | 0 | 39 |
| Large, 32 fl.oz | 220 | 0 | 58 |

*For Complete Menu & Data ~ see CalorieKing.com*

## Manhattan Bagel® (Dec '11)

| *Bagel (East Coast):* Per Bagel | C | F | Cb |
|---|---|---|---|
| Blueberry, 3¾ oz | 300 | 1 | 65 |
| Chocolate Chip, 3¾ oz | 290 | 2.5 | 58 |
| Cinnamon Raisin, 4 oz | 330 | 1 | 70 |
| Egg; Jalapeno Cheddar, avg., 4 oz | 320 | 2 | 67 |
| Everything, 4¼ oz | 350 | 3 | 68 |
| Pizza, 9 oz | 520 | 13 | 78 |
| Poppy, 4¼ oz | 360 | 5 | 69 |
| Pumpernickel, 3½ oz | 240 | 1.5 | 53 |
| Salt, 4¼ oz | 320 | 1 | 68 |
| Sesame Seed, 4½ oz | 360 | 5 | 68 |
| *Cream Cheese:* Plain, 1¼ oz | 120 | 12 | 2 |
| Reduced-Fat, 1¼ oz | 110 | 9 | 4 |

***For Complete Nutritional Data ~ see CalorieKing.com***

## Marie Callender's® (Dec '11)

| *Appetizers:* Per Complete Dish as Served | C | F | Cb |
|---|---|---|---|
| Crispy Chicken Tenders | 940 | 59 | 64 |
| Crispy Green Beans | 810 | 52 | 75 |
| Mozarella Sticks | 690 | 42 | 53 |
| ***Burgers and Sandwiches:*** *With Fries* | | | |
| Original Burger | 1200 | 77 | 84 |
| Albacore Tuna Melt | 1430 | 92 | 99 |
| Grilled Ham Stack | 1260 | 81 | 96 |
| Roasted Turkey Croissant Club | 1450 | 97 | 95 |
| ***Main Meals:*** *Per Complete Meal as Served* | | | |
| **Comfort Classics:** | | | |
| Artichoke & Mushroom Chicken | 980 | 74 | 38 |
| Callender's Fish & Chips | 1280 | 92 | 85 |
| **From The Grill:** Gr. Rosemary Chkn | 780 | 47 | 43 |
| Gr. Atlantic Salmon, Cajun Style | 630 | 39 | 25 |
| St. Louis BBQ Ribs | 1260 | 82 | 58 |
| **Pasta Perfecto:** *Includes Garlic Bread* | | | |
| Chicken & Broccoli Fettuccini | 1480 | 87 | 119 |
| Double Shrimp Pasta | 1490 | 95 | 97 |
| **Pies,** Chicken Pot Pie, w/out Sides | 1140 | 79 | 68 |
| ***Fresh Crisp Salads:*** *Includes Dressing* | | | |
| Chinese Chicken | 810 | 29 | 107 |
| Gorgonzola, Pecan & Field Greens | 780 | 45 | 79 |
| Traditional Caesar | 490 | 35 | 28 |
| *Sides:* Cornbread, 1 piece, 2 oz | 170 | 6 | 26 |
| French Fries, 4 oz | 380 | 20 | 45 |
| Honey Butter, 1 oz | 170 | 16 | 8 |
| ***Desserts:*** *Per Slice Unless Indicated* | | | |
| **Pies:** Apple | 570 | 31 | 70 |
| Banana Cream, with Meringue | 510 | 24 | 66 |
| Chocolate Cream, with Meringue | 570 | 26 | 77 |
| Pumpkin, with Whipped Cream | 530 | 23 | 70 |
| Razzleberry | 660 | 39 | 71 |

***Breakfast & Other Menu Items ~ see CalorieKing.com***

## Max & Erma's® (Dec '11)

| *Appetizers:* | C | F | Cb |
|---|---|---|---|
| Black Bean Roll-Ups w/out dressing | 575 | 10 | 95 |
| ***Entrees:*** *As Served* | | | |
| Caribbean Chicken (lunch) | 535 | 20 | 59 |
| ***Salads:*** *Without Breadstick* | | | |
| Hula Bowl with 3 oz dressing | 585 | 10 | 78 |
| Baby Greens Salad, with dressing | 120 | 11 | 6 |
| ***Sides:*** | | | |
| Fruit Salad, 4½ oz | 55 | 0 | 17 |
| Garlic Breadstick (1) | 150 | 6 | 20 |
| ***Fruit Smoothie*** | 125 | 0.5 | 29 |

## Mazzio's® (Dec '11)

| *Dippin Zone:* Per Serving | C | F | Cb |
|---|---|---|---|
| Cheese Dippers, w/o sauce, ⅓ order | 405 | 18 | 47 |
| Nachos: Beef w/ Jalapenos, ½ order | 485 | 34 | 20 |
| Cheese with Jalapenos, ½ order | 425 | 30 | 19 |
| Rstd. BBQ Tossed Chkn Wings, ⅕ order | 190 | 12 | 7 |
| ***Calzones:*** *Per 1/10 Whole, Without Sauce* | | | |
| Ham Bacon & Cheddar | 245 | 7.5 | 32 |
| Pepperoni | 260 | 10 | 33 |
| ***Pastas:*** *Without Garlic Toast* | | | |
| Fettuccine Alfredo | 1060 | 56 | 107 |
| Spaghetti with Marinara Sauce | 640 | 8 | 120 |
| Lasagna: with Alfredo Sauce | 1265 | 94 | 55 |
| with Meat Sauce | 950 | 52 | 64 |
| ***Sandwiches:*** *Without Chips or Pickle* | | | |
| **Wheatberry:** | | | |
| Chicken, Bacon & Swiss | 1020 | 70 | 48 |
| Ham & Cheddar | 745 | 47 | 47 |
| Mazzio's Sub | 770 | 49 | 45 |
| **Hoagie:** Chicken, Bacon & Swiss | 1360 | 72 | 120 |
| Ham & Cheddar | 1090 | 50 | 119 |
| Mazzio's Sub | 1110 | 52 | 117 |
| Turkey & Swiss | 1060 | 40 | 118 |
| ***Pizzas:*** *Per ⅛ Medium Pizza* | | | |
| Cheese: Original Crust | 235 | 9 | 30 |
| Thin Crust | 180 | 9 | 18 |
| Chicken Club: Original Crust | 260 | 9 | 31 |
| Thin Crust | 205 | 9 | 19 |
| Mazzio's Works: Original Crust | 305 | 14 | 31 |
| Thin Crust | 255 | 15 | 20 |
| Meatbuster: Original Crust | 285 | 13 | 30 |
| Thin Crust | 235 | 13 | 19 |
| Pepperoni: Original Crust | 255 | 11 | 30 |
| Thin Crust | 200 | 11 | 18 |
| Sausage: Original Crust | 275 | 12 | 30 |
| Thin Crust | 225 | 12 | 19 |
| *Sides:* Breadsticks, w/o sce, ¼ order | 150 | 3 | 26 |
| Garlic Toast, w/o sce, 1 pce, 1½ oz | 160 | 10 | 15 |

***For Complete Nutritional Data ~ see CalorieKing.com***

## Mimi's Cafe® (Dec'11)

*Breakfast: With Sides*

| | C | F | Cb |
|---|---|---|---|
| **Gourmet:** Eggs Benedict | 810 | 56 | 36 |
| Eggs Florentine Benedict | 690 | 50 | 36 |
| Quiche Lorraine | 750 | 48 | 49 |
| **Three Egg Omelettes:** | | | |
| Five Alarm Santa Fe | 520 | 32 | 27 |
| Mardi Gras | 620 | 45 | 5 |
| **Chipotle Burrito** | 965 | 44 | 84 |
| **Ciabatta Breakfast Sandwich** | 945 | 53 | 77 |

*Lunch: With Sides*

| | C | F | Cb |
|---|---|---|---|
| **Burgers:** Monterey Chicken Burger | 1130 | 63 | 64 |
| French Quarter | 1580 | 104 | 88 |
| Zesty BBQ Bacon Cheeseburger | 1000 | 57 | 62 |
| **Classics:** Chicken Pot Pie | 1405 | 87 | 86 |
| Oven Fresh Pot Roast | 870 | 54 | 8 |
| **Soups:** Cafe Corn Chowder, 8 fl.oz | 195 | 9 | 28 |
| French Onion, 8 fl.oz | 205 | 12 | 16 |
| **Mimi's Bread Pudding** | 245 | 27 | 36 |

*Dinner: As Served, w/out Soup or Salad*

| | C | F | Cb |
|---|---|---|---|
| **Just Enough Dinner:** | | | |
| Artichoke Asiago Chicken Spaghettini | 1250 | 76 | 81 |
| BBQ Pork Chop with set menu sides | 850 | 40 | 86 |

**For Complete Menu & Data ~ see CalorieKing.com**

## Miami Subs® (Dec'11)

*Burgers:*

| | C | F | Cb |
|---|---|---|---|
| Deluxe Burger | 785 | 59 | 31 |
| Deluxe Cheeseburger | 860 | 65 | 32 |
| Deluxe Bacon Cheeseburger | 920 | 70 | 32 |
| *Platters:* Chicken Breast | 745 | 41 | 57 |
| Gyros | 1420 | 93 | 81 |
| 10 Wings w/ Fries & Blue Cheese | 1020 | 67 | 50 |
| *Salads:* Caesar with Dressing | 460 | 34 | 26 |
| Chicken Caesar with Dressing | 610 | 39 | 28 |
| Chicken Club | 490 | 25 | 23 |
| Greek | 285 | 15 | 24 |
| *Cheesesteaks (6"):* Original | 410 | 11 | 45 |
| Classic | 420 | 11 | 48 |
| Chicken Philly Classic | 550 | 27 | 47 |
| Works | 530 | 23 | 51 |
| *Pitas:* Gyros | 660 | 39 | 47 |
| Chicken | 390 | 13 | 34 |
| *Subs (6"):* Ham & Cheese | 450 | 18 | 49 |
| Italian Deli | 515 | 25 | 49 |
| Meatball | 490 | 22 | 49 |
| Tuna | 470 | 18 | 44 |
| Turkey | 485 | 19 | 51 |
| *Sides:* Mozzarella Sticks | 755 | 57 | 34 |
| Onion Rings | 870 | 68 | 56 |
| **Spicy Fries:** Regular | 530 | 39 | 39 |
| Large | 1040 | 72 | 85 |

## Mr. Goodcents® (Dec'11)

*Cold Sub: Per ½ Sub on Wheat Bread*

| | C | F | Cb |
|---|---|---|---|
| Centsable | 440 | 17 | 57 |
| Italian Sub | 640 | 37 | 55 |
| Mr. Goodcents Original | 510 | 25 | 56 |
| Oven Roasted Chicken Breast | 350 | 6 | 55 |
| Penny Club | 350 | 6 | 57 |
| Pepperoni & Cheese | 700 | 43 | 55 |
| Roast Beef | 350 | 6 | 55 |
| Tuna Salad | 490 | 21 | 63 |
| Veggie Sub | 290 | 4 | 58 |

*Toasted Sub: Per ½ Sub on Wheat Bread w/ Cheese*

| | C | F | Cb |
|---|---|---|---|
| Chicken Bacon Ranch w/ Cheddar | 660 | 27 | 61 |
| Chipotle Cheesesteak | 680 | 31 | 67 |
| Meatball with Mozzarella | 680 | 33 | 67 |

*Pasta:*

| | C | F | Cb |
|---|---|---|---|
| Alfredo Sauce on Mostaccioli | 1290 | 80 | 106 |
| Chicken Alfredo on Mostaccioli | 1370 | 70 | 112 |
| Chicken Parmesan on Mostaccioli | 660 | 10 | 100 |
| Red Sauce on Mostaccioli | 520 | 4 | 100 |

## Mr. Hero® (Dec'11)

*7" Hot Subs & Burgers:*

| | C | F | Cb |
|---|---|---|---|
| **Burgers:** Cheeseburger | 775 | 55 | 47 |
| Romanburger | 860 | 62 | 48 |
| Meatball Sub | 725 | 47 | 47 |
| **Steak Subs:** Tuscan | 625 | 31 | 42 |
| Hot Buttered Cheesesteak | 670 | 42 | 45 |
| Zesty Bacon & Swiss | 615 | 32 | 42 |
| **7" Deli Subs:** Original Italian | 640 | 39 | 47 |
| Tuna & Cheese | 725 | 54 | 44 |
| Turkey | 470 | 20 | 46 |
| Ultimate Italian | 675 | 40 | 46 |
| *4½" Taste Buddies: Per Sandwich* | | | |
| Bacon Cheeseburger | 430 | 30 | 33 |
| Crispy Chicken Wrap | 385 | 23 | 31 |
| Grilled Chicken Wrap | 235 | 10 | 25 |
| Grilled Italiano | 440 | 32 | 32 |
| Tuna 'n Cheese | 485 | 38 | 31 |
| Zesty Chicken | 495 | 25 | 48 |
| *Pasta,* Spag./Rigatoni w/ Meatballs | | | |
| In Marinara Sce & Breadstick | 1115 | 36 | 153 |
| *Sides:* | | | |
| Breadsticks, w/ Marinara Sauce (2) | 445 | 17 | 64 |
| Jalapeno Poppers. 4½ oz | 430 | 28 | 37 |
| Mozzarella Sticks, w/ Marinara Sce | 565 | 43 | 12 |
| Onion Petals, w/ Tangy Sce, 5¾ oz | 695 | 46 | 64 |
| **Fries,** Potato Waffer, 5¾ oz | 430 | 30 | 38 |
| *Desserts:* Oreo Cookie Cheesecake | 260 | 17 | 24 |
| Snickers Cheesecake | 270 | 18 | 23 |
| Strawberry Swirl Cheesecake | 280 | 19 | 22 |

## Mrs Fields Cookies® (Dec'11)

*Brownies:* Per 2.15 oz Brownie

| | C | F | Cb |
|---|---|---|---|
| Butterscotch Blondie | 260 | 10 | 38 |
| Double Fudge | 260 | 13 | 34 |
| Pecan Fudge | 270 | 15 | 32 |
| Special Walnut Fudge & Blondie | 260 | 13 | 35 |
| Toffee Fudge | 260 | 14 | 34 |
| Walnut Fudge | 270 | 15 | 32 |
| *Brownie Bites:* Double Fudge (3) | 200 | 10 | 27 |
| Toffee Fudge (3) | 200 | 11 | 26 |
| *Cake,* Choc. Chip, 1 piece, 2.35 oz | 250 | 12 | 32 |
| *Cookies:* | | | |
| **Bite Size Nibblers:** Cinn. Sugar (3) | 180 | 8 | 25 |
| Debra's Special (3) | 160 | 7 | 22 |
| Peanut Butter (3) | 170 | 9 | 19 |
| Semi-Sweet Chocolate (3) | 170 | 8 | 23 |
| Triple Chocolate (3) | 160 | 8 | 22 |
| White Chunk Macadamia (3) | 180 | 9 | 22 |
| Butter (1) | 200 | 8 | 29 |
| Cut Out (1) | 280 | 11 | 44 |
| Debra's Special (1) | 200 | 9 | 27 |
| Peanut Butter (1) | 200 | 12 | 24 |
| Semi-Sweet: Chocolate (1) | 210 | 10 | 29 |
| With Walnuts(1) | 220 | 11 | 28 |
| Triple Chocolate (1) | 210 | 10 | 28 |
| White Chunk Macadamia (1) | 230 | 12 | 28 |
| *Muffins:* Per 2 oz | | | |
| Blueberry | 190 | 9 | 24 |
| Chocolate Chip | 200 | 10 | 26 |

*For Complete Nutritional Data ~ see CalorieKing.com*

## Nathan's Famous® (Dec'11)

| *Burgers:* | C | F | Cb |
|---|---|---|---|
| Burger with Cheese,10¼ oz | 705 | 43 | 45 |
| Double Burger w/ Cheese, 15½ oz | 1180 | 84 | 45 |
| Bacon Cheeseburger, 10¾ oz | 785 | 50 | 45 |
| Super Cheeseburger, 13½ oz | 985 | 72 | 47 |
| *Nathan's Famous Hot Dogs:* | | | |
| Original, 3½ oz | 295 | 18 | 24 |
| Cheese Dog, 5 oz | 390 | 25 | 30 |
| Chili Dog, 5 oz | 400 | 23 | 33 |
| Corn Dog with Stick, 3¼ oz | 380 | 21 | 39 |
| *Chicken:* | | | |
| Chicken Tenders (3), 6¼ oz | 525 | 39 | 24 |
| Chicken Tender Platter, 17½ oz | 1245 | 90 | 80 |
| Grilled Chicken Breast Platter, 15 oz | 840 | 56 | 58 |

## Nathan's® cont... (Dec'11)

| *Sides:* | C | F | Cb |
|---|---|---|---|
| **Fries:** French: Regular, 6½ oz | 465 | 34 | 35 |
| Large, 9 oz | 635 | 46 | 49 |
| Super, 14 oz | 999 | 73 | 75 |
| Cheese: Regular, 8 oz | 565 | 42 | 41 |
| Large, 11 oz | 735 | 54 | 55 |
| Super, 18 oz | 1200 | 89 | 163 |
| Mozzarella Sticks (3), w/ Sauce, 5½ oz | 390 | 28 | 20 |
| Onion Rings, regular, 5½ oz | 545 | 45 | 36 |
| *Wraps:* | | | |
| Grilled Chicken Caesar | 700 | 34 | 60 |
| Krispy Southwest Chipotle | 750 | 39 | 62 |

## New York Fries
*~ See CalorieKing.com*

## Ninety Nine (Dec'11)

| *Standout Starters:* As Served | C | F | Cb |
|---|---|---|---|
| Boneless Wings & Skins Sampler | 1660 | 110 | 71 |
| Calypso Coconut Shrimp | 600 | 32 | 60 |
| Outrageous Potato Skins | 1130 | 84 | 43 |
| *Sandwiches:* As Served | | | |
| Honey BBQ Chicken Wrap | 930 | 41 | 93 |
| Roast Beef & Cheddar Dip | 680 | 28 | 59 |
| Triple-Decker Turkey Club | 970 | 38 | 106 |
| **Steakburger:** Steakburger | 820 | 47 | 46 |
| With Bacon & Cheese | 980 | 60 | 48 |
| With Cheese | 900 | 53 | 48 |
| *Meals:* Served With Menu Set Sides Unless Indicated | | | |
| Cape Cod Seafood Trio | 650 | 40 | 20 |
| Captain's Combo Platter w/o Chowder | 1840 | 126 | 122 |
| Filet Mignon without Sides | 550 | 31 | 1 |
| Fish & Chips | 1830 | 124 | 120 |
| Hot Buttered Lobster Roll | 1440 | 98 | 98 |
| NY Stip Sirloin without Sides | 680 | 28 | 1 |
| Prime Rib: 12 oz, without Sides | 920 | 72 | 2 |
| 18 oz, without Sides | 1370 | 107 | 2 |
| Smothered Tips | 1010 | 56 | 12 |
| **Salads:** As Served | | | |
| Chicken Caesar | 900 | 57 | 51 |
| Fire Grilled SW Cobb | 920 | 57 | 31 |
| Tropical Chicken | 800 | 42 | 59 |
| *Sides:* | | | |
| Double Bleu Iceberg Wedge | 440 | 40 | 9 |
| Honey Butter Biscuit w/ Honey Butter | 220 | 9 | 29 |
| Loaded Baked Potato | 570 | 33 | 51 |
| *Desserts:* Apple Cinn. Sensation | 560 | 22 | 84 |
| Little Midnight Fudge Hero. | 420 | 22 | 52 |
| White Chocolate Cheesecake | 890 | 65 | 65 |

# Fast - Foods & *Restaurants*

## Noodles & Company® (Dec '11)

*Meals:* Per Regular Bowl

| | C | F | Cb |
|---|---|---|---|
| **American:** Buttered Noodles | 930 | 39 | 114 |
| Mushroom Stroganoff | 790 | 31 | 102 |
| Spaghetti | 660 | 16 | 105 |
| Spaghetti with Meatballs | 970 | 39 | 111 |
| Wisconsin Mac & Cheese | 1030 | 43 | 122 |
| **Asian:** Bangkok Curry | 480 | 14 | 80 |
| Chinese Chop Salad | 370 | 22 | 39 |
| Indonesian Peanut Saute | 830 | 18 | 148 |
| Japanese Pan Noodles | 620 | 15 | 110 |
| Pad Thai | 830 | 18 | 151 |
| **Mediterranean:** Pasta Fresca | 780 | 25 | 114 |
| Penne Rosa | 790 | 35 | 97 |
| Pesto Cavatappi | 800 | 31 | 102 |
| The Med Salad | 320 | 13 | 44 |
| Whole Grain Tuscan Linguine | 680 | 32 | 77 |
| **Proteins:** Braised Beef | 320 | 25 | 0 |
| Chicken Breast | 110 | 3 | 0 |
| Meatballs | 300 | 23 | 6 |
| Organic Tofu | 180 | 11 | 6 |
| Parmesan-Crusted Chicken Breast | 200 | 10 | 8 |
| Sauteed Beef | 340 | 27 | 0 |

*Salads:* Per Side Serving

| | C | F | Cb |
|---|---|---|---|
| Cucumber Tomato | 110 | 0 | 24 |
| Tossed Green with Balsamic | 60 | 6 | 4 |
| *Sides:* Potstickers, without Sce (6) | 340 | 10 | 45 |
| Ciabatta Roll (1) | 120 | 1 | 24 |

*Soups:* Per Regular Serve

| | C | F | Cb |
|---|---|---|---|
| Thai Curry | 470 | 18 | 70 |
| Tomato Basil Bisque | 550 | 38 | 43 |

## Nothing But Noodles® (Dec '11)

*Noodle Bowls:*

| | C | F | Cb |
|---|---|---|---|
| **American:** Beef Stroganoff | 510 | 31 | 33 |
| Buttery Noodles | 650 | 44 | 46 |
| Santa Fe Pasta | 705 | 54 | 40 |
| Southwest Chipotle | 715 | 58 | 41 |
| Spicy Cajun Pasta | 660 | 50 | 44 |
| **Asian:** Pad Thai Noodles | 600 | 10 | 118 |
| Sesame Lo Mein | 410 | 11 | 64 |
| Spicy Japanese Noodles | 420 | 8 | 74 |
| Thai Peanut | 570 | 20 | 89 |
| **Italian:** Basil Pesto | 575 | 42 | 36 |
| Cappelini Primavera | 500 | 28 | 56 |
| Fettuccini Alfredo | 725 | 56 | 36 |
| Margherita Pasta | 475 | 31 | 36 |
| Marinara Pasta | 485 | 11 | 77 |
| Three-Cheese Macaroni | 445 | 21 | 45 |

*For Complete Menu & Data ~ see CalorieKing.com*

## O'Charley's® (Dec '11)

*Appetizers:* As Served

| | C | F | Cb |
|---|---|---|---|
| Chkn Tenders, w/ Chipotle BBQ Sce | 1040 | 37 | 119 |
| Over-Loaded Potato Skins | 1260 | 98 | 44 |
| Southwestern Twisted Chips | 1280 | 89 | 111 |
| Spicy Jack Cheese Wedges (7) | 880 | 60 | 55 |
| Top Shelf Combo Platter | 1890 | 130 | 105 |

*Meals:*

**Chicken & Ribs:** *Without Sides*

| | C | F | Cb |
|---|---|---|---|
| Chkn Tenders w/ Honey Mstrd | 1090 | 61 | 82 |
| O'Charley's Baby Back Ribs: | | | |
| Full Rack | 1480 | 96 | 76 |
| Half Rack | 740 | 48 | 38 |
| Teriyaki Sesame Chicken | | | |
| on Rice Pilaf | 1030 | 25 | 151 |
| **Pasta:** Prime Rib | 1530 | 101 | 90 |
| Shrimp Scampi Pasta | 840 | 33 | 93 |

**Seafood:** *Without Sides*

| | C | F | Cb |
|---|---|---|---|
| Cedar Planked Salmon | 530 | 32 | 2 |
| Gr. Atl. Salmon w/ Chipotle, 9 oz | 610 | 33 | 17 |
| Hand Battered Fish & Chips | 1190 | 85 | 43 |
| Panko Crusted Fried Shrimp, | | | |
| on Rice Pilaf | 570 | 26 | 53 |

**Steak & Combos:** *Per Serving, Without Sides*

| | C | F | Cb |
|---|---|---|---|
| Steak & Chicken Tenders | 1200 | 75 | 53 |
| Steak & Grilled Atl. Salmon | 800 | 50 | 3 |
| Steak & Shrimp Scampi | 770 | 55 | 11 |
| *Sides:* French Fries, per serving | 520 | 33 | 53 |
| Potato: Loaded | 590 | 40 | 52 |
| Smashed | 400 | 14 | 57 |

*Salads:* Without Dressing Unless Indicated

| | C | F | Cb |
|---|---|---|---|
| Black & Bleu Caesar w/ Dressing | 990 | 76 | 22 |
| California Chicken | 700 | 37 | 48 |
| Pecan Chicken Tender | 1020 | 60 | 81 |

*Soup:* Per Cup

| | C | F | Cb |
|---|---|---|---|
| Chicken Harvest | 160 | 8 | 12 |
| Chicken Tortilla | 150 | 9 | 12 |
| Overloaded Potato | 170 | 9 | 16 |
| *Desserts:* Cinnamon Sugar Donuts | 1130 | 54 | 139 |
| Ooey Gooey Caramel Pie, 1 slice | 440 | 21 | 57 |

*For Complete Menu & Data ~ see CalorieKing.com*

## Olive Garden® (Dec '11)

| Appetizers: | C | F | Cb |
|---|---|---|---|
| Bruschetta | 610 | 13 | 100 |
| Muscles di Napoli | 180 | 8 | 13 |
| Sicilian Scampi | 500 | 22 | 43 |
| Stuffed Mushrooms | 280 | 19 | 15 |
| *Entrees:* | | | |
| **Lunch:** Eggplant Parmigiana | 620 | 26 | 70 |
| Fettuccine Alfredo | 800 | 48 | 69 |
| Five Cheese Ziti al Forno | 770 | 32 | 89 |
| Lasagna Classico | 580 | 32 | 35 |
| **Dinner:** Capellini Pomodoro | 840 | 17 | 141 |
| Fettucini Alfredo | 1220 | 75 | 99 |
| Ravioli di Portobello | 670 | 30 | 74 |
| *Garden Fare Selections:* | | | |
| **Lunch:** Capellini Pomodora, 13 oz | 480 | 11 | 78 |
| Linguine alla Marinara | 310 | 4 | 55 |
| Venetian Apricot Chicken | 290 | 4 | 35 |
| **Dinner:** Capellini Pomodora, 21 oz | 840 | 17 | 141 |
| Linguine alla Marinara, 17 oz | 430 | 6 | 76 |
| Shrimp Primavera, 26 oz | 730 | 12 | 110 |
| Venetian Apricot Chicken | 400 | 7 | 34 |
| *Desserts:* Black Tie Mousse Cake | 760 | 48 | 73 |
| Strawb. & White Choc. Cream Cake | 210 | 11 | 27 |
| Tiramisu | 510 | 32 | 48 |

## Old Spaghetti Factory® (Dec '11)

| Appetizers: Per 1 Serving | C | F | Cb |
|---|---|---|---|
| Shrimp, Spinach & Artichoke Dip | 150 | 10 | 10 |
| Sicilian Garlic Cheese Bread | 330 | 19 | 28 |
| Toasted: Beef Ravioli, 1 oz | 50 | 1 | 8 |
| Cheese Ravioli, 1 oz | 50 | 1.5 | 8 |
| *Entrees, Lunch/Dinner:* | | | |
| **Classics:** | | | |
| Spaghetti: With Clam Sauce, 15 oz | 660 | 14 | 104 |
| With Marina Sauce, 15 oz | 560 | 5 | 108 |
| With Meat Sauce, 15 oz | 610 | 9 | 105 |
| With Sicilian Meatballs, 21 oz | 960 | 31 | 114 |
| **Factory Favorites:** | | | |
| Chicken Parmigiana, 19 oz | 810 | 30 | 80 |
| Spinach & Cheese Ravioli, 11 oz | 480 | 16 | 63 |
| Spinach Tortellini w/ Alfredo Sauce | 930 | 55 | 86 |
| **Signature Selection:** Chkn Penne | 830 | 31 | 102 |
| Crab Ravioli, 11 oz | 810 | 45 | 73 |
| Lasagna Vegetariano 20¾ oz | 830 | 48 | 68 |
| Meatloaf, Italian Style, 18½ oz | 1180 | 68 | 83 |

## On the Border® (Dec '11)

| Appetizers: As Served | C | F | Cb |
|---|---|---|---|
| Border Sampler | 2070 | 143 | 102 |
| Fajita Quesadillas: Chicken | 1190 | 84 | 55 |
| Steak | 1220 | 90 | 54 |
| *Burritos: Includes Rice, Without Beans & Sauce* | | | |
| Classic Chicken | 920 | 35 | 105 |
| Classic Shredded Beef | 1020 | 41 | 102 |
| *Chimichangas: Includes Rice, Without Beans & Sauce* | | | |
| Chicken | 1310 | 79 | 105 |
| Ground Beef | 1420 | 90 | 105 |
| *Dinner: Includes Rice, Without Beans* | | | |
| **Enchiladas:** Gr. Pepper Jack Chkn | 1050 | 48 | 106 |
| Ranchiladas | 1250 | 66 | 96 |
| Suiza | 1000 | 45 | 108 |
| *Fajitas, Signature: Without Rice, Beans, Tortillas or Condiments* | | | |
| Monterey Chicken Ranch | 660 | 44 | 13 |
| The Ultimate | 1160 | 96 | 26 |
| *Fresh Grill: Served As Listed* | | | |
| Carne Asada | 970 | 38 | 105 |
| Chicken Salsa Fresca | 520 | 9 | 60 |
| Jalapeno-BBQ Salmon | 590 | 21 | 45 |
| Queso Chicken | 1030 | 41 | 110 |
| Tomatillo Chicken | 850 | 24 | 109 |
| *Salads: Without Dressing* | | | |
| House, side size | 200 | 12 | 20 |
| Lunch Taco Salad: With Ground Beef | 860 | 58 | 57 |
| With Chicken | 800 | 50 | 57 |
| *Sides: Per Serving* | | | |
| Chile con Carne for Buritos/Chimmis | 100 | 5 | 8 |
| Mexican Rice | 280 | 5 | 55 |
| Pico de Gallo | 15 | 1 | 1 |
| Sour Cream for Burritos/Chimmis | 80 | 6 | 5 |
| *Dressings: Per Serving* | | | |
| Ranch Dressing | 230 | 24 | 2 |
| Smoked Jalapeno Vinaigrette | 250 | 24 | 8 |
| ***For Complete Nutritional Data ~ see CalorieKing.com*** | | | |

## Orange Julius® (Dec '11)

| Fruit Drinks: Per Small, 16 fl.oz | C | F | Cb |
|---|---|---|---|
| Bananarilla | 350 | 6 | 75 |
| Blackberry | 380 | 6 | 85 |
| Mango | 250 | 0 | 67 |
| Raspberry | 300 | 0 | 79 |
| Strawberry Banana | 380 | 6 | 83 |
| *Premium Fruit Smoothies: Per Medium, 20 fl.oz* | | | |
| Blackberry Storm | 620 | 6 | 139 |
| Orange Swirl | 460 | 7 | 95 |
| Raspberry Creme | 530 | 6 | 114 |
| Fat Free: Berry Banana Squeeze | 320 | 0 | 82 |
| Strawberry Sensation | 420 | 0 | 99 |
| *Nutrition Boosts:* Banana, 4.45 oz | 110 | 0 | 29 |
| Protein, ¾ oz | 100 | 4 | 9 |

## Outback Steakhouse® (Dec'11)

*Aussie-Tizers:* Per Whole Dish, With Sauce/Dressing

| | C | F | Cb |
|---|---|---|---|
| Alice Springs Chicken Quesadilla: | | | |
| Small, serves 2 | 900 | 59 | 47 |
| Regular, serves 4 | 1495 | 89 | 83 |
| Aussie Cheese Fries: Small, serves 3 | 1290 | 92 | 80 |
| Regular, serves 6 | 1975 | 133 | 139 |
| Bloomin' Onion, serves 6 | 1965 | 160 | 115 |
| Coconut Shrimp, serves 2 | 460 | 25 | 43 |
| Kookaburra Wings, Hot, serves 4 | 2060 | 170 | 18 |
| Seared Ahi Tuna: Small, serves 2 | 360 | 24 | 24 |
| Regular, serves 4 | 500 | 28 | 35 |

*Burgers & Sandwiches:*

| | C | F | Cb |
|---|---|---|---|
| Aged Cheddar Bacon Burger | 1050 | 74 | 36 |
| With Fries | 1435 | 93 | 84 |
| Grilled Chicken & Swiss Sandwich | 710 | 39 | 40 |
| With Fries | 1095 | 58 | 89 |
| The Bloomin Burger | 1030 | 70 | 50 |
| With Fries | 1415 | 89 | 99 |
| The Outbacker Burger | 685 | 40 | 39 |
| With Fries | 1070 | 59 | 87 |

*Steaks:* Without Sides

| | C | F | Cb |
|---|---|---|---|
| New York Strip, 14 oz | 765 | 49 | 0 |
| Outback Special: 6 oz Sirloin | 255 | 13 | 0 |
| 9 oz Sirloin | 380 | 19 | 0 |
| 12 oz Sirloin | 510 | 25 | 0 |
| Prime Rib: 8 oz | 480 | 22 | 2 |
| 16 oz | 950 | 45 | 4 |
| Ribeye, 14 oz | 760 | 49 | 0 |
| Teriyaki Filet Medallions | 690 | 30 | 65 |
| Porterhouse, 20 oz | 1010 | 71 | 4 |
| Victoria's Filet, 6 oz | 220 | 9 | 0 |

*Outback Favorites:* With Set Sides As Per Menu

| | C | F | Cb |
|---|---|---|---|
| Alice Springs Chicken | 1170 | 68 | 61 |
| Baby Back Ribs, full rack | 1540 | 96 | 71 |
| Grilled Chicken on the Barbie | 400 | 8 | 21 |
| New Zealand Rack of Lamb | 1005 | 59 | 45 |
| No Rules Parmesan Pasta | 920 | 52 | 79 |
| With Chicken | 1320 | 71 | 80 |
| With Chicken & Scallops | 1330 | 71 | 84 |
| With Chicken & Shrimp | 1325 | 72 | 81 |
| With Scallops | 1310 | 71 | 87 |
| With Shrimp | 1245 | 72 | 82 |
| Sweet Glazed Rstd Pork Tenderloin | 660 | 28 | 54 |

*Fish & Seafood:* Without Sides Unless Indicated

| | C | F | Cb |
|---|---|---|---|
| Lobster Tails | 450 | 27 | 2 |
| Tilapia with Lump Crab Meat | 515 | 28 | 10 |
| Wood-fired Grilled Ahi Tuna | 520 | 18 | 34 |

## Outback Steakhouse® cont... (Dec'11)

*Perfect Combinations:* Without Sides Unless Indicated

| | C | F | Cb |
|---|---|---|---|
| Filet & Grilled Shrimp On The Barbie | 570 | 39 | 10 |
| Filet, 6 oz & Lobster Tail, 4 oz | 630 | 43 | 3 |

*Sirloin:*

| | C | F | Cb |
|---|---|---|---|
| 6 oz: With Coconut Shrimp | 510 | 25 | 29 |
| With Grilled Shrimp | 505 | 30 | 10 |
| 9 oz: With Coconut Shrimp | 610 | 31 | 22 |
| With Grilled Shrimp | 630 | 36 | 10 |

*Salads:* Without Dressing Unless Indicated

| | C | F | Cb |
|---|---|---|---|
| Aussie Chicken Cobb: Crispy | 845 | 53 | 47 |
| Grilled | 510 | 27 | 17 |
| Chicken Caesar, with dressing | 710 | 42 | 20 |
| Classic Roasted Filet Wedge, with dressing | 745 | 58 | 16 |

*Soups:* Per Bowl

| | C | F | Cb |
|---|---|---|---|
| Creamy Onion | 480 | 36 | 25 |
| Potato | 590 | 34 | 58 |

*Add Ons:*

| | C | F | Cb |
|---|---|---|---|
| Blue Cheese Crumb Crust | 225 | 21 | 4 |
| Grilled Scallops | 210 | 10 | 9 |
| Horseradish Crumb Crust | 215 | 21 | 5 |
| Lobster Tail | 325 | 24 | 2 |
| Sauteed Mushrooms | 205 | 10 | 17 |

*Sides:*

| | C | F | Cb |
|---|---|---|---|
| Aussie Fries | 385 | 19 | 49 |
| Baked Potato: Loaded | 355 | 13 | 50 |
| Plain | 230 | 1 | 49 |
| With Bacon & Sour Cream | 290 | 5 | 51 |
| With Butter | 360 | 15 | 49 |
| With Butter, Cheese & Bacon | 400 | 19 | 49 |
| With Chse, Chives & Sour Cream | 290 | 6 | 51 |
| Blue Cheese Pecan Chopped Salad | 560 | 44 | 28 |
| Fresh Seasonal Mixed Veggies | 95 | 3 | 11 |
| Garlic Mashed Potatoes | 305 | 17 | 32 |
| Sweet Potato: With Honey Butter | 420 | 16 | 66 |
| Without Honey Butter | 320 | 5 | 63 |

*Desserts:* Per Single Serving

| | C | F | Cb |
|---|---|---|---|
| Classic Cheesecake, without Sauce | 165 | 12 | 12 |
| Chocolate Thunder from Down Under | 385 | 26 | 33 |
| Sydney's Sinful Sundae | 420 | 27 | 40 |

*For Complete Menu & Data ~ see CalorieKing.com*

## Panda Express® (Dec'11)

*Appetizers:*

| | C | F | Cb |
|---|---|---|---|
| Chkn Egg Roll, (1), 3 oz | 200 | 12 | 16 |
| Chicken Potsticker (3), 3.3 oz | 220 | 11 | 23 |
| Cream Cheese Rangoon (3), 2.4 oz | 190 | 8 | 24 |
| Veggie Spring Rolls (2), 3.4 oz | 160 | 7 | 22 |

*Beef:*

| | C | F | Cb |
|---|---|---|---|
| Beijing Beef, 5.6 oz | 690 | 40 | 57 |
| Broccoli Beef, 5.4 oz | 130 | 4 | 13 |
| Kobari Beef, 5.3 oz | 210 | 7 | 20 |

## Panda Express® cont... (Dec'11)

### Chicken:

| | C | F | Cb |
|---|---|---|---|
| Black Pepper Chicken, 6.1 oz | 250 | 14 | 12 |
| Kung Pao Chicken, 5.8 oz | 280 | 18 | 12 |
| Mandarin Chicken, 5.8 oz | 310 | 16 | 8 |
| Orange Chicken, 5.7 oz | 420 | 21 | 43 |
| Potato Chicken, 5.2 oz | 220 | 11 | 19 |
| SweetFire Chicken Breast, 5.8 oz | 440 | 18 | 53 |

### Pork & Shrimp:

| | C | F | Cb |
|---|---|---|---|
| BBQ Pork, 4.6 oz | 360 | 19 | 13 |
| Crispy Shrimp (6), 3.5 oz | 260 | 13 | 26 |
| Golden Treasure Shrimp, 5 oz | 390 | 19 | 39 |
| Honey Walnut Shrimp, 3.7 oz | 370 | 23 | 27 |
| Sweet & Sour Pork, 6.2 oz | 390 | 21 | 44 |

### Rice & Noodles: Per Serving

| | C | F | Cb |
|---|---|---|---|
| Chow Mein, 9.4 oz | 500 | 23 | 61 |
| Fried Rice, 9.3 oz | 530 | 16 | 82 |
| Steamed Rice, 8.1 oz | 380 | 0 | 86 |

## Panera Bread® (Dec'11)

### Artisan/Specialty Breads:

| | C | F | Cb |
|---|---|---|---|
| Chocolate Pecan Babka, 5 oz | 570 | 29 | 70 |
| Ciabatta, 2 oz | 150 | 2 | 27 |
| Foccacia, 2 oz | 180 | 4.5 | 28 |

### Bagels: Asiago Cheese

| | C | F | Cb |
|---|---|---|---|
| Asiago Cheese | 330 | 6 | 55 |
| Cinnamon Crunch | 430 | 8 | 80 |

### Breakfast Sandwiches: Power

| | C | F | Cb |
|---|---|---|---|
| Power | 340 | 15 | 31 |
| Asiago Bagel with Sausage | 650 | 2 | 55 |
| Bacon, Egg & Cheese on Ciabatta | 510 | 25 | 43 |
| French Toast Bael with Sausage | 670 | 31 | 69 |

### Hot Paninis: Cuban Chicken

| | C | F | Cb |
|---|---|---|---|
| Cuban Chicken | 860 | 36 | 87 |
| Roasted Turkey Artichoke On Focc | 390 | 17 | 38 |
| Steak & White Cheddar on Baguette | 970 | 33 | 112 |
| Tomato & Mozzarella on Ciabatta | 770 | 29 | 96 |

### Sandwiches: Per Full Sandwich

### Cafe & Signature:

| | C | F | Cb |
|---|---|---|---|
| Asiago Roast Beef, on Asiago Chse | 700 | 27 | 64 |
| Bacon Turkey Bravo on Tom. Basil | 800 | 29 | 83 |
| Chicken Caesar on Three Cheese | 720 | 32 | 69 |
| Italian Combo on Ciabatta | 980 | 41 | 95 |
| Mediterranean Veg. on Tom. Basil | 590 | 13 | 96 |
| Smoked Ham & Swiss on Rye | 590 | 17 | 64 |
| Smoked Turkey Breast on Country | 420 | 3 | 66 |
| Tuna Salad on Honey Wheat | 470 | 16 | 65 |

### Salads: Full Size Without Dressing

| | C | F | Cb |
|---|---|---|---|
| Asian Sesame Chicken, 11¼ oz | 410 | 20 | 31 |
| Caesar, 9¾ oz | 390 | 27 | 25 |
| Greek, 13½ oz | 380 | 34 | 14 |
| Roasted Turkey Harvest | 530 | 36 | 59 |

### Signature Mac & Cheese,

| | C | F | Cb |
|---|---|---|---|
| 1 cup, 7¾ oz | 490 | 30 | 75 |

## Panera Bread® cont... (Dec'11)

### Soups and More: Per Bowl

| | C | F | Cb |
|---|---|---|---|
| Broccoli Cheddar | 300 | 19 | 21 |
| Chili with Cornbread | 510 | 18 | 56 |
| Cream of Chicken & Wild Rice | 310 | 17 | 29 |
| French Onion, with Croutons | 250 | 11 | 30 |
| Low Fat Black Bean | 240 | 2.5 | 50 |

### Cookies, Pastries & Sweet Rolls:

| | C | F | Cb |
|---|---|---|---|
| Apple Pastry, 4¼ oz | 360 | 17 | 46 |
| Bear Claw, 4½ oz | 550 | 28 | 68 |
| Cheese Pastry, 3¾ oz | 400 | 22 | 44 |
| Cinnamon Roll, 6 oz | 630 | 24 | 91 |
| Cobblestone, 7 oz | 650 | 13 | 122 |
| Oatmeal Raisin Cookie, 3¼ oz | 390 | 14 | 62 |
| Pecan Braid, 3¾ oz | 470 | 26 | 53 |
| Pecan Roll, 5½ oz | 740 | 40 | 89 |

### Muffins: Apple Crunch, 5 oz

| | C | F | Cb |
|---|---|---|---|
| Apple Crunch, 5 oz | 450 | 12 | 80 |
| Carrot Walnut, 5 oz | 500 | 21 | 72 |
| Cranberry Orange, 5¼ oz | 480 | 19 | 71 |
| Wild Blueberry Muffin, 4½ oz | 440 | 17 | 66 |

## Papa Gino's® (Dec'11)

### Appetizers: Small, Per Serving

| | C | F | Cb |
|---|---|---|---|
| BBQ Chicken Tenders, 8½ oz | 520 | 18 | 55 |
| Buffalo Chicken Tenders, 9½ oz | 650 | 39 | 39 |
| Cheese Breadsticks, 24¼ oz | 1300 | 47 | 168 |
| Cinnamon Sticks, 7¼ oz | 620 | 19 | 100 |
| Mozzarella Sticks, 15½ oz | 990 | 61 | 79 |

### Pastas: Entree Size

| | C | F | Cb |
|---|---|---|---|
| Papa Platter, Penne; Spag., 26 oz | 1840 | 50 | 285 |
| Ravioli, 16¼ oz | 810 | 30 | 99 |
| Spaghetti & Meatballs, 24 oz | 1680 | 44 | 267 |

### Pizzas:

### Thin Crust: Per Slice of Large Pizza

| | C | F | Cb |
|---|---|---|---|
| Buffalo Chicken | 270 | 8 | 32 |
| Cheese | 230 | 7 | 32 |
| Chicken and Roasted Garlic | 260 | 7 | 34 |
| Meat Combo | 370 | 18 | 32 |
| Papa Roni | 340 | 16 | 32 |
| Pepperoni | 280 | 11 | 32 |
| Super Veggie | 250 | 8 | 35 |
| The Works | 330 | 14 | 34 |

### Subs: Per Small Sub

| | C | F | Cb |
|---|---|---|---|
| BLT | 1010 | 63 | 67 |
| Italian | 610 | 26 | 64 |
| Meatball Parmesan | 870 | 46 | 75 |
| Steak & Cheese | 710 | 33 | 63 |
| Super Steak | 750 | 33 | 72 |
| Tuna | 730 | 39 | 64 |
| Turkey Club | 770 | 35 | 67 |

### Salads: Without Dressing, Includes Bread Stick

| | C | F | Cb |
|---|---|---|---|
| Buffalo Chicken Tender | 540 | 22 | 56 |
| Caesar: Without Chicken | 440 | 19 | 50 |
| With Chicken | 700 | 24 | 53 |

## Papa John's® (Dec'11)

| *Pizzas:* | C | F | Cb |
|---|---|---|---|
| **Original Crust (14"):** *Per ⅛ Pizza* | | | |
| BBQ Chicken & Bacon, 5¼ oz | 350 | 12 | 45 |
| Spicy Italian, 5¼ oz | 380 | 18 | 38 |
| Spinach Alfredo, 4 oz | 280 | 10 | 36 |
| The Meats, 3¾ oz | 370 | 17 | 38 |
| The Works, 5½ oz | 330 | 14 | 39 |
| **Thin Crust (14"):** *Per ⅛ Pizza* | | | |
| BBQ Chicken & Bacon, 4 oz | 290 | 13 | 29 |
| Spicy Italian, 4 oz | 320 | 20 | 22 |
| Spinach Alfredo, 2¾ oz | 220 | 12 | 21 |
| The Meats, 3¾ oz | 310 | 19 | 22 |
| The Works, 4¼ oz | 270 | 15 | 23 |
| ***Wings:*** *Without Sauce* | | | |
| BBQ, 2 wings, 2½ oz | 190 | 12 | 6 |
| Buffalo, 2 wings, 2½ oz | 170 | 13 | 3 |
| Dipping Sauces: Per 1 oz Container | | | |
| Barbeque | 45 | 0 | 11 |
| Blue Cheese | 160 | 16 | 1 |
| Buffalo | 15 | 0.5 | 2 |
| Ranch | 100 | 10 | 1 |
| ***Sides:*** *Without Dipping Sauce* | | | |
| Breadsticks (2) | 290 | 4.5 | 54 |
| Cheesesticks (4), 4¾ oz | 370 | 16 | 41 |
| ChickenStrips (2), 2½ oz | 130 | 4.5 | 10 |

## Papa Murphy's® (Dec'11)

| *Pizzas:* | C | F | Cb |
|---|---|---|---|
| **Original Crust :** *Per 1/12 Family Size* | | | |
| BBQ Chicken | 330 | 12 | 36 |
| Cheese | 270 | 10 | 29 |
| Cowboy | 335 | 16 | 30 |
| Gourmet: Chicken Garlic | 320 | 13 | 30 |
| Classic Italian | 350 | 18 | 31 |
| Vegetarian | 300 | 13 | 31 |
| Hawaiian | 295 | 11 | 33 |
| Murphy's Combo | 350 | 17 | 31 |
| Pepperoni | 320 | 15 | 31 |
| Rancher | 325 | 15 | 30 |
| Specialty of the House, av. | 310 | 14 | 30 |
| Veggie Combo | 280 | 12 | 32 |
| **Stuffed Pizza:** *Per 1/16 Family Size* | | | |
| 5 Meat | 370 | 16 | 38 |
| Big Murphy | 370 | 15 | 39 |
| Chicago Style | 365 | 15 | 39 |
| Chicken and Bacon | 370 | 12 | 38 |

## Papa Murphy's® cont... (Dec'11)

| *Pizzas:* | C | F | Cb |
|---|---|---|---|
| **Thin Crust deLITEs:** *Per 1/10 Large* | | | |
| Cheese | 145 | 7 | 13 |
| Hawaiian | 160 | 7 | 15 |
| Pepperoni | 170 | 9 | 13 |
| Veggie | 160 | 9 | 13 |
| ***Salads:*** *Per Whole Salad, 2 Servings, Without Dressing or Croutons* | | | |
| Club ,13 oz | 280 | 16 | 12 |
| Garden, 14½ oz | 190 | 11 | 15 |
| Italian, 13 oz | 265 | 19 | 13 |

## Pei Wei Asian Diner (Dec '11)

| | C | F | Cb |
|---|---|---|---|
| ***First Tastes:*** *Per Whole Dish, Without Sauce* | | | |
| Crab Wontons (2) | 340 | 20 | 26 |
| Crispy Potstickers (2) | 300 | 16 | 24 |
| Edamame (2) | 320 | 14 | 18 |
| Minced Chicken w/ Lettuce Wraps (2) | 620 | 22 | 72 |
| Vegetable Spring Rolls (1) | 110 | 3.5 | 17 |
| ***Rice & Noodle Bowls:*** *Per Whole Meal, 2 Servings* | | | |
| Dan Dan Noodle, Chicken | 780 | 20 | 106 |
| Fried Rice: Chicken | 1000 | 24 | 132 |
| Steak | 1040 | 32 | 136 |
| Lo Mein Noodles: Chicken | 1120 | 40 | 134 |
| Steak | 1080 | 40 | 134 |
| Pad Thai Noodles: Chicken | 1440 | 40 | 210 |
| Steak | 1580 | 52 | 218 |
| ***Teriyaki Bowl:*** *Includes White Rice* | | | |
| Beef | 1100 | 26 | 162 |
| Chicken | 1120 | 26 | 160 |
| Shrimp | 1060 | 24 | 160 |
| Japanese Chili Ramen: Chicken | 1000 | 32 | 126 |
| Vegetable Tofu | 1080 | 40 | 138 |
| ***Signature Entrees:*** *Per Whole Meal, 2 Servings, W/o Rice* | | | |
| Honey Seared: Chicken | 860 | 30 | 98 |
| Shrimp | 900 | 36 | 98 |
| Sweet & Sour: Chicken | 720 | 20 | 96 |
| Shrimp | 740 | 26 | 94 |
| ***Soup:*** | | | |
| Hot & Sour, 1 Cup, 6 fl.oz | 190 | 8 | 12 |
| Thai Wanton, 1 Cup, 6 fl.oz | 110 | 6 | 5 |
| ***Salads:*** *Per Whole Meal, Serves 2, Without Dressing* | | | |
| Asian Chopped Chicken | 380 | 12 | 26 |
| Spicy Chicken | 1040 | 44 | 116 |
| ***Dressings:*** *Per 2 oz Serving* | | | |
| Lime Vinaigrette | 220 | 20 | 14 |
| Sesame Ginger | 220 | 21 | 6 |
| Sauces: Lettuce Wrap | 50 | 3 | 3 |
| Potsticker | 30 | 1 | 3 |
| Sweet Chile | 130 | 0 | 32 |
| Thai Peanut | 160 | 10 | 16 |

## Pepe's Mexican ~ see CalorieKing.com

Updated Nutrition Data ~ www.CalorieKing.com
Persons with Diabetes ~ See Disclaimer (Page 22)

## Perkin's® (Dec'11)

*Breakfast: W/- Sides Unless Indicated*

| | C | F | Cb |
|---|---|---|---|
| **Benedicts:** Country Cookin', 15.3 oz | 1040 | 82 | 42 |
| Florentine, 12.2 oz | 370 | 11 | 35 |
| N'awlins, 14.2 oz | 750 | 48 | 42 |
| **Classics:** Chkn Biscuit Platter, 19.5 oz | 1400 | 77 | 109 |
| Country Fried Steak & Eggs, 14.5 oz | 780 | 45 | 48 |
| Sausage Biscuit Platter, 17.8 oz | 1310 | 90 | 76 |
| Tremendous 12, w/ Hash Browns | 1620 | 68 | 201 |
| **Griddle Greats:** *With Butter & Syrup Unless Indicated* | | | |
| Belgian Waffle, 9.2 oz | 700 | 33 | 92 |
| Berry Blueb. P'cakes, w/o Butter | 980 | 29 | 163 |
| Buttermilk 5 French Toast, 15.3 oz | 1000 | 44 | 126 |
| Potato Pancakes w/ Applesce, 15 oz | 1240 | 55 | 153 |
| **Omelettes:** Border Grilled Chicken | 240 | 6 | 15 |
| Everything, 13.3 oz | 540 | 40 | 12 |
| Farmer's, 11.1 oz | 710 | 58 | 8 |
| Granny's Country w/ Hash Browns | 1420 | 56 | 184 |
| **Scramblers:** Cheesy Bacon, 6.8 z | 510 | 40 | 4 |
| Southern Fried Chicken, 11.3 oz | 500 | 32 | 22 |
| **Breakfast Sides:** Potatoes, 5 oz | 250 | 12 | 32 |
| Bran Muffin, 5.9 oz | 480 | 15 | 84 |
| Fruit Cup, 3.9 oz | 50 | 0 | 12 |
| Hash Browns, 4.1 oz | 490 | 13 | 87 |
| Short Stack w/ butter/syrup, 10.3 oz | 730 | 35 | 92 |
| *Burgers, Melts, Sandwiches, Wraps: Without Sides* | | | |
| **Burgers:** Pepper Jack, 15.6 oz | 1020 | 65 | 45 |
| Sunrise, 15.9 oz | 1260 | 70 | 83 |
| Tangler, 15.8 oz | 1180 | 80 | 49 |
| **Melts:** Chicken Crisps, 16.3 oz | 1390 | 91 | 87 |
| Country Club, 13.6 oz | 1060 | 64 | 64 |
| Frisco Roast Beef, 15.6 oz | 1050 | 63 | 68 |
| **Sandwiches:** French Dip, 13.3 oz | 610 | 31 | 46 |
| Kickin' Chicken, 13.4 oz | 1030 | 55 | 86 |
| Triple Decker Club, 13.7 oz | 890 | 55 | 54 |
| **Wraps:** Buffalo, 14.5 oz | 1140 | 78 | 73 |
| Chef, 13.7 oz | 840 | 54 | 59 |
| Energizer, 19.4 oz | 630 | 19 | 65 |
| *Appetizers: W/ Dress. & Tortilla Straws Unless Indicated* | | | |
| Dixie Dippers, 13.3 oz | 1230 | 80 | 84 |
| Fried Green Beans, w/o Straws, 11 oz | 890 | 64 | 68 |
| MozzaSticks, 12.3 oz | 900 | 48 | 87 |
| Santa Fe Chimi's, 13.4 oz | 1090 | 66 | 94 |
| *Soups: Per 10 oz Bowl* | | | |
| Broccoli & Cheddar | 280 | 18 | 20 |
| Loaded Baked Potato | 280 | 18 | 25 |
| Chicken Noodle; Vege Beef, average | 150 | 5 | 18 |

## Perkin's® cont... (Dec'11)

*Salads: W/- Dressing or Parmesan Wedges Unless Indicated*

| | C | F | Cb |
|---|---|---|---|
| BLT Chkn w/ Tortilla Wrap, 17.5 oz | 540 | 26 | 26 |
| Chef Deluxe, 18.7 oz | 620 | 39 | 16 |
| Grilled Chicken Chimi, 14.1 oz | 410 | 17 | 34 |
| Honey Mustard Chkn Crunch w drsng | 1060 | 74 | 59 |
| **Dressings:** Per 2.6 oz | | | |
| Blue Cheese | 400 | 43 | 3 |
| Fat-Free Italian | 25 | 0 | 8 |
| Honey Mustard | 380 | 33 | 20 |
| Ranch | 250 | 28 | 3 |
| *Dinner Meals: Per Full Meal As Served* | | | |
| **Favorites:** Chicken Crisp , 23.5 oz | 1820 | 117 | 135 |
| Chicken Pot Pie, 27 oz | 1470 | 106 | 80 |
| Country Fried Steak, 21.5 oz | 1080 | 58 | 95 |
| Down Home Meatloaf, 22.5 oz | 1040 | 65 | 72 |
| Homestyle Pot Roast, 22.6 oz | 820 | 43 | 66 |
| Mushroom 'n Swiss Chkn, 20 oz | 1130 | 45 | 123 |
| **Pasta:** Cavatappi Marinara, 16.4 oz | 960 | 54 | 96 |
| Chkn/Shrimp Monterey, av., 27 oz | 1595 | 110 | 102 |
| **Seafood:** Captain's Catch, 34.3 oz | 2410 | 144 | 222 |
| Island Tilapia, 20 oz | 450 | 6 | 50 |
| Panko-Breaded Cod, 21 oz | 1370 | 82 | 124 |
| Salmon Dijon, 18 oz | 660 | 32 | 46 |
| **Sides:** French Fries, 7 oz | 570 | 36 | 56 |
| Roma Parmesan Wedges (2) | 160 | 9 | 13 |
| **Side Salad:** W/o croutons/drsng | 110 | 4 | 3 |
| With croutons & Ranch, 6.5 oz | 300 | 25 | 15 |
| *Dessert: Per Slice* | | | |
| **Pies:** Caramel Apple, 7.5 oz | 500 | 22 | 68 |
| Chocolate French Silk, 6 oz | 760 | 54 | 66 |
| Peanut Butter Silk, 7.2 oz | 960 | 68 | 73 |
| Strawberry Cheesecake, 7.5 oz | 560 | 33 | 58 |
| Wildberry, no sugar added, 7 oz | 360 | 15 | 50 |
| *Beverages: Per 11.6 fl.oz* | | | |
| Cherry Coke | 160 | 0 | 42 |
| Raspberry Iced Tea | 130 | 0 | 34 |

## Peter Piper Pizza (Dec'11)

*Signature Pizzas: Per Slice*

**Original Crust:** *Per ½ of Extra Large 16" Pizza*

| | C | F | Cb |
|---|---|---|---|
| 5 Meat Supreme | 320 | 13 | 33 |
| California Veggie | 240 | 6 | 33 |
| Chicago Classic | 270 | 9 | 33 |
| NY 3 Cheese/Smokehouse, av. | 340 | 14 | 33 |
| The Werx | 290 | 10 | 33 |

*Continued Next Page ...*

## Peter Piper® cont... (Dec '11)

*Signature Pizzas: Per Slice*  **C**  **F**  **Cb**

**Hand-Tossed Crust:** *Per ½ of Extra Large 16" Pizza*

| | C | F | Cb |
|---|---|---|---|
| 5 Meat Supreme | 320 | 13 | 34 |
| California Veggie | 240 | 6 | 34 |
| Chicago Ckassic | 270 | 9 | 34 |
| NY 3 Cheese/Smokehouse, av | 340 | 14 | 34 |
| The Werx | 280 | 10 | 34 |

**Pan Crust:** *Per ½ of Extra Large 16" Pizza*

| | C | F | Cb |
|---|---|---|---|
| 5 Meat Supreme | 340 | 13 | 39 |
| California Veggie | 260 | 6 | 39 |
| Chicago Classic | 290 | 9 | 39 |
| NY 3 Cheese/Smokehouse, av | 360 | 15 | 39 |
| The Werx | 310 | 10 | 39 |

**Thin Crust:** *Per ¹⁄₁₆ of Extra Large 16" Pizza*

| | C | F | Cb |
|---|---|---|---|
| 5 Meat Supreme | 190 | 9 | 14 |
| California Veggie | 130 | 4 | 14 |
| Chicago Classic | 150 | 6 | 14 |
| NY 3 Cheese/Smokehouse | 200 | 10 | 14 |
| The Werx | 160 | 7 | 14 |

## P.F. Chang's® (Dec '11)

*Starters: Small Plate, Per Serving*

| | C | F | Cb |
|---|---|---|---|
| Crab Wontons, w/o Plum Sauce (2) | 165 | 10 | 13 |
| Egg Roll (1) | 215 | 10 | 21 |
| **Lettuce Wraps:** Chicken (1) | 160 | 7 | 17 |
| Vegetarian (1) | 140 | 7 | 11 |

**Pork Dumplings:** *Without Potsticker Sauce*

| | C | F | Cb |
|---|---|---|---|
| Pan-Fried (1) | 70 | 4 | 6 |
| Steamed (1) | 60 | 2 | 6 |

**Shrimp Dumplings:** *Without Sauce*

| | C | F | Cb |
|---|---|---|---|
| Pan-Fried (1) | 60 | 2 | 6 |
| Steamed (1) | 45 | 0 | 6 |

| | C | F | Cb |
|---|---|---|---|
| **Spare Ribs:** Northern Style (1) | 345 | 19 | 11 |
| Changs BBQ, without Slaw, (1) | 345 | 24 | 7 |
| **Spring Rolls,** without Sauce, (2) | 155 | 8 | 17 |

*Meals: Per Whole Dish, as served, without Rice*

| **Beef:** A La Sichuan, 21 oz | 910 | 36 | 75 |
|---|---|---|---|
| Mongolian, 18 oz | 1010 | 45 | 60 |
| Orange Peel, 15 oz | 850 | 39 | 63 |

**Chicken:**

| | C | F | Cb |
|---|---|---|---|
| Chang's Spicy, 18 oz | 970 | 39 | 69 |
| Kung Pao Chicken, 15 oz | 1150 | 69 | 42 |
| Orange Peel Chicken, 15 oz | 1000 | 45 | 60 |
| Sesame Chicken, 24 oz | 1030 | 42 | 75 |
| Sweet & Sour Chicken, 15 oz | 1110 | 57 | 114 |
| **Duck,** VIP, 12 oz | 1300 | 58 | 110 |

## P.F. Chang's® cont... (Dec '11)

*Meals: Per Whole Dish, w/out Rice*  **C**  **F**  **Cb**

**Seafood:**

| | C | F | Cb |
|---|---|---|---|
| Asian Gr. N'wegian Salmon, 18 oz | 690 | 12 | 76 |
| Crispy Honey Shrimp, 12 oz | 920 | 44 | 110 |
| Shrimp w/ Candied Walnuts, 21 oz | 1130 | 72 | 75 |
| Sichuan Shrimp, 15 oz | 520 | 21 | 30 |

**Vegetarian Plates:**

| | C | F | Cb |
|---|---|---|---|
| Buddha's Feast, steamed, 12 oz | 110 | 0 | 22 |
| Coconut Curry Vegetables, 26 oz | 1020 | 72 | 52 |
| Ma Po Tofu, 30 oz | 1050 | 69 | 51 |

*Lunch Bowls: Per Whole Dish w/ White Rice, w/o Soup*

| | C | F | Cb |
|---|---|---|---|
| Moo Goo Gai Pan, 26 oz | 780 | 22 | 94 |
| Sesame Chicken, 28 oz | 1070 | 30 | 152 |
| Shrimp with Lobster Sauce, 24 oz | 680 | 20 | 90 |

*Sides: Small, Per Whole Dish*

| | C | F | Cb |
|---|---|---|---|
| Garlic Snap Peas, 4½ oz | 95 | 3 | 11 |
| Shanghai Cucumbers, 6 oz | 60 | 3 | 5 |
| Sichuan Asparagus, 7½ oz | 150 | 9 | 15 |
| Spinach Stir-Fried w/ Garlic, 7½ oz | 80 | 4.5 | 8 |

| *Soups:* Hot & Sour: 1 cup, 7 oz | 80 | 3 | 9 |
|---|---|---|---|
| 1 bowl, 34 oz | 390 | 15 | 44 |
| Egg Drop : 1 cup, 7 oz | 60 | 3 | 8 |
| 1 bowl, 34 oz | 290 | 15 | 39 |

| *Desserts:* Banana Spring Rolls (4) | 960 | 40 | 144 |
|---|---|---|---|
| Great Wall of Chocolate Cake (4) | 1440 | 68 | 204 |
| Mini Tiramisu (1) | 180 | 11 | 18 |

## Piccadilly Cafeteria® (Dec '11)

*Meals: Without Sides*

| **Beef:** Angus Chopped Steak, 5¼ oz | 435 | 31 | 0 |
|---|---|---|---|
| 10 oz | 885 | 65 | 5 |
| Liver with Onion Sauce | 365 | 20 | 22 |
| Meatballs & Spaghetti | 815 | 40 | 80 |
| **Chicken:** & Dumplings, 8 oz | 285 | 10 | 7 |
| Breast, Blackened, 1 order | 295 | 14 | 3 |
| Florentine, 8 oz | 465 | 9 | 44 |
| Lemon Pepper, half | 1545 | 105 | 22 |
| Parmigiana, 1 order | 1240 | 36 | 135 |
| Sesame Glaze, 9 oz | 715 | 34 | 57 |
| Tetrazzini, 1 order | 375 | 21 | 18 |
| **Pork Chops:** Smothered, 8 oz | 730 | 34 | 46 |
| Blackened with Fettuccine | 660 | 30 | 35 |
| Southwest, with Mexican Rice | 955 | 31 | 113 |
| **Seafood:** Blcknd Shrimp Fettuccine | 825 | 40 | 73 |
| Cajun Baked Tilapia | 330 | 20 | 4 |
| Crawfish Etoufee | 555 | 14 | 84 |
| Tilapia w/ Shrimp Cream Sauce | 280 | 6 | 10 |
| Mediterranean Tilapia | 240 | 8 | 8 |
| New Orleans Sauteed Shrimp | 835 | 40 | 78 |

# Fast - Foods & Restaurants

## Piccadilly Cafeteria® cont... (Dec '11)

*Salads: Without Dressing*

| | C | F | Cb |
|---|---|---|---|
| Ambrosia, 6½ oz | 285 | 14 | 43 |
| Italian Rotini, 3½ oz | 285 | 19 | 26 |
| Piccadilly Fruit Salad, 5¾ oz | 70 | 0 | 18 |
| Potato, 4 oz | 170 | 7 | 24 |
| Spinach | 95 | 5 | 7 |

*Savory Sides:*

| | | | |
|---|---|---|---|
| Baked Macaroni & Cheese, 5¼ oz | 310 | 17 | 26 |
| Breaded Okra, 3¼ oz | 240 | 13 | 26 |
| Broccoli & Rice, 5 oz | 385 | 17 | 42 |
| Candied Sweet Potatoes, 4½ oz | 305 | 0 | 77 |
| Carrot Souffle, 5 oz | 390 | 17 | 58 |
| Cauliflower with Cheese Sauce | 175 | 10 | 5 |
| Mashed Potatoes, 5 oz | 115 | 4 | 19 |
| Turnip Greens, 1 order | 60 | 2 | 11 |

*Soups: Per Cup:*

| | | | |
|---|---|---|---|
| Seafood Gumbo | 225 | 6 | 32 |
| Shrimp & Corn | 200 | 10 | 19 |
| Tomato-Macaroni | 110 | 1 | 22 |

*Bread:*

| | | | |
|---|---|---|---|
| Corn Sticks (1) | 155 | 9 | 16 |
| Garlic Bread, 1 slice | 205 | 10 | 25 |

*Desserts:*

| | | | |
|---|---|---|---|
| Buttermilk Chess Pie, 1 slice | 635 | 30 | 87 |
| Coconut Cream Pie, 1 slice | 550 | 33 | 59 |
| Peach Cobbler, 8 oz | 545 | 22 | 82 |
| Red Velvet Cake, 1 slice | 835 | 54 | 83 |

## Pita Pit ~ *see CalorieKing.com*

## Pizza Hut® (Dec '11)

*Fit' n Delicious: Per ⅛ of 12" Pizza*

| | | | |
|---|---|---|---|
| Chicken, Mushroom & Jalapeno | 170 | 4.5 | 22 |
| Chicken, Onion & Green Pepper | 180 | 4.5 | 23 |
| Green Pepper, Onion & Tomato | 150 | 4 | 24 |
| Ham, Onion & Mushroom | 160 | 4.5 | 23 |
| Ham, Pineapple & Tomato | 160 | 4.5 | 24 |
| Tomato, Mushroom & Jalapeno | 150 | 4 | 23 |

*Hand-Tossed Style: Per ⅛ of 12" Pizza*

| | | | |
|---|---|---|---|
| Cheese Only | 220 | 8 | 26 |
| Dan's Original | 260 | 12 | 26 |
| Hawaiian Luau | 240 | 9 | 27 |
| Ham & Pineapple | 200 | 6 | 27 |
| Italian Sausage & Onion | 240 | 10 | 27 |
| Meat Lover's | 300 | 16 | 26 |
| Pepperoni | 230 | 9 | 25 |
| Pepperoni & Mushroom | 210 | 8 | 26 |
| Spicy Sicilian | 240 | 11 | 26 |
| Supreme | 260 | 12 | 26 |
| Triple Meat Italiano | 260 | 12 | 26 |
| Veggie Lover's | 200 | 6 | 27 |

## Pizza Hut® cont... (Dec '11)

*Pan: Per ⅛ of 12" Pizza*

| | C | F | Cb |
|---|---|---|---|
| Cheese Only | 240 | 10 | 27 |
| Ham & Pineapple | 230 | 9 | 28 |
| Hawaiian Luau | 260 | 12 | 28 |
| Meat Lover's | 330 | 18 | 27 |
| Pepperoni & Mushroom | 240 | 10 | 27 |
| Supreme | 290 | 14 | 27 |
| Triple Meat Italiano | 290 | 15 | 27 |
| Veggie Lover's | 230 | 9 | 28 |

*Personal Pan: Per 6" Pizza*

| | | | |
|---|---|---|---|
| Cheese Only | 590 | 24 | 69 |
| Ham & Pineapple | 550 | 20 | 71 |
| Meat Lover's | 830 | 46 | 68 |
| Supreme | 720 | 36 | 69 |
| Veggie Lover's | 550 | 20 | 70 |

*P'Zone: Per ½ P'Zone*

| | | | |
|---|---|---|---|
| Classic | 470 | 16 | 61 |
| Meaty | 550 | 23 | 61 |
| Pepperoni | 450 | 15 | 60 |

*Thin 'n Crispy: Per ⅛ of 12" Pizza*

| | | | |
|---|---|---|---|
| Cheese Only | 190 | 8 | 22 |
| Ham & Pineapple | 180 | 6 | 23 |
| Meat Lover's | 280 | 16 | 22 |
| Supreme | 240 | 12 | 23 |
| Veggie Lover's | 180 | 6 | 23 |

*Stuffed Crust: Per ⅛ 14" Pizza*

| | | | |
|---|---|---|---|
| Cheese Only | 340 | 14 | 39 |
| Ham & Pineapple | 330 | 12 | 41 |
| Meat Lover's | 480 | 26 | 39 |
| Supreme | 420 | 20 | 40 |
| Veggie Lover's | 330 | 12 | 41 |

*Appetizers: Breadsticks (1), 1½ oz* ... 140, 5, 19

Cheese Breadsticks (1), 2 oz ... 170, 6, 20

*Wings: Per 2 Pieces without Dipping Sauce*

| | | | |
|---|---|---|---|
| **Bone Out:** Buffalo, all flav., 2½ oz | 190 | 9 | 18 |
| Honey BBQ, 3 oz | 220 | 8 | 27 |

**Crispy Bone In:**

| | | | |
|---|---|---|---|
| Buffalo, all flav., 2½ oz | 230 | 15 | 16 |
| Honey BBQ, 3 oz | 260 | 14 | 24 |
| **Traditional:** All American, 1½ oz | 80 | 5 | 0 |
| Garlic Parmesan, 2 oz | 180 | 16 | 1 |

*Dipping Sauces: Marinara, 3 oz* ... 60, 0, 12

Blue Cheese; Ranch, av., 1½ oz ... 225, 24, 2

*Pastas, Tuscani: Per ½ Pan*

| | | | |
|---|---|---|---|
| Chicken Alfredo | 580 | 32 | 49 |
| Meaty Marinara | 450 | 20 | 44 |

*Desserts:* Cinnamon Sticks (2) ... 160, 4.5, 26

Hershey's: Choc. Dunkers (2) ... 190, 8, 27

With Chocolate Sauce, 1½ oz ... 310, 11, 51

White Icing Dipping Cup, 2 oz ... 170, 0, 44

# Fast - Foods & *Restaurants*

## Pizza Ranch® (Dec'11)

*Pizzas, Medium 12": Per ⅛ Slice*

| | | C | F | Cb |
|---|---|---|---|---|
| **Thin Crust:** Beef; BBQ Chicken | | 130 | 6 | 12 |
| Bacon Cheeseburger | | 140 | 7 | 12 |
| California Chicken | | 165 | 9 | 13 |
| Canadian Bacon | | 120 | 5 | 12 |
| Chicken Broccoli | | 140 | 6 | 12 |
| Prairie (Veggie) | | 130 | 6 | 13 |
| Roundup | | 150 | 8 | 13 |
| Stampede | | 160 | 8 | 13 |
| Texan | | 160 | 7 | 17 |

*Original Crust ~ Add 40 Cals and 9g Carb to Thin Crust*
*Skillet Crust ~ Add 10 Cals & and 2g Carb to Thin Crust*

| *Broasted Chicken:* Breast, 1 piece | 440 | 23 | 4 |
|---|---|---|---|
| Leg, 1 piece | 190 | 12 | 2 |
| Thigh, 1 piece | 370 | 26 | 4 |
| Wing, 1 piece | 190 | 13 | 2 |
| *Sides,* Potato Wedges (1) | 60 | 0 | 13 |

*For Complete Menu & Data ~ see CalorieKing.com*

## Planet Smoothie® (Dec'11)

*Cool Blended Smoothies:*
*Per 22 fl.oz Unless Indicated*

| PB & J | 500 | 16 | 87 |
|---|---|---|---|
| Shag-a-delic | 290 | 0 | 74 |
| The Last Mango | 340 | 1 | 85 |
| Twig & Berries | 280 | 0 | 74 |
| Vinnie del Rocco | 370 | 0 | 92 |

*Energy Smoothies: Per 22 fl.oz Unless Indicated*

| Berry Bada-Bing | 350 | 0.5 | 92 |
|---|---|---|---|
| Chocolate Elvis | 440 | 17 | 72 |
| Frozen Goat | 220 | 0 | 56 |
| Grape Ape | 210 | 0 | 54 |
| Road Runner | 300 | 0 | 75 |
| Spazz | 270 | 0 | 69 |

*Protein Smoothies: Per 22 fl.oz Unless Indicated*

| **Workout Blast:** Big Bang | 260 | 0 | 67 |
|---|---|---|---|
| Chocolate Chimp | 190 | 1.5 | 45 |
| Mr Mongo: Chocolate | 270 | 1.5 | 66 |
| Strawberry | 330 | 0 | 86 |

## Pollo Tropical® (Dec'11)

*Entrees: ¼ Chicken*

| | C | F | Cb |
|---|---|---|---|
| Dark Meat: With skin, 4 oz | 270 | 17 | 0 |
| Without skin, 3 oz | 180 | 9 | 0 |
| White Meat: With skin, 6 oz | 350 | 17 | 0 |
| Without skin, 5 oz | 230 | 7 | 0 |

*Tropichops:*

| Chicken, White Rice/Black Beans: | | | |
|---|---|---|---|
| Regular, 17 oz | 530 | 10 | 90 |
| Large, 30 oz | 1090 | 27 | 142 |
| Chicken, Yellow Rice/Vegetables: | | | |
| Regular, 10 oz | 330 | 5 | 51 |
| Large, 23 oz | 840 | 22 | 93 |
| Pork, White Rice/Black Beans: | | | |
| Regular, 18 oz | 680 | 22 | 92 |
| Large, 31 oz | 1260 | 49 | 145 |
| Pork, Yellow Rice/Vegetables: | | | |
| Regular, 13 oz | 490 | 18 | 54 |
| Large, 24 oz | 1000 | 44 | 97 |
| Vegetarian: Regular, 19 oz | 580 | 12 | 110 |
| Large, 31 oz | 950 | 21 | 178 |

*Fajitas: With Sides, Toppings, Tortillas*

| Chicken; Steak, average | 1145 | 38 | 153 |
|---|---|---|---|
| *Salad,* Caribbean Chicken Cobb | 1190 | 55 | 72 |

*Tropical Favorites:*

| Fried Yuca, 6 pieces | 340 | 16 | 49 |
|---|---|---|---|
| Sweet Plantains, 5 pieces | 430 | 11 | 88 |
| *Wraps:* Chicken Caesar, 5 oz | 370 | 17 | 30 |
| Cuban, 5 oz | 400 | 21 | 29 |

## Popeye's® (Dec'11)

*Chicken: Mild & Spicy with Skin*

| Breast, average | 430 | 27 | 14 |
|---|---|---|---|
| Leg, average | 165 | 10 | 5 |
| Thigh, average | 270 | 20 | 8 |
| Wing, average | 210 | 14 | 8 |
| *Big Easy:* Chicken Po'Boy | 660 | 34 | 61 |
| Chicken Wrap: Loaded | 310 | 12 | 33 |
| Naked | 200 | 6 | 22 |
| *Sides:* Biscuit, 2 oz | 260 | 15 | 26 |
| Cajun Fries, 3 oz | 260 | 14 | 30 |
| Cajun Rice, regular, 4.34 oz | 170 | 5 | 25 |
| Cole Slaw, regular, 4.87 oz | 220 | 15 | 19 |
| Corn on the Cob (1), 7¾ oz | 190 | 2 | 37 |
| Mashed Potatoes, regular, 5 oz | 110 | 4 | 18 |
| Onion Rings (12) | 560 | 38 | 50 |
| Red Beans & Rice, reg., 5.15 oz | 230 | 14 | 23 |
| *Dessert,* Hot Cinn. Apple Pie, 3.53 oz | 320 | 6 | 40 |

## Port of Subs® (Dec '11)

*Figures Based on West Coast Outlets*  **C**  **F**  **Cb**

*Light Submarine S'wiches: Per 5" Sub,*
*(Six Grams of Fat or Less) w/out Cheese, Oil or Mayo*

| | C | F | Cb |
|---|---|---|---|
| #2 Ham Turkey | 305 | 5 | 42 |
| #5 Smoked Ham & Turkey | 320 | 6 | 43 |
| #6 Vegetarian | 250 | 5 | 42 |
| #7 Roast Beef | 315 | 6 | 42 |
| #8 Turkey | 310 | 5 | 44 |
| #9 Peppered Pastrami | 265 | 4 | 41 |
| #10 Roasted Chicken Breast | 300 | 4 | 42 |
| #18 Roast Beef & Turkey | 310 | 5 | 43 |

*Cold Submarine S'wiches: Per 5" Sub with Cheese,*
*Lettuce, Tomato Vinegar, Oil, Salt & Oregano*

| | C | F | Cb |
|---|---|---|---|
| #1 Ham, Salami, Capicolla & Pepperoni with Provolone | 435 | 18 | 42 |
| #2 Ham & Turkey with Provolone | 355 | 9 | 42 |
| #3 Salami & Turkey with Provolone | 390 | 13 | 43 |
| #4 Ham & Salami with Provolone | 385 | 14 | 42 |
| #5 Smkd Ham & Turkey with Cheddar | 370 | 10 | 43 |
| #6 Vegetarian with 3 Cheeses | 450 | 21 | 45 |
| #7 Roast Beef with Provolone | 365 | 10 | 42 |
| #8 Turkey with Provolone | 360 | 8 | 44 |
| #10 Rstd Chicken Brst w./Provolone | 350 | 8 | 42 |
| #11 Ham with American | 405 | 14 | 44 |
| #12 Salami with Provolone | 395 | 16 | 42 |
| #13 Peppered Pastrami Turkey Swiss | 375 | 12 | 43 |
| #15 Salami & Pepperoni w/ Provolone | 405 | 18 | 42 |
| #16 BLT Sandwich | 470 | 26 | 39 |
| #17 Tuna with Provolone | 475 | 25 | 43 |
| #18 Rst Beef & Turkey w. Provolone | 360 | 9 | 43 |

*Wraps: With 12" Flour Tortilla, Cheese, Lettuce,*
*Tomato, Onion, Vinegar, Oil, Salt & Oregano*

| | C | F | Cb |
|---|---|---|---|
| #4 Ham, Salami, Provolone | 600 | 28 | 56 |
| #8 Turkey, Provolone | 565 | 21 | 59 |
| #11 Ham, American | 615 | 27 | 58 |

*Fresh Salads: With Lettuce, Tomato & Onion, w/o Dressing*

| | C | F | Cb |
|---|---|---|---|
| Caesar: With Parmesan, 6 oz | 35 | 0 | 11 |
| Add Grilled Chicken, 10 oz | 190 | 3 | 10 |
| Chefs, 11 oz | 300 | 18 | 10 |
| Garden, 10 oz | 70 | 2 | 11 |
| Grilled Chicken, 10 oz | 190 | 3 | 10 |
| Tuna, 9 oz | 250 | 18 | 9 |

*Salad Dressings: Per 1½ oz package*

| | C | F | Cb |
|---|---|---|---|
| Blue Cheese | 220 | 23 | 2 |
| Caesar | 240 | 23 | 2 |
| Fat Free Ranch | 50 | 0 | 13 |

*Sides: Per Regular, 8 oz*

| | C | F | Cb |
|---|---|---|---|
| Macaroni Salad | 515 | 41 | 44 |
| Potato Salad | 325 | 13 | 52 |

*Desserts:*

| | C | F | Cb |
|---|---|---|---|
| Brownie, 4½ oz | 535 | 12 | 96 |
| Chocolate Chunk Cookie, 4½ oz | 560 | 29 | 72 |

## Pret A Manger® (Dec '11)

*Baguettes: Per Pack*  **C**  **F**  **Cb**

| | C | F | Cb |
|---|---|---|---|
| Caprese | 620 | 25 | 72 |
| Chicken & Smoked Mozzarella | 480 | 10 | 72 |
| Slow Rstd Beef, Arugula & Parmesan | 580 | 17 | 55 |
| Smoked Ham & Roasted Turkey | 530 | 13 | 70 |

*Sandwiches: Per Pack*

| | C | F | Cb |
|---|---|---|---|
| California Club | 530 | 25 | 55 |
| Chicken & Bacon | 480 | 20 | 58 |
| Smoked Ham & Parmesan | 470 | 17 | 49 |
| **Slims:** Chicken Avocado & Balsamic | 260 | 12 | 29 |
| Smoked Ham & Parmesan | 235 | 7 | 25 |
| Sushi, Shrimp & Salmon, 1 pack | 470 | 7 | 77 |

*Wraps: Per Pack*

| | C | F | Cb |
|---|---|---|---|
| Avocado Pine Nut | 440 | 26 | 41 |
| Mandarin 5 Spice Roast Beef | 330 | 7 | 41 |
| Spicy Shrimp & Cilantro | 290 | 7 | 34 |

*Hot Food: Per Pack*

| | C | F | Cb |
|---|---|---|---|
| BBQ Pulled Pork | 410 | 9 | 69 |
| Mozzarella & Pesto Toastie | 400 | 16 | 48 |
| Tuna Melt | 730 | 45 | 44 |
| **Wraps:** Buffalo Chicken | 290 | 11 | 40 |
| Falafel & Red Peppers | 500 | 26 | 53 |
| New York Meatball | 630 | 31 | 58 |

*Salads: Per Pack, Without Dressing*

| | C | F | Cb |
|---|---|---|---|
| Chicken & Avocado | 430 | 28 | 42 |
| The Royal Chef | 290 | 17 | 14 |
| Tricolor | 340 | 26 | 20 |

*Bakery: Per Pack*

| | C | F | Cb |
|---|---|---|---|
| **Cake:** Banana | 420 | 24 | 48 |
| Carrot Cake | 460 | 29 | 46 |
| **Croissants:** Almond | 410 | 23 | 41 |
| Pain au Chocolat | 300 | 15 | 34 |
| **Muffins:** Blueberry | 450 | 24 | 56 |
| Cranberry Orange | 370 | 12 | 62 |

*Beverages: Per Container*

| | C | F | Cb |
|---|---|---|---|
| Apple Cranberry Juice | 120 | 0 | 28 |
| Strawberry Lemonade | 110 | 0 | 27 |

## Pretzelmaker® (Dec '11)

*Pretzels: Each, Unless Indicated*

| | C | F | Cb |
|---|---|---|---|
| **Bites:** Plain, salted, large, 3.5 oz | 250 | 1 | 52 |
| Cinnamon Sugar, 3.8 oz | 330 | 4 | 65 |
| **Pretzel Dogs:** Mini (6) | 300 | 19 | 23 |
| Whirl & Salt | 480 | 29 | 38 |
| **Pretzels:** Caramel Crunch, 4.2 oz | 300 | 4 | 58 |
| Cinnamon Sugar, 3.88 oz | 330 | 4 | 65 |
| Garlic; Salted, 4.2 oz | 310 | 4 | 60 |
| Iced Cinnamon Swirl, 3.88 oz | 330 | 4 | 65 |
| Ranch, 4.2 oz | 320 | 4.5 | 60 |
| Unsalted, 4.2 oz | 280 | 1 | 59 |

*Continued Next Page ...*

# Fast - Foods & Restaurants

## Pretzelmaker® cont... (Dec'11)

*Sauces:* Per Single Portion

| | C | F | Cb |
|---|---|---|---|
| Caramel | 140 | 0 | 35 |
| Cheddar Cheese | 80 | 5 | 4 |
| Cream Cheese | 200 | 20 | 2 |
| Honey Mustard | 80 | 0 | 20 |
| Icing | 180 | 0 | 45 |
| Ketchup | 20 | 0 | 4 |
| Mustard | 10 | 0 | 1 |
| Nacho Cheese | 80 | 5 | 4 |
| Pizza | 20 | 0.5 | 6 |

*Beverages:* Per 20 fl.oz Unless Indicated

**Blended Drinks:**

| | C | F | Cb |
|---|---|---|---|
| Cool Cappuccino | 640 | 21 | 107 |
| Lemon Twist | 540 | 16 | 99 |
| Mango Madness | 520 | 16 | 89 |
| Mocha Mania | 620 | 20 | 106 |
| Power Pomegranate | 490 | 16 | 86 |
| Strawberry Bananaza | 650 | 20 | 115 |
| **Lemonade,** Original, 44 fl oz | 380 | 0 | 91 |

## Qdoba® (Dec'11)

*Burritos:*

*Each, with 3.58 oz Flour Tortilla, Cilantro-Lime Rice, Black Beans, Salsa Verde, Sour Cream and Cheese*

| | C | F | Cb |
|---|---|---|---|
| Grilled Chicken | 1005 | 34 | 118 |
| Ground Beef | 1055 | 41 | 118 |
| Pulled Pork | 975 | 29 | 127 |

**Signature Flavors:** With 3.58 oz Flour Tortilla and Set Menu Toppings

| | | | |
|---|---|---|---|
| Ancho Chile BBQ w/ Pulled Pork | 550 | 14 | 76 |
| Fajita Ranchera, w/ Gr. Chicken | 535 | 19 | 57 |
| Grilled Veggie w/ Ground Beef | 540 | 24 | 51 |
| Mexican Gumbo w/ Pulled Pork | 550 | 16 | 69 |
| Poblamo Pesto w/ Ground Beef | 600 | 29 | 54 |
| Queso with Grilled Chicken | 590 | 25 | 54 |

**Grilled Quesadillas:** Each, with 7.58 oz Soft Flour Tortilla, Cilantro-Lime Rice, Black Beans, Salsa Verde, Sour Cream and Guacamole

| | | | |
|---|---|---|---|
| Grilled Chicken | 1455 | 70 | 126 |
| Shredded Beef | 1455 | 68 | 130 |

**3-Cheese Nachos:** Per Serving, with 3-Cheese Queso, Salsa Roja and Tortilla Chips

| | | | |
|---|---|---|---|
| Grilled Chicken | 955 | 52 | 86 |
| Ground Beef | 1005 | 59 | 86 |
| Pulled Pork | 925 | 47 | 95 |

## Qdoba® cont... (Dec'11)

*Tacos:* Each, with Lettuce, Cheese & Sour Cream

| | C | F | Cb |
|---|---|---|---|
| **Crispy:** Grilled Chicken | 170 | 11 | 9 |
| Ground Beef | 190 | 13 | 9 |
| Pulled Pork | 160 | 9 | 12 |
| Shredded Beef | 170 | 10 | 11 |

*Taco Salads:* With Lettuce, Black Beans, Cheese, Fat Free Picante Dressing & Crunchy Tortilla Bowl

| | | | |
|---|---|---|---|
| Grilled Chicken | 950 | 47 | 78 |
| Ground Beef | 1000 | 54 | 78 |

*Chips & Dip:* Per Small Serve of Tortilla Chips

| | | | |
|---|---|---|---|
| 3- Cheese Queso | 470 | 29 | 43 |
| Guacamole & Salsa Roja | 465 | 27 | 50 |

*Breakfast Items:* With 10" Flour Tortilla

**Breakfast Burrito:** Spicy Chorizo, Egg & Potato

| | | | |
|---|---|---|---|
| With 3-Cheese Queso Sauce | 540 | 26 | 53 |
| With Fajita Ranchero Sauce | 480 | 20 | 52 |

## Quizno's Subs® (Dec'11)

*Subs:*

**Classic:** Per Regular Size, with Standard Menu toppings on Italian Herb Bread

| | | | |
|---|---|---|---|
| Club | 990 | 56 | 68 |
| Italian | 865 | 50 | 67 |
| Honey Bourbon Chicken | 525 | 7.5 | 76 |
| Pork Cuban | 845 | 49 | 60 |
| The Traditional | 800 | 32 | 74 |
| Tuna Melt | 1000 | 66 | 61 |
| Turkey Bacon Guacamole | 840 | 43 | 68 |
| Turkey Ranch Swiss | 650 | 28 | 68 |

**Signature:** Per Regular Size, with Standard Menu Toppings on Italian Herb Bread

| | | | |
|---|---|---|---|
| Baja Chicken | 810 | 36 | 74 |
| Bourbon Grille Steak | 865 | 35 | 80 |
| Chicken Carbonara | 845 | 42 | 62 |
| Double Cheese Cheesesteak | 1030 | 63 | 65 |
| Honey Mustard Chicken | 830 | 41 | 68 |
| Mesquite Chicken | 790 | 39 | 63 |
| Prime Rib and Peppercorn | 920 | 53 | 66 |
| Prime Rib & Blue | 790 | 37 | 66 |

*Toasty Torpedos:* Italian

| | | | |
|---|---|---|---|
| | 920 | 45 | 91 |
| Beef Bacon & Cheddar | 825 | 30 | 93 |
| Pesto Turkey | 705 | 23 | 92 |
| Turkey Club | 850 | 35 | 92 |

*Toasty Bullets:*

| | | | |
|---|---|---|---|
| Beef, Bacon & Cheddar | 395 | 17 | 41 |
| Italian | 455 | 25 | 39 |
| Pesto Turkey | 340 | 13 | 42 |
| Tuna Melt | 470 | 28 | 39 |

## Quizno's Subs® cont... (Dec'11)

*Flatbread Sammies: Includes* **C** **F** **Cb**
*Flatbread and Standard Menu Toppings/Drsings*

| | C | F | Cb |
|---|---|---|---|
| Bistro Steak Melt | 390 | 23 | 31 |
| Chicken Bacon Ranch | 355 | 19 | 28 |
| Italiano | 370 | 21 | 26 |
| Roadhouse Steak | 235 | 4 | 38 |
| Smoky Chipotle Turkey | 355 | 21 | 30 |
| Veggie | 330 | 19 | 28 |
| *Soups: Per Bowl, with 2 Crackers* | | | |
| Broccoli Cheese | 310 | 18 | 26 |
| Chicken Noodle | 160 | 3.5 | 25 |
| Chili | 280 | 7 | 34 |

## Rally's/Checkers® (Dec'11)
*Burgers/Sandwiches:*

| | C | F | Cb |
|---|---|---|---|
| Bacon Double Cheeseburger | 650 | 42 | 32 |
| Big Buford | 670 | 40 | 41 |
| Cheese Double Cheese | 510 | 31 | 31 |
| Chili Cheeseburger | 320 | 15 | 30 |
| Rallyburger | 390 | 22 | 32 |
| *Wings:* Classic Honey BBQ, 5 pieces | 390 | 17 | 18 |
| Extra Hot, 5 pieces | 355 | 21 | 2 |
| Parmesan Garlic, 5 pieces | 480 | 35 | 1 |
| *Fries:* | | | |
| Chili Cheese Fries, 7¾ oz | 550 | 34 | 48 |
| French: Medium, 4 oz | 350 | 21 | 36 |
| Large, 4½ oz | 400 | 24 | 42 |

## Ranch 1® (Dec'11)

| | C | F | Cb |
|---|---|---|---|
| *Sandwiches:* Chicken & Cheese | 390 | 12 | 40 |
| Chicken Philly, 9¼ oz | 410 | 13 | 40 |
| Original: Crispy Chicken, 11½ oz | 640 | 31 | 60 |
| Crispy Spicy Chicken, 11½ oz | 470 | 9 | 68 |
| Grilled Spicy Chicken, 10¼ oz | 360 | 7 | 46 |
| *Bowls:* Chicken Teriyaki, 19¼ oz | 500 | 7 | 86 |
| Chicken Fajita, 10 oz | 540 | 24 | 53 |
| Chicken Platter with Rice, 11.86 oz | 270 | 6 | 28 |
| Popcorn Chicken: Small, 5½ oz | 310 | 10 | 30 |
| Large, 7½ oz | 420 | 14 | 40 |
| Kids, 2 oz | 120 | 4 | 11 |
| *Salads:* Completed | | | |
| Grilled Chicken Caesar, 13¼ oz | 430 | 30 | 14 |
| Southwest Chicken, 17½ oz | 680 | 43 | 44 |
| *Fries:* Medium, 5¾ oz | 380 | 19 | 43 |
| Large, 8 oz | 530 | 27 | 58 |
| Kids, 4¼ oz | 280 | 15 | 31 |
| Cheese: Medium, 7.3 oz | 490 | 27 | 46 |
| Large, 11 oz | 760 | 44 | 66 |

## Red Hot & Blue® (Dec'11)

*Entrees: Per Serving* **C** **F** **Cb**

| | C | F | Cb |
|---|---|---|---|
| Delta Double: With Memphis Chkn | 900 | 54 | 12 |
| With Pulled Pork | 795 | 60 | 9 |
| Five Meat Treat | 935 | 63 | 15 |
| *BBQ Sandwiches: Regular, Without Sides* | | | |
| Beef Brisket | 390 | 15 | 37 |
| Carolina Chopped Pork | 360 | 14 | 34 |
| Pulled Pork | 370 | 15 | 37 |
| *Ribs, Half Slab:* Dry | 935 | 72 | 14 |
| Sweet | 950 | 71 | 22 |
| *Salads: Without Dressing* | | | |
| Grilled Chicken Caesar | 770 | 46 | 47 |
| RH & B Chopped Salad | 850 | 42 | 55 |
| Smokehouse Salad | 670 | 36 | 36 |
| Southern Fried Chicken | 710 | 31 | 60 |
| *Soup,* Memph. Corn Chdr, 1 bowl | 270 | 12 | 23 |
| *Sides:* BBQ Beans | 255 | 2 | 48 |
| Mashed Potatoes with Gravy | 310 | 14 | 44 |
| Potato Salad | 405 | 28 | 33 |

## Red Lobster ● (Dec'11)
**Lunch:**
**Starters:** *As Served*

| | C | F | Cb |
|---|---|---|---|
| Chilled Jumbo Shrimp Cocktail | 120 | 0.5 | 9 |
| Crispy Calamari & Vegetables | 1520 | 97 | 115 |
| Lobster, Crab & Seafood Mushrooms | 330 | 18 | 18 |
| Pan Seared Crab Cakes | 280 | 14 | 13 |
| **Classics:** *Per Lunch Portion Without Sides* | | | |
| Cajun Chicken Linguini Alfredo | 630 | 27 | 45 |
| Crunchy Popcorn Shrimp | 280 | 14 | 26 |
| Sailor's Platter | 330 | 10 | 8 |
| **LightHouse Menu:** *Per ½ Portion, Without Sides/Sauces* | | | |
| Rainbow Trout | 220 | 10 | 6 |
| Salmon | 270 | 9 | 6 |
| Tilapia | 210 | 3 | 9 |
| **Signature Combinations:** | | | |
| Admiral's Feast | 1280 | 73 | 92 |
| Seaside Shrimp Trio | 1010 | 55 | 65 |
| Ultimate Feast | 600 | 28 | 25 |
| **Dinner:** | | | |
| **Starters:** *As Served* | | | |
| Lobster, Artichoke & Seafood Dip | 1200 | 74 | 101 |
| Parrot Isle Coconut Shrimp | 530 | 36 | 34 |
| Shrimp Nachos | 1090 | 64 | 94 |
| **Lobster & Crab Entrees:** *Without Sides* | | | |
| Lobster & Shrimp Pasta, full serve | 1020 | 50 | 86 |
| New England Lobster Rolls | 590 | 34 | 47 |
| Snow Crab Legs Meat, 3½ oz | 180 | 2 | 0 |
| **Sides:** Fries | 330 | 17 | 40 |
| Creamy Lobster Mashed Potatoes | 370 | 22 | 30 |
| Home-Style Mashed Potatoes | 210 | 10 | 27 |

*Continued Next Page ...*

## Red Lobster® cont... (Dec'11)

*Salads: Includes Dressing*

| | C | F | Cb |
|---|---|---|---|
| Caesar Salad with Chicken | 670 | 52 | 14 |
| Caesar Salad with Shrimp | 620 | 51 | 14 |

*Dipping Sauces: Per 1½ oz*

| | | | |
|---|---|---|---|
| Cocktail Sauce | 40 | 0 | 9 |
| Honey Mustard | 280 | 26 | 12 |
| Tartar Sauce | 190 | 19 | 6 |
| 100% Pure Melted Butter | 350 | 38 | 2 |

*For Complete Nutritional Data ~ see CalorieKing.com*

## Red Robin® (Dec'11)

*Nutritional Information varies between restaurants. Please refer to their website for further information*

*Appetizers: As Served*

| | | | |
|---|---|---|---|
| Chili Chili con Queso | 1370 | 88 | 109 |
| Creamy Spinach & Artichoke Dip | 1115 | 60 | 101 |
| Guacamole, Salsa & Chips | 780 | 46 | 87 |
| Just-in-Quesadilla | 1136 | 60 | 78 |
| Nachos: Chili | 1965 | 129 | 132 |
| With Chicken | 2090 | 131 | 133 |
| RR's Buzzard Wings | 1075 | 84 | 4 |
| Towering Onion Rings | 1770 | 112 | 171 |

*Entrees: With Sides, Dressings & Sauce*

| | | | |
|---|---|---|---|
| Arctic Cod Fish & Chips | 1115 | 67 | 83 |
| Clam Strips | 1440 | 84 | 139 |
| Classic Creamy Mac 'N' Cheese | 1230 | 73 | 91 |
| Clucks & Fries: Regular Style | 1450 | 92 | 100 |
| Buffalo Style | 1695 | 121 | 100 |
| Ensenada Chicken Platter, 1 piece | 580 | 36 | 24 |
| Jumbo Shrimp & Slaw Platter | 1255 | 56 | 148 |
| Prime Rib Dip | 1010 | 55 | 74 |
| Southwest Chicken Pasta | 1170 | 45 | 128 |
| Triple S Riblet Basket | 1430 | 85 | 59 |

*Sandwiches & Burgers: With Standard Components*

**Gourmet Burgers:**

| | | | |
|---|---|---|---|
| A.1. Peppercorn | 1030 | 59 | 69 |
| All American Patty Melt | 1315 | 98 | 60 |
| Bacon Cheeseburger | 1035 | 69 | 52 |
| Burnin' Love | 930 | 60 | 54 |
| Guacamole Bacon | 1050 | 64 | 56 |
| Pub | 955 | 55 | 57 |
| Royal | 1125 | 83 | 52 |
| Sauteed 'Shroom | 960 | 56 | 58 |
| The Banzai | 1035 | 62 | 68 |
| Whiskey River BBQ | 1120 | 68 | 72 |

**Sandwiches:**

| | | | |
|---|---|---|---|
| Chicken: Blackened | 685 | 33 | 52 |
| Bruschetta | 670 | 30 | 55 |
| California | 830 | 43 | 53 |
| Caprese | 675 | 29 | 52 |
| Teriyaki | 900 | 47 | 65 |

## Rocky Rococo® (Dec'11)

*Pastas: Per Serving*

| | C | F | Cb |
|---|---|---|---|
| Can't Decide, 14 oz | 465 | 9 | 77 |

Fettuccine with Alfredo Sauce:

| | | | |
|---|---|---|---|
| Regular, 14 oz | 460 | 14 | 66 |
| Light, 7 oz | 230 | 7 | 33 |

**Spaghetti with Meatballs:**

| | | | |
|---|---|---|---|
| Regular, 15 oz | 630 | 16 | 89 |
| Light, 7½ oz | 315 | 8 | 45 |

**Spaghetti with Tomato Sauce:**

| | | | |
|---|---|---|---|
| Regular, 14 oz | 470 | 4 | 87 |
| Light, 7 oz | 235 | 2 | 44 |

*Pizzas: Per Slice, ⅛ Pizza*

| | | | |
|---|---|---|---|
| Cheese | 380 | 9 | 54 |
| Garden | 390 | 10 | 56 |
| Pepperoni | 425 | 13 | 54 |
| Sausage | 495 | 19 | 54 |

*Sides:*

| | | | |
|---|---|---|---|
| **Breadsticks:** With Marinara Sce (6) | 420 | 7 | 72 |
| With Jalapeno Cheese Sauce (6) | 530 | 18 | 72 |
| Wheat Muffin (1) | 200 | 4 | 38 |

## Roly Poly® (Dec'11)

| | C | F | Cb |
|---|---|---|---|

*Wraps: Per 6" White Wrap Unless Indicated*

**Ham & Smoked Pork:**

| | | | |
|---|---|---|---|
| Italian Classic | 335 | 12 | 32 |
| Key West Cuban Mix | 330 | 9 | 44 |
| Peachtree Melt | 310 | 11 | 27 |
| Pork Melt | 310 | 11 | 26 |
| Porky's Nightmare | 320 | 12 | 28 |
| **Chicken:** Basil Cashew Chicken | 300 | 10 | 30 |
| Catalina Chicken | 315 | 11 | 28 |
| Chicken Caesar | 310 | 11 | 30 |
| Chicken Fajita | 315 | 9 | 28 |
| Cobb Salad | 255 | 12 | 27 |
| Delhi Chicken | 325 | 12 | 33 |
| Hickory Chicken | 350 | 10 | 25 |
| Oriental Chicken | 270 | 4 | 29 |
| Santa Fe Chicken | 305 | 11 | 28 |
| **Tuna:** Popeye's Tuna On Wheat | 305 | 4 | 31 |
| Classic Tuna Melt | 340 | 17 | 26 |
| Texas Tuna Melt | 310 | 12 | 30 |
| Thai Hot Tuna | 340 | 11 | 30 |

## Round Table Pizza® (Dec'11)

*Appetizers:*

| | C | F | Cb |
|---|---|---|---|
| Buffalo Wings, 6 pieces | 420 | 30 | 6 |
| Garlic Bread: 6 pieces | 420 | 21 | 54 |
| With Cheese, 6 pieces | 600 | 36 | 54 |
| Garlic Parmesan Twists, 3 pieces | 510 | 15 | 78 |
| Honey BBQ Wings, 6 pieces | 480 | 27 | 12 |

*Pizzas (Large 14"): Per Slice, ½ Pizza*

| | | | |
|---|---|---|---|
| **Original Crust:** Cheese | 230 | 9 | 25 |
| Chicken & Garlic Gourmet | 250 | 11 | 25 |
| Chicken Smokehouse | 270 | 12 | 26 |
| Gourmet Veggie | 240 | 10 | 27 |
| Guinevere's Garden Delight | 220 | 8 | 26 |
| Hawaiian | 220 | 8 | 27 |
| Italian Garlic Supreme | 270 | 14 | 25 |
| King Arthur Supreme | 270 | 13 | 26 |
| Maui Zaui, with Polynesian Sce | 260 | 10 | 29 |
| Montague's All Meat Marvel | 290 | 15 | 25 |
| Pepperoni | 240 | 11 | 24 |
| Smokehouse Combo | 290 | 14 | 26 |
| **Pan Crust:** Cheese | 300 | 11 | 38 |
| Chicken & Garlic Gourmet | 340 | 13 | 39 |
| Chicken Smokehouse | 360 | 14 | 40 |
| Gourmet Veggie | 320 | 12 | 41 |
| Guinevere's Garden Delight | 300 | 10 | 39 |
| Hawaiian | 300 | 10 | 40 |
| Italian Garlic Supreme | 360 | 16 | 39 |
| King Arthur Supreme | 340 | 14 | 39 |
| Maui Zaui w/ Polynesian Sauce | 340 | 12 | 43 |
| Montague's All Meat Marvel | 360 | 15 | 38 |
| Pepperoni | 320 | 13 | 38 |
| **Skinny Crust:** Cheese | 190 | 9 | 18 |
| Chicken & Garlic Gourmet | 220 | 11 | 18 |
| Chicken Smokehouse | 240 | 12 | 19 |
| Gourmet Veggie | 200 | 10 | 20 |
| Guinevere's Garden Delight | 180 | 8 | 19 |
| Hawaiian | 190 | 8 | 20 |
| Italian Garlic Supreme | 240 | 14 | 18 |
| King Arthur Supreme | 240 | 13 | 19 |
| Maui Zaui with Polynesian Sauce | 220 | 10 | 22 |
| Montague's All Meat Marvel | 260 | 15 | 18 |
| Pepperoni | 210 | 11 | 18 |

*Sandwiches:*

| | | | |
|---|---|---|---|
| Chicken Club | 800 | 43 | 59 |
| Ham Club | 740 | 40 | 60 |
| RT Veggie | 630 | 32 | 65 |
| Turkey Club | 720 | 38 | 59 |
| Turkey Sante-Fe | 730 | 40 | 57 |

*For Complete Nutritional Data ~ see CalorieKing.com*

## Rubio's Mexican Grill® (Dec'11)

*Burritos: Each, With Flour Tortilla, Without Chips*

| | C | F | Cb |
|---|---|---|---|
| **Baja:** Grill Chicken | 630 | 28 | 55 |
| Steak | 650 | 32 | 55 |
| Bean & Cheese | 760 | 37 | 78 |
| Beer-Battered Fish | 810 | 48 | 70 |
| **Grilled:** Mesquite Shrimp | 730 | 34 | 75 |
| Ono | 670 | 31 | 60 |
| Veggie | 770 | 35 | 83 |
| **Big Burrito Especial:** Chicken | 820 | 31 | 102 |
| Steak | 840 | 34 | 102 |
| **Health Mex:** *With Whole Grain Tortilla* | | | |
| Chicken | 520 | 12 | 72 |
| Grilled Vege | 510 | 12 | 78 |
| *Nachos:* Grande | 1270 | 78 | 112 |
| Grande Chicken | 1340 | 78 | 114 |
| *Quesadillas:* Three Cheese | 1120 | 70 | 87 |
| Three Cheese Chicken | 1200 | 70 | 89 |
| *Tacos: Per 1 Corn Tortilla* | | | |
| **From The Land:** | | | |
| Grilled Gourmet: Chicken | 130 | 1 | 22 |
| Steak | 330 | 19 | 24 |
| **Health Mex,** Grilled Chicken | 130 | 11 | 22 |
| **Street:** Carnitas | 100 | 4 | 8 |
| Grilled: Chicken | 90 | 2.5 | 9 |
| Steak | 90 | 4 | 9 |
| **From The Sea:** Blackened Ono | 230 | 10 | 26 |
| Chili-Lime Wild Salmon | 230 | 9 | 25 |
| Fish: Original | 300 | 17 | 27 |
| Especial | 360 | 22 | 29 |
| Gr. Gourmet Garlic Herb Shrimp | 340 | 19 | 23 |
| Health Mex, Grilled Ono | 150 | 2 | 21 |
| *Salads: Includes Dressing/Sauce* | | | |
| Chicken Balsamic & Roasted Vege | 310 | 11 | 29 |
| Chicken Chipotle Ranch | 450 | 31 | 22 |
| Chicken Chopped | 460 | 24 | 36 |
| Chicken Grilled Grande Bowl | 630 | 27 | 62 |
| *Salsas: Per 1 oz* | | | |
| Picante | 20 | 1 | 2 |
| All Other Varieties | 5 | 0 | 1 |
| *Dessert,* Churro, 1½ oz | 170 | 8 | 22 |

## Ruby Tuesday® (Dec '11)

| Appetizers: Serves 4, w/out Sauce | C | F | Cb |
|---|---|---|---|
| Asian Dumplings | 455 | 20 | 48 |
| Fried Mozzarella | 580 | 24 | 52 |
| Jumbo Lump Crab Cake | 365 | 24 | 20 |
| Southwestern Spring Rolls | 630 | 32 | 72 |
| Thai Phoon Shrimp | 765 | 52 | 44 |

*Burgers: Without Sides*

| | C | F | Cb |
|---|---|---|---|
| **Handcrafted:** Alpine Swiss | 1050 | 62 | 71 |
| Boston Blue | 1200 | 71 | 88 |
| Ruby's Classic | 930 | 55 | 66 |
| Smokehouse | 1230 | 72 | 91 |
| **Premium:** Avocado Turkey Burger | 885 | 55 | 52 |
| Buffalo Chicken Burger | 790 | 41 | 64 |
| Chicken BLT | 800 | 40 | 64 |
| Turkey Burger | 700 | 40 | 50 |
| **Prime:** Triple Prime | 1115 | 82 | 49 |
| Triple Prime Bacon Cheddar | 1335 | 101 | 49 |
| Triple Prime Cheddar | 1275 | 96 | 49 |

*Premium Seafood: Without Sides*

| | C | F | Cb |
|---|---|---|---|
| Asian Glazed Salmon | 415 | 24 | 12 |
| Crab Cake Dinner | 450 | 34 | 21 |
| Creole Catch | 210 | 8 | 7 |
| Herb-Crusted Tilapia | 400 | 24 | 11 |
| New Orleans Seafood | 375 | 20 | 3 |
| Salmon Florentine | 485 | 30 | 7 |

*Ribs & Platters: Without Sides*

| | C | F | Cb |
|---|---|---|---|
| Asian Sesame Glazed, Half | 505 | 29 | 16 |
| Classic BBQ, Half | 500 | 24 | 29 |
| Memphis Dry Rub, Half | 460 | 29 | 6 |

*Smart Eating: Without Sides*

| | C | F | Cb |
|---|---|---|---|
| Creole Catch | 210 | 8 | 7 |
| Grilled Salmon | 340 | 20 | 0 |

*Steaks & Chicken: Without Sides*

| | C | F | Cb |
|---|---|---|---|
| BBQ Grilled Chicken | 275 | 4 | 12 |
| Chef's Cut 12 oz Sirloin | 740 | 50 | 2 |
| Chicken Bella | 385 | 14 | 10 |
| Chicken Florentine | 380 | 14 | 9 |
| Rib Eye | 820 | 63 | 2 |
| Top Sirloin | 390 | 22 | 2 |

## Ruby Tuesday® cont... (Dec '11)

| Pasta Classics: Without Sides | C | F | Cb |
|---|---|---|---|
| Chicken & Broccoli | 1550 | 96 | 94 |
| Chicken & Mushroom Alfredo | 1230 | 61 | 90 |
| Lobster Carbonara | 1425 | 95 | 80 |
| Parmesan Chicken | 1420 | 77 | 111 |
| Parmesan Shrimp | 1050 | 57 | 88 |
| Spaghetti Squash Marinara | 230 | 9 | 29 |

*Petite Plates: Without Sides*

| | C | F | Cb |
|---|---|---|---|
| Chicken Fresco | 435 | 25 | 26 |
| Grilled Salmon | 470 | 32 | 25 |
| Sliced Sirloin | 400 | 24 | 20 |
| Trout Almondine | 560 | 38 | 28 |

*Garden Fresh Salads: Without Dressing*

| | C | F | Cb |
|---|---|---|---|
| Carolina Chicken | 705 | 38 | 39 |
| Garden | 395 | 17 | 50 |
| Grilled Chicken | 690 | 26 | 46 |
| Grilled Salmon | 710 | 37 | 44 |

*Petite Salads:*

| | C | F | Cb |
|---|---|---|---|
| Carolina Chicken | 435 | 23 | 30 |
| Grilled Chicken | 355 | 13 | 26 |

*Dressing: Per 1 oz*

| | C | F | Cb |
|---|---|---|---|
| Blue Cheese | 180 | 19 | 1 |
| Balsamic Vinaigrette | 40 | 2 | 5 |
| Honey Mustard | 90 | 8 | 5 |
| Italian | 60 | 6 | 2 |
| Ranch | 100 | 11 | 1 |
| Signature Parmesan | 150 | 16 | 1 |
| Thousand Island | 70 | 7 | 3 |

| *Fresh, Fresh Sides:* French Fries | 425 | 18 | 63 |
|---|---|---|---|
| **Baked Potato:** Plain | 260 | 2 | 52 |
| Loaded Baked Potato | 570 | 28 | 54 |
| Brown-Rice Pilaf | 245 | 8 | 37 |
| Creamy Mashed Cauliflower | 135 | 8 | 14 |
| Garlic Cheese Biscuit | 100 | 5 | 13 |
| Onion Rings | 340 | 19 | 37 |
| Sauteed Baby Portob, Mshsrms | 100 | 4 | 10 |
| White Cheddar Mashed Potatoes | 225 | 14 | 21 |
| *Desserts:* Blondie for One | 630 | 27 | 88 |
| Italian Cream Cake | 990 | 56 | 110 |
| New York Cheesecake | 735 | 60 | 84 |
| **Cookies:** Chocolate Chip | 180 | 9 | 24 |
| White Choc. Macadamia Nut | 200 | 12 | 23 |
| *Drinks:* Peach Fruit Tea | 135 | 2 | 9 |
| **Lemonade:** Pomegranate | 195 | 0 | 12 |
| Blackberry; Wild Berry | 205 | 0 | 9 |

*For Complete Menu ~ see CalorieKing.com*

## Runza® (Dec '11)

### Burgers:

| | C | F | Cb |
|---|---|---|---|
| Legendary: ¼ lb Cheeseburger Runza | 430 | 21 | 32 |
| ½ lb Double Cheeseburger Runza | 640 | 32 | 37 |
| ¼ lb Bacon Cheeseburger | 510 | 29 | 36 |
| ¼ lb Legend Supreme | 770 | 37 | 62 |
| ¼ lb Swiss Mushroom | 450 | 25 | 36 |
| Junior: Cheeseburger | 330 | 17 | 28 |
| Cheeseburger Runza | 310 | 14 | 30 |
| Swiss Mushroom | 380 | 21 | 26 |

### Sandwiches:

| | C | F | Cb |
|---|---|---|---|
| BBQ Chicken, grilled | 390 | 9 | 46 |
| Buffalo Chicken grilled | 440 | 13 | 36 |
| Cheese Runza | 560 | 21 | 66 |
| Deluxe Chicken, crispy | 480 | 19 | 51 |
| Original Runza | 500 | 17 | 65 |
| Polish Dog | 420 | 26 | 30 |
| Smothered Chicken, grilled | 380 | 10 | 41 |
| Swiss Mushroom Runza | 590 | 25 | 68 |

### French Fries: Small, 3 oz

| | C | F | Cb |
|---|---|---|---|
| French Fries: Small, 3 oz | 280 | 15 | 31 |
| Medium, 4½ oz | 410 | 23 | 46 |
| Large, 7 oz | 630 | 35 | 70 |
| **Frings,** 6½ oz | 540 | 28 | 64 |
| **Onion Rings:** Medium, 4 oz | 370 | 20 | 41 |
| Large, 6½ oz | 590 | 32 | 66 |
| **Onion Ring Dip,** 2 oz | 90 | 6 | 4 |

### Salads: Without Dressing

| | C | F | Cb |
|---|---|---|---|
| Tossed, with Crispy Chicken | 440 | 27 | 29 |
| Tossed, with Grilled Chicken | 280 | 13 | 13 |
| **Dressings:** Caesar | 410 | 45 | 3 |
| Fat-Free Hidden Valley Ranch | 60 | 0 | 15 |

### Soups: Per Bowl

| | C | F | Cb |
|---|---|---|---|
| Boston Clam Chowder | 320 | 23 | 33 |
| Broccoli Cheese | 360 | 27 | 35 |
| Cauliflower Cheese | 330 | 26 | 32 |
| Chicken Noodle | 170 | 5 | 21 |
| Homemade Chili | 310 | 10 | 26 |
| Potato with Bacon | 310 | 20 | 40 |
| Vegetable Cheese | 330 | 22 | 28 |
| Wisconsin Cheese | 430 | 35 | 36 |

### Kids Meals: Includes Small Fries, Without Drink

| | C | F | Cb |
|---|---|---|---|
| Mini Corn Dogs (5) | 550 | 32 | 56 |
| Chicken Strips (2) | 460 | 25 | 42 |
| Jr Hamburger | 500 | 24 | 55 |
| Kids Runza Sandwich | 530 | 24 | 64 |

### Desserts & Drinks:

| | C | F | Cb |
|---|---|---|---|
| Chocolate Chip Cookie (1) | 310 | 16 | 34 |
| Shakes: Cappuccino, reg., 12 floz | 470 | 18 | 65 |
| Vanilla, regular, 12 fl.oz | 470 | 16 | 69 |
| Pepsi Runza Slushie, med., 18 fl.oz | 220 | 0 | 60 |

## Ryan's Grill Buffet & Bakery® (Dec '11)

### Entrees: Without Sides

| | C | F | Cb |
|---|---|---|---|
| **Beef:** BBQ'd, 4 oz | 140 | 5 | 16 |
| Country Fried Steak w/ gravy, 2.6 oz | 230 | 14 | 16 |
| Meatloaf, 3 oz | 180 | 11 | 7 |
| Perfect Pot Roast, 4.95 oz | 160 | 7 | 9 |
| Roasted, carved, 3 oz | 230 | 15 | 0 |
| Salisbury Steak, 3.53 oz | 150 | 9 | 8 |
| Sirloin Steak, 3 oz | 180 | 9 | 0 |

### Chicken:

| | C | F | Cb |
|---|---|---|---|
| Breasts: Country BBQ, 5.8 oz | 310 | 16 | 6 |
| Rotisserie, 5.3 oz | 310 | 17 | 1 |
| Traditional, Baked, 5.3 oz | 310 | 17 | 0.5 |
| Chicken & Dumplings, 4.95 oz | 160 | 5 | 17 |
| New Orleans Bourbon Street, 3 oz | 180 | 8 | 9 |
| Orange Chicken, 3 oz | 340 | 22 | 26 |

### Fish/Seafood:

| | C | F | Cb |
|---|---|---|---|
| **Fish/Seafood:** Baked Fish, 2 oz | 90 | 4.5 | 0 |
| Butter Crumb Alaskan Pollock, 1¾ oz | 110 | 5 | 2 |
| Butterfly Shrimp (6), 2.3 oz | 210 | 9 | 24 |
| Carved Salmon Filet, 3 oz | 190 | 11 | 0 |
| Clam Strips, 3 oz | 320 | 20 | 28 |
| Fried: Fish, 3 pieces, 3 oz | 240 | 12 | 27 |
| Shrimp (22), 3 oz | 240 | 12 | 24 |
| Wood Seared Salmon, 1 pce, 3 oz | 220 | 16 | 0 |

### Pasta/Spaghetti: Per 1 Spoonful, 4.95 oz

| | C | F | Cb |
|---|---|---|---|
| Country Pasta Gratine | 160 | 4 | 24 |
| Creamy Penne Carbonara | 260 | 17 | 17 |
| Fire Grilled Chicken Alfredo | 220 | 14 | 14 |
| Grilled Italian Sausage Penne | 180 | 11 | 14 |

### Pork:

| | C | F | Cb |
|---|---|---|---|
| Carved: Grilled Loin, 3 oz | 140 | 10 | 0 |
| Ham, 3 oz | 100 | 5 | 0 |
| Honey Glazed Baked, 1 sl, 3 oz | 120 | 5 | 1 |
| Ribs, BBQ/County-Style, (3), 3½ oz | 420 | 27 | 15 |
| Steak: Grilled, 2 oz | 140 | 9 | 0 |
| BBQ, grilled, 2 oz | 150 | 9 | 3 |

### Salads: Without Dressing Unless Indicated

| | C | F | Cb |
|---|---|---|---|
| Asian Chopped, 3.55 oz | 90 | 4 | 13 |
| Caesar, 1 cup, 2½ oz | 70 | 6 | 4 |
| Greek, 2.65 oz | 120 | 8 | 10 |
| Seafood, 4.15 oz | 310 | 26 | 15 |

### Sides:

| | C | F | Cb |
|---|---|---|---|
| Baked Potato, plain, 4½ oz | 150 | 0 | 36 |
| BBQ Baked Beans, 3 oz | 130 | 3 | 26 |
| Cauliflower Aut Gratin, 3 oz | 50 | 2 | 8 |
| French Fries, 2 oz | 170 | 9 | 23 |
| Fried Okra, 3 oz | 220 | 12 | 28 |
| Mashed Potatoes, 4 oz | 70 | 0.5 | 13 |

### Desserts:

| | C | F | Cb |
|---|---|---|---|
| **Desserts:** Cheesecake, plain, 1 sl. | 190 | 8 | 25 |
| Key Lime Pie, scratch, 1 sl., 2½ oz | 220 | 9 | 31 |
| Lemon Cream Pie, 2¼ oz | 130 | 4.5 | 34 |

**235**

## 7-Eleven® (Dec '11)

*Breakfast:*

| | C | F | Cb |
|---|---|---|---|
| **Bites:** Big Bite Frank, no bun, 2 oz | 180 | 17 | 1 |
| ¼ lb Big Bite, no bun, 4 oz | 360 | 34 | 2 |
| Cheeseburger Bite, no bun, 4.2 oz | 410 | 36 | 4 |
| Smokie Bite, no bun, 3.2 oz | 270 | 24 | 2 |
| **Burrito Rollers:** | | | |
| Chicken & Pepper Jack Cheese | 230 | 9 | 23 |
| Sausage, Bacon, Egg & Cheese | 290 | 16 | 24 |
| **Sandwiches:** | | | |
| Biscuit, Sausage, Egg & Cheese | 500 | 30 | 41 |
| Croissant, Egg, Ham & Cheese | 360 | 23 | 25 |
| Muffin: English | 390 | 25 | 24 |
| Sausage, Egg & Cheese | 360 | 23 | 25 |
| **Donuts:** | | | |
| Glazed: Plain, 2.9 oz | 280 | 10 | 43 |
| Chocolate, 3.6 oz | 350 | 13 | 54 |

*Fresh:*

| | C | F | Cb |
|---|---|---|---|
| **Big Eats Sandwiches:** *Per Sandwich* | | | |
| Egg Salad on White Bread | 520 | 29 | 42 |
| Ham & Havarti Chse on Onion Roll | 420 | 15 | 43 |
| Smoked Turkey: | | | |
| With Jack Cheese on Wheat Bread | 460 | 22 | 42 |
| With Southwest Mayo | 540 | 26 | 49 |
| Tuna Salad on Wheat Bread | 450 | 19 | 48 |
| Turkey & Swiss on Pita Bread | 460 | 14 | 64 |

*Hot:*

| | C | F | Cb |
|---|---|---|---|
| **7 Select Burritos:** | | | |
| Beef & Bean; Red Hot Beef, av., 5 oz | 350 | 16 | 43 |
| Beef & Bean, 10 oz | 720 | 31 | 89 |
| Red Hot Beef, 10 oz | 670 | 30 | 83 |
| **Chicken:** Tender (1) | 160 | 5 | 11 |
| Wings, Asian Haban; Buffalo (1), av. | 60 | 1.5 | 7 |
| **Pizza:** Chse; Pepperoni., av., 4 oz sl. | 290 | 13 | 30 |
| **Rollers:** Corn Dog Roller | 320 | 21 | 23 |
| Southwest Burrito Roller | 230 | 8 | 30 |
| **Taquitos:** Bacon, Egg, Chse & Potato | 190 | 8 | 23 |
| Buffalo Chicken | 180 | 8 | 22 |

*Beverages: Per 8 fl.oz*

| | C | F | Cb |
|---|---|---|---|
| Fr. Vanilla/Mocha Iced Cappuccino | 140 | 3 | 26 |
| Hershey's S'Mores Cocoa | 200 | 7 | 36 |

*Fountain Drinks: (Assumes ⅓ Ice)*

| | C | F | Cb |
|---|---|---|---|
| **Coca-Cola/Pepsi/Dr.Pepper/7Up:** | | | |
| Gulp, 20 oz | 195 | 0 | 51 |
| Big Gulp, 32 oz | 310 | 0 | 82 |
| Super Gulp, 44 oz | 430 | 0 | 112 |
| **Diet Coke/Diet Pepsi,** 16 oz | 1 | 0 | 0 |

*Slurpees:* Average All Flavors,

| | C | F | Cb |
|---|---|---|---|
| 12 oz size | 95 | 0 | 24 |
| 22 oz size | 175 | 0 | 44 |
| 28 oz size | 220 | 0 | 56 |
| Hawaiian Punch; Dr Pepper, av. | | | |
| 12 oz size | 180 | 0 | 48 |
| 22 oz size | 330 | 0 | 88 |

## Saladworks® (Dec '11)

*Salads: Without Dressing*

| | C | F | Cb |
|---|---|---|---|
| Autumn Harvest | 300 | 12 | 40 |
| Bently | 245 | 10 | 11 |
| Buffalo Bleu | 250 | 7 | 24 |
| Chicken Caesar | 285 | 4 | 19 |
| Cobb | 270 | 16 | 13 |
| Fire Roasted Cabo Jack | 390 | 19 | 31 |
| Garden Deluxe | 240 | 2 | 92 |
| Greek | 185 | 10 | 18 |
| Mandarin Chicken | 230 | 7 | 37 |
| Nuevo Nicoise | 230 | 5 | 73 |
| Sophie's Salad | 310 | 14 | 35 |
| Tivoli | 430 | 20 | 74 |

*Focaccia Fusion: Without Spread*

| | C | F | Cb |
|---|---|---|---|
| BLT | 345 | 13 | 32 |
| Chicken Monterey | 385 | 12 | 35 |
| Fajitalicious | 380 | 12 | 33 |
| Turkey Ranch | 365 | 10 | 33 |

*Dressings: Per 1 oz Ladle*

| | C | F | Cb |
|---|---|---|---|
| Balsamic: Regular | 170 | 18 | 4 |
| Fat Free | 20 | 0 | 5 |
| Classic French | 130 | 12 | 6 |
| Dijon Lemon Capri | 130 | 13 | 4 |
| Green Goddess | 150 | 15 | 3 |
| Oriental Sesame | 90 | 4.5 | 12 |
| Parmesan Caesar | 150 | 17 | 1 |
| Rustic Thousand Island | 140 | 13 | 5 |

*Extra Menu Items ~ See CalorieKing.com*

## Sandella's® (Dec '11)

*Wraps:*

| | C | F | Cb |
|---|---|---|---|
| Buffalo Chicken | 400 | 7 | 51 |
| Chicken Fajita | 520 | 20 | 53 |
| Pacific Chicken | 550 | 23 | 57 |
| Pesto Turkey | 460 | 15 | 54 |
| Sweet & Spicy Chicken | 490 | 14 | 62 |
| *Paninis:* Chicken Delicato | 490 | 18 | 51 |
| Spinach, Ham & Swiss | 550 | 20 | 61 |
| Turkey & Mozzarella | 520 | 13 | 62 |
| Tuscan Chicken | 540 | 21 | 55 |
| *Quesadillas:* California | 500 | 23 | 53 |
| Chicken Fajita | 510 | 19 | 52 |
| Mediterranean | 400 | 13 | 53 |
| *Grilled Flatbread:* Brazilian Bacon | 650 | 24 | 78 |
| Brazilian Chicken | 510 | 10 | 73 |
| Pesto Chicken | 610 | 28 | 56 |
| Spinach & Bacon | 750 | 45 | 51 |
| Vegetable Confetti | 510 | 21 | 61 |
| *Salads:* Fiesta, without Dressing | 360 | 8 | 54 |
| Greek, without Dressing | 310 | 15 | 37 |
| *Rice Bowls:* Black Bean & Rice | 840 | 20 | 130 |
| Chicken Fajita | 750 | 20 | 104 |

*For Complete Menu & Data ~ see CalorieKing.com*

## Sarku Japan® (Dec '11)

### D'Lite Meals:

| | C | F | Cb |
|---|---|---|---|
| Rice & Chicken Tempua15 oz | 970 | 58 | 81 |
| Rice & Shrimp Tempura, 11 oz | 540 | 21 | 70 |
| Vegetarian, 14 oz | 360 | 0.5 | 79 |
| Vegetarian Soba Noodle, 14 oz | 710 | 24 | 106 |

### Combos:

| | C | F | Cb |
|---|---|---|---|
| **Tempura:** Chicken, 23 oz | 1270 | 78 | 102 |
| Chicken & Shrimp, 20 oz | 980 | 53 | 95 |
| **Teriyaki:** Beef, 19 oz | 570 | 10 | 85 |
| Beef & Shimp, 21 oz | 630 | 11 | 85 |
| Chicken, 22 oz | 640 | 13 | 90 |
| Chicken & Shrimp, 24 oz | 700 | 14 | 90 |
| Shrimp, 19 oz | 500 | 2.5 | 83 |
| *Sauce,* Teriyaki, 1.5 oz | 45 | 0 | 9 |
| *Sides:* Maki Roll, 2 oz | 140 | 11 | 9 |
| **Rice:** Steamed, 9 oz | 290 | 0 | 64 |
| Fried, 9 oz | 330 | 4.5 | 62 |
| Tempura Chicken, 1 piece, 2 oz | 230 | 19 | 8 |
| Tempura Shrimp, 1 piece, 0.8 oz | 90 | 7 | 4 |

## Schlotzsky's® (Dec '11)

| | C | F | Cb |
|---|---|---|---|
| *Oven-Toasted Sandwiches: Per Medium Sandwich* | | | |
| **Angus:** Beef & Provolone | 815 | 33 | 84 |
| Corned Beef Reuben | 910 | 40 | 79 |
| Corned Beef | 580 | 13 | 78 |
| Pastrami Reuben | 910 | 39 | 79 |
| Pastrami & Swiss | 905 | 36 | 83 |
| BLT | 670 | 30 | 73 |
| Chicken & Pesto | 570 | 13 | 75 |
| Chicken Breast | 515 | 5 | 80 |
| Chipotle Chicken | 550 | 13 | 70 |
| Homestyle Tuna | 600 | 18 | 73 |
| Santa Fe Chicken | 650 | 16 | 78 |
| Smoked Turkey Breast | 520 | 9 | 77 |
| Smoked Turkey Reuben | 895 | 38 | 84 |
| Turkey & Guacamole | 570 | 13 | 82 |
| Turkey Bacon Club | 830 | 35 | 77 |
| **Original Style:** The Original | 770 | 34 | 77 |
| Cheese | 795 | 38 | 76 |
| Ham & Cheese | 735 | 27 | 79 |
| Turkey | 835 | 35 | 79 |
| **Panini:** Classic Swiss & Tomato | 625 | 26 | 63 |
| Grilled Chicken Romano | 570 | 15 | 63 |
| Italiano | 605 | 22 | 65 |
| Mozzarella & Portobello | 515 | 17 | 64 |
| Smoked Turkey & Guacamole | 625 | 23 | 70 |
| **Wraps:** Asian Chicken | 540 | 11 | 81 |
| Feta & Portobello | 705 | 46 | 58 |
| Grilled Chicken & Guacamole | 700 | 36 | 62 |
| Homestyle Tuna | 480 | 18 | 55 |
| Parmesan Chicken Caesar | 600 | 23 | 62 |

## Schlotzsky's® cont... (Dec '11)

### 8" Pizzas: Per Pizza

| | C | F | Cb |
|---|---|---|---|
| BBQ Chicken & Jalapeno | 705 | 16 | 109 |
| Baby Spinach Salad | 445 | 6 | 80 |
| Bacon, Tomato & Portobello | 685 | 29 | 76 |
| Combination Special | 650 | 26 | 77 |
| Double Cheese | 595 | 21 | 74 |
| Fresh Tomato & Pesto | 555 | 18 | 73 |
| Grilled Chicken & Pesto | 650 | 19 | 76 |
| Mediterranean | 560 | 20 | 74 |
| Pepperoni & Double Cheese | 725 | 33 | 74 |
| Smoked Turkey & Jalapeno | 650 | 20 | 78 |
| Thai Chicken | 730 | 22 | 87 |
| Vegetarian Special | 570 | 20 | 75 |

### Salads: Without Dressing/Croutons Unless Indicated

| | C | F | Cb |
|---|---|---|---|
| Baby Spinach & Feta | 155 | 11 | 6 |
| Caesar Salad with Croutons | 130 | 6 | 10 |
| Chicken | 320 | 15 | 14 |
| Garden | 50 | 1 | 12 |
| Greek | 135 | 8 | 13 |
| Grilled Chicken Caesar with Croutons | 250 | 8 | 14 |
| Ham & Turkey Chef | 255 | 13 | 15 |
| Pasta | 70 | 3 | 12 |
| Potato | 240 | 13 | 29 |
| Turkey Chef | 310 | 18 | 15 |

### Soup: Per Bowl

| | C | F | Cb |
|---|---|---|---|
| Boston Clam Chowder | 260 | 17 | 29 |
| Broccoli Cheese | 280 | 22 | 19 |
| Timberline Chili | 415 | 14 | 47 |
| Wisconsin Cheese | 395 | 30 | 30 |

### Chips:

| | C | F | Cb |
|---|---|---|---|
| Original: Baked; Mesquite BBQ | 140 | 3 | 25 |
| Kettle | 190 | 11 | 18 |
| All other varieties | 220 | 12 | 25 |

### Kid's Meals: Without Cookie or Drink

| | C | F | Cb |
|---|---|---|---|
| Cheese Pizza | 480 | 13 | 73 |
| Cheese Sandwich | 445 | 19 | 49 |
| Ham & Cheese Sandwich | 475 | 20 | 50 |
| Pepperoni Pizza | 525 | 17 | 73 |
| Turkey Sandwich | 300 | 5 | 49 |

### Desserts:

| | C | F | Cb |
|---|---|---|---|
| Brownie | 415 | 22 | 54 |
| Carrot Cake | 715 | 42 | 80 |
| New York Style Cheesecake | 350 | 23 | 30 |
| **Cookies:** Choc./Fudge Choc. Chip | 160 | 8 | 22 |
| Oatmeal Raisin | 150 | 6 | 22 |
| Sugar | 160 | 7 | 22 |
| White Chocolate Macadamia | 170 | 9 | 21 |

## Second Cup® ~ see CalorieKing.com

## Shakey's® (Dec '11)

*Pizzas: Per Slice, ½ Large Pizza*

| | C | F | Cb |
|---|---|---|---|
| **Cheese:** Pan Crust | 185 | 6 | 26 |
| Thin Crust | 150 | 5.5 | 18 |
| **Firehouse:** Pan Crust | 255 | 12 | 27 |
| Thin Crust | 220 | 12 | 19 |
| **Garden Veggie:** Pan Crust | 185 | 5.5 | 27 |
| Thin Crust | 150 | 5 | 19 |
| **Margherita:** Pan Crust | 175 | 5 | 26 |
| Thin Crust | 135 | 4.5 | 18 |
| **Rustic Garlic Chicken:** Pan Crust | 190 | 5.5 | 26 |
| Thin Crust | 155 | 5.5 | 18 |
| **Shakey's Special:** Pan Crust | 210 | 6.5 | 31 |
| Thin Crust | 195 | 10 | 18 |
| **Texas BBQ Chicken:** Pan Crust | 205 | 5 | 29 |
| Thin Crust | 170 | 5 | 21 |
| **Ultimate Meat:** Pan Crust | 280 | 14 | 26 |
| Thin Crust | 245 | 13 | 18 |
| **Additional Toppings:** Beef | 35 | 3 | 0 |
| Cheese | 15 | 1 | 0.5 |
| Chicken | 15 | 0.5 | 0 |
| Ham | 10 | 0.5 | 0 |
| Pepperoni | 25 | 2.5 | 0 |
| Sausage | 45 | 4 | 0.5 |

*Sharables: Per Serving Unless Indicated*

| | C | F | Cb |
|---|---|---|---|
| Chicken Strips (5) | 620 | 31 | 48 |
| Mojo Potatoes (5) | 215 | 11 | 25 |
| Mojo Supreme, serves 4-6 | 1950 | 120 | 160 |
| Shakey's Spicy Wings (6) | 495 | 29 | 27 |

*Shakey's Famous Chicken: Per Piece*

| | C | F | Cb |
|---|---|---|---|
| **Fried Chicken:** Breast | 475 | 26 | 16 |
| Leg | 170 | 19 | 6 |
| Thigh | 350 | 24 | 10 |
| Wing | 130 | 9 | 3.5 |

## Sheetz® (Dec '11)

*Breakfast: Plain Bagel, Without Ad d Ons or Dressing Unless Indicated*

| | C | F | Cb |
|---|---|---|---|
| **Shmagelz:** Bacon & Egg | 530 | 27 | 53 |
| Egg & American Cheese | 440 | 19 | 50 |
| Egg, Ham & Provolone | 525 | 21 | 55 |
| **Shmiscuitz:** Bacon & Egg | 540 | 35 | 39 |
| Egg & American Cheese | 450 | 27 | 36 |
| Egg, Ham & Swiss Cheese | 550 | 30 | 41 |
| Egg, Sausage & American Cheese | 625 | 44 | 36 |
| **Shmuffins:** Bacon & Egg | 410 | 25 | 29 |
| Egg & American Cheese | 320 | 17 | 26 |
| Egg & Ham | 310 | 11 | 30 |
| Egg, Sausage & Cheddar Cheese | 495 | 34 | 26 |
| Egg & Steak | 395 | 16 | 27 |

*Continued Next Page ...*

## Sheetz® cont... (Dec '11)

*Cold Subz: Per 6" White Sub, Without Add Ons or Dressing*

| | C | F | Cb |
|---|---|---|---|
| American Cheese | 350 | 11 | 45 |
| BLT | 455 | 19 | 50 |
| Chicken Salad | 490 | 23 | 54 |
| Italian | 365 | 10 | 47 |
| Roast Beef | 280 | 4 | 46 |
| Tuna Salad | 455 | 18 | 54 |
| Turkey | 295 | 4 | 47 |

*Hot Subz: Per 6" White Sub, W/out Add Ons or Dressing*

| | C | F | Cb |
|---|---|---|---|
| Chicken | 360 | 6 | 45 |
| Meatball | 370 | 13 | 48 |
| Pepperoni | 440 | 20 | 45 |
| Steak | 425 | 10 | 46 |

*Add Ons:*

| | C | F | Cb |
|---|---|---|---|
| Bacon | 150 | 12 | 2 |
| Black Olives | 10 | 1 | 0.5 |
| Cheeses: American; Cheddar; Swiss | 110 | 9 | 0 |
| Hot Pepper; Provolone | 100 | 8 | 1 |
| Parmesan | 5 | 0.5 | 0.5 |
| Green/Jalapeno Peppers | 5 | 0 | 0.5 |
| Onions; Peppers, cooked, average | 25 | 1 | 2 |
| Shredded Lettucce; Diced Onions, av. | 5 | 0 | 1 |
| Tomatoes, sliced | 5 | 0.5 | 1 |
| Dressings/Sauces: Honey Mustard | 15 | 0 | 4 |
| Italian Romano | 55 | 6 | 2 |
| Marinara | 10 | 0.5 | 1 |
| Mayo; Ranch, average | 145 | 16 | 1 |
| *Hot Dogz,* with Chili & Onions | 310 | 19 | 27 |
| *Nachoz,* | | | |
| Bueno/Grande, w/ Nacho Cheese | 515 | 23 | 65 |

*Saladz: Without Dressing*

| | C | F | Cb |
|---|---|---|---|
| Chef with Shredded Cheese | 250 | 12 | 13 |
| Crispy Chicken w/ Shredded Chse | 370 | 16 | 31 |
| Garden with Shredded Cheese | 130 | 8 | 8 |
| Grilled Chicken | 145 | 4 | 7 |
| Steak | 210 | 8 | 8 |
| Taco with Shredded Cheese | 355 | 18 | 39 |

*Sidez:*

| | C | F | Cb |
|---|---|---|---|
| Chili, Mac & Cheese, 6.7 oz | 130 | 6 | 14 |
| Cole Slaw, 5 oz | 200 | 9 | 28 |
| **Fryz:** Bag, 3.2 oz | 160 | 6 | 23 |
| Cup, 5 oz | 260 | 10 | 36 |
| Cheese, 14.4 oz | 670 | 32 | 81 |
| Smokehouse, 15.38 oz | 985 | 53 | 103 |
| *Beverages,* Hot Chocolate, med. | 290 | 1 | 56 |

Updated Nutrition Data ~ www.CalorieKing.com
Persons with Diabetes ~ See Disclaimer (Page 22)

## Shoney's® (Dec '11)

### Breakfast:

| | C | F | Cb |
|---|---|---|---|
| *Off The Grill: Per Plate* | | | |
| Bacon, Egg & Cheddar Croissant | 790 | 57 | 30 |
| Sirloin Steak & Eggs | 580 | 36 | 3 |
| Platters: Pancakes, with Bacon | 665 | 11 | 110 |
| With Sausage Patties | 775 | 21 | 110 |
| Skillets: Big Biscuit | 980 | 56 | 93 |
| Fiesta | 1030 | 76 | 42 |
| Sunrise Special | 1470 | 62 | 191 |

### Lunch/Dinner:

| | C | F | Cb |
|---|---|---|---|
| **Starters:** Angus Steak Chili | 620 | 37 | 50 |
| Chicken Enchilada Soup | 445 | 22 | 50 |
| Chicken Strips | 1270 | 84 | 87 |
| Onion Rings, Jumbo | 980 | 69 | 102 |
| **Burgers:** *Without Sides* | | | |
| All American | 1160 | 93 | 40 |
| BBQ Bacon Cheeseburger | 1470 | 117 | 45 |
| Classic | 1360 | 111 | 40 |
| Mushroom Swiss | 1195 | 89 | 42 |
| **Chicken:** *Without Sides* | | | |
| **Sandwiches:** Blackened Chicken | 720 | 36 | 40 |
| Grilled Chicken Sandwich | 720 | 36 | 40 |
| Croissant, Chicken Salad | 645 | 33 | 39 |
| **Classic Sandwiches:** *Without Sides* | | | |
| Philly Cheese Steak | 1140 | 74 | 61 |
| Reuben | 835 | 45 | 44 |
| Slim Jim | 695 | 36 | 57 |
| Turkey Club | 1250 | 83 | 60 |
| Croissant, BLT | 580 | 48 | 26 |
| *Entrees: With Standard Sides Unless Indicated* | | | |
| **Chicken:** Blackened w/ BBQ Sauce | 585 | 18 | 39 |
| With Honey Mustard | 785 | 44 | 33 |
| Chicken Strips | 1320 | 88 | 91 |
| Grilled with BBQ Sauce | 450 | 20 | 14 |
| With Honey Mustard | 650 | 46 | 22 |
| **Fish:** Fish & Chips Basket | 1310 | 74 | 102 |
| Fish Sandwich, without sides | 1190 | 63 | 105 |
| Grilled Salmon | 515 | 34 | 27 |
| Pan-Blackened Catfish Fry | 915 | 60 | 66 |
| Southern Catfish Fry | 1465 | 78 | 137 |
| **Pasta:** Baked Spaghetti | 1460 | 54 | 145 |
| Lasagna: Half Portion | 730 | 44 | 58 |
| Full Portion | 1140 | 65 | 93 |
| **Skillets:** | | | |
| Artichoke & Crabmeat Casserole | 1410 | 80 | 134 |
| Lemon Chicken w/ Mshrm & Rice | 1220 | 67 | 91 |
| Slow-Cooked Pot Roast | 835 | 45 | 57 |

## Shoney's® cont... (Dec '11)

| *Entrees (Cont): W/ Standard Sides* | C | F | Cb |
|---|---|---|---|
| **Steak:** Half-O-Pound | 1325 | 103 | 62 |
| Porterhouse Steak, 16 oz | 2170 | 136 | 97 |
| Ribeye, 10 oz | 1485 | 90 | 97 |
| Smothered Liver & Onions | 775 | 46 | 48 |
| Steakhouse Sirloin, 8 oz | 1380 | 83 | 97 |
| T-Bone, 12 oz | 1725 | 110 | 100 |
| *Salads:* Entrée Fried Chicken | 1095 | 70 | 93 |
| Grilled Chicken | 1060 | 56 | 70 |
| Salmon | 870 | 60 | 49 |
| *Kid's Menu:* Cheeseburger | 790 | 56 | 41 |
| Fish Wrap | 490 | 32 | 25 |
| Grilled Cheese | 450 | 32 | 24 |
| Mac & Cheese | 965 | 54 | 83 |
| *Sides:* Baked Potato, plain | 225 | 0 | 51 |
| Biscuit (1) | 190 | 9 | 23 |
| Fries: Chili Cheese Fries | 680 | 42 | 61 |
| French | 520 | 30 | 56 |
| Homefries | 120 | 6 | 15 |
| Fruit Bowl | 60 | 0 | 15 |
| Garlic Grecian Bread, 1 slice | 330 | 24 | 23 |
| Loaded Potato Mix | 115 | 13 | 8 |
| Mashed Potatoes | 240 | 11 | 31 |
| Onion Rings | 490 | 35 | 51 |
| Wild Rice | 150 | 4 | 25 |
| *Desserts:* Apple Crisp | 810 | 38 | 81 |
| Hot Fudge Cake | 710 | 30 | 101 |
| Key Lime Cheesecake | 830 | 58 | 74 |
| Pies: Peanut Butter, 1 slice | 570 | 35 | 57 |
| Strawberry, 1 slice | 350 | 13 | 53 |
| Sundaes: Banana Split | 545 | 21 | 93 |
| Hot Fudge | 535 | 25 | 68 |
| Peach | 370 | 17 | 46 |
| Strawberry | 375 | 17 | 47 |

## Sizzler® (Dec '11)

| *Burgers & Sandwiches:* | C | F | Cb |
|---|---|---|---|
| **Burgers:** Mega Bacon Chseburger | 1010 | 61 | 48 |
| Sizzler Burger: ⅓ lb | 620 | 30 | 47 |
| ½ lb | 760 | 40 | 47 |
| **Sandwiches:** Grilled Chicken Club | 665 | 31 | 48 |
| Malibu Chicken | 705 | 37 | 59 |
| *Hot Entrees: Without Sides, Dipping Sauces &* | | | |
| *Condiments Unless Indicated* | | | |
| **Chicken:** Hibachi Chkn Breast (1) | 200 | 7 | 7 |
| With Hibachi Sauce, 1 oz | 245 | 7 | 17 |
| Lemon-Herb Chicken Breast | 220 | 12 | 2 |
| With Lemon Herb Sauce, 1 oz | 265 | 16 | 3 |

*Continued Next Page ...*

## Sizzler® cont... (Dec '11)

*Hot Entrees (Cont): Without Sides, Dipping Sauces & Condiments Unless Indicated*

| | C | F | Cb |
|---|---|---|---|
| **Seafood:** Fish 'n Chips | 1035 | 49 | 111 |
| Fisherman's Platter | 820 | 34 | 82 |
| Gr. Salmon w/ Rice Pilaf | 530 | 20 | 40 |
| Gr. Shrimp Fettuccine Alfredo | 985 | 55 | 64 |
| Shrimp: Grilled Skewers (2) | 545 | 26 | 42 |
| Shrimp Fry (12) | 435 | 12 | 48 |
| Shrimp, Shrimp, Shrimp | 970 | 41 | 92 |
| **Steaks:** Bacon Wrapped Sirloin | 555 | 35 | 5 |
| Classic, 8 oz | 320 | 14 | 2 |
| Chopped Steak, 8 oz | 255 | 12 | 2 |
| Porterhouse, 18 oz | 1365 | 107 | 1 |
| Rib Eye, 12 oz | 950 | 62 | 1 |
| **Steak Combos:** Classic Trio | 835 | 40 | 37 |
| Ultimate Sizzlin' Trio | 1415 | 86 | 74 |

*Prepared Salads: Per 4oz Serving w/out Dressing*

| | C | F | Cb |
|---|---|---|---|
| Ambrosia | 125 | 4 | 22 |
| Caesar | 50 | 4 | 2 |
| Carrot Raisin | 110 | 6 | 12 |
| Creamy Cole Slaw | 70 | 4 | 6 |
| Greek | 50 | 4.5 | 2 |
| Macaroni | 225 | 12 | 27 |
| Potato | 325 | 27 | 18 |
| Seafood | 160 | 11 | 11 |

*Salad Dressings: Per 2 Tbsp, 1 oz*

| | C | F | Cb |
|---|---|---|---|
| Honey Mustard | 110 | 8 | 9 |
| Italian, Low Fat | 40 | 3 | 3 |
| Ranch | 115 | 12 | 1 |
| Signature Blue Cheese | 105 | 11 | 1 |
| Thousand Island | 95 | 9 | 5 |

*Salad Bar Items:* Bacon Bits, 2 oz

| | C | F | Cb |
|---|---|---|---|
| Bacon Bits, 2 oz | 110 | 6 | 6 |
| Cottage Cheese, 2 oz | 50 | 2 | 2 |
| Garbanzo Beans, 2 oz | 50 | 0 | 8 |
| Kidney Beans, 2 oz | 50 | 0 | 8 |
| Peas, 2 oz | 30 | 0 | 6 |
| Turkey Ham, 2 oz | 75 | 6 | 2 |

*Sides: W/out Condiments/Toppings*

| | C | F | Cb |
|---|---|---|---|
| Baked Potato | 265 | 4 | 51 |
| Broccoli, 5 oz | 50 | 1 | 7 |
| Cheese Toast, 1 slice | 240 | 19 | 13 |
| French Fries, 5 oz | 285 | 13 | 42 |
| Fresh Baked Roll | 165 | 1 | 33 |
| Rice Pilaf, 5 oz | 225 | 5 | 40 |
| **Kids:** Cheese Pizza, 4 slices | 390 | 16 | 47 |
| Classic Steak, 6 oz | 255 | 12 | 2 |
| Dino Chicken Nuggets | 285 | 16 | 17 |
| Grilled Cheese | 400 | 26 | 28 |
| Macaroni & Cheese | 490 | 16 | 68 |
| Sizzler Burger, ⅓ lb | 620 | 30 | 47 |

*For Complete Menu & Data ~ see CalorieKing.com*

## Skyline Chili® (Dec '11)

*Burritos:*

| | C | F | Cb |
|---|---|---|---|
| All Chili Burrito | 560 | 30 | 37 |
| All Chili Deluxe Burrito | 650 | 35 | 45 |
| *Meals: Per Regular Serving* | | | |
| Black Bean & Rice, 3-Way | 800 | 40 | 74 |
| Black Bean & Rice, 4-Way | 810 | 40 | 77 |
| Black Bean & Rice, 5-Way | 880 | 40 | 89 |
| Black Bean & Rice, Spaghetti | 490 | 12 | 79 |
| **Bowls:** Chili | 270 | 16 | 6 |
| Chili Bean | 270 | 12 | 17 |
| Chili Cheese | 440 | 30 | 6 |
| Coney | 870 | 69 | 9 |
| Loaded Chili | 580 | 40 | 18 |
| Vegetarian Black Beans & Rice | 320 | 9 | 46 |
| **Chili Spaghetti:** Regular | 450 | 18 | 43 |
| With Beans | 520 | 17 | 61 |
| With Beans & Onions | 530 | 17 | 64 |
| **Coneys:** Regular, without cheese | 220 | 12 | 17 |
| With Cheese | 340 | 22 | 17 |
| **Steamed Potatoes:** Plain | 310 | 0 | 72 |
| Cheddar | 740 | 41 | 72 |
| Chili | 440 | 8 | 74 |

*Salads: Without Dressing*

| | C | F | Cb |
|---|---|---|---|
| Buffalo/Classic Chicken, average | 150 | 7 | 7 |
| Garden | 80 | 5 | 6 |
| Greek Chicken | 170 | 8 | 9 |
| Greek | 60 | 3.5 | 5 |
| Southwestern Chicken w/ Tortilla Chips | 760 | 44 | 66 |

*Wraps: Without Dressing*

| | C | F | Cb |
|---|---|---|---|
| Buffalo/Classic Chicken, average | 520 | 21 | 55 |
| Greek Chicken | 510 | 21 | 54 |
| Southwest Chicken | 670 | 30 | 65 |
| *Sides:* Cheese | 230 | 19 | 1 |
| Chili | 130 | 8 | 3 |
| Crackers, 1 bowl | 100 | 3 | 20 |
| French Fries | 630 | 33 | 79 |

*For Complete Nutritional Data ~ see CalorieKing.com*

## Smoothie King® (Dec '11)

*Fruit Smoothies: Per 20 fl.oz Cup Figures Include Turbinado. Without Turbinado, deduct 100 calories and 23 carbs.*

| | C | F | Cb |
|---|---|---|---|
| **Get Energy:** Acai Adventure | 435 | 5 | 92 |
| Go Goji | 435 | 0 | 104 |
| Green Tea Tango | 280 | 3 | 52 |
| **Shape Up, High Protein Smoothies:** | | | |
| Almond Mocha | 365 | 9 | 42 |
| Banana | 320 | 9 | 32 |
| Chocolate | 365 | 9 | 42 |

Updated Nutrition Data ~ www.CalorieKing.com
Persons with Diabetes ~ See Disclaimer (Page 22)

## Smoothie King® cont... (Dec '11)

*Fruit Smoothies: Per 20 fl.oz Cup*

**Figures Include Turbinado. Without Turbinado, deduct 100 calories and 23 carbs.**

| | C | F | Cb |
|---|---|---|---|
| **Snack Right:** Banana Berry Treat | 365 | 0 | 86 |
| Berry Punch | 360 | 0 | 91 |
| Fruit Fusion | 355 | 1 | 76 |
| Grape Expectations | 400 | 0 | 95 |
| **Stay Healthy:** Cranberry Cooler | 495 | 0 | 120 |
| Cranberry Supreme | 555 | 1 | 130 |
| Mangosteen Madness | 385 | 0 | 94 |
| Orange KA-BAM | 465 | 0 | 117 |
| **Trim Down:** Blackberry Dream | 365 | 1 | 68 |
| MangoFest | 285 | 0 | 72 |
| Muscle Punch | 365 | 1 | 84 |
| Passion Passport | 395 | 0 | 96 |
| Peach Slice | 315 | 0 | 72 |
| Raspberry Collider | 340 | 0 | 86 |
| Raspberry Sunrise | 390 | 0 | 95 |
| Slim-N-Trim: Chocolate | 295 | 2 | 57 |
| Orange Vanilla | 215 | 1 | 46 |
| Strawberry | 375 | 1 | 84 |
| Strawberry Kiwi Breeze | 375 | 0 | 90 |
| The Shredder: Chocolate | 310 | 3 | 36 |
| Strawberry | 355 | 1 | 56 |
| Youth Fountain | 255 | 0 | 61 |

*32 fl.oz Cup: Multiply 20 fl.oz figures by 1.5*
*40 fl.oz Cup: Multiply 20 fl.oz figures by 2*

**Kids Kup Smoothies:**

| | C | F | Cb |
|---|---|---|---|
| Berry Interesting | 275 | 0 | 69 |
| Choc-A-Laka | 245 | 3 | 44 |
| Gimme-Grape | 265 | 0 | 64 |
| Smarti Tarti | 200 | 0 | 49 |

## Snappy Tomato (Dec '11)

*Pizza: Per Slice , ⅛ of Pizza*

| | C | F | Cb |
|---|---|---|---|
| Buffalo Grilled Chicken | 250 | 5 | 32 |
| Cheese | 220 | 7 | 30 |
| Hawaiian | 370 | 18 | 33 |
| Meat Topper | 430 | 23 | 31 |
| Pepperoni | 340 | 17 | 31 |
| Ranch | 370 | 21 | 31 |
| Snapperoni | 390 | 22 | 31 |
| Supreme | 340 | 17 | 32 |
| Ultimate | 460 | 26 | 33 |
| Veggie | 240 | 8 | 33 |

*Oven Baked Hoagie Sandwiches, W/o Toppings, Sauce/Dressing*

| | | | |
|---|---|---|---|
| Grilled Chicken | 490 | 11 | 71 |

*Snappetizers, Without Sauce,*

| | | | |
|---|---|---|---|
| Snappy Wings (3), Plain, 2.6 oz | 160 | 11 | 0 |

## Sonic Drive-In® (Dec '11)

*Burgers: With Standard Toppings*

| | C | F | Cb |
|---|---|---|---|
| Green Chili Cheeseburger | 770 | 43 | 55 |
| Jr. | 310 | 15 | 30 |
| Jr. Deluxe | 350 | 20 | 28 |
| Veggie with Mustard | 500 | 14 | 75 |
| **Sonic:** With Mayonnaise | 800 | 49 | 55 |
| With Mustard | 700 | 38 | 54 |
| Bacon Cheeseburger with Mayo | 930 | 60 | 56 |
| Cheeseburger, with Mayonnaise | 860 | 54 | 55 |
| Super Sonic: | | | |
| Bacon Dble Cheeseburger w/ Mayo | 1370 | 96 | 55 |
| Dble Cheeseburger w/ Mayo | 1270 | 87 | 56 |
| *Coneys:* | | | |
| All Beef Chili Cheese | 430 | 26 | 33 |
| Footlong, ¼ pound | 830 | 53 | 55 |
| *Toaster Sandwiches:* Chkn Club | 790 | 48 | 55 |
| Bacon Cheeseburger | 820 | 51 | 51 |
| *Wraps:* Crispy Chicken | 490 | 23 | 49 |
| Grilled Chicken | 390 | 14 | 39 |
| *Chicken:* Chicken Strip Dinner (4) | 970 | 45 | 106 |
| Jumbo Popcorn Chicken: | | | |
| Small, without Sauce, 4 oz | 380 | 22 | 27 |
| Large, without Sauce, 6 oz | 560 | 32 | 41 |
| *Sides: Per Medium Serving* | | | |
| French Fries: Plain, 4 oz | 330 | 13 | 48 |
| With Cheese, 5½ oz | 460 | 23 | 55 |
| With Chili & Cheese, 7¼ oz | 540 | 28 | 59 |
| Mozzarella Sticks, w/o sauce, 5 oz | 440 | 22 | 40 |
| Onion Rings, 5½ oz | 440 | 21 | 55 |
| Tater Tots: Plain, 2½ oz | 200 | 13 | 20 |
| With Cheese, 3½ oz | 300 | 21 | 21 |
| With Chili & Cheese, 5½ oz | 390 | 27 | 25 |
| *Breakfast:* | | | |
| **Burritos:** Bacon, Egg & Cheese | 470 | 28 | 37 |
| Sausage, Egg & Cheese | 500 | 31 | 37 |
| Steak & Egg | 590 | 33 | 45 |
| SuperSonic | 590 | 36 | 47 |
| French Toast Sticks: With Syrup (4) | 590 | 31 | 71 |
| Without Syrup (4) | 500 | 31 | 49 |
| **Sandwiches:** | | | |
| Breakfast Bagel: With Bacon | 590 | 24 | 68 |
| With Sausage | 680 | 34 | 68 |
| CroiSonic: Bacon, Egg & Cheese | 510 | 36 | 28 |
| Sausage, Egg & Cheese | 600 | 46 | 28 |

*Continued Next Page ...*

## Sonic Drive-In® cont... (Dec '11)

*Desserts:*

| | C | F | Cb |
|---|---|---|---|
| Banana Split | 490 | 18 | 76 |
| **Single Topping Sundaes:** | | | |
| Chocolate | 500 | 22 | 69 |
| Hot Fudge | 520 | 27 | 63 |
| Pineapple | 440 | 22 | 55 |
| **Sonic Blasts:** Oreo; Snickers, av. | 680 | 37 | 77 |
| Vanilla Cone | 250 | 13 | 31 |

*Beverages: Per Regular Size, 14 oz*

**Floats/Blended:**

| | C | F | Cb |
|---|---|---|---|
| Diet Coke; Diet Dr Pepper | 260 | 14 | 29 |
| Coca-Cola | 330 | 14 | 49 |
| **Malts:** Chocolate | 600 | 27 | 81 |
| Hot Fudge | 630 | 32 | 75 |
| Strawberry | 530 | 27 | 65 |
| **Shakes:** Banana | 520 | 27 | 63 |
| Chocolate | 590 | 27 | 79 |
| Pineapple; Strawberry, average | 525 | 27 | 64 |

*For Complete Nutritional Data ~ see CalorieKing.com*

## Souplantation® (Dec '11)

*Soups: Per Cup*

**Regular Soup:**

| | C | F | Cb |
|---|---|---|---|
| Chesapeake Corn Chowder | 290 | 17 | 30 |
| Classical Minestrone | 120 | 2 | 20 |
| Cream of Mushroom | 290 | 24 | 15 |
| New Orelans Jambalaya | 210 | 11 | 18 |
| Vegetarian Harvest | 200 | 10 | 23 |
| *Breads:* Sourdough | 150 | 0.5 | 27 |
| Buttermilk Cornbread, 1 piece | 140 | 2 | 27 |
| *Focaccia,* Garlic Asiago | 160 | 8 | 19 |

*Hot Tossed Pastas: Per Cup*

| | | | |
|---|---|---|---|
| Creamy Bruschetta | 360 | 16 | 43 |
| Garden Vegetable with Meatballs | 310 | 10 | 44 |
| Vegetarian Marinara with Basil | 260 | 4 | 44 |

*Prepared Salads: Per ½ Cup*

| | | | |
|---|---|---|---|
| BBQ Potato | 170 | 9 | 21 |
| Carrot Raisin | 90 | 3 | 17 |
| Dijon Potato with Garlic Dill Vinegar | 150 | 12 | 9 |
| Greek Couscous w/ Feta & Pinenuts | 210 | 10 | 25 |
| Thai Noodle with Peanut Sauce | 190 | 10 | 19 |

*Dressing & Croutons: Per 2 Tbsp*

| | | | |
|---|---|---|---|
| Balsamic Vinaigrette | 180 | 19 | 1 |
| Blue Cheese Dressing | 130 | 13 | 3 |
| Honey Mustard Dressing: Regular | 150 | 13 | 8 |
| Fat Free | 25 | 0 | 7 |
| Italian Dressing, Fat-Free | 45 | 0 | 10 |
| Ranch Dressing: Regular | 150 | 15 | 4 |
| Fat Free | 50 | 0 | 2 |
| Thousand Island Dressing | 90 | 9 | 3 |
| **Croutons,** Garlic Parmesan, 5 pcs | 80 | 5 | 6 |

## Souplantation® cont... (Dec '11)

*Bakery:*

| | C | F | Cb |
|---|---|---|---|
| Chocolate Brownie | 180 | 8 | 26 |
| Chocolate Chip Cookie, small | 75 | 3 | 10 |
| Chocolate Lava Cake, ½ cup | 330 | 8 | 62 |
| Fruit Medley Bran | 130 | 0.5 | 29 |

*Desserts: Per ½ Cup*

| | | | |
|---|---|---|---|
| Apple Cobbler | 360 | 10 | 67 |
| Apple Medley | 70 | 0 | 18 |
| Banana Royale | 80 | 0 | 20 |
| Rice Pudding | 110 | 2 | 20 |

*For Complete Nutritional Data ~ see CalorieKing.com*

## Southern Tsunami® (Dec '11)

*Rolls:*

| | C | F | Cb |
|---|---|---|---|
| **With White Rice:** Berry, 6 oz | 230 | 5 | 44 |
| Blueberry: Salmon, 8 oz | 350 | 15 | 45 |
| Shrimp, 8 oz | 330 | 12 | 45 |
| Done Deal, 7 oz | 365 | 17 | 39 |
| Happy Mango, 8 oz | 445 | 21 | 53 |
| Jalapeno, 8 oz | 307 | 7 | 48 |
| Mango Shrimp, 6 oz | 365 | 19 | 41 |
| Red Rock/Fujisan, 7 oz | 400 | 15 | 42 |
| Spicy Mango Roll, 8 oz | 400 | 17 | 46 |
| Ultimate Chili, 6 oz | 285 | 9 | 41 |
| Chef Samplers: A, 9.5 oz | 410 | 2 | 65 |
| B, 7.5 oz | 355 | 6 | 57 |
| **Plus Rolls:** *Per Two Servings* | | | |
| California, 6 oz | 230 | 5 | 44 |
| Cream Cheese Plus: Salmon, 6 oz | 290 | 11 | 39 |
| Shrimp, 6 oz | 260 | 8 | 39 |
| Tuna, 6 oz | 285 | 8 | 39 |
| Eel, 6 oz | 300 | 8 | 46 |
| Seaside Plus: Eel, 6 oz | 380 | 15 | 47 |
| Salmon, 6 oz | 290 | 7 | 45 |
| Shrimp, 6 oz | 235 | 1 | 45 |
| Steelhead, 6 oz | 280 | 4 | 45 |
| Tuna, 6 oz | 280 | 1 | 45 |
| Spicy Plus: Salmon, 6 oz | 275 | 9 | 39 |
| Shrimp, 6 oz | 235 | 5 | 39 |
| Steelhead, 6 oz | 270 | 7 | 39 |
| Tuna, 6 oz | 265 | 5 | 39 |
| Vegetable, 6 oz | 225 | 4 | 46 |

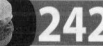

## Southern Tsunami® cont... (Dec'11)

### Rolls (Cont)

| | C | F | Cb |
|---|---|---|---|
| **With Brown Rice: Berry, 6 oz** | 200 | 6 | 33 |
| Blueberry: Salmon, 8 oz | 315 | 15 | 34 |
| Steelhead, 8 oz | 310 | 14 | 34 |
| Crunchy: Dragon, Hot, 6 oz | 265 | 10 | 30 |
| Tempura, 6 oz | 260 | 7 | 37 |
| Jalapeno , 8 oz | 270 | 7 | 35 |
| Mango Shrimp, 6 oz | 345 | 19 | 33 |
| Red Rock/Fujisan, 7 oz | 370 | 16 | 31 |
| Ultimate Chli Combo, 6 oz | 255 | 10 | 30 |
| *Wraps:* Avocado Salad Roll, 4.6 oz | 125 | 5 | 21 |
| Berry, 4.6 oz | 175 | 8 | 25 |
| California, 6.6 oz | 270 | 17 | 28 |
| Smoked Salmon Salad, 4.6 oz | 205 | 10 | 21 |
| *Salads: Without Dressing* | | | |
| Edamame, 4 oz | 125 | 7 | 9 |
| Seared Tuna, 9 oz | 205 | 8 | 18 |
| *Dressings/Sauces:* Eel Sauce, 1 T. | 35 | 0 | 8 |
| Ginger Dresing, 2 Tbsp | 50 | 2 | 8 |
| Peanut Sauce, 2 Tbsp | 30 | 1 | 6 |
| Sweet Chili, 3 fl.oz | 300 | 0 | 72 |
| Wasabe Dressing, 2 Tbsp | 30 | 2 | 2 |

## Starbucks® (Dec'11)

*Brewed Coffee:*
*Figures based on 16 fl.oz Grande without Whipped Cream*

| | C | F | Cb |
|---|---|---|---|
| **Caffe Misto (Au Lait):** W/ Whole Milk | 130 | 7 | 10 |
| With Nonfat Milk | 70 | 0 | 10 |
| With Soy Milk | 100 | 3 | 13 |
| *Hot Espresso Beverages:* | | | |
| **Caffe Latte:** With Whole Milk | 220 | 11 | 18 |
| With Nonfat Milk | 130 | 0 | 19 |
| With Soy Milk | 170 | 4.5 | 23 |
| **Caffe Mocha:** WithWhole Milk | 290 | 12 | 42 |
| With Nonfat Milk | 220 | 2.5 | 43 |
| With Soy Milk | 260 | 7 | 46 |
| **Cappuccino:** With Whole Milk | 140 | 7 | 12 |
| With Nonfat Milk | 80 | 0 | 12 |
| With Soy Milk | 120 | 3.5 | 16 |
| **Caramel Macchiato:** W/ Whole Milk | 270 | 11 | 34 |
| With Nonfat Milk | 190 | 1 | 35 |
| **Cinn. Dolce Latte:** With Whole Milk | 300 | 10 | 40 |
| With Nonfat Milk | 210 | 0 | 40 |
| **Cocoa Cappuccino:** W/ Whole Milk | 220 | 9 | 33 |
| With Nonfat Milk | 170 | 2 | 34 |
| With Soy Milk | 200 | 5 | 36 |
| **Espresso:** 1 doppio, 2 fl.oz | 10 | 0 | 2 |
| 1 solo, 1 fl.oz | 5 | 0 | 1 |
| Con Panna, 1 fl.oz | 30 | 2.5 | 2 |

## Starbucks® cont... (Dec'11)

| *Hot Chocolate:* | C | F | Cb |
|---|---|---|---|
| With Whole Milk | 330 | 13 | 47 |
| With Nonfat Milk | 240 | 2.5 | 48 |
| With Soy | 290 | 7 | 51 |
| *Iced Espresso: Per 16 fl.oz Grande, without Whipped Cream* | | | |
| **Caffe Latte:** With Whole Milk | 150 | 7 | 13 |
| With Nonfat Milk | 90 | 0 | 13 |
| With Soy Milk | 130 | 3.5 | 17 |
| **Caffe Mocha:** With Whole Milk | 220 | 8 | 36 |
| With Nonfat Milk | 170 | 2.5 | 37 |
| With Soy Milk | 200 | 5 | 39 |
| **White Choc. Mocha:** W/ Whole Milk | 360 | 11 | 55 |
| With Nonfat Milk | 310 | 6 | 56 |
| With Soy Milk | 340 | 8 | 58 |
| *Frappuccino Blended Coffee: Cold, per16 fl.oz Grande with Whole Milk, without Whipped Cream* | | | |
| Caffe Vanilla | 310 | 3 | 68 |
| Caramel | 280 | 3.5 | 60 |
| Cinnamon Dolce | 240 | 3 | 51 |
| Coffee | 240 | 3 | 50 |
| Double Chocolaty Chip | 290 | 8 | 53 |
| Espresso | 230 | 2.5 | 50 |
| Java Chip | 340 | 7 | 67 |
| Mocha | 290 | 4 | 61 |
| White Chocolate Mocha | 330 | 5 | 66 |
| *Frappuccino Blended Creme: Cold, per 16 fl.oz Grande, with Whole Milk and Whipped Cream* | | | |
| Cinnamon Dolce Creme | 350 | 16 | 49 |
| Tazo Green Tea Creme | 430 | 16 | 68 |
| Vanilla Bean Creme | 400 | 16 | 59 |
| White Chocolate Creme | 420 | 18 | 59 |
| *Tazo Teas: Per 16 fl.oz Grande, with Whole Milk* | | | |
| **Hot Tea Latte:** Awake | 210 | 7 | 31 |
| Chai | 270 | 7 | 45 |
| Earl Grey | 200 | 7 | 29 |
| Green Tea | 390 | 13 | 57 |
| **Iced Tea Latte:** Awake | 120 | 2 | 24 |
| Chai | 260 | 7 | 44 |
| Green Tea | 320 | 9 | 51 |
| *Vivanno Smoothies: Per16 fl.oz Grande, with 2% Milk, without Whipped Cream* | | | |
| Chocolate | 300 | 5 | 53 |
| Orange Mango | 270 | 1.5 | 53 |
| Strawberry | 300 | 2 | 60 |
| *Kid's Drinks & Others:* | | | |
| Apple Juice, Cold, 12 fl.oz | 190 | 0 | 49 |
| Apple Juice, Steamed, 8 fl.oz | 110 | 0 | 28 |

*Continued Next Page ...*

## Starbucks® cont... (Dec '11)

| Drink Extras: | C | F | Cb |
|---|---|---|---|
| **Caramel Drizzle,** 1 teaspoon | 15 | 0.5 | 3 |
| **Flavored Syrup:** 1 Tbsp | 35 | 0 | 9 |
| Sugar-Free, 1 Tbsp | 0 | 0 | 0 |
| **Mocha Sauce,** 1 Tbsp | 25 | 0.5 | 6 |
| **Sweetened Whipped Cream:** | | | |
| Grande/Venti, cold drinks, average | 115 | 11 | 3 |
| Grande/Venti, hot drinks | 70 | 7 | 2 |
| *Breakfast Specialities:* | | | |
| Bacon, Gouda & Egg Fritata | | | |
| on Artisan Roll | 350 | 18 | 30 |
| Egg White, Spinach, Feta Wrap | 280 | 10 | 33 |
| Egg White/Turkey Bacon | | | |
| and Cheese on Muffin | 320 | 7 | 43 |
| Oatmeal: 1¼ oz, without sugar | 140 | 2.5 | 25 |
| With brown sugar, ½ oz | 190 | 2.5 | 38 |
| *Bistro Boxes:* | | | |
| Cheese & Fruit, 5.29 oz | 480 | 28 | 39 |
| Chicken & Hummus, 6.3 oz | 270 | 8 | 29 |
| Chicken & Lettuce Wraps, 7.3 oz | 360 | 19 | 32 |
| Sesame Noodles, 8.3 oz | 350 | 11 | 50 |
| Tuna Salad, 5.89 oz | 380 | 21 | 24 |
| *Sandwiches, Panini & Wraps:* | | | |
| Ham & Swiss Panini | 360 | 9 | 43 |
| Roasted Tomato & Mozz. Panini | 380 | 18 | 40 |
| Roasted Vegetable Panini | 350 | 12 | 48 |
| Tarragon Chicken Salad Sandwich | 420 | 13 | 46 |
| Turkey & Swiss Sandwich | 390 | 13 | 36 |
| **8-Grain Roll,** Plain | 350 | 8 | 67 |
| **Bagels:** Everything with Cheese | 280 | 2 | 56 |
| Multigrain | 300 | 3 | 60 |
| Plain | 280 | 1 | 59 |
| *Bars & Brownies:* Blueberry Oat Bar | 370 | 14 | 47 |
| Double Chocolate Brownie | 410 | 24 | 46 |
| Marshmallow Dream Bar | 210 | 4 | 43 |
| *Cakes:* Per Slice | | | |
| Banana Nut Loaf, 4.27 oz | 490 | 19 | 75 |
| Pumpkin Bread, 4.27 oz | 390 | 14 | 61 |
| **Pound:** Iced Lemon, 4½ oz | 490 | 23 | 67 |
| Marble, 3¾ oz | 350 | 13 | 54 |
| Starbuck's Classic Coffee, 4 oz | 440 | 19 | 63 |
| **Reduced Fat Cakes:** | | | |
| Banana Chocolate Chip Coffee | 400 | 8 | 80 |
| Cinnamon Swirl | 340 | 9 | 62 |
| Very Berry Coffee | 350 | 10 | 59 |
| *Cookies:* Chocolate Chunk | 380 | 17 | 51 |
| Outrageous Oatmeal | 370 | 14 | 56 |
| *Croissants:* Butter | 310 | 18 | 32 |
| Chocolate | 300 | 17 | 34 |
| *Doughnuts,* Old-Fashioned Glazed | 420 | 21 | 57 |

## Starbucks® cont... (Dec '11)

| Muffins: | C | F | Cb |
|---|---|---|---|
| Apple Bran | 350 | 9 | 64 |
| Blueberry Streusel | 360 | 11 | 59 |
| Zucchini Walnut | 490 | 28 | 52 |
| *Sweet Rolls & Danish:* | | | |
| Apple Fritter | 420 | 20 | 59 |
| Cheese Danish | 420 | 25 | 39 |
| Morning Bun | 350 | 16 | 45 |
| *Parfaits:* Dark Cherry Yogurt, 8.1 oz | 310 | 4 | 61 |
| Greek Yogurt Honey, 6 oz | 300 | 12 | 44 |
| Strawberry & Blueb. Yogurt, 8.1 oz | 300 | 3.5 | 60 |
| *Petites:* Cake Pops, average, 1.5 oz | 175 | 9 | 22 |
| P'nut Butter Mini Cupcakes, 1.5 oz | 180 | 10 | 21 |
| Red Velvet Whoopie Pie, 1.4 oz | 190 | 11 | 21 |
| *Ice Cream ~ See Page 107* | | | |
| *Bottled Drinks ~ See Page 37* | | | |
| *Coffee Mix (VIA) ~ See Page 35* | | | |

## Steak Escape® (Dec '11)

| *Burgers:* With Set Menu Board Toppings, without Condiments | C | F | Cb |
|---|---|---|---|
| Single | 590 | 32 | 48 |
| Double | 860 | 50 | 52 |
| Double Philly | 700 | 35 | 43 |
| Double Char | 870 | 50 | 49 |
| *Sandwiches:* With Set Menu Board Toppings, without Condiments | | | |
| 6": Classic Italian | 600 | 33 | 46 |
| Turkey Club | 360 | 9 | 42 |
| Wild West BBQ | 460 | 13 | 49 |
| 12": Buffalo Chicken | 1080 | 44 | 126 |
| Fire Escape | 880 | 26 | 90 |
| Triple Cheesesteak | 1220 | 57 | 89 |
| *Wraps:* With Set Menu Board Toppings, without Condimdents | | | |
| French Onion | 630 | 28 | 56 |
| Ragin Cajun | 470 | 17 | 50 |
| Teriyaki Chicken | 520 | 18 | 55 |
| *Salads:* Without Dressing | | | |
| **Grilled:** Chicken; Steak, average | 425 | 25 | 15 |
| Ham | 360 | 22 | 17 |
| *Sides:* | | | |
| **Fresh Cut Fries:** Small | 510 | 26 | 61 |
| Regular | 700 | 36 | 84 |
| Regular: Cheddar & Bacon | 910 | 52 | 91 |
| Ranch & Bacon | 1160 | 82 | 86 |
| **Killer Potatoes:** Chicken | 470 | 15 | 54 |
| Ham; Turkey, average | 420 | 12 | 56 |
| **Loaded:** Bacon & Ranch | 670 | 46 | 51 |
| Cheddar & Bacon | 430 | 17 | 56 |

*For Complete Nutritional Data ~ see CalorieKing.com*

## Steak 'n Shake® (Dec '11)

| The Original Steakburgers: | C | F | Cb |
|---|---|---|---|
| Single | 280 | 11 | 30 |
| Double 'n Cheese | 440 | 25 | 31 |
| Triple | 510 | 30 | 30 |
| Bacon 'n Cheese Double | 480 | 28 | 31 |
| Cheesy Cheddar | 480 | 27 | 32 |
| Guacamole | 700 | 48 | 47 |
| Spicy Chipotle | 640 | 41 | 42 |
| *Chili Bowls:* 3-Way (1) | 830 | 36 | 94 |
| 5-Way (1) | 1170 | 63 | 99 |
| Deluxe (1) | 1220 | 74 | 81 |
| *Sandwiches:* Grilled Chicken | 400 | 15 | 51 |
| Spicy Chicken | 490 | 21 | 51 |
| Turkey Club | 420 | 16 | 45 |
| *Signature Steak Franks:* Regular | 380 | 27 | 22 |
| Cheesy Cheddar | 490 | 36 | 24 |
| Chicago Style | 420 | 27 | 30 |
| Chili Cheese | 620 | 44 | 31 |
| *Salads: Without Dressing* | | | |
| Apple Pecan Grilled Chicken | 330 | 8 | 39 |
| Fried Chicken | 470 | 26 | 34 |
| Grilled Chicken | 270 | 10 | 30 |
| *French Fries:* Regular | 440 | 21 | 60 |
| Large | 640 | 30 | 87 |
| **Cheese:** Regular | 610 | 34 | 67 |
| Large | 810 | 43 | 94 |
| *Breakfast:* | | | |
| **Bagels Sandwich:** With Bacon | 450 | 16 | 51 |
| With Sausage | 570 | 29 | 50 |
| **Biscuits:** Bacon, Egg & Cheese | 520 | 35 | 32 |
| Egg and Cheese | 450 | 30 | 31 |
| Sausage & Egg | 600 | 44 | 31 |
| Sausage, Egg & Cheese | 650 | 48 | 31 |
| With Sausage Gravy: Half order | 540 | 37 | 43 |
| Full Order | 1070 | 74 | 86 |
| **Hash Browns:** Shredded | 290 | 23 | 19 |
| Side order, 5 pieces | 260 | 17 | 23 |
| **Perfect Start Oatmeal** | 340 | 11 | 57 |
| **Skillets:** Country | 1230 | 93 | 63 |
| Portobello & Swiss | 1040 | 87 | 27 |
| *Hand Dipped Shakes: Per Regular* | | | |
| Banana; Mocha | 700 | 23 | 111 |
| Butterfinger | 910 | 31 | 146 |
| Chocolate; Vanilla, average | 700 | 23 | 112 |
| Cookies 'n Cream | 1010 | 34 | 163 |

## Subway® (Dec '11)

*6" Sandwiches (6g Fat or Less):* Figures based on 9-grain wheat bread, lettuce, tomatoes, onions, green peppers and cucumbers. Cheese, oil or mayo not included.

| | C | F | Cb |
|---|---|---|---|
| Black Forest Ham | 290 | 4.5 | 46 |
| Oven Roasted Chicken | 320 | 5 | 47 |
| Roast Beef | 320 | 5 | 45 |
| Subway Club | 310 | 4.5 | 46 |
| Sweet Onion Chicken Teriyaki | 380 | 4.5 | 59 |
| Turkey Breast | 280 | 3.5 | 46 |
| Turkey Breast & Black Forest Ham | 280 | 4 | 46 |
| Veggie Delite | 230 | 2.5 | 44 |

*6" Flatbread Sandwich (7g Fat or Less):* Figures based on 6" flatbread, lettuce, tomatoes, onions, green peppers and cucumbers. Cheese, oil or mayo not included.

| | | | |
|---|---|---|---|
| Black Forest Ham | 300 | 7 | 44 |
| Oven Roasted Chicken | 330 | 7 | 45 |
| Roast Beef | 330 | 7 | 43 |
| Subway Club | 320 | 7 | 44 |
| Sweet Onion Chicken Teriyaki | 390 | 7 | 57 |
| Turkey Breast | 290 | 6 | 44 |
| Turkey Breast & Black Forest Ham | 290 | 6 | 44 |
| Veggie Delite | 240 | 4.5 | 42 |

*6"Toasted Sandwiches:* Figures based on 9-grain wheat bread, lettuce, tomatoes, onion, green peppers, cucumbers and cheese. Oil or mayo not included.

| | | | |
|---|---|---|---|
| Big Philly Cheesesteak | 500 | 17 | 51 |
| BLT | 320 | 9 | 43 |
| Chicken & Bacon Ranch Melt | 570 | 28 | 47 |
| Italian B.M.T. | 410 | 16 | 46 |
| Meatball Marinara | 480 | 18 | 59 |
| Spicy Italian | 480 | 24 | 46 |
| Steak & Cheese | 380 | 10 | 48 |
| Subway Melt | 370 | 11 | 47 |

*Low-Fat Footlong Sandwiches:* Figures based on 9-grain wheat bread, lettuce, tomatoes, onions, green peppers and cucumbers. Oil or mayo not included.

| | | | |
|---|---|---|---|
| Black Forest Ham | 570 | 9 | 92 |
| Oven Roasted Chicken | 640 | 10 | 95 |
| Roast Beef | 630 | 10 | 90 |
| Subway Club | 630 | 9 | 92 |
| Sweet Onion Chicken Teriyaki | 750 | 9 | 117 |
| Turkey Breast & Black Forest Ham | 570 | 8 | 92 |
| Veggie Delite | 460 | 4.5 | 87 |

*Kids Meal Sandwiches:* Figures based on 9-grain wheat bread, lettuce, tomatoes, onions, green peppers and cucumbers. Oil or mayo not included.

| | | | |
|---|---|---|---|
| Black Forest Ham | 180 | 2.5 | 30 |
| Roast Beef | 200 | 3 | 30 |
| Turkey Breast | 180 | 2 | 30 |
| Veggie Delite | 150 | 1.5 | 29 |

*Continued next page...*

## Subway® cont... (Dec '11)

*Breakast:*

**Egg Muffin Melts:** *Figures based on light wheat English muffin, cheese & regular egg.*

| | C | F | Cb |
|---|---|---|---|
| Breakfast B.M.T. | 240 | 10 | 25 |
| Bacon, Egg & Cheese | 200 | 7 | 24 |
| Egg & Cheese | 170 | 6 | 24 |
| Egg & Cheese with Ham | 190 | 6 | 24 |
| Steak, Egg & Cheese | 200 | 6 | 25 |
| Sunrise Melt | 230 | 8 | 26 |

**6" Breakfast Omelet Sandwiches:** *Figures based on 9-grain bread, cheese & regular egg.*

| | C | F | Cb |
|---|---|---|---|
| Bacon, Egg & Cheese | 410 | 16 | 45 |
| Egg & Cheese | 360 | 12 | 44 |
| Egg & Cheese with Ham | 390 | 13 | 45 |
| Steak, Egg & Cheese | 430 | 15 | 47 |
| Sunrise Melt | 470 | 17 | 48 |

**Regular Egg On Mornin' Flatbreads:** *Figures based on flatbread, cheese and regular egg.*

| | C | F | Cb |
|---|---|---|---|
| Egg & Cheese | 190 | 7 | 21 |
| Breakfast B.M.T. | 250 | 12 | 22 |
| Bacon, Egg & Cheese | 210 | 9 | 21 |
| Steak, Egg & Cheese | 210 | 8 | 22 |
| Sunrise Melt | 240 | 10 | 23 |

*Salads (6g Fat or Less):* *Figures based on lettuce, tomatoes, onions, green peppers, olives & cucumbers. Dressing or croutons not included.*

| | C | F | Cb |
|---|---|---|---|
| Black Forest Ham | 110 | 3 | 11 |
| Grilled Chicken & Baby Spinach | 130 | 2.5 | 10 |
| Oven Roasted Chicken Breast | 130 | 2.5 | 9 |
| Roast Beef; Subway Club, av | 140 | 3.5 | 10 |
| Turkey Breast/Ham, average | 110 | 2.5 | 11 |
| Veggie Delite | 50 | 1 | 9 |

*Salad Dressing:* Fat Free Italian, 2 oz

| | C | F | Cb |
|---|---|---|---|
| Fat Free Italian, 2 oz | 35 | 0 | 7 |
| Ranch, 2 oz | 320 | 35 | 3 |

*Condiments & Sauces for 6" Subs or Flatbreads:*

**Cheese:** American, 2 triangles, ¼ oz

| | C | F | Cb |
|---|---|---|---|
| American, 2 triangles, ¼ oz | 40 | 3.5 | 1 |
| Cheddar, 2 triangles,¼ oz | 60 | 5 | 0 |
| Swiss, 2 triangles, ¼ oz | 50 | 4.5 | 0 |

**Dressings:**

| | C | F | Cb |
|---|---|---|---|
| Chipotle Southwest, 0.74 oz | 100 | 10 | 1 |
| Honey Mustard, Fat-Free, 0.74 oz | 30 | 0 | 7 |
| Mayonnaise: 1 Tbsp, ½ oz | 110 | 12 | 0 |
| Light, 1 Tbsp, ½ oz | 50 | 5 | 0.5 |
| Mustard, Yellow or Deli Brown. 2 tsp | 5 | 0 | 0.5 |
| Olive Oil Blend, 1 tsp | 45 | 5 | 0 |
| Ranch Dressing, 0.74 oz | 110 | 11 | 1 |
| Ranch Dressing on Wrap, 0.14 oz | 5 | 2.5 | 0 |
| Sweet Onion, Fat-Free, 0.74 oz | 40 | 0 | 9 |
| **Meat:** Bacon Strips (2) | 45 | 3.5 | 0 |
| Chicken Strips, 2.5 oz | 80 | 1.5 | 0 |

## Subway® cont... (Dec '11)

*Soups:* Per 10 oz Bowl

| | C | F | Cb |
|---|---|---|---|
| Chicken Tortilla | 110 | 1.5 | 11 |
| Chili Con Carne | 280 | 8 | 35 |
| Chipotle Chicken Corn Chowder | 130 | 2.5 | 22 |
| Creamy Potato with Bacon | 250 | 14 | 26 |
| Fire-Roasted Tomato Orzo | 130 | 1 | 24 |
| Golden Broccoli & Cheese | 180 | 11 | 16 |
| Minestrone | 90 | 1 | 15 |
| New England Style Clam Chowder | 150 | 5 | 20 |
| Roasted Chicken Noodle | 110 | 2 | 15 |
| Rosemary Chicken & Dumpling | 90 | 1.5 | 14 |
| Spanish Style Chkn & Rice | 110 | 2.5 | 16 |
| Tomato Garden Vegetable w/ Rotini | 90 | 0 | 20 |
| Vegetable Beef | 100 | 2 | 15 |
| Wild Rice with Chicken | 220 | 12 | 22 |

*Cookies & Desserts:*

| | C | F | Cb |
|---|---|---|---|
| Apple Slices, 1 package, 2½ oz | 35 | 0 | 9 |
| Chocolate Chip Cookie, 1½ oz | 210 | 10 | 30 |
| Oatmeal Raisin Cookie, 1½ oz | 200 | 8 | 30 |
| Raspberry Cheesecake, 1.6 oz | 200 | 9 | 29 |

## Sweet Tomatoes®

**Same Menu & Data as Souplantation ~ See Page 242**

## Swiss Chalet® (Dec '11)

*Starters:*

| | C | F | Cb |
|---|---|---|---|
| Garlic Loaf, without Cheese | 700 | 40 | 73 |
| Chalet Chicken Wings (8), with sauce | 550 | 34 | 23 |
| Cheese Perogies (7) | 420 | 10 | 69 |
| Caesar Salad without Dressing | 90 | 3 | 13 |

*From The Grill:* *Without Sides*

| | C | F | Cb |
|---|---|---|---|
| **Burgers:** Classic Hamburger | 710 | 39 | 43 |
| Classic Bacon & Cheese | 890 | 54 | 46 |
| Veggie | 330 | 12 | 52 |
| **BBQ Ribs:** Half Rack | 650 | 42 | 6 |
| Full Rack | 1300 | 85 | 11 |

*Rotisserie Chicken:* *Meat Only*

| | C | F | Cb |
|---|---|---|---|
| Double Leg with Skin | 630 | 38 | 4 |
| Half Chicken, with Skin | 610 | 31 | 5 |
| Quarter Chicken: | | | |
| Dark meat, without Skin | 160 | 8 | 0 |
| Dark meat with Skin | 240 | 16 | 0 |
| White meat without Skin | 220 | 6 | 0 |
| White meat with Skin | 290 | 11 | 0 |
| **Chicken Pot Pie**, 1 pie | 510 | 24 | 42 |

*Sandwiches:* *Without Sides*

| | C | F | Cb |
|---|---|---|---|
| Classic Hot Chicken, white meat | 500 | 14 | 51 |
| Flatbread: Hickory Chicken | 700 | 35 | 68 |
| Southwest Chicken | 710 | 38 | 65 |

## Swiss Chalet® cont...(Dec'11)

| Stir-Frys: | C | F | Cb |
|---|---|---|---|
| Chicken: With Rice | 750 | 30 | 89 |
| Without Rice | 430 | 26 | 26 |
| Vegetable, with Rice | 660 | 28 | 94 |
| *Wrap,* Rotisserie Chicken Club | 820 | 40 | 58 |
| *Entree Salads: Without Dressing* | | | |
| Bacon Ranch Chicken | 380 | 17 | 19 |
| Chalet Chopped | 340 | 12 | 25 |
| Spinach Chicken Salad | 340 | 13 | 28 |
| *Dressing/Sauce:* | | | |
| Caesar Dressing, 1 oz | 180 | 18 | 2 |
| Chalet Dressing, 1 Tbsp, 1oz | 160 | 14 | 6 |
| Chalet Dipping Sauce, 3½ oz | 25 | 1 | 5 |
| Greek Dressing, 1 oz | 140 | 14 | 2 |
| *Sides:* Oven-Baked Potato, 10 oz | 220 | 0 | 48 |
| Gravy, 4 oz | 45 | 1.5 | 7 |
| Mashed Potatoes, 5 oz | 150 | 4 | 27 |
| Sauteed Mushrooms, 6 oz | 140 | 1 | 30 |
| Seasoned Rice, 6 oz | 240 | 3.5 | 48 |
| *Desserts/Pies:* Apple Pie | 440 | 19 | 65 |
| Coconut Cream Pie | 540 | 33 | 57 |
| Lemon Meringue Pie | 400 | 11 | 73 |
| Old Fashioned Carrot Cake | 260 | 16 | 24 |
| Pecan Pie | 590 | 29 | 79 |

## Taco Bell® (Dec'11)

| Burritos: | C | F | Cb |
|---|---|---|---|
| **Regular:** ½ lb Comb | 460 | 18 | 53 |
| ½ lb Cheesy Potato | 540 | 26 | 59 |
| 7-Layer | 500 | 18 | 69 |
| Cheesy Bean & Rice | 480 | 21 | 60 |
| Chili Cheese | 380 | 17 | 41 |
| **Fresco Style,** Bean | 350 | 8 | 57 |
| **XXL Grilled Stuft:** | | | |
| Beef | 880 | 42 | 95 |
| Chicken | 840 | 35 | 92 |
| Steak | 820 | 36 | 92 |
| **Supreme:** Beef | 420 | 16 | 53 |
| Chicken | 400 | 12 | 51 |
| Steak | 390 | 13 | 51 |
| *Chalupas:* | | | |
| **Baja:** Beef | 410 | 26 | 30 |
| Chicken | 390 | 23 | 28 |
| Steak | 380 | 23 | 28 |
| **Nacho Cheese:** Beef | 360 | 22 | 31 |
| Chicken | 340 | 18 | 30 |
| Steak | 330 | 19 | 30 |

## Taco Bell® cont...(Dec'11)

| Gorditas: | C | F | Cb |
|---|---|---|---|
| **Baja:** Beef | 340 | 18 | 30 |
| Chicken | 310 | 15 | 28 |
| Steak | 310 | 15 | 28 |
| **Nacho Cheese:** Beef | 290 | 14 | 31 |
| Chicken | 270 | 10 | 29 |
| Steak | 260 | 11 | 29 |
| **Supreme:** Beef | 300 | 14 | 31 |
| Chicken | 270 | 10 | 29 |
| Steak | 270 | 11 | 29 |
| *Nachos:* Regular | 330 | 20 | 31 |
| BellGrande | 770 | 42 | 79 |
| Supreme | 440 | 25 | 42 |
| *Tacos:* | | | |
| **Crunchy:** Regular | 170 | 10 | 12 |
| Supreme | 200 | 12 | 15 |
| **Double Decker:** Regular | 320 | 13 | 37 |
| Supreme | 350 | 15 | 40 |
| **Fresco:** Regular, crunchy | 150 | 8 | 13 |
| Chicken, soft | 150 | 3.5 | 18 |
| **Soft:** Beef | 210 | 9 | 21 |
| Supreme | 230 | 11 | 22 |
| Chicken | 180 | 6 | 18 |
| Crispy Potato | 270 | 13 | 31 |
| Fresco Chicken | 150 | 3.5 | 18 |
| *Specialities:* | | | |
| Cheese Roll-Up | 190 | 9 | 18 |
| Chilli Cheese Burrito | 380 | 17 | 41 |
| Crunchwrap Supreme | 540 | 21 | 71 |
| **Enchiritos:** Beef | 360 | 17 | 34 |
| Chicken | 340 | 14 | 32 |
| Steak | 330 | 14 | 32 |
| MexiMelt | 270 | 14 | 21 |
| Mexican Pizza | 540 | 30 | 47 |
| **Quesadillas:** Cheese | 480 | 27 | 40 |
| Chicken | 530 | 28 | 41 |
| Steak | 520 | 28 | 41 |
| Taquitos, Grilled Chicken | 320 | 11 | 37 |
| Tostada | 250 | 10 | 30 |
| *Taco Salads:* Chicken Fiesta | 730 | 35 | 70 |
| Express with Chips | 580 | 29 | 59 |
| Fiesta | 770 | 42 | 74 |
| Steak Fiesta | 710 | 36 | 70 |
| *Volcano Menu:* Burrito | 780 | 41 | 80 |
| Nachos | 980 | 60 | 89 |
| Taco | 230 | 16 | 14 |

*Continued next page...*

## Taco Bell® cont... (Dec '11)

### Sides:

| | C | F | Cb |
|---|---|---|---|
| Cheesy Fiesta Potatoes, 4¾ oz | 270 | 16 | 28 |
| Mexican Rice, 3 oz | 120 | 3.5 | 20 |
| Pintos 'n Cheese | 170 | 6 | 20 |
| **Condiments:** Guacamole, 1½ oz | 70 | 6 | 4 |
| Salsa, 1½ oz | 10 | 0 | 2 |
| Sour Cream, Reduced Fat, 1½ oz | 60 | 4 | 4 |

### Why Pay More!™:

| | C | F | Cb |
|---|---|---|---|
| Burritos: Bean | 370 | 10 | 56 |
| Beefy 5-Layer | 540 | 22 | 68 |
| Caramel Apple Empanada | 310 | 15 | 39 |
| Cinnamon Twists | 170 | 7 | 26 |

Note: Nutritional data in New York outlets may vary slightly. Please check Taco Bell website

## Taco Cabana® (Dec '11)

### Burritos:

| | C | F | Cb |
|---|---|---|---|
| Bean & Cheese | 730 | 35 | 77 |
| Black Bean | 450 | 8 | 82 |
| Stewed Chicken | 660 | 25 | 73 |

*Flameante Chicken: Includes Rice, Beans, Lettuce, pico de gallo & 2 Flour Tortillas*

| | C | F | Cb |
|---|---|---|---|
| ¼ Chicken Dark Dinner | 950 | 41 | 87 |
| ¼ Chicken White Dinner | 800 | 23 | 87 |
| ½ Chicken Dinner | 1620 | 63 | 146 |

*Sizzling Fajitas: Includes all Standard Toppings & 2 Flour Tortillas*

| | C | F | Cb |
|---|---|---|---|
| Chicken | 740 | 20 | 98 |
| Steak | 760 | 24 | 98 |

### Tacos:

| | C | F | Cb |
|---|---|---|---|
| **Crispy:** Ground Beef | 180 | 10 | 11 |
| Stewed Chicken | 160 | 7 | 13 |
| **Soft:** Bean & Cheese | 300 | 14 | 32 |
| Beef | 230 | 9 | 22 |
| Black Bean | 200 | 4 | 34 |
| Carne Guisada | 190 | 6 | 21 |
| Chicken, stewed | 210 | 7 | 23 |

### Sides & Add-Ons: Per Serving

| | C | F | Cb |
|---|---|---|---|
| Black Beans | 80 | 0 | 14 |
| Borracho Beans | 140 | 3 | 20 |
| Guacamole, 3 oz | 110 | 9 | 7 |
| Queso, 3 oz | 200 | 15 | 5 |
| Refried Beans | 250 | 13 | 24 |
| Rice | 120 | 0.5 | 25 |
| **Salsa:** Fuego; Roja, 1 oz | 5 | 0 | 1 |
| Ranch, 1 oz | 35 | 4 | 1 |
| Verde, 1 oz | 10 | 0 | 1 |
| Sour Cream, 3 oz | 160 | 14 | 3 |
| Southwest Ranch Dressing, 1 oz | 110 | 11 | 2 |
| **Tortillas:** 6" Corn | 70 | 1 | 15 |
| 6" Flour | 120 | 3 | 19 |

## Taco Del Mar® (Dec '11)

### Baja Bowls: As Served

| | C | F | Cb |
|---|---|---|---|
| **Mondo:** Carne Asada Steak | 490 | 15 | 62 |
| Chicken; Shredded Beef | 520 | 17 | 62 |
| Fish | 570 | 34 | 46 |
| Ground Beef | 570 | 23 | 62 |
| Pork | 500 | 15 | 61 |
| Vegan | 360 | 8 | 64 |

### Burritos: As Served

**Mondito:** *Per 9.6 oz Unless Indicated*

| | C | F | Cb |
|---|---|---|---|
| Carne Asada Steak | 440 | 13 | 65 |
| Chicken; Shredded Beef | 460 | 14 | 65 |
| Fish, 10.7 oz | 510 | 23 | 61 |
| Ground Beef | 480 | 17 | 65 |
| Pork | 450 | 13 | 65 |
| Vegan, 9.3 oz | 380 | 9 | 66 |

**Mondo:** *Per 18.45 oz Unless Indicated*

| | C | F | Cb |
|---|---|---|---|
| Carne Asada Steak | 820 | 23 | 118 |
| Chicken; Shredded Beef | 860 | 25 | 118 |
| Fish, 19 oz | 900 | 42 | 102 |
| Ground Beef | 900 | 32 | 118 |
| Pork | 840 | 24 | 117 |
| Vegan, 17.88 oz | 700 | 16 | 120 |

### Platters: As Served

**Enchilada:** *Per 2 Enchiladas*

| | C | F | Cb |
|---|---|---|---|
| Carne Asada Steak | 780 | 28 | 104 |
| Cheese | 870 | 38 | 104 |
| Chicken; Shredded Beef, average | 820 | 30 | 104 |
| Ground Beef | 860 | 36 | 105 |
| Pork | 800 | 28 | 103 |

**Enchilada/Taco:** *Per 1 Enchilada/1 Taco*

| | C | F | Cb |
|---|---|---|---|
| Carne Asada Steak | 820 | 30 | 109 |
| Chicken; Shredded Beef | 850 | 32 | 108 |
| Ground Beef | 900 | 38 | 109 |
| Pork | 830 | 30 | 108 |

**Quesadillas:** *As Served*

| | C | F | Cb |
|---|---|---|---|
| Carne Asada Steak | 1170 | 49 | 135 |
| Chicken; Shredded Beef | 1200 | 51 | 135 |
| Ground Beef | 1250 | 57 | 136 |
| Pork | 1180 | 50 | 134 |

**Nachos:** *As Served*

| | C | F | Cb |
|---|---|---|---|
| 6 Layer Cheese | 1050 | 62 | 96 |
| Super: Carne Asada Steak | 1140 | 65 | 98 |
| Chicken; Shredded Beef, av. | 1170 | 67 | 98 |
| Ground Beef | 1220 | 74 | 98 |
| Pork | 1150 | 66 | 97 |

**Salads:** *As Served*

| | C | F | Cb |
|---|---|---|---|
| **Cabo:** Chicken; Shredded Beef | 420 | 19 | 36 |
| Fish | 450 | 22 | 47 |
| Pork | 400 | 18 | 36 |
| **Taco:** Carne Asada Steak | 610 | 29 | 59 |
| Ground Beef | 690 | 37 | 60 |

## Taco John's® (Dec '11)

| Burritos: | C | F | Cb |
|---|---|---|---|
| Bean Burrito | 370 | 11 | 53 |
| Beef Grilled Burrito | 600 | 32 | 53 |
| Beefy Burrito | 440 | 21 | 42 |
| Chicken & Potato Burrito | 480 | 21 | 56 |
| Chicken Grilled Burrito | 590 | 30 | 50 |
| Combination Burrito | 410 | 16 | 47 |
| Crunchy Chicken & Potato Burrito | 580 | 27 | 67 |
| Meat & Potato Burrito | 520 | 25 | 57 |
| Super Burrito | 450 | 20 | 50 |
| *Tacos:* Soft Shell, Chicken | 190 | 6 | 21 |
| Taco Bravo | 330 | 13 | 38 |
| Taco Burger | 280 | 12 | 29 |
| **10 Grams of Fat or Less:** *Without Cheese* | | | |
| Bean | 310 | 7 | 52 |
| Chili | 150 | 6 | 16 |
| Crispy, with Beef | 170 | 10 | 11 |
| *Specialties:* | | | |
| Taco Salad w/o dressing | 540 | 33 | 40 |
| Chicken Taco Salad w/o dressing | 500 | 27 | 39 |
| Crunchy Chicken Taco Salad w/o dress. | 630 | 36 | 53 |
| Super Nachos: Small | 440 | 27 | 38 |
| Regular | 790 | 47 | 72 |
| Super Potato Oles: Small | 660 | 40 | 60 |
| Regular | 1090 | 67 | 98 |
| Quesadilla Melt: Cheesy | 450 | 24 | 40 |
| Fajita Beef | 550 | 29 | 46 |
| Fajita Chicken | 520 | 25 | 45 |
| Crunchy Chicken without sauce | 370 | 18 | 29 |
| *Snacks:* Chips & Queso | 430 | 25 | 43 |
| Cini-Sopapilla Bites | 200 | 8 | 34 |
| *Sides:* Potato Oles: Small | 480 | 27 | 52 |
| Medium | 670 | 38 | 73 |
| Large | 860 | 49 | 94 |
| Refried Beans: With Cheese | 320 | 7 | 46 |
| Without Cheese | 260 | 2.5 | 45 |
| Mexican Rice | 250 | 6 | 45 |
| *Condiments:* Nacho Cheese, 3 oz | 110 | 9 | 5 |
| Salsa, 2 oz | 10 | 0 | 2 |
| Sour Cream, 2 oz | 120 | 10 | 3 |
| House Dressing, 1½ oz | 70 | 7 | 2 |
| Ranch Dressing, 1½ oz | 140 | 16 | 2 |
| *Desserts:* Apple Grande | 260 | 11 | 39 |
| Choco Taco | 390 | 21 | 48 |
| Churro | 200 | 9 | 29 |

## Taco Mayo® (Dec '11)

| Burritos: | C | F | Cb |
|---|---|---|---|
| Bean | 495 | 16 | 71 |
| Beef | 490 | 23 | 41 |
| Super Beef | 540 | 23 | 57 |
| Super Chicken | 405 | 16 | 39 |
| *Melts:* Tamale | 620 | 34 | 50 |
| Tostada | 525 | 32 | 35 |
| *Quesadillas:* Chicken | 680 | 37 | 46 |
| Fajita Chicken | 700 | 39 | 47 |
| Fajita Steak | 725 | 40 | 47 |
| *Tacos:* Crispy Taco, Beef | 160 | 9 | 10 |
| Soft Taco: Beef | 230 | 11 | 17 |
| Chicken | 185 | 6 | 16 |
| *Salads:* Acapulco: Chicken | 680 | 50 | 35 |
| Steak | 705 | 51 | 35 |
| SalsaLita Steak | 305 | 8 | 33 |
| Taco Steak | 445 | 25 | 30 |
| *Sides:* Mexicali Rice | 160 | 1 | 36 |
| Refried Beans | 295 | 9 | 43 |
| Potato Locos, Small | 380 | 24 | 36 |

## Taco Time® (Dec '11)

| Burritos: | C | F | Cb |
|---|---|---|---|
| Beef, Bean & Cheese | 490 | 17 | 55 |
| Chicken B.L.T. | 690 | 39 | 43 |
| **Big Juan:** Chicken | 580 | 16 | 70 |
| Ground Beef | 630 | 23 | 73 |
| **Casita:** Chicken | 490 | 17 | 42 |
| Ground Beef | 540 | 24 | 46 |
| **Crisp Burrito:** Chicken | 380 | 17 | 33 |
| Ground Beef | 430 | 21 | 36 |
| Pinto Bean | 360 | 14 | 47 |
| **Soft Burrito:** Beef | 430 | 16 | 43 |
| Pinto Bean | 370 | 10 | 54 |
| Veggie | 520 | 17 | 73 |
| *Tacos:* | | | |
| **Soft Tacos:** *Per 7 oz Unless Indicated* | | | |
| Chicken | 360 | 9 | 40 |
| Ground Beef | 420 | 16 | 43 |
| **Super Soft Wheat Taco:** Beef | 590 | 23 | 63 |
| Chicken | 530 | 16 | 60 |
| *Other Favorites:* Cheddar Melt | 250 | 12 | 25 |
| Nachos Grande | 930 | 43 | 96 |
| **Tostada:** Bean | 230 | 13 | 21 |
| Chicken | 320 | 13 | 22 |
| Ground Beef | 380 | 20 | 25 |
| Cheddar Fries, medium, 7 oz | 500 | 35 | 39 |
| Mexi Fries, medium, 6 oz | 390 | 26 | 38 |
| Mexi-Rice, 3½ oz | 80 | 0.5 | 17 |
| Stuffed Fries, medium, 7 oz | 460 | 28 | 42 |
| Refritos, with Chips, 6 oz | 230 | 7 | 29 |

*Continued next page...*

**249**

## Taco Time® cont... (Dec '11)

| Salads: | C | F | Cb |
|---|---|---|---|
| Regular: Chkn Taco, 9½ oz | 310 | 13 | 22 |
| Ground Beef Taco, 9 oz | 370 | 20 | 24 |
| Tostada Delight: Chicken, 9 oz | 450 | 19 | 35 |
| Ground Beef, 9 oz | 490 | 26 | 36 |
| *Salsas, Sauces & Dressings:* | | | |
| Chipotle Ranch Dressing, 1 oz | 170 | 18 | 1 |
| Guacamole, 1 oz | 50 | 4.5 | 2 |
| Salsa Fresca, 1 oz | 10 | 0 | 2 |
| *Desserts:* Churro: Plain | 210 | 16 | 17 |
| With Cinnamon & Sugar | 250 | 16 | 27 |
| Crustos | 290 | 6 | 58 |
| Empanada, average | 240 | 7 | 41 |

## Target Food Court (Dec '11)

| *Entrees:* Per Order | C | F | Cb |
|---|---|---|---|
| Beef Hot Dog | 380 | 23 | 27 |
| Chicken Alfredo Pasta | 540 | 36 | 33 |
| Chicken Tenders | 270 | 10 | 18 |
| Italian Sausage | 440 | 29 | 27 |
| Kids: Chicken Nuggets | 180 | 12 | 9 |
| Macaroni & Cheese | 310 | 12 | 39 |
| *Pizza (Market Pantry):* Per Order | | | |
| Cheese | 400 | 13 | 54 |
| Pepperoni | 450 | 17 | 54 |
| *Sandwiches:* Ham & Swiss, 7 oz | 410 | 13 | 46 |
| 6.1 oz | 370 | 10 | 40 |
| Turkey & Provolone | 410 | 14 | 44 |
| Turkey Club | 590 | 28 | 48 |
| Pitta Melts: Chicken Parmesan | 240 | 10 | 23 |
| Honey Mustard Chicken | 250 | 9 | 27 |
| Toasted Flatbeads: Chkn Marinara | 180 | 8 | 15 |
| Chicken Spinach Artichoke | 160 | 7 | 17 |
| *Salads:* Chicken Caesar | 550 | 36 | 20 |
| Harvest Chicken | 550 | 29 | 39 |
| *Soups:* Chicken Noodle | 130 | 1 | 18 |
| Tomato Basil | 180 | 11 | 15 |
| *Snacks:* French Fries | 230 | 9 | 33 |
| Nachos with Cheese & Jalapenos | 530 | 25 | 89 |
| Popcorn | 300 | 16 | 33 |
| Yogurt Parfait | 270 | 6 | 46 |
| *Treats:* Brownie | 410 | 18 | 57 |
| Chocolate Chip Cookie | 510 | 26 | 68 |
| Pretzels: Bavarian, with Butter | 490 | 6 | 93 |
| And Cinnamon Sugar | 520 | 6 | 102 |
| *Smoothies:* Mango | 220 | 0 | 54 |
| Strawberry | 240 | 0 | 60 |

*For Complete Nutritional Data ~ see CalorieKing.com*

## TCBY® (Dec '11)

| *Soft Serve Froz. Yogurt:* Per 4 fl.oz | C | F | Cb |
|---|---|---|---|
| Golden Vanilla | 120 | 2 | 23 |
| Peanut Butter | 130 | 2 | 26 |
| Average other flavors | 110 | 2 | 23 |
| **No Sugar Added, Fat Free,** | | | |
| average all flavors | 80 | 0 | 22 |
| *Sorbet,* | | | |
| average all flavors, 4 fl.oz | 100 | 0 | 25 |
| *Hand-Scooped Frozen Yogurt:* | | | |
| **Butter Pecan:** Kid's, 4 fl.oz | 150 | 7 | 17 |
| Small, 6.4 fl.oz | 240 | 11 | 27 |
| Regular, 12.8 fl.oz | 480 | 22 | 54 |
| **Choc. Chunk Cookie Dough:** | | | |
| Kid's, 4 fl.oz | 150 | 6 | 23 |
| Small, 6.4 fl.oz | 240 | 10 | 37 |
| Regular, 12.8 fl.oz | 480 | 19 | 74 |
| **Peaches/Strawberries & Cream:** | | | |
| Kid's, 4 fl.oz | 110 | 2.5 | 18 |
| Small, 6.4 fl.oz | 175 | 4 | 29 |
| Regular, 12.8 fl.oz | 350 | 8 | 58 |
| **Peanut Butter Delight:** Kid's, 4 fl.oz | 170 | 8 | 21 |
| Small, 6.4 fl.oz | 270 | 13 | 34 |
| Regular, 12.8 fl.oz | 540 | 26 | 68 |
| **Vanilla Bean:** Kid's, 4 fl.oz | 110 | 3 | 18 |
| Small, 6.4 fl.oz | 175 | 5 | 29 |
| Regular, 12.8 fl.oz | 350 | 10 | 58 |
| *Cakes:* Per ⅒ Cake | | | |
| Choc. & Van. Yogurt Dble Crunch | 350 | 18 | 43 |
| White Choc. Mousse Yog. w/ Choc. | 310 | 14 | 42 |
| *Pies:* Per ⅒ Pie | | | |
| Chocolate Decadence | 330 | 13 | 49 |
| Cookies & Creme | 320 | 15 | 42 |

## TGI Friday® (Dec '11)

| | C | F | Cb |
|---|---|---|---|
| *Appetizers:* Per Individual Serving | | | |
| Crispy Green Bean Fries | 840 | 56 | 73 |
| Fried Mozzarella | 770 | 44 | 56 |
| Pan Seared Potstickers | 830 | 52 | 72 |
| Sesame Jack Chicken Strips | 1150 | 37 | 158 |
| **To Share:** | | | |
| Ale House Shrimp & Chips | 1210 | 64 | 127 |
| Loaded Potato Skins | 2070 | 135 | 162 |
| Tostada Nachos | 1700 | 117 | 57 |
| Tuscan Spinach Dip | 1080 | 70 | 85 |
| **Dressings:** Per 3 oz | | | |
| Bleu Cheese | 490 | 51 | 3 |
| Ranch | 480 | 50 | 4 |

## TGI Friday® cont... (Dec '11)

| Black Angus Burgers: With Fries | C | F | Cb |
|---|---|---|---|
| Burger | 1140 | 57 | 111 |
| Cheeseburger | 1220 | 68 | 106 |
| Jack Daniel's Burger | 1680 | 84 | 162 |
| Kansas City BBQ Burger | 1380 | 75 | 103 |
| NY Cheddar & Bacon Burger | 1500 | 87 | 120 |
| Southwest Burger | 1690 | 109 | 123 |
| Turkey Burger | 1000 | 44 | 107 |

*Sandwiches: With Sides Unless Indicated*

| | C | F | Cb |
|---|---|---|---|
| California Club without sides | 920 | 58 | 53 |
| Caribbean Chicken with Fries | 1250 | 47 | 145 |
| Jack Daniel's Chicken w/out sides | 1290 | 60 | 117 |
| Ultimate Sicillian w/out sides | 1000 | 61 | 48 |

*Entrees: Without Sides Unless Indicated*

**Black Angus Steaks:**

| | C | F | Cb |
|---|---|---|---|
| Black Angus Brew House w/ sides | 1030 | 71 | 43 |
| Flat Iron | 510 | 33 | 2 |
| Sirloin: Petite | 490 | 30 | 3 |
| With Half Rack Ribs | 960 | 49 | 46 |
| With Salmon | 1080 | 72 | 3 |
| Sirloin: 10 oz | 540 | 38 | 4 |
| With Grilled Shrimp Scampi | 920 | 69 | 8 |

**Chicken & Pasta:**

| | C | F | Cb |
|---|---|---|---|
| Chicken Fingers with Fries | 1120 | 62 | 102 |
| Dragonfire Chicken with sides | 520 | 12 | 68 |
| Pasta: Bruschetta Chicken | 950 | 42 | 96 |
| Cajun Shrimp & Chicken | 1430 | 88 | 96 |
| Chicken Piccata | 930 | 40 | 94 |

**Jack Daniels Grill:**

| | C | F | Cb |
|---|---|---|---|
| Chicken | 490 | 5 | 76 |
| Chicken & Shrimp | 590 | 11 | 77 |
| Flat Iron Steak | 840 | 34 | 77 |
| Ribs & Shrimp with sides | 1840 | 72 | 199 |
| Sirloin & Shrimp | 990 | 31 | 102 |

*Salads: Includes Dressing*

| | C | F | Cb |
|---|---|---|---|
| Caribbean Passion with Tuna | 1130 | 66 | 85 |
| Chipotle Yucatan Chicken | 940 | 64 | 45 |
| Pecan-Crusted Chicken | 980 | 57 | 76 |
| Southwest Wedge | 490 | 25 | 38 |

*Sides: Ginger-Lime Slaw*

| | C | F | Cb |
|---|---|---|---|
| Ginger-Lime Slaw | 110 | 5 | 2 |
| Mashed Potatoes | 390 | 17 | 50 |
| Potato Salad | 300 | 20 | 27 |
| Seasoned Fries | 370 | 15 | 54 |
| Thick Cut Steak Fries | 410 | 23 | 44 |

## TGI Friday® cont... (Dec '11)

| Soups: Per 10 oz Bowl | C | F | Cb |
|---|---|---|---|
| Broccoli Cheese | 500 | 38 | 26 |
| French Onion | 250 | 15 | 18 |
| **Soup Of The Day:** Chicken Noodle | 230 | 9 | 24 |
| New England Clam Chowder | 560 | 33 | 53 |
| Tomato Basil | 310 | 23 | 23 |
| Tortilla | 340 | 17 | 36 |
| **Desserts:** Brownie Obsession, ½ serve | 360 | 20 | 45 |
| Ice Cream Strawb. Shortcake, ½ serve | 210 | 10 | 30 |
| Oreo Madness | 520 | 13 | 97 |
| Vanilla Bean Cheesecake | 990 | 61 | 93 |

*Signature Slushes: Per 22 oz Tumbler*

| | C | F | Cb |
|---|---|---|---|
| Blue Rasperry | 310 | 0 | 75 |
| Mango Peach Lemonade | 150 | 0 | 41 |
| Red Bull Passion | 220 | 0 | 54 |
| Ruby Red Bull | 200 | 0 | 51 |
| Strawberry Lemonade | 200 | 0.5 | 58 |

## Thundercloud Subs® (Dec '11)

| Subs: Small, w/ Standard Toppings | C | F | Cb |
|---|---|---|---|
| **Classic:** BLT | 405 | 17 | 40 |
| Roast Beef | 315 | 4 | 40 |
| Smoked Chicken | 295 | 4 | 40 |
| Turkey | 280 | 4 | 41 |
| **Hot Subs:** Meatball | 650 | 32 | 56 |
| Hot Pastrami | 430 | 13 | 41 |
| **Signature Subs:** Club | 480 | 19 | 43 |
| California Club | 510 | 23 | 45 |
| NY Italian | 570 | 30 | 42 |
| Office Favorite | 850 | 40 | 81 |
| Texas Tuna | 700 | 45 | 44 |
| Veggie Delite, with Hummus | 360 | 10 | 53 |

## Tim Hortons® (Dec '11)

| Breakfast: | C | F | Cb |
|---|---|---|---|
| **Sandwiches:** *Regular Size* | | | |
| Bagel BELT with Cheese | 460 | 16 | 59 |
| Bacon, Egg & Cheese | 440 | 25 | 35 |
| Breakfast Sausage & Biscuit | 420 | 27 | 32 |
| Egg & Cheese | 390 | 21 | 35 |
| **English Muffins:** Bacon, Egg & Chse | 330 | 15 | 33 |
| Sausage, Egg & Cheese | 450 | 27 | 33 |
| **Wraps:** Bacon | 270 | 16 | 18 |
| Egg & Cheese | 220 | 12 | 17 |
| Sausage | 390 | 28 | 18 |
| **Hashbrowns,** 1¾ oz | 100 | 5 | 12 |

*Continued next page...*

## Tim Horton's® cont... (Dec'11)

**Sandwiches:** Regular, on White Bun **C** **F** **Cb**
with Standard Ingredients

| | C | F | Cb |
|---|---|---|---|
| BLT | 420 | 18 | 47 |
| Chicken Salad | 350 | 9 | 48 |
| Ham & Swiss | 400 | 12 | 48 |
| Toasted Chicken Club | 390 | 7 | 52 |
| Turkey Bacon Club | 380 | 7 | 55 |
| **Wrap Snackers:** | | | |
| BBQ Chicken, 3.5 oz | 180 | 6 | 30 |
| Chicken Ranch, 3.5 oz | 190 | 8 | 35 |
| **Soups:** Per Small 10 oz Bowl | | | |
| Beef Barley w/ Portobello Mshrm | 110 | 2 | 18 |
| Chicken Noodle | 110 | 2.5 | 19 |
| Cream of Broccoli | 160 | 10 | 15 |
| Hearty Potato Bacon | 230 | 13 | 23 |
| Split Pea with Ham | 160 | 2.5 | 28 |
| Turkey & Wild Rice | 120 | 1.5 | 24 |
| **Baked Goods:** Each | | | |
| **Cookies:** Chocolate Chunk | 230 | 9 | 35 |
| Oatmeal Raisin Spice | 220 | 8 | 35 |
| Peanut Butter | 280 | 16 | 27 |
| Triple Chocolate | 250 | 13 | 31 |
| **Donuts:** | | | |
| Cake: Chocolate Glazed | 260 | 10 | 39 |
| Old Fashioned Plain | 260 | 19 | 20 |
| Sour Cream Plain | 270 | 17 | 27 |
| Filled: Blueberry | 230 | 8 | 36 |
| Boston Cream | 250 | 9 | 37 |
| Canadian Maple | 260 | 9 | 41 |
| Strawberry | 230 | 8 | 36 |
| Honey Cruller | 320 | 19 | 37 |
| Yeast, Apple Fritter | 300 | 11 | 49 |
| **Timbits:** Low-Fat | | | |
| Cake, Glazed: Chocolate | 70 | 2.5 | 10 |
| Sour Cream | 90 | 4.5 | 12 |
| Old Fashion, Plain | 70 | 5 | 5 |
| Filled, all varieties | 60 | 2 | 10 |
| Yeast: Apple Fritter | 50 | 1.5 | 9 |
| Honey Dip | 60 | 2 | 9 |
| **Desserts:** Per 6 oz Container | | | |
| Low Fat Yogurt: Creamy Vanilla | 160 | 2.5 | 32 |
| Strawberry | 150 | 2.5 | 28 |
| **Beverages:** | | | |
| Cafe Mocha, 10 fl.oz | 170 | 6 | 27 |
| Coffee w/med. sugar/cream, 10 fl.oz | 75 | 3.5 | 9 |
| Hot Chocolate, 10 fl.oz | 240 | 6 | 45 |
| **Iced Cappuccinos:** Per Small, 12 fl.oz | | | |
| Original: With milk | 180 | 1.5 | 39 |
| With cream | 300 | 15 | 41 |
| Mocha: With milk | 300 | 7 | 55 |
| With cream | 410 | 21 | 54 |

## T.J. Cinnamons® (Dec'11)

**Bakery:**

| | C | F | Cb |
|---|---|---|---|
| Cinnamon Roll, 5¼ oz | 505 | 10 | 73 |
| Cinnamon Twist (1), 2½ oz | 260 | 14 | 33 |
| Pecan Sticky Bun: (1), 6½ oz | 690 | 22 | 91 |
| 4-Pack | 2750 | 90 | 363 |
| Sticky Bun Smear w/ Pecans, 1¼ oz | 180 | 12 | 18 |
| T.J. Cream Cheese Icing, 1 oz | 115 | 5 | 18 |
| **Beverages:** Per 12 fl.oz Serving | | | |
| **Mocha Chill:** W/o Whipped Cream | 265 | 4 | 46 |
| With Whipped Cream | 305 | 7 | 48 |

## Togo's Eatery® (Dec'11)

**Sandwiches:** **C** **F** **Cb**
**Cold:** Per Regular White Bread with Standard Toppings
without Dressing

| | C | F | Cb |
|---|---|---|---|
| Albacore Tuna | 550 | 17 | 73 |
| Black Forest Ham & Provolone | 520 | 15 | 66 |
| Roast Beef & Avocado | 570 | 13 | 69 |
| The Italian | 780 | 34 | 71 |
| Turkey & Avocado | 530 | 15 | 74 |
| Turkey Bacon Club | 530 | 16 | 67 |
| **Vegetarian:** Avocado & Provolone | 630 | 29 | 73 |
| Avocado & Cucumber | 450 | 11 | 75 |
| Egg Salad & Cheese | 640 | 28 | 70 |
| **Hot:** BBQ Beef | 670 | 19 | 85 |
| Chicken | 480 | 4 | 71 |
| French Dip | 690 | 17 | 66 |
| Pastrami | 770 | 37 | 66 |
| Roast Beef | 580 | 9 | 66 |
| **Toasted Sandwiches:** Per Regular Size with Menu Board Featured Bread | | | |
| Clubhouse | 660 | 23 | 80 |
| Pepper Jack Pastrami | 980 | 57 | 68 |
| Uncle Toby's Italian | 880 | 47 | 73 |
| **Salad Wraps:** Includes Whole Wheat Wrap, Standard Toppings & Dressings | | | |
| Asian Chicken with Asian Dressing | 670 | 32 | 74 |
| BBQ Chicken Ranch w/ Buttmlk Ranch | 630 | 26 | 77 |
| Chicken Caesar w/ Caesar Drssng | 550 | 20 | 67 |
| Santa Fe Chicken with Spicy Pepitas | 800 | 44 | 75 |
| **Salads:** Per Full Salad, without Dressing | | | |
| Asian Chicken | 200 | 9 | 17 |
| BBQ Chicken Ranch | 390 | 20 | 32 |
| Chicken Caesar | 210 | 6 | 17 |
| Santa Fe Chicken | 370 | 16 | 33 |

## Tropical Smoothie Cafe® (Dec'11)

### Breakfast:

| | C | F | Cb |
|---|---|---|---|
| **Wraps:** Early Bird | 740 | 34 | 61 |
| All American | 620 | 26 | 53 |

### Bistro Sandwiches: Without Cheese & Sauce

| | C | F | Cb |
|---|---|---|---|
| Cranberry Walnut Chicken Salad | 730 | 39 | 70 |
| Hummus Veggie | 630 | 24 | 84 |
| The Italian | 410 | 13 | 37 |
| Turkey Bacon Ranch | 440 | 14 | 37 |
| Ultimate Club | 460 | 16 | 39 |
| **Toasted Wraps:** Buffalo Chicken | 620 | 22 | 60 |
| Jamaican Jerk Chicken | 700 | 18 | 86 |
| King Caesar | 650 | 29 | 57 |
| Sesame Chicken | 700 | 24 | 84 |
| Totally Turkey | 580 | 20 | 56 |

### Gourmet Salads: Includes Standard Dressing

| | C | F | Cb |
|---|---|---|---|
| Cranberry Walnut Chicken | 490 | 38 | 23 |
| Sesame Chicken | 530 | 25 | 49 |
| Thai Chicken | 400 | 11 | 43 |
| TSC Signature | 350 | 12 | 38 |

### Low Fat Smoothies: With Turbinado

| | C | F | Cb |
|---|---|---|---|
| Blimey Limey | 480 | 0 | 124 |
| Blue Lagoon | 310 | 1 | 79 |
| Hawaiian Breeze | 370 | 0 | 93 |
| Rockin Raspberry | 380 | 1 | 99 |
| Strawberry Beach | 440 | 1 | 113 |
| Sunrise Sunset | 420 | 0 | 109 |

### Supercharged: With Turbinado

| | C | F | Cb |
|---|---|---|---|
| Health Nut | 490 | 6 | 97 |
| Lean Machine | 420 | 1 | 111 |
| Muscle Blaster | 430 | 3 | 89 |
| Stress Defender | 480 | 1 | 120 |

### Simply Indulgent Smoothies: With Turbinado

| | C | F | Cb |
|---|---|---|---|
| Beach Bum | 510 | 5 | 123 |
| Chocolate Chiller | 530 | 7 | 118 |
| Peanut Butter Cup | 650 | 21 | 117 |
| Tropi-Colada | 460 | 1 | 129 |

**With Splenda, deduct 200 calories & 50g carbs**

## Tubby's® (Dec'11)

### Subs: Per Regular Sandwich

| | C | F | Cb |
|---|---|---|---|
| **Burger Subs:** Big Tub | 475 | 45 | 41 |
| Burger Special | 625 | 41 | 42 |
| Cheeseburger | 590 | 41 | 36 |
| Pizza Burger | 605 | 41 | 38 |

## Tubby's® Cont... (Dec'11)

### Subs (Cont): Per Regular Sandwich

| | C | F | Cb |
|---|---|---|---|
| **Deli Subs:** Club Sub | 480 | 29 | 36 |
| Ham & Cheese | 400 | 22 | 38 |
| Famous | 465 | 28 | 39 |
| Turkey Club | 475 | 27 | 36 |
| **Specialty Subs:** BLT | 465 | 31 | 35 |
| Cold Veggie | 265 | 5 | 45 |
| Italian Sausage | 510 | 32 | 40 |
| Tuna | 295 | 13 | 33 |
| Veggie Stir Fry | 375 | 19 | 42 |
| **Chicken Subs:** | | | |
| Chicken & Broccoli | 480 | 19 | 38 |
| Chicken & Cheddar | 470 | 18 | 37 |
| Chicken Fajita | 370 | 7 | 38 |
| Grilled Chicken | 300 | 2 | 34 |
| **Steak Subs:** | | | |
| Mushroom Steak | 580 | 39 | 37 |
| Pepper Steak | 575 | 39 | 37 |
| Steak & Cheese | 570 | 39 | 36 |
| Steak Special | 605 | 39 | 42 |

## Uno Chicago Grill® (Dec'11)

### Appetizers: Per Single Serve

| | C | F | Cb |
|---|---|---|---|
| Crispy Cheese Dippers (1), 3¾ oz | 280 | 16 | 27 |
| Pizza Skins, ⅛ pizza, 5 oz | 410 | 28 | 29 |
| Shrimp & Crab Fondue, 3¼ oz | 220 | 16 | 13 |

### Burgers: Without Sides

| | C | F | Cb |
|---|---|---|---|
| BBQ with Bacon & Cheddar (1) | 1020 | 72 | 34 |
| Cheddar (1) | 900 | 62 | 30 |
| Uno (1) | 780 | 54 | 28 |

### Entrees: Per Whole Dish, without Sides or Breadstick

| | C | F | Cb |
|---|---|---|---|
| Baked Stuffed Chicken | 360 | 18 | 6 |
| Chicken Milanese | 860 | 58 | 42 |
| Chicken Thumb Platter | 480 | 18 | 34 |

### Steak & Seafood: Per Whole Dish w/out Sides or Breadstick

| | C | F | Cb |
|---|---|---|---|
| Baked Haddock | 580 | 34 | 12 |
| Grilled Shrimp & Sirloin | 640 | 30 | 8 |
| Lemon Basil Salmon | 480 | 34 | 0 |
| The Chop House Classic | 400 | 14 | 0 |

### Thin Crust Pizza: Per ⅓ Pizza

| | C | F | Cb |
|---|---|---|---|
| Mediterranean, Traditional Crust | 310 | 16 | 32 |
| Pepperoni, Flatbread Base | 330 | 16 | 33 |
| Roasted Eggplant, Spinach & Feta, Traditional Crust | 290 | 11 | 38 |
| **Sides:** French Fries, 7.6 oz | 450 | 33 | 36 |
| Red Bliss Mashed Potatoes | 270 | 14 | 34 |
| Roasted Seasonal Veges, 7.2 oz | 80 | 4.5 | 10 |
| Steamed Seasonal Veges, 6.25 oz | 100 | 7 | 9 |

# Fast - Foods & *Restaurants*

## Villa Fresh Italian® (Dec '11)

*Pizza (18"): Per Slice (⅙ Pizza)*

| | C | F | Cb |
|---|---|---|---|
| **Neapolitan:** Cheese | 405 | 13 | 49 |
| Sausage and Cheese | 545 | 26 | 51 |
| Pepperoni and Cheese | 480 | 20 | 49 |
| **Stuffed:** Meat | 840 | 41 | 75 |
| Spinach and Broccoli | 755 | 35 | 79 |
| **Sicilian,** Deluxe | 540 | 24 | 58 |
| *Stromboli:* | | | |
| Sausage and Cheese | 675 | 25 | 78 |
| Pepperoni and Cheese | 840 | 40 | 77 |
| *Pasta & Italian Specialties:* | | | |
| Baked Ziti | 595 | 23 | 66 |
| Meat Lasagna | 695 | 21 | 94 |
| Spinach and Cheese Lasagna | 995 | 45 | 106 |
| Spaghetti | 755 | 34 | 94 |
| Chicken Cacciatore | 805 | 56 | 42 |
| Italian Sausage and Peppers | 380 | 31 | 16 |
| Sauteed Fresh Vegetables | 520 | 50 | 18 |

## Vocelli Pizza® (Dec '11)

*Pizze: Per ⅛ Slice Medium Pizza*

| | C | F | Cb |
|---|---|---|---|
| **Gourmet:** Chicken Alfredo Spinaci | 230 | 8 | 27 |
| Deluxe | 260 | 10 | 29 |
| Meat Steak | 270 | 12 | 27 |
| *Pasta:* Chicken Alfredo, 18 oz | 1080 | 55 | 100 |
| Chicken Parmesan, 20 oz | 1030 | 35 | 132 |
| Chicken Pesto, 18 oz | 1110 | 59 | 99 |
| *Hot Subs:* | | | |
| Chicken Florentine, 8½ oz | 480 | 21 | 40 |
| Chicken Pesto, 7½ oz | 410 | 17 | 34 |
| Chicken Parmesan on Ciabatta | 440 | 18 | 45 |
| *Salads: Per Regular Size* | | | |
| Antipasta, 16 oz | 270 | 16 | 17 |
| Chicken Caesar, 8 oz | 130 | 3 | 5 |
| Mediterranean, 16 oz | 270 | 18 | 17 |
| Tuscan Chicken | 290 | 13 | 12 |
| *Appetizers:* | | | |
| Bruschetta, 1 slice, 4⅔ oz | 230 | 11 | 25 |
| Buffalo Wings, bone in, 9 oz | 720 | 54 | 2 |
| BBQ Wings, bone in, 9 oz | 760 | 53 | 14 |
| Garlic Bread, 1¾ oz | 230 | 11 | 27 |
| *Dessert:* Cannoli (1), with cream | 150 | 7 | 17 |
| Tiramisu, 4 oz | 340 | 21 | 34 |

## Wahoo's Fish Taco® (Dec '11)

*Bowls: With White Rice & Black Beans*

| | C | F | Cb |
|---|---|---|---|
| #7 Blackened/Charbroiled Chkn, av. | 860 | 15 | 127 |
| # 8 Charbroiled/Teriyaki Fish, av. | 930 | 22 | 126 |
| #9 Veggie | 760 | 11 | 141 |
| #10 Carnitas/Kahlua Pig, average | 1025 | 25 | 131 |
| *Classic Burrito, A la Carte:* | | | |
| Carne Asada | 480 | 19 | 53 |
| Carnitas | 605 | 25 | 54 |
| *Charbroiled/Blackened:* | | | |
| Fish, average | 545 | 23 | 53 |
| Chicken, average | 495 | 18 | 52 |
| Mushroom | 405 | 16 | 55 |
| Shrimp | 400 | 16 | 53 |
| Veggie, w/ White Rice & Black Beans | 635 | 19 | 98 |
| *Tacos, A la Carte:* | | | |
| Blackened Chicken | 185 | 5 | 22 |
| Carne Asada | 180 | 5 | 22 |
| Carnitas | 235 | 8 | 23 |
| Veggie w/ White Rice & Black Beans | 215 | 4 | 36 |
| *Sides:* Brown Rice | 350 | 7 | 64 |
| White Beans | 285 | 3 | 54 |
| *Salads: Chips Not Included* | | | |
| Blackened Chicken | 415 | 22 | 14 |
| Carne Asada | 400 | 23 | 16 |
| Charbroiled Fish | 485 | 29 | 14 |

**For Complete Nutritional Data ~ see CalorieKing.com**

## WAWA® (Dec '11)

*Breakfast:*

| | C | F | Cb |
|---|---|---|---|
| **Bagels:** Plain | 290 | 1 | 60 |
| Plain, with Butter | 490 | 23 | 60 |
| Cinnamon Raisin | 290 | 1 | 63 |
| Cinnamon, with Cream Cheese | 410 | 13 | 65 |
| Everything | 310 | 6 | 56 |
| **Bowls:** *Per Bowl, without Syrup* | | | |
| Creamed Chipped Beef On White | 290 | 10 | 40 |
| Pancake: Without Syrup | 330 | 10 | 56 |
| With Bacon | 370 | 12 | 57 |
| With Sausage | 490 | 24 | 57 |
| With Turkey Sausage | 420 | 16 | 57 |
| Scrambled Egg: With Bacon | 370 | 25 | 9 |
| With Sausage | 500 | 38 | 9 |
| **Ciabatta Melts:** *On Shorti Roll, without Extras* | | | |
| Scrambled Eggs: With Bacon | 530 | 20 | 58 |
| With Beef Cheesesteak | 640 | 21 | 60 |
| With Ham & Swiss | 670 | 27 | 62 |
| Italian Style | 640 | 26 | 60 |
| **Sizzlis:** *Without Hashbrowns* | | | |
| Bagels: Bacon, Egg & Cheese | 370 | 15 | 42 |
| Pork Roll, Egg & Cheese | 400 | 16 | 43 |

## WAWA® cont... (Dec '11)

| Lunch: | C | F | Cb |
|---|---|---|---|
| **Bagel Sandwiches:** *With Plain Bagel, w/o Toppings* | | | |
| BLT | **390** | 8 | 62 |
| Chicken Salad | **630** | 29 | 66 |
| Egg Salad | **630** | 31 | 66 |
| **Cold Hoagies:** *On Shorti Roll, without Toppings* | | | |
| Egg Salad | **540** | 32 | 46 |
| Tuna Salad | **620** | 38 | 48 |
| Turkey | **320** | 5 | 46 |
| **Soups:** *Per Medium Serving* | | | |
| Cream of Broccoli | **220** | 13 | 19 |
| Maryland Crab | **120** | 1 | 20 |
| Minestrone | **140** | 3.5 | 23 |
| **Sides:** *Per Medium Serving* | | | |
| Chili | **250** | 8 | 32 |
| Macaroni & Cheese | **500** | 25 | 49 |
| Mashed Potatoes | **530** | 33 | 52 |
| Meatballs in a Cup | **360** | 25 | 20 |
| Shepherd's Pie | **540** | 23 | 36 |
| Stuffing | **400** | 23 | 42 |
| *Dinner:* | | | |
| **Breaded Chicken Strips:** | | | |
| 3 piece | **240** | 13 | 16 |
| 5 piece | **400** | 22 | 27 |
| **Hot Dogs:** *Without Toppings, Mustard or Sauce* | | | |
| Regular | **230** | 15 | 21 |
| ¼ Pound | **400** | 27 | 21 |
| Big Bacon Cheese Dog | **640** | 40 | 41 |
| **Hot Hoagies:** *On Shorti Roll, without Toppings* | | | |
| Beef Cheesesteak | **360** | 7 | 42 |
| Chicken Cheesesteak | **340** | 6 | 42 |
| Meatballs | **560** | 28 | 60 |
| **Sides:** *Per Medium Serving,* | | | |
| Beef Stew | **620** | 15 | 23 |
| **Soups:** *Per Medium Serving* | | | |
| Italian Wedding | **130** | 4.5 | 16 |
| Loaded Potato | **410** | 26 | 28 |
| **Toasted Flatbreads:** *Without Sour Cream* | | | |
| Buffalo Chicken | **520** | 18 | 56 |
| Salsa Chicken | **560** | 19 | 58 |
| *Bakery:* | | | |
| **Croissant,** Plain | **280** | 14 | 35 |
| **Muffins:** Banana Walnut | **670** | 34 | 83 |
| Blueberry | **610** | 30 | 78 |
| Chocolate Chip | **680** | 34 | 86 |
| Corn | **640** | 29 | 87 |
| *Beverages: Per 24 oz* | | | |
| Hot Cappuccinos: Original | **370** | 13 | 63 |
| English Toffee | **340** | 9 | 63 |
| Smoothie, Strawberry Banana | **690** | 0 | 180 |

## Wendy's® (Dec '11)

| Burgers: *With Standard Toppings* | C | F | Cb |
|---|---|---|---|
| ¼ lb Single | **580** | 33 | 42 |
| ½ lb Double | **800** | 48 | 42 |
| ¾ lb Triple | **1060** | 67 | 42 |
| Baconator Double | **970** | 63 | 40 |
| Bacon Deluxe Double | **890** | 56 | 42 |
| Cheeseburger Deluxe | **350** | 19 | 27 |
| Double Stack | **400** | 21 | 26 |
| Jr. Bacon Cheeseburger | **400** | 24 | 25 |
| Jr. Cheeseburger | **290** | 13 | 26 |
| *Sandwiches: With Standard Toppings* | | | |
| Asiago Ranch Club | **690** | 36 | 56 |
| Crispy Chicken | **380** | 20 | 37 |
| Homestyle Chicken | **510** | 21 | 54 |
| Spicy Chicken | **520** | 22 | 55 |
| Ultimate Chicken Grill | **390** | 10 | 42 |
| *Go Wraps:* Homestyle Chicken | **320** | 16 | 30 |
| Grilled Chicken | **260** | 10 | 25 |
| Spicy Chicken | **330** | 16 | 31 |
| *Natural Cut Fries:* Value | **230** | 11 | 30 |
| Small, 4 oz | **320** | 16 | 42 |
| Medium, 5 oz | **420** | 21 | 55 |
| Large, 6½ oz | **530** | 25 | 68 |
| *Crispy Chicken Nuggets:* 5 pieces | **220** | 14 | 13 |
| 10 pieces | **450** | 29 | 26 |
| *Sauces:* Barbecue Nugget | **45** | 0 | 11 |
| Heartland Ranch Dipping | **120** | 12 | 3 |
| *Garden Sensations Salads: Full, Without Dressing* | | | |
| Apple Pecan Chicken | **450** | 21 | 34 |
| Baja | **630** | 37 | 45 |
| BLT Cobb | **450** | 25 | 9 |
| Spicy Chicken Caesar | **540** | 28 | 39 |
| *Dressings:* Classic Ranch, 1 pkt | **100** | 10 | 2 |
| Italian Vinaigrette, 1 pkt | **70** | 6 | 4 |
| Thousand Island, 1 pkt | **160** | 15 | 5 |
| *Sides:* | | | |
| **Chili,** Large, 16 oz | **310** | 9 | 31 |
| **Hot Stuffed Baked Potatoes:** Plain | **270** | 0 | 61 |
| Bacon & Cheese | **520** | 20 | 65 |
| Broccoli & Cheese | **410** | 10 | 67 |
| Sour Cream & Chives | **320** | 3.5 | 63 |
| *Frosty:* Chocolate/Vanilla, small | **255** | 7 | 42 |
| *Frosty Shakes: Per Large 24 oz, With Whipped Cream* | | | |
| Caramel | **1020** | 19 | 198 |
| Chocolate | **890** | 18 | 168 |
| Strawberry | **820** | 15 | 156 |
| Vanilla Bean | **890** | 16 | 172 |

*For Complete Nutritional Data ~ see CalorieKing.com*

## Whataburger® (Dec '11)

| Burgers/Sandwiches: | C | F | Cb |
|---|---|---|---|
| **Burgers:** Justaburger | 290 | 15 | 26 |
| Whataburger: Burger | 620 | 30 | 58 |
| With Bacon & Cheese | 780 | 43 | 59 |
| Double Meat | 870 | 49 | 58 |
| Triple Meat | 1120 | 68 | 58 |
| Jr. | 300 | 15 | 28 |
| **Sandwiches:** Grilled Chicken | 470 | 19 | 49 |
| Whatacatch | 450 | 24 | 44 |
| Whatachick'n | 550 | 27 | 57 |
| *French Fries:* Small, 3 oz | 320 | 18 | 36 |
| Medium, 4½ oz | 480 | 27 | 55 |
| Large, 6 oz | 640 | 36 | 73 |
| *Onion Rings:* Medium, 4¼ oz | 400 | 25 | 37 |
| Large, 6½ oz | 600 | 38 | 56 |
| *Chicken Strips,* (2 pieces) | 300 | 16 | 22 |
| *Salads: Without Dressing* | | | |
| Chicken Strips Salad | 350 | 16 | 33 |
| With Shredded Cheddar Cheese | 520 | 29 | 34 |
| Garden Salad | 50 | 0 | 11 |
| With Shredded Cheddar Cheese | 220 | 13 | 12 |
| Grilled Chicken Salad | 220 | 7 | 18 |
| With Shredded Cheddar Cheese | 390 | 20 | 19 |
| *Sauces: Per 2oz* | | | |
| Buttermilk | 310 | 33 | 3 |
| Honey Mustard | 250 | 21 | 15 |
| Thousand Island | 150 | 13 | 10 |
| *Malts:* | | | |
| Choc.; Strawb.: Small, av.,12.63 oz | 520 | 13 | 94 |
| Medium, average, 15.75 oz | 670 | 15 | 123 |
| Vanilla: Small, 12.63 oz | 470 | 13 | 77 |
| Medium, 15.75 oz | 600 | 17 | 98 |
| *Shakes:* | | | |
| Choc.; Strawb.: Small, 12.63 oz | 500 | 13 | 86 |
| Medium, average, 15.75 oz | 630 | 16 | 111 |
| Vanilla: Small, 12.63 oz | 440 | 14 | 69 |
| Medium, 15.75 oz | 560 | 17 | 87 |
| *Breakfast:* Cinnamon Roll | 390 | 9 | 71 |
| Hash Brown Sticks (4) | 200 | 12 | 60 |
| Texas Toast, 1 slice | 150 | 7 | 20 |
| **Biscuits:** Plain | 300 | 17 | 32 |
| With Bacon | 350 | 20 | 32 |
| With Gravy | 560 | 33 | 54 |
| With Sausage | 540 | 37 | 32 |
| Honey Butter Chicken | 560 | 34 | 50 |
| **Biscuit Sandwiches:** | | | |
| With Egg & Cheese | 450 | 28 | 33 |
| With Bacon, Egg & Cheese | 500 | 32 | 33 |
| With Sausage, Egg & Cheese | 690 | 49 | 33 |

## Whataburger® cont... (Dec '11)

| Breakfast (Cont): | C | F | Cb |
|---|---|---|---|
| **Breakfast On A Bun:** With Bacon | 360 | 21 | 25 |
| With Sausage | 550 | 38 | 25 |
| **Breakfast Platter (Biscuit/Eggs/Hash Brown):** | | | |
| With Bacon | 730 | 45 | 93 |
| With Sausage | 920 | 63 | 93 |
| **Pancakes:** Plain (3) | 540 | 7 | 104 |
| With Bacon | 580 | 11 | 104 |
| With Sausage | 780 | 28 | 104 |
| **Taquito:** With Bacon & Egg | 380 | 21 | 27 |
| With Bacon, Egg & Cheese | 420 | 24 | 27 |
| With Potato & Egg | 430 | 23 | 57 |
| With Potato, Egg & Cheese | 470 | 27 | 57 |
| With Sausage & Egg | 410 | 24 | 27 |
| With Sausage, Egg & Cheese | 450 | 28 | 27 |
| *Dessert,* Hot Apple Pie, 3 oz | 250 | 12 | 31 |

## White Castle® (Dec '11)

| Burgers: | C | F | Cb |
|---|---|---|---|
| **Cheeseburger:** Single | 170 | 9 | 15 |
| Double | 300 | 17 | 20 |
| *Sliders:* Original | 140 | 6 | 13 |
| Double | 240 | 12 | 21 |
| Chicken Ring with Cheese | 380 | 30 | 16 |
| Chicken Breast with Cheese | 390 | 28 | 20 |
| Fish with Cheese | 340 | 24 | 18 |
| Surf & Turf with Cheese, 6 oz | 540 | 38 | 27 |
| *Sides:* | | | |
| Chicken Rings: 6 rings, 5 oz | 530 | 47 | 12 |
| 9 rings, 7½ oz | 790 | 71 | 18 |
| Clam Strips, regular, 4½ oz | 210 | 17 | 5 |
| Fish Nibblers, regular, 5 oz | 320 | 16 | 28 |
| French Fries, 5.6 oz | 370 | 25 | 33 |
| Mozzarella Cheese Sticks, 3 sticks | 440 | 33 | 22 |
| Onion Chips, 6.1 oz | 670 | 50 | 46 |
| Onion Rings, Homestyle, 5 oz | 480 | 33 | 40 |
| *Sauces & Condiments: Per Packet* | | | |
| Ketchup, 1 pkt | 10 | 0 | 2 |
| Mayonnaise, 1 pkt | 60 | 7 | 0 |
| Ranch Dressing, 1 oz | 150 | 17 | 1 |
| **Sauces:** BBQ, 1 pkt | 10 | 0 | 3 |
| Seafood, 1 oz | 30 | 0 | 7 |
| White Castle Zesty Zing, 1 oz | 120 | 11 | 4 |

## Wienerschnitzel® (Dec '11)

*Hot Dogs:* | **C** | **F** | **Cb**

**Original:** *On Standard Bun*

| | C | F | Cb |
|---|---|---|---|
| Chili | 290 | 13 | 31 |
| Chili Cheese | 340 | 17 | 31 |
| Deluxe | 270 | 12 | 30 |
| Kraut | 260 | 12 | 28 |
| Plain | 270 | 13 | 28 |
| Stadium | 370 | 20 | 32 |

**Original:** *On Pretzel Bun*

| | C | F | Cb |
|---|---|---|---|
| Chili | 430 | 16 | 57 |
| Kraut; Mustard; Plain | 400 | 15 | 54 |
| Stadium | 510 | 23 | 58 |

**Big Original:** *On Standard Bun*

| | C | F | Cb |
|---|---|---|---|
| Plain | 370 | 22 | 39 |
| BBQ Bacon | 480 | 30 | 44 |
| Chicago | 430 | 22 | 52 |
| Pastrami | 520 | 33 | 40 |

**Angus All Beef:** *On Pretzel Bun*

| | C | F | Cb |
|---|---|---|---|
| Chicago | 600 | 27 | 69 |
| Chili Cheese | 680 | 37 | 59 |
| **Corn Dogs:** Regular | 250 | 17 | 15 |
| Mini (6 pack) | 320 | 22 | 22 |
| *Sides:* Chili Cheese Fries | 540 | 38 | 39 |
| **Fries:** Regular | 300 | 22 | 25 |
| Large | 430 | 31 | 35 |
| Jalapeno Poppers (3) | 210 | 11 | 21 |

*Breakfast:*

| | C | F | Cb |
|---|---|---|---|
| **Biscuits:** Egg, Bacon, Cheese | 440 | 25 | 36 |
| Egg, Sausage, Cheese | 540 | 34 | 40 |
| **Burritos:** Egg, Bacon, Cheese | 490 | 25 | 39 |
| Egg, Sausage, Cheese | 590 | 34 | 43 |
| French Toast Sticks | 490 | 29 | 49 |
| Syrup, 1 oz | 120 | 0 | 31 |

*Desserts:*

| | C | F | Cb |
|---|---|---|---|
| **Cones:** Plain, 6 oz. | 300 | 11 | 49 |
| Chocolate Dipped, 6 oz. | 490 | 29 | 57 |
| **Floats:** Mountain Dew; Root Beer, av. | 440 | 12 | 84 |
| Tropicana Strawberry Lemonade | 450 | 12 | 82 |
| **Freezees:** Butterfinger | 620 | 24 | 100 |
| Oreo; M&M | 630 | 25 | 99 |
| Reese's Peanut Butter Cup | 630 | 26 | 97 |
| **Sundaes:** Caramel; Hot Fudge avg. | 400 | 15 | 65 |
| Chocolate | 390 | 14 | 64 |
| Pineapple; Strawberry | 370 | 14 | 59 |
| **Shakes,** average all flavors | 650 | 23 | 110 |

*Drinks: 16 fl.oz, without ice*

| | C | F | Cb |
|---|---|---|---|
| Lipton Raspberry Iced Tea | 180 | 0 | 45 |
| Mountain Dew | 230 | 0 | 61 |
| Mug Root Beer | 210 | 0 | 57 |
| Pepsi | 200 | 0 | 55 |

## Winchell's® (Dec '11)

*Donuts:* Per Donut | **C** | **F** | **Cb**

| | C | F | Cb |
|---|---|---|---|
| Buttermilk Bars: Choc Iced; Glazed | 420 | 19 | 61 |

Jelly Filled:

| | C | F | Cb |
|---|---|---|---|
| Apple with Cinnamon Crumb | 370 | 15 | 53 |
| Raspberry with Glaze | 390 | 13 | 61 |
| Strawberry with Sugar | 380 | 13 | 60 |
| Old Fashioned, Glazed; Maple Iced | 410 | 17 | 60 |
| Raised Ring: Choc. Iced | 270 | 10 | 41 |
| Sugared | 230 | 9 | 34 |

## WingStreet (Dec '11)

*Chicken:* | **C** | **F** | **Cb**

**Crispy Bone In Wings:** *Per 2 Pieces*

| | C | F | Cb |
|---|---|---|---|
| All American, 2 oz | 200 | 14 | 8 |
| Buffalo, Mild/Med./Hot, 2¾ oz | 230 | 15 | 16 |
| Garlic Parmesan, 2½ oz | 300 | 25 | 9 |
| Honey BBQ, 3 oz | 260 | 14 | 24 |

**Bone Out Wings:** *Per 2 Pieces*

| | C | F | Cb |
|---|---|---|---|
| All American, 2 oz | 150 | 8 | 11 |
| Buffalo, Mild/Medium, 2½ oz | 190 | 9 | 18 |
| Garlic Parmesan, 2½ oz | 260 | 19 | 11 |
| Honey BBQ, 3 oz | 220 | 8 | 27 |

**Traditional Wings:** *Per 2 Pieces*

| | C | F | Cb |
|---|---|---|---|
| All American, 1¼ oz | 80 | 5 | 0 |
| Buffalo, Medium/Hot, 2 oz | 110 | 6 | 8 |
| Garlic Parmesan, 2 oz | 180 | 16 | 1 |
| Spicy Asian, 2.3 oz | 130 | 5 | 13 |
| *Sides:* Apple Pies, 2 pies, 3 oz | 330 | 17 | 40 |
| Fried Cheese Sticks (4), 4.2 oz | 380 | 24 | 29 |
| Wedge Fries, side order, 4.35 oz | 320 | 18 | 35 |

## Woody's Bar-B-Q® (Dec '11)

*Starters:* | **C** | **F** | **Cb**

| | C | F | Cb |
|---|---|---|---|
| Breaded Wings (10) | 700 | 47 | 13 |
| Beef Chili Cheese Fries | 805 | 38 | 63 |
| Super Sampler | 720 | 31 | 83 |

*Dinner Entrees: Without Sides*

| | C | F | Cb |
|---|---|---|---|
| ½ Chicken | 840 | 56 | 0 |
| Baby Back Ribs, ½ Rack, side order | 260 | 20 | 1 |
| Beef Prime Rib | 760 | 62 | 1 |

*Sandwiches: Per Regular, Without Sides*

| | C | F | Cb |
|---|---|---|---|
| Beef | 390 | 14 | 28 |
| Pork | 490 | 26 | 29 |

*Wraps: Without Sides*

| | C | F | Cb |
|---|---|---|---|
| Beef BBQ | 380 | 13 | 31 |
| Pork | 440 | 21 | 31 |
| *Dogs:* Chili Cheese | 630 | 48 | 26 |
| Slaw | 580 | 44 | 32 |

*For Complete Nutritional Data ~ see CalorieKing.com*

## Yoshinoya® (Dec '11)

*Bowls: With Sauce*

| | C | F | Cb |
|---|---|---|---|
| **Beef Bowl:** Regular | 685 | 27 | 81 |
| Large | 1040 | 38 | 131 |
| With Vegetables, regular | 605 | 20 | 84 |
| Beef & Chicken Combo, large | 1070 | 30 | 146 |
| **Chicken Bowl:** Regular | 610 | 12 | 94 |
| Large | 980 | 18 | 155 |
| **Shrimp Bowl,** Grilled | 505 | 3 | 96 |
| **Vegetable Bowl,** regular | 390 | 2.5 | 86 |
| **Kids,** Chicken | 360 | 7 | 53 |

*BBQ Style Plates:*

| | C | F | Cb |
|---|---|---|---|
| **Beef Plate:** W/ Fried Rice & Noodles | 850 | 35 | 98 |
| With Fried Rice | 830 | 38 | 89 |
| With Steamed Rice | 800 | 31 | 100 |
| **Chicken Plate:** W/ Fried Rice & Ndles | 700 | 23 | 79 |
| With Fried Rice | 720 | 24 | 84 |
| With Steamed Rice | 690 | 17 | 94 |

*Feast: Serves 4-5*

| | C | F | Cb |
|---|---|---|---|
| Beef & Chicken Combo | 4200 | 140 | 515 |
| Beef with Vegetables | 4000 | 150 | 490 |
| Chicken | 4400 | 130 | 535 |
| *Sushi:* Salmon Lover: Regular | 250 | 5 | 34 |
| Large | 485 | 9 | 72 |
| California Rolls: Regular | 215 | 5 | 36 |
| Large | 425 | 10 | 72 |
| *Dessert,* Cheese Cake | 330 | 19 | 35 |

## Z Pizza® (Dec '11)

*Pizzas: Small, Per Slice*

| | C | F | Cb |
|---|---|---|---|
| **Creations:** Berkeley Vegan | 180 | 8 | 19 |
| California | 150 | 6 | 19 |
| Casablanca | 190 | 9 | 18 |
| Greek | 150 | 6 | 17 |
| Italian; Mexican; Napoli, av. | 180 | 8 | 18 |
| Provence | 160 | 7 | 20 |
| Santa Fe | 180 | 7 | 20 |
| Thai | 170 | 6 | 19 |
| Tuscan | 160 | 7 | 18 |
| ZBQ | 170 | 5 | 21 |
| **Rusticas:** *Per Slice* | | | |
| Chicken Sausage | 105 | 3 | 11 |
| Curry Chicken & Yam | 135 | 4 | 17 |
| Mediterranean | 145 | 8 | 12 |
| Moroccan | 120 | 6 | 13 |
| Pear & Gorgonzola | 135 | 5 | 13 |
| *Calzones:* Meat Calzone | 760 | 36 | 75 |
| Veggie Calzone | 600 | 22 | 80 |
| *Salads: Small w/o Dressing* | | | |
| Arugula | 450 | 37 | 23 |
| Caesar Side | 200 | 17 | 8 |
| California | 90 | 5 | 13 |
| Pear and Gorgonzola | 530 | 44 | 25 |

## Zaxby's® (Dec '11)

*Zappetizers: With Sauce*

| | C | F | Cb |
|---|---|---|---|
| Fried White Cheddar Bites, 6 oz | 820 | 52 | 38 |
| Onion Rings, 5 oz | 780 | 56 | 59 |
| Spicy Fried Mushroom, 5.7 oz | 620 | 46 | 43 |
| Tater Chips, 5.2 oz | 940 | 68 | 72 |

*Meal Dealz: With Sauce , wihout Drink Unless Indicated*

| | C | F | Cb |
|---|---|---|---|
| Big Zax Snak | 950 | 52 | 82 |
| Buffalo Wings, without sauce | 900 | 56 | 51 |
| Chicken Finger Nibbler | 1330 | 71 | 137 |

*Most Popular: As Served*

| | C | F | Cb |
|---|---|---|---|
| Chicken Finger Plate: Regular | 1260 | 72 | 99 |
| Large | 1775 | 105 | 129 |

*Sandwich Baskets: Includes Fries*

| | C | F | Cb |
|---|---|---|---|
| Cajun Club | 1140 | 58 | 98 |
| Club | 1250 | 73 | 99 |

*Wings & Fingerz: With Sauce*

| | C | F | Cb |
|---|---|---|---|
| Buffalo Fingerz: 5 pieces | 630 | 42 | 15 |
| 10 pieces | 1050 | 65 | 27 |
| Buffalo Wings: 5 pieces | 540 | 40 | 3 |
| 10 pieces | 880 | 60 | 4 |
| Chicken Fingerz: 5 pieces | 610 | 39 | 19 |
| 10 pieces | 1230 | 80 | 36 |

*Zax Kidz: Without Drink*

| | C | F | Cb |
|---|---|---|---|
| Kiddie Cheese | 490 | 29 | 49 |
| Kiddie Finger | 570 | 36 | 40 |
| Kiddie Nibbler | 610 | 33 | 61 |

*Zalads: With Texas Toast, without Dressing*

| | C | F | Cb |
|---|---|---|---|
| **Blue,** with Blackened Chicken | 605 | 29 | 34 |
| **Caesar Zalad:** | | | |
| With Fried Chicken | 730 | 39 | 39 |
| With Grilled Chicken | 570 | 26 | 29 |
| **House Zalad:** With Fried Chicken | 765 | 42 | 44 |
| With Grilled Chicken | 605 | 29 | 34 |

*Salad Dressings:*

| | C | F | Cb |
|---|---|---|---|
| Blue Cheese, 1 packet, 1¼ oz | 180 | 19 | 2 |
| Honey French, 1¼ oz | 150 | 12 | 9 |
| Honey Mustard, 1¼ oz | 150 | 13 | 6 |
| Lite Ranch, 1¼ oz | 90 | 8 | 3 |
| Mediterranean, 1¼ oz | 140 | 14 | 4 |
| Ranch, 1¼ oz | 160 | 16 | 2 |
| Thousand Island | 230 | 24 | 3 |
| *Sides:* Celery Basket, with sauce | 220 | 20 | 7 |
| Cole Slaw, 2.2 oz | 140 | 11 | 12 |
| Crinkle Fries, regular, 5 oz | 360 | 16 | 48 |
| Texas Toast, 3 wedges, 4.3 oz | 440 | 20 | 60 |

## Zero Sub's® ~ *see CalorieKing.com*

# Fats & Cholesterol Guide

## Notes on Cholesterol

- **Cholesterol** is a white waxy substance produced mainly by our liver. It is also found in animal food products. Plant foods have no cholesterol.

- **Cholesterol is essential to life.** It is a structural part of every body cell wall and is the building block for vitamin D, sex hormones, and bile acids which help in the digestion of dietary fats.

- **The body makes sufficient cholesterol** for its needs and does not rely on cholesterol in the diet. Dietary fats have a major influence on blood cholesterol levels - more so than dietary cholesterol.

- **A high blood cholesterol level increases** the risk of atherosclerosis - the thickening of arteries that can reduce or block blood flow to the heart, brain, eyes, kidneys, sex organs and other body parts.

  **This in turn increases the risk of heart attack,** stroke, blindness, kidney failure, impotence and other blood circulatory problems.

  **Other risk factors which increase the risk of atherosclerosis include high blood pressure, smoking, obesity and uncontrolled diabetes.**

### HEART ATTACK WARNING SIGNALS

Many victims die before reaching the hospital by ignoring warning signals and delaying medical help.

**Symptoms vary and commonly include:**

- **Chest pain,** vice-like squeezing or burning sensation in center of the chest or between the shoulder blades, or in the mid-back. Pain may even feel like severe indigestion.
- **Pain** may be felt in the arms, shoulders, neck or jaw.
- **Shortness of breath** often occurs with or before chest discomfort.
- **Other signs,** with or without pain, include a cold sweat, nausea or light-headedness.

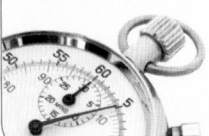

*If you experience any of the above symptoms call IMMEDIATELY for medical help. Every minute counts.*

*Call 9-1-1 or your emergency number*

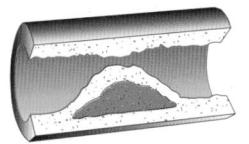

▲ **Atherosclerosis can clog arteries and impede blood flow to the heart or other body organs.**

▼ **A thrombus (blood clot) can form on unstable, festering athero-sclerotic plaque and rapidly block blood flow. A heart attack or stroke can result.**

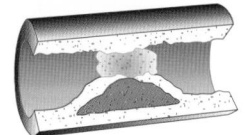

# Fats & Cholesterol Guide

The amount and type of dietary fat has the greatest influence on blood cholesterol levels.

**Fats in food are a mixture of 3 basic types:** saturated, monounsaturated, and polyunsaturated. Animal fats are mainly saturated while plant oils and fish oils are mainly mono- and polyunsaturated.

**Saturated fats** have subgroups known as long-chain, medium-chain, and short-chain fats. Most of the long chain fats raise blood cholesterol, and increase the risk of blood clots and thrombosis leading to artery blockage.

Long-chain saturated fats are found mainly in full-cream milk, cheese, butter, cream, fatty meats and sausages, and processed foods.

**Monounsaturated fats** tend to more selectively lower 'bad' LDL cholesterol and maintain the protective 'good' HDL cholesterol in the bloodstream – but only if they replace saturated fats in the diet.

Foods rich in monounsaturates include canola and olive oils, canola margarine, peanuts, and avocados.

**Polyunsaturated fats** consist of two main classes. **Omega-6** polyunsaturates tend to lower blood cholesterol. Rich sources include safflower, sunflower and corn oils.

**Omega-3** polyunsaturated fats can lower blood cholesterol; significantly lower blood triglycerides; and reduce the rise of thrombosis, heart arrythmmia, and artery spasm.

**Best practical omega-3 sources** include canola oil and margarine, soybean oil and fish.

**A balanced intake** of the two omega classes is important for optimal health. For most Americans, slightly increasing omega-3 intake would help attain a more ideal balance.

**Trans fats** from hydrogenated vegetable oils and shortenings should also be avoided. They are common in commercial baked and fried food products such as cakes, muffins, pastries, doughnuts, fried snacks and french fries.

> Note: All fats are high in calories and need to be limited for weight control.

## DIETARY FATS COMPARISON

■ Saturated Fat  ■ Monounsaturated Fat
Polyunsaturated Fats:
■ Linoleic (Omega-6)  ■ Alpha-Linolenic (Omega-3)

### OILS — PERCENTAGE CONTENT

| Oil | Saturated Fat | Monounsaturated Fat | Linoleic (Omega-6) | Alpha-Linolenic (Omega-3) |
|---|---|---|---|---|
| CANOLA OIL | 7 | 63 | 20 | 10 |
| LINSEED/FLAX OIL | 9 | 19 | 17 | 55 |
| SAFFLOWER OIL | 9 | 14 | 77 | |
| GRAPESEED OIL | 10 | 22 | 68 | |
| SUNFLOWER OIL | 11 | 23 | 66 | |
| CORN OIL | 14 | 32 | 52 | 2 |
| OLIVE OIL | 14 | 76 | 10 | |
| SOYBEAN OIL | 15 | 23 | 54 | 8 |
| PEANUT OIL | 19 | 45 | 34 | 2 |
| COTTONSEED OIL | 26 | 16 | 58 | |
| PALM OIL | 51 | 39 | 10 | |

### SPREADS & FATS

Saturated Fat includes 'Trans Fats'    ☐ WATER CONTENT

| Spread/Fat | Saturated Fat | Monounsaturated Fat | Linoleic (Omega-6) | Alpha-Linolenic (Omega-3) | Water Content |
|---|---|---|---|---|---|
| LIGHT MARGARINE | 14 | 14 | 21 | | 51 |
| CANOLA MARGARINE | 18 | 45 | 12 | 6 | 19 |
| POLYUNSATURATED MARG | 24 | 20 | 36 | | 20 |
| BUTTER | 57 | 18 | 2 | | 24 |
| LARD | 41 | 47 | | | 12 |
| BEEF FAT | 44 | 37 | 4 | | 15 |

## GOOD SOURCES OF OMEGA-3 FATS

| Plant Sources | Omega-3 Fats (Grams) |
|---|---|
| Canola Oil, 1 Tbsp, ½ fl.oz | 1.5g |
| Flaxseed Oil, 1 Tbsp | 8g |
| Soybean Oil, 1 Tbsp | 1.2g |
| Canola Margarine, 1 Tbsp, ½ oz | 1g |
| Soybeans, cooked, ½ cup, 4 oz | 0.5g |
| Walnuts, ½ oz | 0.5g |

**FISH** - *Per 4 oz Serving*

**High Content:** Salmon (Chinook), Tuna, Trout (Lake), Sardines, Herring, Mackerel — **3g**, **3g**

**Medium Content:**
Salmon, (Pink/Red/Coho), 4 oz — **2g**

**Fair Content:** *Per 4 oz Serving*
Bass, Catfish, Cod, Grouper, Hake, Halibut, Kingfish, Perch, Pollock, Shark, Trout (Rainbow), Tuna, Crab, Oysters, Blue Mussels, Shrimp, Squid — **0.5-1g**

## How Much Is Needed?

**As little as 1-2 grams daily of omega-3 fats** may benefit general health. High doses of fish-oil supplements should only be taken as directed by your doctor.

## Dietary Cholesterol

Cholesterol in food varies in its effect on blood cholesterol level (BCL) from person to person. Much depends on the amount and type of fat and fiber eaten at the same meal.

Any elevating effect of dietary cholesterol on BCL is more likely to occur when the diet is high in saturated fat. Little elevation, if any, generally occurs when dietary fats are balanced in favor of monounsaturated and polyunsaturated fats (including omega-3 fats).

For example, while fish does contain cholesterol, the omega-3 fats can prevent any increase in BCL. Conversely, a meal containing no cholesterol but rich in saturated fat may result in a significant increase in BCL.

**Consequently, the need to be overly concerned about dietary cholesterol is being de-emphasized in favor of the approach of limiting total fat, saturated fat, and trans fat in particular – and substituting unsaturated fats.**

The liver usually cuts back its own cholesterol production in response to cholesterol in the diet. Many people can consume normal amounts of high-cholesterol foods without concern.

However, it is difficult to identify just who is at risk - the so-called 'hyper-responders'. Because over 50% of Americans have a BCL above ideal levels, the **American Heart Association** advises all Americans to be prudent and limit their cholesterol intake to less than 300mg daily, as well as to adopt a heart-healthy diet.

This limitation still allows the inclusion of most foods that are regularly eaten – even the overly maligned egg.

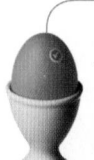

Eggs contain a modest 5 grams of fat per large egg. Barely 2 grams is saturated, the rest being monounsaturated or polyunsaturated.

By comparison, a cup of whole milk has 8g fat of which almost 5g is saturated.

## CHOLESTEROL COUNTER

Cholesterol is found only in foods of animal origin. Plant foods contain no cholesterol.

| | Cholesterol mg |
|---|---|
| **Meat** - Average all types: | |
| Lean Meat, cooked, 120g | 100 |
| Fatty Meat, cooked, 120g | 100 |
| Fat, thick strip, 60g | 40 |

*Note: While lean meat and fat have similar amounts of cholesterol, choose lean meat to limit fat intake.*

| | |
|---|---|
| **Chicken/Turkey,** average, 120g | 100 |
| **Organ Meats:** Liver, fried, 4 oz | 500 |
| Brains, beef, pan fried, 3 oz | 1700 |
| **Sausages:** Frankfurter, 40g | 25 |
| Salami, 2 slices, 55g | 40 |
| **Bacon:** 3 slices, cooked, 30g | 20 |
| **Fish:** Fish fillets, average, ckd, 120g | 70 |
| Tuna/Salmon, canned, 100g | 50 |
| Scallops, 9 medium, 3 oz | 30 |
| Prawns, raw, 100g | 110 |
| Oysters, raw, 6 medium, 85g | 45 |
| Crayfish, Crab, cooked, 100g | 70 |
| **Eggs** (Chicken), 1 large | 210 |
| 1 medium | 180 |
| Egg White, *Scramblers* | 0 |
| **Milk/Yoghurt:** Whole, 1 cup, 250ml | 30 |
| Light/low-fat Milk (1%), 1 cup | 10 |
| Skim/Non-fat, 1 cup | 10 |
| **Soy Milk, Tofu, Tempeh** | 0 |
| **Cheese:** Natural/Hard/Cream, 30g | 30 |
| Cottage, low-fat, 2 Tbsp, 40g | 5 |
| Cream Cheese, 30g | 25 |
| **Fats:** Butter, 1 Tbsp, 20g | 45 |
| Margarine, Oils (vegetable) | 0 |
| Mayonnaise, 1 Tbsp | 10 |
| **Cream:** Heavy, whipping, 2 Tbsp, 40g | 40 |
| Light/Sour, 2 Tbsp | 10 |
| **Ice Cream:** Full-fat (10-11%), 100ml/50g | 20 |
| Low-fat (less than 4%), 50g | 5 |
| **Fruit, Vegetables,** Avocados | 0 |
| **Nuts, Seeds, Grains** | 0 |
| **Coffee, Tea, Beer, Wine** | 0 |

*For Comprehensive Food Listings ~ see CalorieKing.com*

## DIETARY HINTS TO LOWER BLOOD CHOLESTEROL

**1. Maintain a healthy weight.**
If overweight, lose weight with a low-fat meal plan and daily exercise.

**2. Reduce saturated fat intake by:**
**(a) eating less dairy fat.** Choose low-fat or fat-reduced varieties of milk, yogurt, soy drinks, cheese, and ice cream.

**(b) replacing saturated fats** with fats and oils rich in monounsaturated and polyunsaturated fats. Choose vegetable oils such as canola, olive, sunflower and soybean. Avoid solid frying fats.

**Take Control and Benecol** (spreads) contain plant stanol esters which can lower total and LDL cholesterol.

**(c) eating less fat from meat and poultry**. Choose lean cuts of meat and skinless chicken. Go easy on lunch meats, salami and fatty sausages. Enjoy fish.

**(d) eating less saturated and trans fats** from baked and fried fast-foods. Avoid deep-fried foods. Avoid donuts, cakes, pastries and cookies unless made with healthier fats and oils.

**3. Increase your soluble fiber intake.**
Foods rich in soluble fiber include beans, lentils, chick peas, hummus, nuts, seeds, psyllium-seed husks and psyllium-fiber supplements. Oat bran, rice bran and barley are also good sources, as are fruit, veggies and avocados. (*See Fiber Guide - Page 264-269*).

**4. Eat more soy bean products** such as: soy drinks, tofu, tempeh (cultured soy beans), soy flour and soy vegetarian foods.
Soy protein in place of animal protein can significantly decrease high blood cholesterol levels as well as 'bad' LDL cholesterol and blood triglycerides while 'good' HDL cholesterol is maintained. For best results, eat at least 25g of soy protein per day (from 3-4 servings).

**5. Eat more fruit, vegetables, and whole grains** in place of high-fat foods. Aim for 2 fruits and 5 servings of vegetables per day. They also contain valuable antioxidants. The fat of avocados (and most nuts) is mainly unsaturated and can lower blood cholesterol levels.

**6. Limit cholesterol to 300mg per day.** (Extra Notes ~ See Previous Page)

**7. Avoid brewed unfiltered coffee** (espresso; plunger-style). Several cups per day may raise blood cholesterol. Filtered coffee is fine.

**8. Spread your food intake over the day.** Have 5-6 small meals per day rather than just 2-3 large meals. Nibbling, versus gorging, favors lower blood cholesterol.

## ALCOHOL – WINE

Alcohol is a mixed bag. Moderate amounts of 1-2 drinks daily appear to reduce the risk of heart attack and ischemic stroke in older persons.

However, larger amounts increase the risk of high blood pressure, obesity, heart failure and hemorrhagic stroke, and can aggravate hypertriglyceridemia: as well as many other health hazards. (*See Alcohol Guide – Page 23*)

The speculative benefits of moderate alcohol intake have been overstated in the media. The overriding harmful effects of excess alcohol do not allow its recommendation for any aspects of health promotion.

*Fruit, Vegetables & Tea Also Protect:*
**Red wine and red grapes (more so than white) contain antioxidants which may help protect cholesterol in the blood from becoming oxidized.**

**Many fruits, vegetables, grains, nuts and tea also contain protective antioxidants.**

Fats in the diet affect more than blood cholesterol levels. They can also strongly influence blood clot formation and thrombosis, as well as blood flow and ultimate oxygen delivery to body parts and organs.

While advanced atherosclerosis can impede blood flow to the heart and other organs, it is thrombosis (complete blockage by blood clots) or arterial spasm which commonly results in a heart attack or stroke.

**Plant and fish oils rich in omega-3 fats** lessen the risk of blood clots, thrombus formation, and artery spasm by reducing platelet stickiness and adhesion to artery walls. This reduces the risk of atherosclerotic plaque becoming unstable and reactive.

**Omega-3 fats also improve blood flow** by reducing blood viscosity and increasing the flexibility of red blood cells (RBC) that need to flex and twist on themselves in order to squeeze through tiny narrow capillaries often half their diameter.

**A diet high in saturated fats** has the opposite effect by stiffening RBC membranes and increasing blood viscosity, thereby hindering blood flow. The stiffening of the RBC membrane also reduces its ability to release vital oxygen to body cells and take up carbon dioxide.

Stiff red blood cells may also form aggregates that resemble coin stacks. In narrow blood vessels, this further impedes blood flow and impairs oxygen release through the much-lessened surface area of red blood cell membranes exposed to blood. (Smoking, lack of exercise, and stress can have similar adverse effects on thrombosis, red blood cell flexibility, and blood flow.).

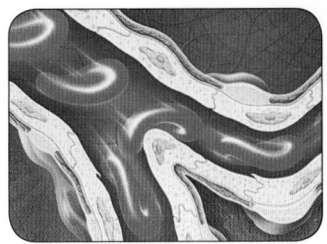

▲ **Picture of Healthy Blood Flow**

*Flexible red blood cells twist and slide through tiny capillaries - often half the diameter of red blood cells.*

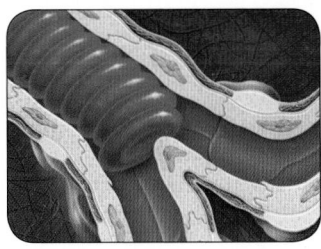

▲ **A Not-So-Healthy Picture!**

*Red blood cells have lost their flexibility and ability to twist and slip through capillaries. They are stacked up, thereby impeding blood flow.*

*A diet high in saturated fats can contribute to this picture - as can smoking, lack of exercise, and stress.*

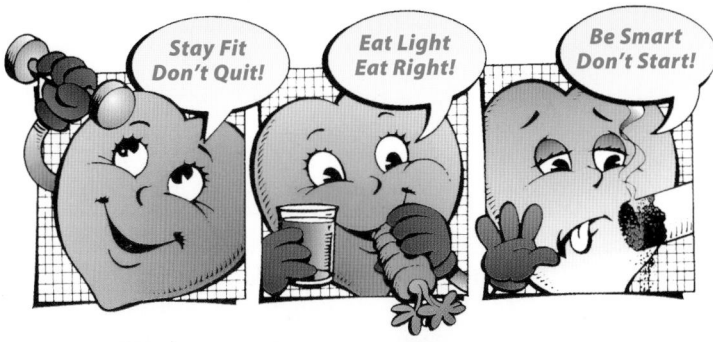

# Fiber Guide

## Introduction

`Fiber`

Fiber is the general term for those parts of plant food that we cannot digest (although bacteria in the large bowel partly digests fiber through fermentation). It is not found in foods of animal origin (meats, dairy products).

Fiber promotes intestinal health, bowel regularity, can benefit diabetes and blood cholesterol levels, and may help prevent colon cancer. High-fiber foods also assist weight control.

Most Americans don't eat enough fiber – less than 20 grams/day - instead of a healthier 25 to 35 grams/day.

## Types of Fiber

Plant foods contain a mixture of different fibers in varying proportions. Insoluble and soluble fiber categories are based on their solubility in water. All types of fiber are beneficial to the body.

◆ **Insoluble fibers** (cellulose, hemi-celluloses, lignin) make up the structural parts of plant cell walls.

> **Best food sources** are wheat bran, corn bran, rice bran, wholegrain cereals and breads, beans and peas, nuts, seeds, and the skins of fruits and vegetables.

These fibers absorb many times their own weight in water. They create a soft bulk and hasten the passage of waste products through the intestines.

**They promote bowel regularity,** and aid in the prevention and treatment of uncomplicated forms of **constipation, diverticulosis and hemorrhoids.**

**The risk of colon cancer** may also be reduced by fiber's diluting effect on potentially harmful substances.

◆ **Soluble fibers** (pectin, gums, mucilages) are found mainly within plant cells, soy milk (whole bean) and products.

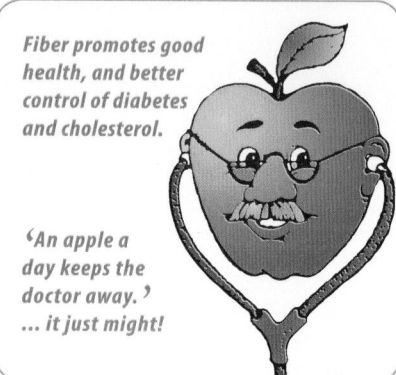

*Fiber promotes good health, and better control of diabetes and cholesterol.*

'*An apple a day keeps the doctor away.*'
... it just might!

## Types of Fiber (Cont)

**Best Sources of Soluble Fiber:**
Fruits and vegetables, oat bran, barley, beans and peas, prunes, psyllium and flax seed.

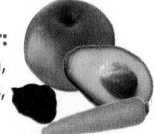

These fibers form a gel which slows both stomach emptying and the absorption of sugars from the intestines. **This helps to control blood sugar levels.**

**Weight control** is also aided by the slower emptying of the stomach and the feeling of **fullness provided by soluble fiber.**

Some soluble fibers can lower **blood cholesterol** by binding bile acids and excreting them. More body cholesterol must then be broken down to supply bile acids for emulsification of dietary fats. **Rice bran, while not high in soluble fiber, can also lower blood cholesterol.**

◆ **Resistant starch** is that part of starchy foods (approx. 10%) which is tightly bound by fiber and resists normal digestion. Friendly bacteria in the large bowel ferment and change the resistant starch into short-chain fatty acids, which are important to bowel health and may protect against colon cancer.

Starchy foods include bread, cereals, rice, pasta, potatoes and legumes.

# Fiber Guide

## Fiber & Weight Control

**Fiber can assist weight control** in several ways. Fiber-rich foods such as fresh fruit and vegetables, potatoes and wholegrain bread contain few calories for their large volume (due to their low-fat, high-water content).

**Their bulk fills the stomach** and satisfies the appetite much sooner than fiber-depleted foods. The extra chewing time also contributes to satiety, and gives the stomach time to register a feeling of fullness. Excessive calories are less likely to be consumed.

**Fiber-depleted foods and drinks** are more concentrated in calories; e.g. fats, sugar, candy, soft drinks, fruit juices, alcohol. They require little or no chewing. Large amounts with excessive calories can be consumed before the appetite is satisfied.

**Example:** Whereas one fresh apple might satisfy the appetite, an apple juice drink with the equivalent sugars and calories of 2-3 apples only minimally satisfies the appetite. (See illustration below.)

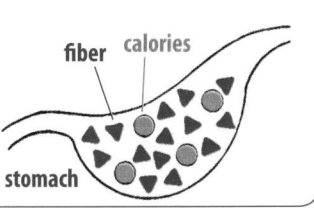

**High-fiber foods fill the stomach. Fewer calories are consumed.**

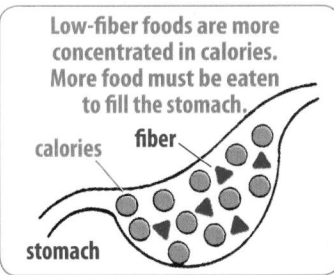

**Low-fiber foods are more concentrated in calories. More food must be eaten to fill the stomach.**

## EFFECTS OF REMOVING FIBER FROM FOOD

**2-3 pieces of fresh fruit produces 1 glass of fruit juice. The removal of fiber concentrates the sugar and calories.**

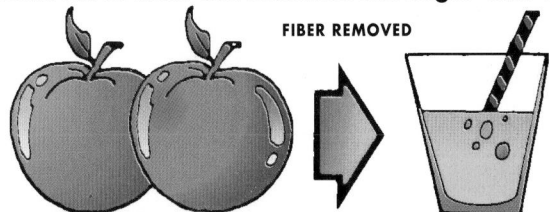

FIBER REMOVED

| Fresh Fruit | | Fruit Juice |
|---|---|---|
| High Fiber | ← | Negligible Fiber |
| Low Calorie Density | ← | High Calorie Density |
| Long Eating Time | ← | No Eating Time (Drink) |
| Satisfies Hunger | ← | Does Not Satisfy Hunger |
| Sugar Slowly Absorbed | ← | Sugar More Quickly Absorbed |
| Less Insulin Required | ← | More Insulin Required |

# Fiber Guide ~ Constipation

## Constipation

**Constipation** can reasonably be defined as a failure to have a bowel movement at least every second day – and just as importantly, without straining or pain.

Typically, constipated stools are too hard, too narrow and too small.

The **main cause** is simply a lack of dietary fiber. Other contributing factors include insufficient fluids, too little exercise, emotional stress, gastrointestinal disease, lack of proper dentition to chew high-fiber foods, and some medications (e.g. some antacids, antidepressants, pain medications).

**Note:** Check with your doctor to rule out any underlying medical problem – especially if you have a change in bowel habits in middle-age or later years.

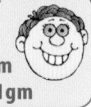

### DESIRABLE FIBER INTAKE

**Adults: 25-35gm per day**
**Children (under 18): Age + 5gm**
**Example: 6-year old (6 + 5)= 11gm**

### SAMPLE FOOD QUANTITIES
For 35 Grams of Fiber/Day

| | Fiber |
|---|---|
| Breakfast Cereal (higher-fiber) | 5g |
| **plus** 4 slices wholegrain Bread | 6g |
| **plus** 3 servings fresh Fruit | 9g |
| **plus** 1 medium Potato (w. skin) | |
| **or** 1 cup Brown Rice | 4g |
| **or** ½ cup wholegrain Pasta | |
| **plus** 3-4 servings Veggies/Salad | 6g |
| **plus** 1 cup Bean Soup | |
| **or** ¼ cup Baked/Soy Beans | |
| **or** ½ cup Corn/Peas/Lentils | 5g |
| **or** 1¼ oz Almonds (natural) | |
| **or** 3 medium Figs | |

## HINTS TO INCREASE FIBER AND AVOID CONSTIPATION

**①** **Breakfast is an important** contributor to daily fiber intake. Eat high-fiber breakfast cereals (bran-based cereals, oatmeal etc.). Add 1-2 tablespoons of unprocessed bran.

Dried fruits, chopped nuts, soy grits, and seeds are also excellent additions to cereals.

*Note:* A gradual increase in fiber will prevent bloating, gas or pain. People intolerant to bran may benefit from psyllium-based fiber supplements and cereals.

**②** **Drink adequate water daily.** Fiber works by absorbing many times its own weight in water.

**③** **Eat wholegrain breads,** or fiber-enriched breads. They have over double the fiber of regular white bread.

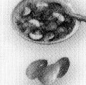

**④** **Enjoy fruit as fresh fruit** with skin rather than as fruit juice. Enjoy wholegrain pasta, barley, brown rice, nuts and seeds.

**⑤** **Eat more vegetables,** salads and legumes – especially cooked beans, lentils, potatoes with skins, avocado, broccoli, brussels sprouts, cabbage, carrots, celery, and peas.

**⑥** **Add bran** (barley/rice/wheat) or soy grits to soups, casseroles, yogurt, desserts, cookies, cakes. Also use whole-meal flour or soy flour in place of white flour. Use nuts, seeds, and ground linseed.

**⑦** **Snack** on fresh or dried fruits, carrot or celery sticks, popcorn, nuts or seeds, wholegrain crackers, high-fiber bars (low-fat). Limit amounts if overweight.

**⑧** **Exercise regularly** to strengthen abdominal muscles and stimulate the gut. Keep up water intake, especially in warm weather.

**⑨** **Avoid** indiscriminate and regular use of harsh laxatives. They can overstimulate the intestinal muscles and may make normal bowel activity impossible. It may take several weeks to restore normal bowel function.

> **FOODS WITH ZERO FIBER**
> - **Dairy Products (Milk, Cheese, etc)**
> - **Meats, Poultry, Fish, Eggs**
> - **Fats/Oils, Sugar/Syrups**
>
> (Only foods of plant origin contain fiber.)

## Breakfast Cereals

| | Fiber |
|---|---|
| ***General Mills:*** | |
| Basic 4, 1 cup, 2 oz | 3 |
| Cheerios (Honey Nut; Multigrain), 1 c., 1 oz | 2 |
| Fiber One, ½ cup, 1.1 oz | 14 |
| Multi-Bran Chex, 1 cup, 2 oz | 7 |
| Oatmeal Crisp Almond, 1 cup, 2 oz | 4 |
| Raisin Nut Bran, 1¼ cup, 2 oz | 6 |
| Total, average all types, ¾ cup, 1 oz | 3 |
| Wheat Chex, 1 cup, 2 oz | 6 |
| Wheaties ¾ cup, 1 oz | 3 |
| ***Health Valley:*** | |
| Amaranth Flakes, ¾ cup, 1 oz | 3 |
| Crunches & Flakes, ¾ cup, 1.9 oz | 4 |
| Fiber 7 Flakes, ¾ cup, 1 oz | 7 |
| Golden Flax, ¾ cup, 1.9 oz | 6 |
| Granola (Low-Fat), ⅔ cup, 2 oz | 6 |
| Healthy Fiber Flakes, ¾ cup, 1.1 oz | 4 |
| Oat Bran Flakes, all types, ¾ cup, 1 oz | 2 |
| Oat Bran O's, ¾ cup, 1 oz | 3 |
| Real Oat Bran, ½ cup, 1.7 oz | 5 |
| ***Kellogg's:*** All-Bran, ½ cup, 1.1 oz | 10 |
| All-Bran w. Extra Fiber, ½ cup, 1 oz | 13 |
| All-Bran Bran Buds, ⅓ cup, 1.1 oz | 13 |
| Corn Flakes, Fruit Loops, Smacks 1 cup, 1 oz | 1 |
| Cocoa/Rice Krispies Treats, 1¼ cup, 1 oz | 0 |
| Complete: Wheat Flakes, ¾ c., 1 oz | 5 |
| Oat Bran Flakes, ¾ cup, 1.1 oz | 4 |
| Corn Pops, 1 cup, 1.1 oz | 0 |
| Cracklin' Oat Bran, ¾ cup, 1.7oz | 6 |
| FiberPlus Antioxidants: | |
| Berry Yogurt Crunch, 1 c., 1.9 oz | 10 |
| Cinnamon Oat Crunch ¾ c., 1.1 oz | 9 |
| Frosted Mini Wheats, 24 bisc., 2 oz | 5 |
| Granola w. Raisins, ⅔ cup, 2.1 oz | 3 |
| Raisin Bran, 1 cup, 2.1 oz | 7 |
| Smart Start, Strong Heart, Cinnamon Raisin, 1 cup, 1.8 oz | 4 |
| Special K, 1 cup, 1.1 oz | 0.5 |

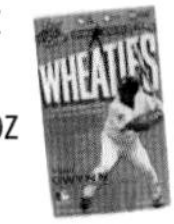

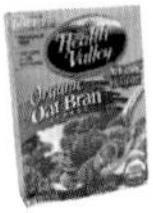

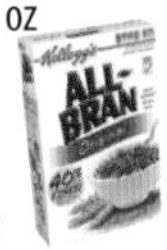

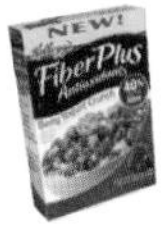

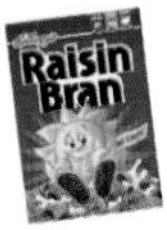

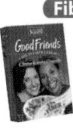

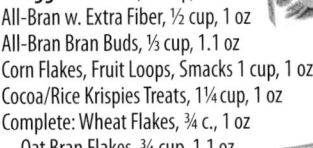

**Fiber** ~ Fiber (grams)

## Breakfast Cereals (Cont)

| | Fiber |
|---|---|
| ***Kashi:*** GoLEAN Cereal, 1 cup, 1.8 oz | 10 |
| GoLEAN Crunch!, 1 cup, 1.9 oz | 8 |
| GoLEAN Bars, avg. (1) | 6 |
| Good Friends: Original, 1 cup, 1.9 oz | 12 |
| Cinna-Raisin Crunch, 1 cup, 1.8 oz | 8 |
| Heart to Heart, ¾ cup, 1.2 oz | 5 |
| 7 Whole Grain Pilaf, ½ cup, cooked, 5 oz | 7 |
| 7 Whole Grain Puffs, 1 cup, 0.7 oz | 1 |
| ***Quaker:*** Cap'n Crunch, ¾ cup, 1 oz | 1 |
| 100% Natural Granola, avg., ½ cup, 1.8 oz | 3 |
| Crunchy Corn Bran, 1 cup, 1 oz | 5 |
| Life Cereal, ¾ cup, 1.1 oz | 2 |
| Oat Bran, ½ cup, 1.4 oz | 6 |
| Oatmeal, average, 1 packet | 3 |
| ***Post:*** 100% Bran, ⅓ cup, 1 oz | 9 |
| Alpha Bits, 1 cup, 1 oz | 2 |
| Blueberry Morning, 1 cup, 1.9 oz | 5 |
| Cocoa/Fruity Pebbles, 1 cup, 1 oz | 0 |
| Cranberry Almond Crunch, 1 cup, 1.8 oz | 3 |
| Fruit & Bran, 1 cup, 1.9 oz | 6 |
| Grape-Nuts, ½ cup, 2 oz | 7 |
| Great Grains, ⅔ cup, 1.9 oz | 5 |
| Honey Bunches of Oats, ¾ cup, 1.1 oz | 2 |
| Shredded Wheat & Bran, ½ cup, 2 oz | 8 |

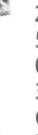

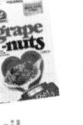

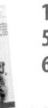

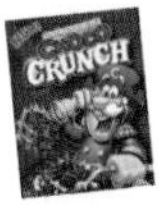

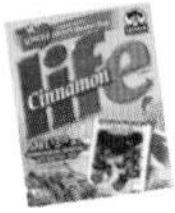

## Brans & Supplements, Metamucil

| | Fiber |
|---|---|
| **Oat Bran:** 1 Tbsp (level) | 1 |
| ⅓ cup, (5⅓ Tbsp), 1 oz | 5 |
| **Rice Bran,** raw. ¼ cup, 1 oz | 6 |
| **Wheat Bran** (unprocessed): | |
| Raw, 1 Tbsp | 1.5 |
| 2 Tbsp (level), ¼ oz | 3 |
| ¼ cup, (4 Tbsp), ½ oz | 6 |
| **Wheat Germ:** Raw, ¼ cup, 1 oz | 4 |
| **Psyllium** Seed Husks, 2 Tbsp | 8 |
| ***Fibersure,*** 1 heaping tsp | 5 |
| ***Metamucil:*** Orange, 1 rnd Tbsp, 11g | 3 |
| Fiber Wafers (2) | 6 |

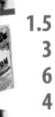

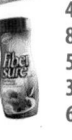

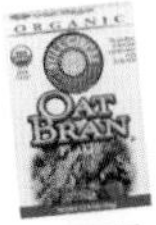

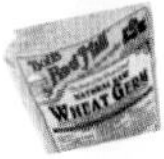

## Hot Cereals, Oatmeal

| | Fiber |
|---|---|
| Bulgur (cracked Wheat), ckd, 1 cup | 8 |
| Corn/Hominy Grits, dry, 3 Tbsp, 1 oz | 0.5 |
| Cream of Wheat, cooked, ¾ cup | 1 |
| **Oatmeal** (uncooked ⅓ cup), ckd, ⅔ cup | 3 |

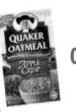

# Fiber Counter

## Breads & Crackers

| | Fiber |
|---|---|
| **Bread:** White, 1 slice, 1 oz | 0.6 |
| Whole-wheat, 1 slice, 1 oz | 1.5 |
| Wholegrain, 1 slice, 1 oz | 2 |
| Rye, Pumpernickel, 1 oz | 1.5 |
| Bagel/Roll/Bun, 1 medium, 2 oz | 1.5 |
| Pita, whole wheat, 6½" pocket | 4.5 |
| **Crackers:** Graham, average, 2 | 0.4 |
| Saltine, 4 crackers | 0.4 |
| **Crispbreads** (Rye), average, 2 | 4 |
| **Matzo** 1 board, 1 oz | 1 |
| **Rice Cakes,** average, 1 cake | 0.3 |
| **Tortilla:** Regular, 6" | 0.5 |
| Whole-wheat, 6" | 1.3 |

## Barley, Pasta, Rice & Flours

| | Fiber |
|---|---|
| **Barley,** pearled, raw, ¼ cup, 1.7 oz | 8 |
| **Rice:** White, cooked, 1 cup | 0.6 |
| Brown, cooked, 1 cup | 3.5 |
| *Rice-A-Roni,* average, 1 cup, prepared | 1.5 |
| **Spaghetti/Noodles:** Cooked, 1 cup | 2 |
| Whole-Wheat, cooked, 1 cup | 4 |
| **Flour:** Wheat, All-purpose, 1 cup, 4½ oz | 3.5 |
| Whole-Wheat, 1 cup, 4½ oz | 15 |
| Cornmeal, stone ground, 1 cup, 4½ oz | 13 |
| Carob Flour, 1 cup, 3½ oz | 41 |
| Rye Flour, 1 cup, 3½ oz | 15 |
| Soy Flour: Defatted, 1 cup, 3½ oz | 17 |
| Full-fat, raw, 1 cup, 3 oz | 8 |
| Soy Meal, defatted, 1 cup, 4½ oz | 14 |

## Frozen Entrees & Dinners

| | Fiber |
|---|---|
| ***Average All Brands:*** *Per Serving* | |
| Beans/Chili base, average | 6-10 |
| Potato/Pasta base, average | 4-6 |
| Vegetable base, average | 3 |
| Meat/Chicken base, average | 2-3 |
| **Pizzas,** ¼ large, average | 3 |
| **Vegetarian Soy Burgers,** 1 pattie | 4 |

## Soups

| | Fiber |
|---|---|
| Chicken Noodle, 1 cup | 0.5 |
| Tomato Soup, average, 1 cup | 0.5 |
| Vegetable Soup, average, 1 cup | 3 |
| ***Health Valley:*** *Per 1 Cup Serving* | |
| Black Bean; Minestrone | 8 |
| Tomato | 1 |
| 5-Bean Vegetable; Lentil & Carrots | 10 |
| Mushroom Barley; Vegetable | 4 |
| Split Pea | 8 |

## Fast Foods & Restaurants

| | Fiber |
|---|---|
| **Hamburgers:** Small, average | 1.5 |
| Large/Whopper, average | 2.5 |
| **Hot Dog,** Regular | 1.5 |
| **French Fries:** Small serving, 2½ oz | 2.5 |
| Regular/Medium, 3½ oz | 3.5 |
| **Chicken Nuggets,** 6 pack | 0.5 |
| **Chicken Sandwich,** average | 2 |
| **Taco,** average | 4 |
| **Sundaes, Shakes,** Soft Drinks | 0 |
| ***Arby's:*** Baked Potato w. Broc. & Cheese | 8 |
| Roast Beef Sandwich, regular | 2 |
| ***Denny's:*** Grilled Chicken Salad, no bread | 4 |
| Classic Burger, no fries | 4 |
| Club Sandwich, no fries | 2 |
| Grilled Chicken Sandwich, no fries | 4 |
| ***Domino's* (12"):** Classic/Thin, 1 slice | 1 |
| Deep Dish, 1 slice | 3 |
| Feast Pizza, Classic/Thin, 1 slice | 3 |
| ***McDonald's:*** Big Mac | 3 |
| Hamburger; Quarter Pounder | 1 |
| Egg McMuffin | 2 |
| Grilled Chicken Caesar Salad | 3 |
| ***Pizza Hut:*** *Per 1 Slice, Medium* | |
| Pan Pizza: Cheese, Pepperoni | 1 |
| Supreme | 2 |
| Thin 'n Crispy, Supreme | 2 |
| Hand-Tossed, average all varieties | 2 |
| ***Subway:*** Sandwich, white roll, av. | 4 |
| w. Honey Wheat Roll, average | 3.2 |
| Salads, average | 4 |

## Cakes, Cookies, Snack Bars

| | Fiber |
|---|---|
| **Apple/Fruit Pie,** 1 serving, 4 oz | 2 |
| **Cake:** w. plain flour, 1 serving, 3.4 oz | 1.5 |
| w. whole-wheat flour, 1 serving | 3 |
| **Carrot Cake,** 4 oz | 4 |
| **Cookies,** oatmeal, (3 small/1 large) | 1 |
| **Donuts,** Medium, 1.7 oz | 0.7 |
| **Fruit Cake,** 1 serving, 1½ oz | 2 |
| **Fig Bars,** 1 cookie, ½ oz | 0.7 |
| **Muffins,** Oat Bran (2 small, 1 large), 4 oz | 5 |
| **Granola Bars,** average, 1 bar | 2 |
| *Atkins Advantage Bars,* average | 7 |
| *Clif Bars,* 2.5 oz | 5 |
| *Curves,* Chocolate Peanut Bar, 25g | 5 |
| *Fi-Bar Chewy & Nutty* 1 bar | 1 |
| *Fiber One* (Gen. Mills), 1.4 oz bar | 9 |
| *FiberPlus,* all bars, 1.2 oz | 9 |
| *Health Valley:* Fruit/Granola Bars | 3 |
| Cereal Bars | 1 |
| *Luna Bars,* avg., 1.7 oz | 3 |
| *Special K,* Protein Meal Bar, 1.6 oz | 5 |

## Chocolate, Chips, Popcorn | Fiber

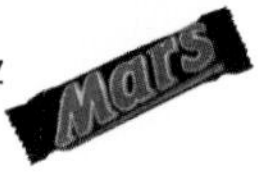

| | |
|---|---|
| **Cheese Balls/Curls/Twists** | 1 |
| **Chocolate, Hard Candy,** 1 oz | 0 |
| **Chocolate with nuts/fruit,** 2 oz bar | 1.5 |
| *Mars Bar,* 1.8 oz | 1 |
| **Potato Chips, corn chips,** 1 oz | 1 |
| **Popcorn,** 3 cups | 3 |
| **Pretzels,** Twists (6) | 1 |

## Nuts, Seeds

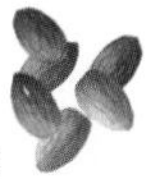

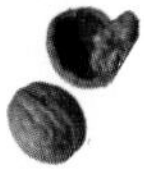

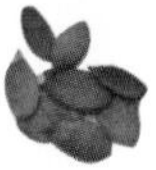

| | |
|---|---|
| **Almonds:** Natural, 25 nuts, 1 oz | 3.5 |
| Blanched (skins removed), 1 oz | 3 |
| **Cashews,** Filberts, Pecans, 1 oz | 1.7 |
| **Peanuts,** Mixed Nuts, Coconut, 1 oz | 2.5 |
| **Peanut Butter,** 2 Tbsp, 1 oz | 2 |
| **Pistachio Nuts,** dried, shelled, 1 oz | 3 |
| **Walnuts,** Black/English, dried, 1 oz | 2 |
| **Seeds:** Amaranth, 2½ Tbsp, 1 oz | 3.5 |
| Flax Seeds, 3 Tbsp, 1 oz | 7 |
| Psyllium Seed Husks, 5 Tbsp, 1 oz | 20 |
| Quinoa Seeds, 3 Tbsp, 1 oz | 1.7 |
| Sesame Seeds, whole, 1 oz | 3.4 |
| Sesame Butter/Tahini, 2 Tbsp, 1.1 oz | 1.4 |
| Sunflower kernels, ¼ cup, 1 oz | 3.8 |
| Teff Seeds, 1 oz | 3.8 |

## Fruit – Fresh

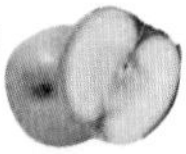

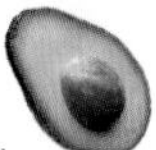

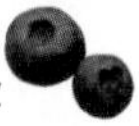

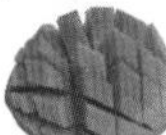

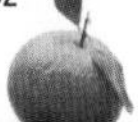

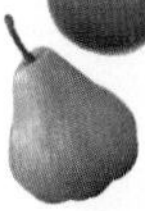

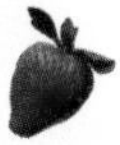

| | |
|---|---|
| **Apples:** 1 medium, 5½ oz (whole) | |
| with skin + core | 3.7 |
| with skin, no core | 3.2 |
| without skin, no core | 1.7 |
| **Apricots,** 2 medium, 4 oz | 1.5 |
| **Avocado,** average, ½ medium | 6.7 |
| **Banana,** 1 medium, 6 oz (w. skin) | 3 |
| **Blueberries,** raw, ½ cup, 2½ oz | 1.7 |
| **Cherries,** sweet, raw, 8 fruits, 1.6 oz | 1 |
| **Grapefruit,** average, ½ fruit, 10 oz | 1.4 |
| **Grapes,** 1 medium bunch, seedless, 7 oz | 2 |
| **Kiwifruit,** 1 medium, 2.7 oz | 2.3 |
| **Mango,** 1 medium, 11 oz (whole) | 1.6 |
| **Melons,** Cantaloupe, 4 oz (edible) | 1 |
| **Nectarine,** 1 medium, 4 oz | 1.9 |
| **Olives,** average all types, 7 jumbo, 2 oz | 1.5 |
| **Oranges,** 1 medium (7-8 oz w. skin) | |
| 5½ oz (peeled) | 3.8 |
| **Passionfruit,** 2 medium, 2½ oz | 5 |
| **Peaches,** 1 large, 6 oz | 2 |
| **Pears,** raw, 1 medium, 6 oz | 4.5 |
| **Pineapple,** 1 slice, 3 oz | 1.2 |
| **Plums,** 2 medium, 6 oz | 1.8 |
| **Strawberries,** 6 medium/3 large, 2 oz | 1 |
| **Watermelon,** 4 oz (edible) | 0.5 |

## Fruit – Dried, Juice | Fiber

| | |
|---|---|
| **Dried Fruit:** Apricots, 8 halves, 1 oz | 2.2 |
| Dates (3 med); Raisins (2 Tbsp), 1 oz | 1.5 |
| Figs, 3 medium,1½ oz | 5 |
| Prunes, 4 medium, 1 oz | 2 |
| **Fruit Juice:** Orange/Apple etc, 1 glass | <0.5 |
| Prune Juice, 5 oz | 1.4 |
| Carrot Juice, 8 oz | 1.8 |

## Vegetables

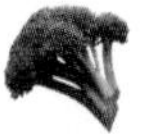

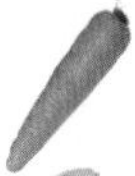

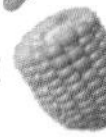

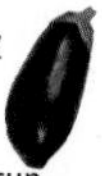

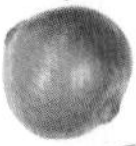

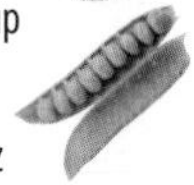

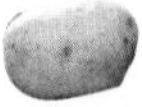

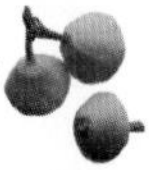

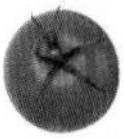

| | |
|---|---|
| **Asparagus,** 4 medium spears | 1.3 |
| **Bean Sprouts,** ½ cup, 2 oz | 1 |
| **Beans:** Snap/Green, ½ cup, 2 oz | 2 |
| Baked Beans in Tom Sce, ½ c, 4½ oz | 5 |
| Dried Beans, ckd, average, ½ cup | 7 |
| **Beets,** ckd, slices, ½ cup, 3 oz | 1.7 |
| **Broccoli,** cooked, ½ cup, 3 oz | 2.4 |
| **Brussels Sprouts,** ckd, ½ cup, 3 oz | 3.5 |
| **Cabbage:** White, ckd, ½ cup, 2½ oz | 1 |
| Red, ckd, ½ cup, 2½ oz | 2 |
| **Carrots,** 1 medium (7½"), ½ cup, 3 oz | 2.5 |
| **Cauliflower,** cooked, 3 flowerets, 2 oz | 1.5 |
| **Celery,** raw, diced, 1 cup, 3½ oz | 1.6 |
| **Chick Peas** (Garbanzos), ckd, ½ c., 3 oz | 6.5 |
| **Corn:** Kernels, cooked, ½ cup, 2½ oz | 2.5 |
| Corn on the Cob, 1 ear, 5 oz | 4 |
| **Cucumber/Lettuce/Mushrooms,** 2 oz | 0.5 |
| **Eggplant,** raw, sliced, ½ cup , 1½ oz | 2 |
| **Lentils,** cooked, ½ cup, 3½ oz | 8 |
| **Mixed Vegetables,** frozen, cooked, ½ cup | 3 |
| **Onions,** Raw, 1 medium, 4 oz | 1.5 |
| Spring Onions, chop., ¼ cup, 1 oz | 0.7 |
| **Peas:** Green, Raw, 2½ oz | 3.7 |
| Cowpeas (Black-eyed), ckd, ½ cup | 10 |
| Split Peas, ckd, ½ cup, 3½ oz | 8 |
| **Peppers,** sweet, raw, 1 large, 6 oz | 3 |
| **Potatoes:** 1 medium, with skin, 5 oz | 4 |
| without skin | 2.5 |
| ½ cup mashed, 3½ oz | 1.5 |
| French Fries, small, 2.6 oz | 3 |
| **Spinach,** cooked, ½ cup, 3 oz | 2.2 |
| **Squash:** Summer, cooked, ½ cup, 3 oz | 2.5 |
| Winter, cooked, ½ cup, 3½ oz | 2.4 |
| **Tomatoes:** 1 medium, 4½ oz | 1.5 |
| Tomato Sauce, 1 cup | 0.3 |
| **Soybean Products:** Miso, ½ c., 5 oz | 7.4 |
| Tempeh, cooked, 1 piece, 3 oz | 2 |
| Tofu, ½ cup, 4.4 oz | 0.4 |
| **Salads: Side Salad,** average | 1 |
| **Bean Salad,** ½ cup | 5 |
| **Coleslaw,** ½ cup | 1 |
| **Potato Salad,** ½ cup | 2 |

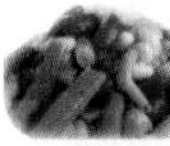

# Protein Guide

## General Notes

- **Protein has many important body functions.** It builds and repairs muscle, and is the basis of our body's organs, hormones, enzymes, and antibodies to fight infection.

- **Protein is also an emergency fuel** in the absence of sufficient carbohydrate and fats. For this reason, weight loss should be gradual so as to preserve protein levels in muscle, the heart and other body organs.

- **It is easy to obtain sufficient protein,** even if vegetarian. **Plant proteins are not inferior to animal proteins.** In fact, eating more soy and other plant proteins, and less animal protein, may help to build stronger bones and prevent osteoporosis, and may help to control blood cholesterol levels.

- **When changing to a vegetarian diet,** include soybeans, and other beans, soy milk drinks (calcium-enriched), lentils, tofu, tempeh, nuts and wholegrain breads and cereals. Milk, yogurt, cheese and eggs can enhance nutrient intake.

## Protein & Muscle

- Although muscles are built of protein, protein is not a special fuel for working muscle cells – carbohydrates and fats are.

- In fact, a diet high in protein (and fat) and low in carbohydrate can significantly reduce the performance of endurance sports athletes. **Carbohydrates** are the best fuel for muscles exercised for long periods.

- Any **extra protein** required by athletes and body-builders can easily be obtained from the extra food eaten to satisfy hunger and energy needs.

- Remember, **excessive protein** intake will not build bigger muscles. Any excess is converted and stored as fat. Excess protein can also strain the kidneys, which excrete the waste products of protein metabolism.

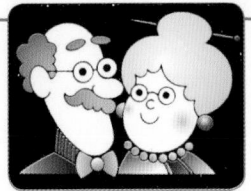

Elderly people (and dieters) must eat sufficient food to ensure adequate protein intake.

Inadequate protein leads to a drop in immune response with greater susceptibility to illness and infections. Muscle strength and muscle mass also drop.

Protein needs are easily met with sensible eating. Athletes who eat enough food for their energy needs can obtain sufficient protein.

### RECOMMENDED DAILY PROTEIN INTAKE ~ HEALTHY RANGE ~
(Lower figure is RDA)

| | | PROTEIN |
|---|---|---|
| Children: | 1-3 yrs | 13g-26g |
| | 4-8 yrs | 19g-38g |
| | 9-13 yrs | 34g-64g |
| Males: | 14-18 yrs | 52g-120g |
| | 19+ | 56g-120g |
| Females: | 14+ | 46g-110g |
| Pregnancy: | | 71g-120g |
| Breastfeeding: | | 71g-120g |

**Note:** On lower-calorie diets, aim for higher amounts of protein within the Healthy Range.

## Pro ~ Protein (grams)

### Meat

| | Pro |
|---|---|
| **Steak:** *Average all cuts, lean (no fat)* | |
| Small (4 oz raw/3 oz ckd) | 23 |
| Medium (6 oz raw/4¼ oz ckd) | 34 |
| Large (10 oz raw/7¼ oz ckd) | 57 |
| **Roast Beef,** lean, 2 slices, 3 oz | 24 |
| **Ground Beef patty,** lean, ckd, 3 oz | 21 |
| **Lamb chop,** broiled, 3 oz | 22 |
| **Liver,** cooked, 3 oz | 23 |
| **Veal cutlet,** 1 medium | 23 |
| **Pork,** cooked, lean, 3 oz | 24 |
| Bacon, 3 medium slices | 6 |
| **Ham,** roasted, 2 pieces, 3 oz | 18 |
| **Ham, luncheon,** 2 slices, 1½ oz | 7 |
| **Pastrami** *(Oscar Mayer),* 3 sl., 1¾ oz | 10 |
| **Sausages:** Bologna, 2 sl., 2 oz | 7 |
| Braunschweiger, 2 sl., 2 oz | 8 |
| Pork link, thick, 2 oz | 6 |
| Frankfurter, 1⅓ oz | 5 |
| Salami, hard, 3 slices, 1 oz | 7 |
| **Vegetarian** *(Boca Burger),* 1 pattie | 13 |
| **Chicken/Turkey:** *Without Skin* | |
| **Chicken,** ckd; Breast, Roasted, 4 oz | 36 |
| Leg/Thigh,Roasted, 2 oz | 14 |
| ½ Whole Chicken | 60 |
| Drumstick, Rstd, 1 med., 3 oz | 13 |
| **Turkey,** cooked: Light meat, 3 oz | 28 |
| Dark meat, lean, 3 oz | 24 |

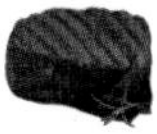

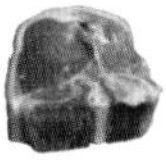

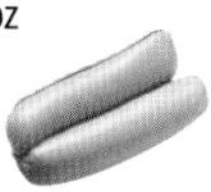

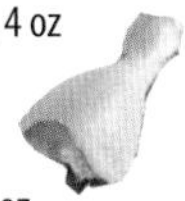

### Fish

| | Pro |
|---|---|
| **Fresh Fish:** *Per 4 oz, cooked* | |
| Cod, Flounder/Sole, Pollock | 28 |
| Catfish, Haddock, Halibut, M/Mahi | 28 |
| Ocean Perch, Swordf., Orange Roughy | 28 |
| **Canned Fish:** Tuna, Light, 3 oz | 25 |
| White, 3 oz | 23 |
| Salmon, pink, 3 oz | 17 |
| Salmon, red, 3 oz | 17 |
| Sardines, 3 whole (3"), 1¼ oz | 9 |
| Anchovies, 1 can, 1½ oz | 13 |
| **Shellfish:** Crabmeat, 3 oz | 17.5 |
| Clams, raw, 4 large/9 sml, 3 oz | 11 |
| Crayfish, cooked, 3 oz | 20 |
| Lobster, cooked, 3 oz | 17 |
| Oysters, raw, 6 medium, 3 oz | 7 |
| Scallops, 2 lge/5 small, 1 oz | 5 |
| Shrimp, raw, 6 large, 1½ oz | 8.5 |
| **Fish Products:** Fish Sticks, 4 sticks | 10 |
| Fish Portions, in batter, 4 oz | 13 |
| Gefilte Fish, 1 medium ball, 2 oz | 8 |

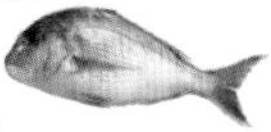

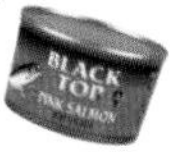

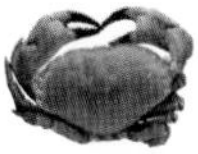

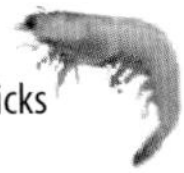

### Eggs

| | Pro |
|---|---|
| **1 Large Egg,** whole | 6 |
| Egg Yolk | 3 |
| Egg White | 3 |
| **Omelet:** Plain, 2 eggs | 13 |
| Ham & cheese | 17 |
| **Egg Substitutes** (liquid): | |
| *Egg Beaters,* ¼ cup, 2 oz | 4.5 |
| *Better 'n Eggs/Scramblers,* ¼ cup, 2 oz | 6 |

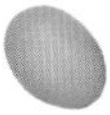

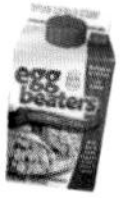

### Milk, Yogurt, Ice Cream

| | Pro |
|---|---|
| **Milk:** Whole: 2%, 1 cup | 8 |
| Low-Fat (1%); Fat-Free, 1 cup | 8.5 |
| **Chocolate Milk,** 1 cup | 8 |
| **Thick Shake,** Chocolate, 10 oz | 9 |
| Vanilla, 10 oz | 11 |
| **Soymilk** (fortified), average, 1 cup | 7 |
| *Soy Dream* Enriched, shelf-stable, 1 cup | 7 |
| **Yogurt:** Plain, 6 oz | 10 |
| Fruit flavors: 6 oz | 8 |
| 8 oz | 11 |
| **Ice** Cream: Rich, ½ cup | 2 |
| Regular, Vanilla, ½ cup | 2.5 |
| **Sherbet,** ½ cup | 1 |
| **Custard,** baked, ½ cup | 7 |

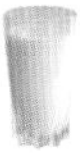

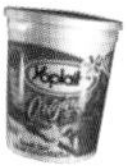

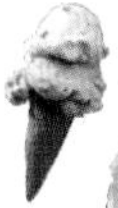

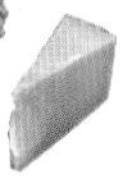

### Cheese

| | Pro |
|---|---|
| **Hard Cheeses,** average, 1 oz | 7 |
| **Cottage Cheese,** ½ cup | 13 |
| **Cream Cheese,** avg., 1 oz | 2 |
| **Ricotta,** part skim, ½ cup | 14 |

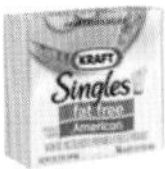

### Bread, Bagels, Biscuits

| | Pro |
|---|---|
| **Bread** (w. enriched flour): 1 slice, 1 oz | 2 |
| 4 thin slices, 4 oz | 8 |
| 4 thick slices, 6 oz | 1.2 |
| **Bagel,** plain 2 oz | 6 |
| **Biscuits,** 1 oz | 2 |
| **Pita Bread,** 1 pita, 1½ oz | 4 |
| **Pumpernickel,** 1 slice, 1 oz | 3 |

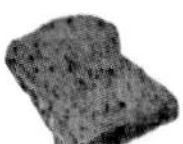

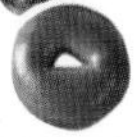

### Infant/Baby Foods

| | Pro |
|---|---|
| **Infant Formula Milk:** | |
| *Enfamil/Gerber/Similac* | |
| Regular/Low Iron , 5 fl.oz | 2.2 |
| With Iron, 5 fl.oz | 2.2 |
| *Isomil/Nursoy/ProSobee* | 3 |
| **Baby Cereals:** | |
| *Average all brands* | |
| Dry, 4 Tbsp, ½ oz | 1 |
| Jars (w. fruit), 4½ oz | 1 |

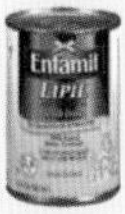

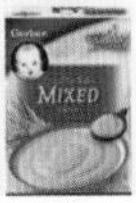

# Protein Counter

## Breakfast Cereals `Pro`

**Hot Cereals, cooked:**

| | |
|---|---|
| **Bulgur,** cooked, 1 cup, 5 oz | 9 |
| **Oatmeal:** Reg., non-fortified, 1 cup | 6 |
| Instant, fortified, avg., 1 pkt | 4 |
| *Quaker,* all flavors, ½ cup | 5 |
| **Corn/Hominy Grits:** 1 cup | 3 |
| *Quaker:* Reg., 3 Tbsp, 1 oz | 2 |
| Instant White, 1 packet | 2 |
| **Cream of Wheat,** 1 cup | 4 |

**Brands ~ Ready-To-Eat**

| | |
|---|---|
| *Arrowhead:* Average all varieties, 1 oz | 3 |
| *General Mills:* Basic 4, 1 cup, 2 oz | 4 |
| Cheerios, Original, 1 cup, 1 oz | 3 |
| Cocoa Puffs, 1 cup, 1 oz | 1 |
| Kix, 1⅓ cups, 1 oz | 2 |
| Multi-Bran Chex, 1 cup, 2 oz | 4 |
| Country Corn Flakes, 1 cup, 1.2 oz | 2 |
| Total Raisin Bran, 1 cup, 2 oz | 3 |
| Wheaties ¾ cup, 1 oz | 3 |
| *Health Valley:* Oat Bran O's, ¾ cup, 1 oz | 3 |
| Amaranth Flakes, ¾ cup, 1 oz | 3 |
| Bran Flakes w. Raisins, ¾ cup, 1.1 oz | 5 |
| Low-Fat Granola, ⅔ cup, 2 oz | 5 |
| Real Oat Bran Alm. Crunch, ½ cup, 1.7 oz | 6 |
| Golden Flax, ¾ cup, 1.9 oz | 6 |
| *Kashi:* Friends, 1 cup, 1.9 oz | 5 |
| GoLean Crunch!, 1 cup, 1.9 oz | 9 |
| 7 Whole Grain Flakes, 1 c., 1.8 oz | 6 |
| *Kellogg's:* All-Bran: ½ cup, 1 oz | 4 |
| Complete Oat Flakes, ¾ c., 1.1 oz | 3 |
| Cocoa Krispies, ¾ cup, 1 oz | 1 |
| Corn Flakes, 1 cup, 1 oz | 2 |
| Low-fat Granola w. Raisins ⅔ c., 2.1 oz | 4 |
| Product 19, 1 cup, 1 oz | 2 |
| Raisin Bran, 1 cup, 2 oz | 7 |
| Rice Krispies, 1¼ cup, 1.2 oz | 2 |
| Smart-Start Healthy Heart, 1 c., 1.8 oz | 6 |
| Special K: Regular, 1 c., 1.1 oz | 6 |
| Protein Plus, ¾ cup, 1 oz | 10 |
| *Post:* Raisin Bran, ⅔ cup, 2 oz | 4 |
| Grape Nuts, ½ cup, 2 oz | 6 |
| *Quaker:* Crunchy Corn Bran, 1 cup, 1 oz | 2 |
| 100% Natural Granola, ½ cup, 1.7 oz | 5 |
| Life, ¾ cup, 1.1 oz | 3 |
| Cap'n Crunch, ¾ cup, 1 oz | 1 |
| Oat Bran, ½ cup, 1.4 oz | 7 |

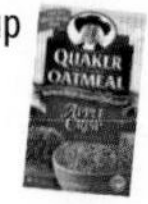

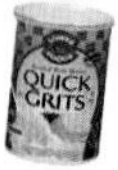

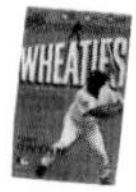

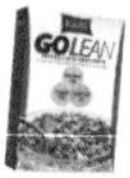

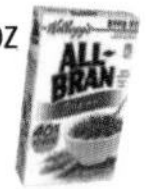

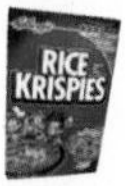

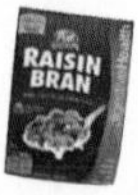

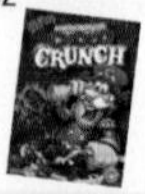

## Brans & Wheatgerm `Pro`

| | |
|---|---|
| **Oat Bran,** raw, 1 Tbsp | 2 |
| **Rice Bran,** raw, 2 Tbsp | 1 |
| **Wheat Bran,** unprocessed, 2 T. | 1 |
| **Wheat Germ,** 2 Tbsp, ½ oz | 4 |

## Grains & Flours, Yeast

| | |
|---|---|
| **Amaranth,** ½ cup, 3.4 oz | 14 |
| **Barley,** ½ cup, 3.2 oz | 12 |
| **Buckwheat Flour:** Whole-groat, 1 cup | 15 |
| **Carob Flour,** 1 cup, 3.6 oz | 5 |
| **Corn Flour,** 1 cup, 4 oz | 11 |
| **Corn Meal,** 1 cup, 4½ oz | 8 |
| **Flour:** White, 1 cup, 5.6 oz | 9 |
| Wholegrain, 1 cup, 4¼ oz | 16 |
| **Millet,** wholegrain, 1 cup, 3½ oz | 12 |
| **Rye Flour:** Dark, 1 cup, 4½ oz | 18 |
| Light, 1 cup, 3½ oz | 9 |
| **Soy Flour,** full fat, 1 cup, 3 oz | 29 |
| **Yeast:** Brewers, 2 Tbsp, ½ oz | 8 |
| Nutritional Yeast Flakes *(Red Star)*, 1 heaping Tbsp, ½ oz | 8 |

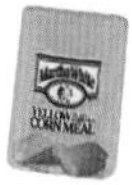

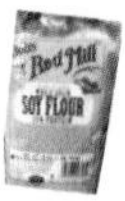

## Rice, Spaghetti, Macaroni

| | |
|---|---|
| **Rice:** Brown/White, average 1 cup cooked, 6½ oz | 5 |
| **Spaghetti/Macaroni/Noodles (enriched):** | |
| Cooked, 1 cup, 4½ oz | 7 |
| Canned: in Tomato Sce, ½ cup | 2 |
| w. Meatballs, 1 cup, 8 oz | 10 |
| Macaroni & Cheese, 1 cup, 9 oz | 8 |

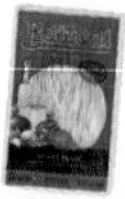

## Soups

| | |
|---|---|
| With Noodles/Vegetables, 1 cup | 3 |
| With Meat/Beans/Peas, 1 cup | 8 |

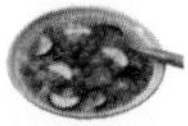

## Fruit

**Fresh/Canned:**

| | |
|---|---|
| Average, all types 1 medium/2 small fruit | 1 |
| **Avocado,** ½ medium | 2 |
| **Dried Fruit:** Apricots, 8 halves, 1 oz | 1 |
| Dates, 6 dates, 2 oz | 1.5 |
| Figs, 4 medium figs, 2 oz | 2 |
| Prunes, 5 medium, 1½ oz | 1 |
| Raisins, 1 oz | 1 |
| **Fruit Juice:** Average, 1 cup | 0.5 |
| Prune Juice, 6 fl.oz | 1 |
| Tomato Juice, 1 cup, 8 fl.oz | 1.5 |

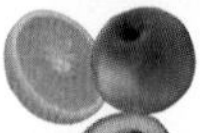

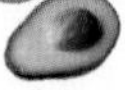

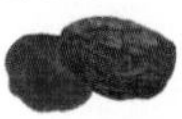

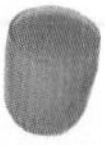

## Vegetables | Pro

**Beans:** Snap/green, ½ cup, 2 oz — 1
  Dried: Average all types, cooked, ½ cup — 7
  Baked Beans, ½ cup 4½ oz — 5
**Bean Sprouts,** mung, 1 c., 4 oz — 3
**Broccoli,** 3raw, ½ cup, 1½ oz — 1.5
**Cabbage; Cauliflower,** raw, 1 c. 3 oz — 1.5
**Corn,** raw, ½ cup kernels, 3 oz — 2.5
  1 ear trimmed to 3½" — 2
**Lentils,** cooked, ½ cup, 3½ oz — 9
**Mushrooms,** raw, ½ c., sliced — 1
**Peas:** Green, raw, ½ c., 2½ oz — 4
  Split Peas, cooked, 1 cup, 7 oz — 16
**Potatoes,** cooked:
  1 medium, with skin, 5 oz — 3.3
    without skin, 4 oz — 2.3
  French Fries, small, 2.6 oz — 2
**Potato Salad,** ½ cup, 4 oz — 3.5
**Pumpkin,** ½ cup mashed, 4.3 oz — 1
**Seaweed,** kelp, 1 oz — <1
**Spinach,** cooked, ½ cup, 3 oz — 2.7
**Squash,** ckd, all types, ½ cup — 1
**Tomatoes,** 1 medium, 4½ oz — 1
**Vegetables,** mixed, ckd, 1 cup — 2.5
**Soybeans,** cooked, ½ cup, 3 oz — 14

### Tofu, Tempeh, Miso

Tofu, raw, firm, ½ cup, 4½ oz — 10
Tempeh, ½ cup, 3 oz — 16
Miso, ½ cup, 5 oz — 16
Miso Soup, 1 cup — 3
**Soybean Protein** (TVP), 1 oz — 18

### Cakes, Pastries, Pies

(Made with enriched flour)
Carrot w. cream cheese frosting, 4 oz — 4
Cheesecake, 1 piece, 4 oz — 6
Chocolate, 1 piece, 2 oz — 2
Fruitcake, 1 piece, 3 oz — 4
Plain, 1 piece, 3 oz — 4
**Croissant,** plain, 2 oz — 5
**Danish Pastry,** 1 pastry, 2¼ oz — 4
**Donuts,** average, 2 oz — 4
**Muffins,** average, 1 med., 1½ oz — 3
**Pancakes,** 4" diam., two, 2 oz — 4
**Pies:** Fruit, 1 piece, 5½ oz — 4
  Pecan, 1 piece, 5 oz — 7
**Puddings,** average, ½ cup, 4½ oz — 4
**Waffles,** 1 large, 2½ oz — 7

## Peanut Butter | Pro

**Regular:** 2 Tbsp, 1.1 oz — 8
  *Peter Pan* Plus, 2 Tbsp, 1.1 oz — 8

### Sugar, Honey, Jam

**Sugar:** White — 0
  Brown, 1 Tbsp — 0
**Molasses:** Light/Med., 1 Tbsp — 0
  Blackstrap, 1 Tbsp, ¾ oz — 0
**Corn Syrup,** 1 Tbsp, ¾ oz — 0
**Honey, Jams, Jelly** — 0

### Candy, Chocolate, Carob

**Candy,** sugar-based — 0
**Chocolate:** Plain, 2 oz bar — 4
  with nuts, 2 oz bar — 6
**Carob,** plain, 2 oz — 6

### Cookies, Crackers, Chips

**Cookies,** average, 4 cookies — 2
**Crackers,** Graham, 2½" sq., (2) — 1
**Rice Cakes,** average, one — 1
**Corn/Potato Chips,** 1 oz — 2
**Nuts:** Almonds, shelled, 20-25 nuts — 6
Brazil Nuts, 7-8 medium nuts, 1 oz — 4
Cashews, 12-16 nuts, 1 oz — 5
Macadamias, 1 oz — 2
Peanuts, dry rsted, 40 nuts, 1 oz — 6
Pecans, 24 halves, 1 oz — 2
Walnuts, 15 halves, 1 oz — 4
**Seeds:** Sesame Seeds, dry, 1 Tbsp — 2
Pumpkin Kernels, dry, hulled, 1 oz — 7
Sunflower Seeds, dried, hulled, 1 oz — 6
Tahini, 1 Tbsp, ½ oz — 2.5

### Granola & Food/Protein Bars

**Granola Bars,** avg., 1 bar, 2 oz — 2
*Anytime Health,*
  Meal Bars, 80g — 20
  Snack Bars, 50g — 12
*Balance* Bars, Orig. 1.76 oz — 14
*Bariatrix* Proti-Bars (1), 1.4 oz — 15
*Dr Soy* Protein Bars, 1.76 oz — 11
*GeniSoy* Protein Bar, 1.6 oz — 15
*Jenny Craig* Bars, 1.8 oz — 4
*Met-Rx* "Big 100", 3.5 oz — 27
*Myoplex Carb Sense* Bar, 2.5 oz — 26
*Optifast* Peanut Butter, 1.59 oz — 8
*PowerBar:* Harvest — 10
  Performance Bar, 2.3 oz — 10
  ProteinPlus, 1 bar, avg., 2.75 oz — 24
*Slim-Fast:* High Protein Meal, 1.7 oz — 15
  Optima Meal, 2 oz bar — 8
*Special K*: Protein Meal, 1.6 oz — 10
  Protein Snack, 0.9 oz — 4

# Protein Counter

## High Protein Drinks    **Pro**

*Anytime* Health:
| | |
|---|---:|
| Whey Protein Isolate, All flavors, 1 oz | 25 |
| *Atkins* Shakes, 11 fl.oz can | 18 |
| *Boost* High Protein, 8 oz | 10 |
| *Carnation* Instant Breakfast, 10 oz | 13 |
| *Curves* Protein Drink, 2 scoops, dry | 15 |
| *dotFIT:* FirstString, 4 scoops, 5.2 oz | 42 |
| Meal Replacement, Chocolate, 2 scoops, 2.2 oz | 20 |
| WheySmooth, Choc., 2 scoops, 2.2 oz | 40 |
| *Ensure* Plus, 8 oz can | 13 |
| *Gatorade:* Nutrition Shake, 11 oz | 20 |
| Protein Recovery Shake, 11 oz | 20 |
| *GeniSoy* Shake, 1 scoop, 1.2 oz | 14 |
| *Kashi GoLean Shake,* 2 sc., 2.1 oz | 21 |
| *Met-Rx* RTD 40 | 40 |
| *Myoplex,* Original Nutrition Shake, 1 pkt | 42 |
| *Optifast 800,* made up, 8 fl oz | 14 |
| *Resource (Novartis)* Standard, 8 fl.oz | 15 |
| *Slim-Fast Shakes:* Meal, 11 oz can | 10 |
| High Protein, 11 oz can | 15 |
| Optima, 11 oz can | 10 |
| *Special K₂0* Protein Water, 16 fl.oz | 5 |
| *Walgreens* Slim For Less, 11 oz can | 10 |
| *Weider* Mass 1000, 4 scoops, 7 oz | 34 |

## Coffee, Tea, Soda
| | |
|---|---:|
| **Coffee, Coffee Substitutes,** 1 cup, 8 fl.oz | 0 |
| Coffee w. 2 oz milk, 1 cup, 8 fl.oz | 2 |
| Caffe latte, large, 16 fl.oz | 12 |
| Cappuccino, large, 16 fl.oz | 8 |
| Frappuccino, avg., 16 fl.oz | 6 |
| **Hot Chocolate,** with milk, 1 cup, 8 fl.oz | 8 |
| **Soft Drinks/Soda** | 0 |
| **Tea** (all types) | 0 |

## Beer, Wine, Spirits
| | |
|---|---:|
| Beer, 12 fl.oz | 1 |
| Wines, red/white, 1 glass | 0 |
| Spirits/Liquor | 0 |

## Fast-Foods/Burgers
| | |
|---|---:|
| **Pancakes:** Average all outlets, 3 | 8 |
| **Shakes,** Chocolate, 16 fl.oz | 12 |
| **Sundaes:** Average all outlets | 7 |
| *Arby's:* Roast Beef Sandwich, regular | 20 |
| Chicken Club Salad | 32 |
| Roast Beef Sandwich, Super | 21 |
| *Burger King:* Whopper S/wich | 29 |
| Bacon Double Cheeseburger | 32 |
| BK Big Fish Sandwich | 24 |

## Fast Foods/Burgers (Cont)    **Pro**

*Carl's Jr:*
| | |
|---|---:|
| Famous Star Hamburger w/ Cheese | 27 |
| Charbroiled Chicken Club Sandwich | 39 |
| Super Star Hamburger w/ Cheese | 47 |
| *Domino's Pizza:* Deep Dish (12") | |
| Beef, 2 slices | 10 |
| Cheese, 2 slices | 12 |
| Pepperoni, Sausage, 1 sl. | 10 |
| *KFC:* Original, Breast | 42 |
| Crispy Strips, 3 strips | 33 |
| Snacker, Regular | 15 |
| *McDonald's:* Big Mac | 25 |
| Cheeseburger | 15 |
| Chicken McNuggets (6) | 14 |
| Crispy Chicken Classic Burger | 28 |
| Filet-O-Fish | 15 |
| Hamburger | 12 |
| Quarter Pounder w. Cheese | 29 |
| French Fries: Small, 2.5 oz | 3 |
| Large, 5.4 oz | 6 |
| Salads w. Chicken, average | 30 |
| Triple Shake, average, 16 fl.oz | 16 |
| **Breakfast:** Egg McMuffin | 18 |
| Bacon, Egg & Cheese McGriddles | 15 |
| Sausage Burrito | 12 |
| Sausage McMuffin w. Egg | 21 |
| *Pizza Hut:* Per Medium, 1 slice, ⅛ Pizza | |
| Thin 'n Crispy, Supreme | 10 |
| Pan Pizzas, average | 11 |
| Hand Tossed, Pepperoni | 10 |
| Fit n' Delicious, Ham/Pineapple/Tomato | 7 |
| *Subway* (6" Subs): Roast Beef | 26 |
| Meatball Marinara | 24 |
| Roast Chicken Breast | 23 |
| Subway Club | 26 |
| Sweet Onion Chicken Teriyaki | 26 |
| *Taco Bell:* Bean Burrito | 12 |
| Chicken Quesadilla | 28 |
| Chicken/Steak Enchirito | 21 |
| Gordita Baja Beef | 13 |
| Steak Burrito Supreme | 18 |
| Taco Supreme | 11 |
| *Wendy's:* ¼ lb Single Burger | 27 |
| Chicken Club | 37 |
| Jr Hamburger | 13 |

## High Blood Pressure

**Many American adults** have hypertension (high blood pressure), and are unaware of it. It is generally symptomless, so **have your blood pressure checked annually** – particularly if it runs in the family.

**Untreated hypertension** overworks the heart, damages arteries and promotes atherosclerosis. This in turn greatly increases the risk of heart disease, stroke, blindness, kidney disease and impotence. The earlier hypertension is detected, the sooner it can be brought under control.

### BLOOD PRESSURE CLASSIFICATION

*For Adults Age 18 & Older ~ Not Acutely ill or on Medication (American Heart Association)*

|  | **DIASTOLIC** |  | **SYSTOLIC** |
|---|---|---|---|
| Normal ➤ | Below 80 | and | Below 120 |
| Prehypertension ➤ | 80-89 | or | 120-139 |
| **Hypertension:** | | | |
| Stage 1 ➤ | 90-99 | or | 140-159 |
| Stage 2 ➤ | 100 or more | or | 160 or more |

## Treating Hypertension

**Prehypertension** (in the chart above) means you don't have high blood pressure now but are likely to develop it in the future.

**You can take steps to lessen the risk by adopting healthy lifestyle habits such as:**
  • reducing sodium intake
  • eating adequate fruit and vegetables
  • losing weight if overweight
  • limiting alcohol to 2 drinks or less daily
  • quitting smoking
  • exercising regularly, managing stress.

**Stage 1 hypertension** can often be treated with the above lifestyle changes.

**Stage 2 hypertension** usually requires drug therapy. However, salt restriction, abstaining from alcohol, and the above lifestyle changes will improve the success of drug therapy, and enable smaller drug doses to be prescribed.

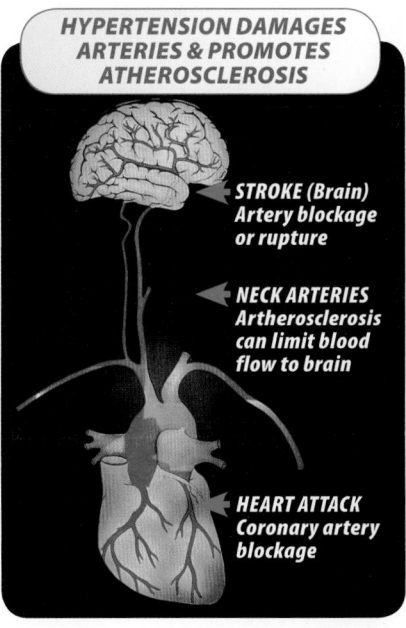

**HYPERTENSION DAMAGES ARTERIES & PROMOTES ATHEROSCLEROSIS**

**STROKE (Brain)**
**Artery blockage or rupture**

**NECK ARTERIES**
**Artherosclerosis can limit blood flow to brain**

**HEART ATTACK**
**Coronary artery blockage**

### STROKE
#### KNOW THE WARNING SIGNS

**Stroke is a medical emergency! If you notice one or more of these signs, call 9-1-1 or your doctor immediately.**

These signs may be signalling a possible stroke or transient ischemic attack:

• **Sudden weakness** or numbness in your face, arm, or leg on one side of your body

• **Sudden confusion,** trouble speaking or understanding

• **Sudden trouble seeing,** in one or both eyes

• **Sudden trouble walking,** dizziness, loss of balance or coordination

• **Sudden severe headache** - 'a bolt out of the blue' – with no apparent cause

# Salt & Sodium Guide

## Salt & Sodium

- **Sodium is a mineral element** most commonly found in salt (sodium chloride). It also occurs naturally in much smaller amounts in animal and plant foods, and water – normally sufficient for our needs without having to add salt to our diet.

- **Sodium is required** for nerve and muscle function, as well as to balance the amount of fluid in our tissues and blood.
  Sodium acts like a sponge to attract and hold fluids in body tissues.

- **Excess sodium** can cause water retention, and increase the risk of developing hyper-tension. Very high salt intake may also increase the risk of stomach cancer.

- **Too little sodium** may cause low blood pressure (hypotension), and decrease blood flow to the heart, brain and kidneys – especially during exercise. (A certain blood volume is required to sustain the blood pressure needed for adequate blood flow in the capillaries).

## Salt-Sensitive Persons

- **Normally, our kidneys** excrete excess dietary sodium. The thirst we feel after a salty meal is the body calling for water to dilute the sodium, and enable the kidneys to flush out excess sodium.

- **However, 'salt - sensitive'** persons (up to 70% of adults) tend to retain excess sodium (above approximately 3000mg daily) instead of excreting it. Such persons are more likely to develop hypertension and would benefit most from sodium restriction. Assume you are susceptible if there is a family history of hypertension.

- **Although not everyone will benefit, all Americans are being asked to moderate their salt and sodium intake** as a public health measure – particularly because so many do not know whether or not they have hypertension, and also because we do not know just who is salt-sensitive.

### SAFE SODIUM LEVELS

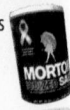
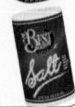

The American Heart Association recommends a **maximum sodium intake of 1500mg per day** for adults with normal blood pressure.

**Persons with hypertension** and kidney ailments are usually restricted to as little as **1000mg sodium per day**. Your doctor will discuss the correct sodium level for you.

### FINDING HIDDEN SODIUM

On average, **less than one third of our sodium intake comes from the salt shaker.**
The rest is hidden in processed foods that have salt added during manufacture.

Sodium compounds added to food or medicinals can also contribute significant sodium.

**Sodium bicarbonate** in particular is widely used in antacid tablets (such as *Alka Seltzer*) and powders. Sodium bicarbonate contains 27% sodium by weight. Each gram contributes 270mg sodium. Large amounts of sodium can be unwittingly consumed – up to 600mg per tablet. (See Antacids ~ Page 280)

**Example:** 2 *Alka-Seltzer* Tablets = 1000mg sodium

**Other sodium compounds** include monosodium glutamate (MSG), sodium ascorbate, sodium nitrite, and sodium citrate.

### POTASSIUM BALANCES SODIUM

Potassium helps to balance sodium by helping the kidneys to excrete excess sodium. Fruit and vegetables are rich sources of potassium - another reason to ensure you have your 5-7 servings every day.

Nuts also provide potassium as well as magnesium and other heart-healthy nutrients and anti-oxidants. Eat them unsalted.

*Note: This info is only for people with normal kidney function. Also not for persons on potassium-sparing diuretics.*

### ALCOHOL DANGER

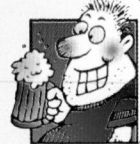

*Excessive alcohol intake contributes to hypertension. Susceptible persons should limit alcohol intake to 1-2 drinks per day.*

Sodium accounts for only 40% of the weight of salt (sodium chloride). Examples:
**1 gram (1000mg) Salt has 400mg Sodium**
**1 teaspoon (5g) Salt has 2000mg Sodium**

## HINTS TO REDUCE SODIUM

- **Cut down use of the salt shaker.** Start with an easy 50% cut in sodium by using Lite Salt (*Morton*) or *Cardia* Salt. Then gradually cut back until you can leave the salt shaker off the table. Sea salt is still high in sodium.

- **Use fresh herbs,** and salt-free seasonings to add flavor to food.

- **Choose low-sodium,** sodium-free, and reduced-sodium products in place of regular, salted products.

- **Check food labels for sodium levels.** FDA Guidelines for sodium descriptors are:
  - **Reduced Sodium:** At least 25% less sodium than the original product
  - **Low Sodium:** 140 mg or less/serving
  - **Very Low Sodium:** 35mg or less/serving
  - **Sodium Free:** Less than 5mg/serving
  - **No Salt Added:** Made without the salt normally added, but still contains the sodium that is a natural part of the food

- **Use reduced-sodium breads,** butter and margarine. Regular varieties are considered high in sodium in view of their significant contribution to our diet.

- **Go easy on salty condiments and sauces** such as ketchup, mustard, soy sauce, spaghetti sauces, and salad dressings. Use low-sodium varieties.

- **Limit pizzas and salty fast-foods.** Check the *CalorieKing.com* food database.

- **Avoid salty snack foods** such as potato chips, corn chips, salted nuts, pretzels and cheesy-flavored snacks. **Choose unsalted** popcorn, nuts or seeds. Eat more fruit.

- **Don't salt children's food** to your taste.

- **Avoid antacids with** sodium bicarbonate (such as *Alka-Seltzer*). They are high in sodium. Look for low-sodium alternatives.

### FOODS HIGH IN SODIUM

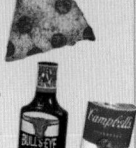

- Cheese, Butter, Margarine
- Pickles, Sauerkraut, Olives
- Condiments, Sauces
- Salad Dressings
- Canned vegetables/salads/beans
- Deli Salads (with dressing)
- Frozen/Packaged Meals/Entrees
- Soups: Canned/dry; bouillon cubes
- Meats: Ham, bacon, sausage, luncheon meats, smoked meats
- Canned Fish (in brine/salt)
- Sea Salt, Garlic/Celery Salt
- Snack Foods (potato chips, pretzels)
- Tomato Juice (Canned), V8 Vegetable Juice
- Fast Foods: Pizza, Burgers, Chicken
- *Alka-Seltzer* Antacid
- Bread (regular)

### MODERATE SODIUM

- **Meat, Fish, Poultry - Unprocessed**
- **Milk, Yogurt, Soy Drinks, Eggs**
- **Peanut Butter**
- **Breakfast Cereals** (less than 200mg/serving)
- **Chocolate Candy, Fruit/Nut Bars**
- *Reduced Sodium & Low Sodium* Products

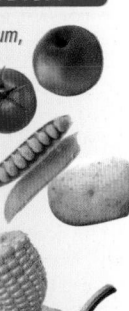

### FOODS LOW IN SODIUM

- Products labelled *Very Low Sodium*, or *Sodium Free*
- Bread (No Salt Added)
- Fresh fruits and vegetables
- Canned and Dried Fruits
- Potatoes, Rice, Pasta
- Dried Beans & Lentils, Tofu
- Nuts & Seeds (unsalted)
- Corn & Popcorn (unsalted)
- Pepper, Spices, Herbs
- Jam, Honey, Syrup
- Candy, Gum
- Hard & Jelly Candy
- Coffee, Tea, Alcohol
- Fresh Fruit Juices, Water

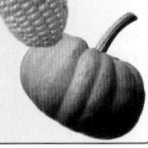

# Sodium Counter

**Sodium** ~ Sodium (mg)

## Milk & Dairy Products

| | Sodium |
|---|---|
| **Milk:** Whole/lowfat/skim, average | |
| 1 cup, 8 fl.oz | 120 |
| Whole, low sodium, 1 cup | 5 |
| **Choc Milk,** 1 cup | 130 |
| **Soy Milk,** 8 fl.oz | 30 |
| **Buttermilk,** cultured, 8 fl.oz | 250 |
| **Dry/Powder,** skim, ¼ cup, 1 oz | 110 |
| **Yogurt,** with fruit average, 8 oz | 130 |
| **Cheese:** Bleu, 1 oz | 330 |
| Parmesan, 1 oz | 450 |
| *Kraft* Cheddar, 2% milk, 1 oz | 230 |
| *Philadelphia* Cream Cheese, 1 oz | 90 |
| Process Cheese., average,1 oz | 430 |
| Swiss, 1 oz | 40 |
| Cottage Cheese, ½ cup, 4 oz | 450 |
| Ricotta Cheese, ½ cup, 4 oz | 150 |

## Ice Cream, Frozen Yogurt

| | |
|---|---|
| Icecream, average, ½ cup | 50 |
| Frozen Yogurt, ½ cup | 50 |

## Fats/Oils

| | |
|---|---|
| **Butter/Margarine:** | |
| Regular, 2 Tbsp, 1 oz | 230 |
| Unsalted, reg., 2 Tbsp, 1 oz | 5 |
| **Mayonnaise,** aver., 2 Tbsp, 1 oz | 160 |
| **Oils/Lard/Drippings** | 0 |
| **Cream,** average, 1 Tbsp | 5 |
| *Coffee-Mate:* Powdered, 1 tsp | 2 |
| Liquid, 1 Tbsp | 5 |

## Eggs

| | |
|---|---|
| **Whole,** 1 large | 70 |
| **Omelet,** 2 egg, plain | 220 |
| w. cheese | 400 |
| *Egg Beaters:* Original, ¼ cup | 115 |
| Flavors, average, ¼ cup | 230 |

## Meats

| | |
|---|---|
| **Meat,** average all types, cooked | |
| (Beef/Lamb/Veal/Pork), 4 oz | 80 |
| **Corned Beef,** cooked, 3 oz | 800 |
| **Bacon,** cooked, 2 sl., ½ oz | 270 |
| **Ham,** 3 oz | 1100 |

## Chicken & Turkey

| | |
|---|---|
| **Chicken/Turkey,** cooked, unsalted, 4 oz | 80 |
| **Stuffing Mixes,** average., ½ cup | 500 |
| *KFC ~ See Page 281 (Fast-Foods)* | |

## Sausages & Meats

| | Sodium |
|---|---|
| Bologna, 1 oz | 280 |
| Frankfurter, 2 oz | 640 |
| Ham, chopped, ¾ oz slice | 290 |
| Liverwurst (Braunschweiger), 1 oz | 320 |
| Pepperoni, 5 slices, 1 oz | 570 |
| Salami, cooked, 1 oz | 350 |
| dry/hard, 1 oz | 600 |
| Sausage, 1 oz link | 220 |
| Pork, 2 oz patty | 260 |
| *Spam:* Classic, 2 oz | 790 |
| 25% Less Sodium, 2 oz | 580 |
| Turkey Roll, 1 oz | 160 |

| **Fish:** Fresh Fish, average, plain | |
|---|---|
| Cooked, 4 oz (no bone) | 60 |
| Broiled w. butter, 4 oz | 150 |
| Breaded & fried, 4 oz | 320 |
| Fish fillets, batter-dipped 3 oz | 350 |
| Fish sticks, 1 oz stick | 160 |
| Gefilte Fish (w. broth), 1 pce, 1½ oz | 220 |
| Herring, pickled, 2 pces, 1 oz | 260 |
| Lobster, meat only, 4 oz | 180 |
| Oysters, fresh, 6 med., 3 oz | 95 |
| **Salmon:** Canned, 3 oz | 460 |
| No Salt Added, 3 oz | 65 |
| **Smoked fish,** average, 3 oz | 650 |
| **Tuna:** Canned, regular, 3 oz | 330 |
| No Added Salt, 3 oz | 40 |
| Spicy Flavored, 5 oz can | 550 |

## Entrees & Meals

| | |
|---|---|
| **Frozen Meals,** average | 600-900 |
| *Lean Cuisine,* average | 700 |
| *Stouffer's,* average | 580 |
| **Dinners,** average | 900-1200 |
| **Side Dishes,** average | 400-600 |
| **Pizza,** frozen, ¼ large, 6 oz | 800-1200 |
| **Microwave** Cup Meals | 900-1200 |
| **Cup O'Noodles,** average | 1500 |

*Pizza ~ See Page 281 (Pizza Hut)*

**More Sodium Counts:**
**www.CalorieKing.com**

## Soups

**Sodium**

| | |
|---|---|
| **Condensed,** average, 1 cup, 8 oz | 800-1000 |
| Low Sodium, average | 70 |
| **Chicken Noodle,** average, 1 cup | 900 |
| **Bouillon Cube,** average | 950 |
| **Ramen Noodle Soup,** av., 3 oz pkg | 1500 |
| **Soup Cups,** average | 850 |
| **Soup Mixes,** average, 1 cup | 900 |

### Condiments, Sauces, Dressings

| | |
|---|---|
| **A-1 Sauce,** 1 Tbsp | 280 |
| **Barbecue** Sauce, 1 Tbsp | 130 |
| **Bragg's** Liquid Aminos, 1 tsp | 220 |
| **Chili Sauce,** 1 Tbsp | 230 |
| **Ketchup:** Tomato, 1 Tbsp | 180 |
| Low Sodium, 1 Tbsp | 20 |
| **Mayonnaise,** 1 Tbsp | 80 |
| **Mustard,** 1 tsp | 70 |
| **Pizza Sauce,** ½ cup | 700 |
| **Salad Dressings,** 2 Tbsp, 1 oz | 160-400 |
| **Spaghetti Sauce,** ½ cup | 500 |
| **Soy Sauce:** 1 Tbsp | 900 |
| Lite *(Kikkoman)*, 1 Tbsp | 600 |
| **Sweet & Sour,** ½ cup | 250 |
| **Tabasco,** 1 tsp | 25 |
| **Vinegar,** Lemon Juice | 0 |
| **Worcestershire,** 1 Tbsp | 200 |
| **Tomato:** Sauce, 1 cup | 1200 |
| Paste/Puree (salted), ½ cup | 1000 |
| No Salt Added, ½ cup | 25 |

### Salt & Salt Substitutes

| | |
|---|---|
| **Table Salt:** 1 teaspoon, 6g | 2400 |
| Single Serve package, 1 g | 400 |
| *Cardia Salt,* 1 teaspoon | 1080 |
| **Lite Salt** *(Morton)*, 1 teaspoon, 6g | 1200 |
| *Morton/No Salt* **Substitute, 1 tsp** | 5 |
| **Garlic/Onion/Seasoned Salt,** 1 tsp, 4g | 1350 |
| **Garlic/Seasoned Salt** 1 teaspoon, 4g | 1300 |
| **Sea Salt,** 1 teaspoon, 5g | 2250 |

### Seasonings, Herbs & Spices

| | |
|---|---|
| Baking Powder, 1 tsp, 3g | 340 |
| Baking Soda (Sodium bicarb), 1 tsp, 3g | 810 |
| *Accent* (Flavor Enhancer), 1 tsp | 600 |
| Chili Powder, 1 tsp, 3g | 25 |
| Curry Powder | 0 |
| Lemon Pepper *(Lawry's)*, 1 tsp | 340 |
| Meat Tenderizer, 1 tsp, 5g | 1750 |
| MSG (Monosodium glutamate), 5g | 500 |
| *Mrs Dash* Blends/Marinades | 0 |
| *Old Bay,* Seasoning (Less Sodium), 1 teaspoon, 2.4g | 380 |
| Pepper, Mustard (dry), 1 tsp | 1 |
| Yeast, Nutritional, 1 Tbsp | 10 |

## Breakfast Cereals

**Sodium**

**Kellogg's:**

| | |
|---|---|
| All-Bran, ½ cup, 1 oz | 80 |
| Special K, 1 cup, 1.1 oz | 220 |
| Corn Flakes, 1 cup, 1 oz | 200 |
| Just Right, ¾ cup, 2 oz | 240 |
| Mini Wheats Frosted, 24 bisc., 1.8 oz | 5 |
| *Health Valley Cereals,* 1 serving | 5 |
| *Quaker:* Cap'n Crunch, ¾ cup, 1 oz | 200 |
| Crunchy Corn Bran, ¾ cup, 1 oz | 230 |
| 100% Natural Granola, ½ cup, 1 oz | 15 |
| Puffed Rice/Wheat, 2 cups, 1 oz | 1 |
| *General Mills:* Total, ¾ cup, 1 oz | 190 |
| **Oatmeal:** Regular, ¾ cup | 1 |
| Instant *(Quaker)*, ⅔ cup (1 pkt) | 270 |

### Breads, Bagels, Crackers

| | |
|---|---|
| **Bread:** Thin Slice, average 1 oz | 140 |
| Thick Slice, 1½ oz | 210 |
| Low Sodium, 1 oz | 10 |
| **Bagels:** Plain, medium, 2 oz | 200 |
| Large, take-out, average, 4 oz | 550 |
| *Sara Lee,* 3.4 oz | 500 |
| **Biscuits,** average, 1 oz | 180 |
| **Bun/Roll:** 1 medium, 1½ oz | 200 |
| Large, 4 oz | 560 |
| **Crackers:** Saltine, 2 crackers | 70 |
| Low Salt *(Premium)*, 2 | 25 |
| Graham, 2 regular | 50 |
| **Croissant,** Plain, average, 2 oz | 280 |
| **Rice Cakes,** average | 25 |
| **Ritz Crackers,** Low-Sodium, 1 oz | 60 |
| **Ry-Krisp** Crispbread, Sesame, 2 | 100 |

### Cookies, Cakes, Desserts

| | |
|---|---|
| **Cookies:** Average, 2-3 cookies, 1 oz | 100 |
| Average, 2½ oz | 180 |
| **Baked Custard,** ½ cup | 100 |
| **Brownie,** 1½ oz | 130 |
| **Carrot Cake,** 8 oz | 650 |
| **Cheesecake,** 7 oz | 350 |
| **Cinnamon Sweet Roll,** 2 oz | 250 |
| **Danish,** Apple/Fruit | 250 |
| **Donut,** average | 150 |
| **Muffins:** 1 medium, 2 oz | 150 |
| 1 extra large, 4 oz | 300 |
| **Pancakes,** (4"), x 3 | 360 |
| **Fruit Pies,** average, 7 oz | 600 |
| **Pudding:** Average, ½ cup | 160 |
| *Jell-O* (Mix), Instant, ½ cup | 400 |
| **Waffles:** Home-made, 7", 2½ oz | 350 |
| Frozen: Average, 1¼ oz | 260 |
| *Aunt Jemima,* avg, 2½ oz | 565 |

# Sodium Counter

## Fruit & Juices

| | Sodium |
|---|---|
| **Fresh Fruit,** average all types, 1 serving | 1 |
| **Dried/Canned Fruit,** ½ cup | 1 |
| **Fruit Juice:** Fresh, sqz'd, 6 fl.oz | 1 |
| Commercial, aver., 6 fl.oz | 20 |
| **Tomato Juice** *(Campbell's)*, 6 fl.oz | 570 |
| Low Sodium (No Salt Added) | 20 |
| **V8 Vegetable** *(Campbell's)*: 5.5 fl.oz can | 290 |
| 12 fl.oz bottle | 630 |
| Low Sodium, 5.5 fl.oz can | 95 |

## Vegetables

**Fresh/Frozen (No Salt Added):** *Per ½ Cup*

| | |
|---|---|
| Asparagus, Bean Sprouts, Corn | 3 |
| Beets, Carrots, Celery, ½ cup | 40 |
| Broccoli, Cabbage, Cauliflower | 10 |
| Cucumber, Green Beans, Mushroom, Okra | 3 |
| Onions, Peas, Potato, Pumpkin, Squash | 3 |
| Peppers, Hot Chili, raw, each | 3 |
| Spinach, Turnips, ½ cup, ckd | 40 |
| Tomato, 1 medium, 5 oz | 10 |
| **Canned:** Asparagus, 4 spears | 300 |
| Beans, baked in tomato sauce | 450 |
| Beets, ½ cup, 3 oz | 240 |
| Corn Kernels, ½ cup, 3 oz | 190 |
| Creamed, ½ cup, 4½ oz | 330 |
| Mushrooms w. butter sce, 2oz | 550 |
| Peas, ½ cup, 3 oz | 250 |
| Sauerkraut, ½ cup, 4 oz | 750 |

## Pickles, Olives

| | |
|---|---|
| **Olives,** pickled: Green, 1 large | 90 |
| Ripe/black, 1 large | 40 |
| **Pickles:** Bread & Butter, 4 sl., 1 oz | 200 |
| Dill, 1 pickle, 2½ oz | 900 |
| Sweet, 1 gherkin, ½ oz | 130 |

## Soybean Products

| | |
|---|---|
| **Miso** (Soy Paste), ¼ c., 2½ oz | 2500 |
| Soybean Protein Isolate, 1 oz | 280 |
| **Tempeh,** Natural, ½ cup, 3 oz | 5 |
| **Tofu,** average, ½ cup, 4 oz | 5 |

## Jam, Honey, Syrups

| | |
|---|---|
| **Jam/Jelly,** 1 Tbsp | 2 |
| **Honey/Maple Syrup,** 1 Tbsp | 1 |
| *Log Cabin* Syrup, 1 fl.oz | 35 |
| Lite, 1 fl.oz | 90 |

## Peanut Butter

| | |
|---|---|
| Peanut Butter: Regular, 2 Tbsp, ½ oz | 190 |
| Low Sodium *(Jif)*, 2 Tbsp | 65 |
| Unsalted *(Trader Joe's)*, 2 Tbsp | 5 |

## Snacks, Nuts

| | Sodium |
|---|---|
| **Cheese Balls/Curls,** 1 oz | 280 |
| **Cheetos,** 1 oz | 290 |
| **Corn/Tortilla Chips,** average, 1 oz | 220 |
| *Fritos,* Lightly Salted, 1 oz | 80 |
| **Granola bars,** average, 1 bar | 80 |
| **Nuts:** Plain, unsalted, 1 oz | 1 |
| Lightly salted, 1 oz | 80 |
| Salted or Honey Roasted, 1 oz | 160 |
| **Popcorn:** Plain (unsalted), 1 cup | 1 |
| Flavored, average, 1 cup | 60 |
| Salt added, 1 cup | 180 |
| **Potato Chips:** Plain, 1 oz | 160 |
| *Lay's,* Lightly Salted, 1 oz | 90 |
| Flavored, average, 1 oz | 250 |
| **Pretzels:** Regular, 3, 1 oz | 450 |
| Soft, salted, large | 1000 |

## Candy, Chocolate

| | |
|---|---|
| **Chocolate,** milk, 1 oz | 30 |
| **Fudge,** chocolate, 1 oz | 55 |
| **Candy Bars,** average, 1½ oz | 60 |
| **Hard Candy,** Jelly Beans, 1 oz | 10 |
| **Licorice,** 1 oz | 30 |

## Beverages, Alcohol

| | |
|---|---|
| **Coffee, Tea,** 1 cup | 1 |
| **Cocoa,** dry, plain, 1 Tbsp | 0 |
| Mix, average, 1 envelope | 120 |
| **Quik** *(Nestle)*, 2 tsp | 35 |
| **Soft Drinks,** average, 8 fl.oz | 20 |
| **Mineral Water,** Perrier, 8 fl.oz | 5 |
| **Gatorade** Thirst Quencher, 8 fl.oz | 110 |
| **Red Bull,** 8½ fl.oz can | 200 |
| **Water,** Average, 1 cup, 8 fl.oz | 5 |
| **Alcohol:** Beer, average, 12 fl.oz | 15 |
| Wines, average, 4 fl.oz | 10 |
| Spirits (distilled), 1½ fl.oz | 1 |

## Antacids ~ Alka-Seltzer

| | Sodium |
|---|---|
| *Alka-Seltzer (Per Tablet):* | |
| Original; Heartburn | 570 |
| Extra Strength | 590 |
| Lemon Lime | 500 |
| Gold | 310 |
| *Alka-Mints,* chewable | 0 |
| *Bromo Seltzer,* ¾ capful | 760 |
| *Picot,* 1 packet, 5g | 670 |
| *Rolaids,* All types | 0 |
| *Tums,* Regular/Extra Strength | 0 |

## Cold & Flu ~ Alka-Seltzer Plus

| | |
|---|---|
| Effervescents, average, 1 tablet | 480 |
| Fast Crystal Packs; Liquid Gels | 0 |

## Fast-Foods & Restaurants — Sodium

**Burger King:**

| | |
|---|---|
| **Burgers**: A1 Steakhouse XT | 1930 |
| Cheeseburger | 740 |
| Double Bacon Cheeseburger | 1180 |
| Hamburger | 520 |
| **Whoppers**: Original | 1020 |
| With Cheese | 1450 |
| Whopper Jr. with Cheese | 750 |
| **Chicken,** Original | 1390 |
| **Sides**: French Fries, medium, salted | 670 |
| Onion Rings, medium | 630 |
| **Breakfast**, Ham, Egg & Cheese Croissanwich | 1110 |

**Denny's:**

| | |
|---|---|
| **Better Burgers**: Classic Cheeseburger | 1410 |
| Western | 1820 |
| **Sandwiches**: Club | 1530 |
| Spicy Buffalo Chicken Melt | 3820 |
| **Steak & Seafood**: Lemon Pepper Tilapia | 1520 |
| T-Bone & Breaded Shrimp | 1490 |
| **Soups, Salads & Sides**: Chicken Noodle, 12 oz | 1300 |
| Clam Chowder, 12 oz | 1820 |
| **Breakfast**: Buttermilk Pancakes (3) | 1770 |
| Ham & Cheddar Omelette | 1330 |
| Southwestern Sizzlin Skillet | 2140 |
| **Sides**: Coleslaw, 3 oz | 520 |
| Everything H. Browns w/ Onions, Cheese & Gravy | 3820 |
| Garlic Bread, 2 pieces | 350 |
| Hash Browns, 5 oz | 650 |
| Vegetable Rice Pilaf, 5 oz | 820 |
| **Desserts**: Carrot Cake, 8 oz | 660 |
| Hershey's Chocolate Cake, 5 oz | 400 |

**Jack In The Box:**

| | |
|---|---|
| **Burgers**: Bacon Untimate Cheeseburger | 1840 |
| Hamburger | 570 |
| Jumbo Jack with Cheese | 1250 |
| **Sandwiches**: Homestyle Ranch Chicken Club | 1940 |
| Turkey, Bacon & Cheddar | 2130 |

**KFC:**

| | |
|---|---|
| **Chicken Breast**: Original | 710 |
| Extra Crunchy | 1010 |
| Grilled | 460 |
| **Popcorn Chicken**: Individual, 4 oz | 1160 |
| Value Box | 1900 |
| **Strips**, Crispy, 3 pieces | 1280 |
| **Wings**, Boneless Honey BBQ, 3 wings | 1020 |
| **Sandwiches**: Grilled Filet | 850 |
| Grilled Twister | 1300 |
| **Snackers**, average all varieties | 700 |
| **Sides**: Macaroni & Cheese | 880 |
| Mashed Potatoes with Gravy | 530 |
| Potato Wedges | 740 |

## Fast-Foods & Restaurants — Sodium

**McDonalds:**

| | |
|---|---|
| **Burgers**: Angus Bacon & Cheese | 2070 |
| Big Mac | 1040 |
| Cheeseburger | 750 |
| Double | 1150 |
| Hamburger | 520 |
| McChicken | 830 |
| Quarter Pounder with Cheese | 1190 |
| **McNuggets**: 6 pieces | 600 |
| **BBQ Sauce,** 1 package, 1 oz | 260 |
| **Sandwich**, Prem. Grilled Chicken Ranch BLT | 1440 |
| **French Fries**: Small, 2.5 oz | 160 |
| Medium, 4.1 oz | 270 |
| Large, 5.4 oz | 350 |
| **Ketchup**, 1 package, 10g | 110 |
| **Breakfast**: Egg McMuffin | 820 |
| Big Breakfast, reg. size Biscuit | 1560 |
| Hash Browns, 2 oz | 310 |
| Hotcakes, with Syrup & Whipped Margarine | 665 |
| McSkillet Burrito, with Sausage | 1390 |
| **Happy Meal**: Cheeseburger/Fries/Choc. Milk | 1060 |
| **Desserts/Shakes**: Hot Fudge Sundae | 180 |
| Chocolate Triple Thick Shake, 16 fl.oz | 250 |

**Pizza Hut:**

| | |
|---|---|
| **Pan Pizza, 12"**: *Per ½ Pizza, 4 Slices* | |
| Meat Lovers | 3300 |
| Cheese; Ham & Pineapple; Veggie, average | 2100 |
| Pepperoni; Hawaiian Luau; Dan's Original, av | 2400 |
| Supreme; Triple Meat; Spicy Sicilian, average | 2800 |
| **Thin 'N Crispy** ~ *Add an extra 100mg to above figures* | |

**Subway:**

| | |
|---|---|
| **6" Lowfat Sandwich**: *W/o Condiments/Dressings/Cheese* | |
| Roast Beef/Chicken, average | 800 |
| Subway Club; Turkey; Ham | 1150 |
| Sweet Onion Chicken Teriyaki | 1000 |
| Veggie Delite | 400 |
| **6" Sandwiches**: *Without Condiments* | |
| BLT; Tuna, average | 950 |
| Philly Chsestk; Meatball Mar.; Subway Melt | 1550 |
| Italian B.M.T.; Spicy Italian, average | 1800 |
| **12" Footlong** ~ *Double above figures* | |

**Taco Bell:** *Per Single Item*

| | |
|---|---|
| **Burritos**: ½ lb Combo | 1640 |
| Supreme: Beef; Chicken; Steak, average | 1400 |
| **Chapulas; Gorditas**: Average | 750 |
| **Nachos**: Regular | 520 |
| BellGrande | 1300 |
| **Specialties,** Cheese Quesadillas | 1120 |
| **Tacos**: Chicken, Soft | 660 |
| Crunchy; Supreme, average | 340 |

*Other Restaurants ~ www.CalorieKing.com*

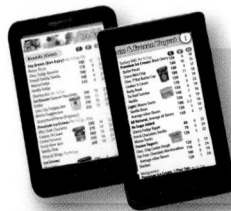

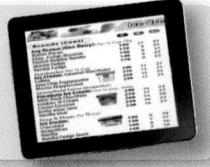

## FAST-FOODS INDEX
## ~ PAGE 175 ~

FAST-FOODS INDEX
~ PAGE 175 ~

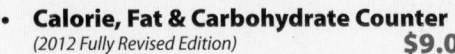
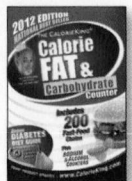
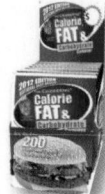
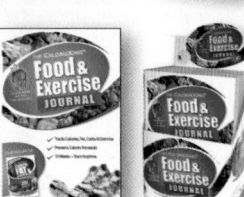
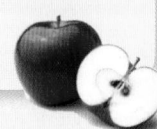
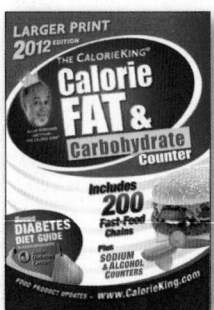
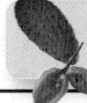
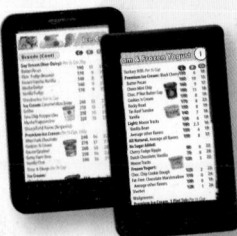
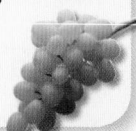
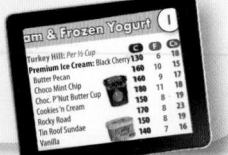